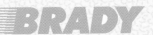

Paramedic Care
Principles & Practice
INTRODUCTION TO ADVANCED PREHOSPITAL CARE

SECOND EDITION

BRYAN E. BLEDSOE, D.O., F.A.C.E.P., EMT-P

Emergency Physician
Midlothian, Texas
and
Adjunct Associate Professor of Emergency Medicine
The George Washington University Medical Center
Washington, DC

ROBERT S. PORTER, M.A., NREMT-P

Senior Advanced Life Support Educator
Madison County Emergency Medical Services
Canastota, New York
and
Flight Paramedic
AirOne, Onondaga County Sheriff's Department
Syracuse, New York

RICHARD A. CHERRY, M.S., NREMT-P

Clinical Assistant Professor of Emergency Medicine
Assistant Residency Director
Upstate Medical University
Syracuse, New York

PEARSON
Prentice
Hall

Brady
Prentice Hall Health
Upper Saddle River, NJ 07458

Library of Congress Cataloging-in-Publication Data
Bledsoe, Bryan E., (date)
    Paramedic care: principles & practice / Bryan E. Bledsoe, Robert S. Porter, Richard
A. Cherry. — 2nd ed.
        p.; cm.
    Includes bibliographical references and index.
    ISBN 0–13–117819–9 (v. 1 : alk. paper)
    1. Emergency medicine. 2. Emergency medical technicians. I. Porter, Robert S.,
1950- . II. Cherry, Richard A. III. Title.
    [DNLM: 1. Emergencies. 2. Emergency Medical Technicians. 3. Emergency
Treatment. WB 105 B646pa 2005]
    RC86.7.B5964 2005
    616.02′5—dc22   2004012985

Publisher: Julie Levin Alexander
Publisher's Assistant: Regina Bruno
Executive Editor: Marlene McHugh Pratt
Senior Managing Editor for Development: Lois Berlowitz
Editorial Assistant: Matthew Sirinides
Project Manager: Sandy Breuer
Managing Photography Editor: Michal Heron
Director of Marketing: Karen Allman
Executive Marketing Manager: Katrin Beacom
Senior Channel Marketing Manager: Rachele Strober
Marketing Coordinator: Michael Sirinides
Director of Production and Manufacturing: Bruce Johnson
Managing Editor for Production: Patrick Walsh
Production Liaison: Faye Gemmellaro
Production Editor: Lynn Steines, Carlisle Publishers Services
Manufacturing Manager: Ilene Sanford
Manufacturing Buyer: Pat Brown
Creative Director: Cheryl Asherman
Senior Design Coordinator: Christopher Weigand
Cover Design: Christopher Weigand
Cover Image: Eddie Sperling
Cover Image Manipulation: Studio Montage
Interior Photographers: Michael Gallitelli, Michal Heron, Richard Logan
Interior Illustrations: Rolin Graphics
Interior Design: Jill Little
Media Project Manager: John J. Jordan
Manager of Media Production: Amy Peltier
New Media Project Manager: Stephen J. Hartner
Composition: Carlisle Publishers Services
Printing and Binding: Courier/Kendallville
Cover Printer: Phoenix Color

Notices

It is the intent of the authors and publishers that
this textbook be used as part of a formal paramedic
education program taught by a qualified instructor
and supervised by a licensed physician. The care
procedures presented here represent accepted
practices in the United States. They are not offered
as a standard of care. Paramedic-level emergency
care is to be performed only under the authority
and guidance of a licensed physician. It is the
reader's responsibility to know and follow local care
protocols as provided by medical advisors directing
the system to which he or she belongs. Also, it is the
reader's responsibility to stay informed of
emergency care procedure changes.

Notice on Drugs and Drug Dosages

Every effort has been made to ensure that the drug
dosages presented in this textbook are in accordance
with nationally accepted standards. When
applicable, the dosages and routes are taken from
the American Heart Association's *Advanced Cardiac
Life Support Guidelines.* The American Medical
Association's publication *Drug Evaluations,* the
Physicians' Desk Reference, and the *Prentice Hall
Health Professional's Drug Guide* are followed with
regard to drug dosages not covered by the American
Heart Association's guidelines. It is the responsibility
of the reader to be familiar with the drugs used in
his or her system, as well as the dosages specified by
the medical director. The drugs presented in this
book should only be administered by direct order,
whether verbally or through accepted standing
orders, of a licensed physician.

Notice on Gender Usage

The English language has historically given
preference to the male gender. Among many words,
the pronouns "he" and "his" are commonly used to
describe both genders. Society evolves faster than
language and the male pronouns still predominate
in our speech. The authors have made great effort
to treat the two genders equally, recognizing that a
significant percentage of paramedics and patients
are female. However, in some instances, male
pronouns may be used to describe both male and
female paramedics and patients solely for the
purpose of brevity. This is not intended to offend
any readers of the female gender.

Notice on Photographs

Please note that many of the photographs
contained in this book are taken of actual
emergency situations. As such, it is possible that
they may not accurately depict current,
appropriate, or advisable practices of emergency
medical care. They have been included for the sole
purpose of giving general insight into real-life
emergency settings.

Notice on Case Studies

The names used and situations depicted in the case
studies throughout this textbook are fictitious.

10 9 8 7 6 5 4 3 2

ISBN 0-13-117819-9

DEDICATION

This edition of *Paramedic Care: Principles & Practice* is dedicated to the memory and life of Jim Page. Few people have had such a positive impact on EMS and society in general. Jim was many things—attorney, publisher, EMT, firefighter, visionary, advocate, fire chief, and friend. Most of all, he was humble. He never knew how important he really was. Jim had the unique talent of remembering names and always made you feel that, regardless of what was going on around him, you had his undivided attention and ear. We mourn his passing and miss his warm handshake and booming voice. Each of the three authors of this textbook called Jim a close friend, and we are forever grateful for his years of advice, counsel, and friendship. An old Spanish proverb says, "Good men must die, but death cannot kill their names." We hope that every paramedic student who reads these textbooks will periodically turn to this page and quietly reflect on the impact this important yet humble man had on EMS and the fire service.

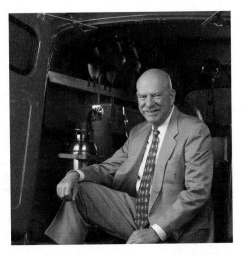

Tom Page/Jems Communications

James O. Page
1936–2004

No one's death comes to pass without making some impression, and those close to the deceased inherit part of the liberated soul, and thus become richer in their humaneness.

Robert Oxton Bolt

Content Overview

Volume I Introduction to Advanced Prehospital Care

Below is a brief content description of each chapter in Volume 1, *Introduction to Advanced Prehospital Care.*

continued

Content Overview

Volume I Introduction to Advanced Prehospital Care (continued)

Content Overview

Volume 2 Patient Assessment

Below is a brief content description of each chapter in Volume 2, *Patient Assessment.*

Chapter 1   The History 2

★ Provides the basic components of a complete health history
★ Discusses how to effectively conduct an interview
★ Provides suggestions for communicating with difficult patients, hostile patients, and patients with language barriers

Chapter 2   Physical Exam Techniques 26

★ Presents the techniques of conducting a comprehensive physical exam
★ Includes in each section a review of anatomy and physiology

Chapter 3   Patient Assessment in the Field 172

★ Offers a practical approach to conducting problem-oriented history and physical exams

Chapter 4   Clinical Decision Making 236

★ Provides the basic steps for making clinical decisions
★ Discusses how to think critically in emergency situations

Chapter 5   Communications 252

★ Discusses communication, the key component that links every phase of an EMS run
★ Includes several examples of typical radio medical reports

Chapter 6   Documentation 276

★ Describes how to write a prehospital care report (PCR)
★ Offers examples of the various narrative writing styles

Content Overview

Volume 3 Medical Emergencies

Below is a brief content description of each chapter in Volume 3, *Medical Emergencies.*

Content Overview

Volume 3 Medical Emergencies

Content Overview

Volume 4 Trauma Emergencies

Below is a brief content description of each chapter in Volume 4, *Trauma Emergencies*.

Chapter 1 Trauma and Trauma Systems 2

★ Discusses the nature of trauma and its costs to society
★ Introduces the concept of trauma care systems
★ Outlines the role of the paramedic in trauma care
★ Introduces trauma triage protocols

Chapter 2 Blunt Trauma 16

★ Describes the physics of blunt trauma and the effects of blunt trauma on the body
★ Outlines how to evaluate the mechanism of injury in cases of blunt trauma in order to determine likely injuries

Chapter 3 Penetrating Trauma 54

★ Describes the physics of penetrating trauma and the effects of penetrating trauma on the body
★ Outlines how to evaluate the mechanism of injury in cases of penetrating trauma in order to determine likely injuries

Chapter 4 Hemorrhage and Shock 78

★ Describes the anatomy, physiology, and pathophysiology of the cardiovascular system as they apply to hemorrhage and shock
★ Discusses the assessment and management of hemorrhage and shock

Chapter 5 Soft-Tissue Trauma 126

★ Reviews the anatomy and physiology of the integumentary system
★ Discusses the pathophysiology of soft-tissue trauma
★ Discusses the assessment and management of soft-tissue trauma, including a discussion of bandaging

Chapter 6 Burns 176

★ Describes the anatomy, physiology, and pathophysiology of burn injuries
★ Discusses the assessment and management of burns

Chapter 7 Musculoskeletal Trauma 216

★ Reviews the anatomy and physiology of the musculoskeletal system
★ Discusses the various types of injuries and conditions that can affect the musculoskeletal system
★ Discusses the assessment and management of musculoskeletal trauma, including discussions of realignment, splinting, and pain control

Content Overview

Volume 4 Trauma Emergencies

Content Overview

Volume 5 Special Considerations/Operations

Below is a brief content description of each chapter in Volume 5, *Special Considerations/Operations*.

Chapter 1 **Neonatology 2**

★ Introduces the specialized world of neonatology
★ Discusses how size and anatomy affect assessment and treatment
★ Emphasizes neonatal resuscitation in the field setting

Chapter 2 **Pediatrics 38**

★ Provides an overview of common and uncommon pediatric emergencies encountered in a field setting
★ Emphasizes that children are not "small adults"
★ Presents specialized pediatric assessment techniques and field emergency procedures

Chapter 3 **Geriatric Emergencies 138**

★ Reviews the anatomy and physiology of aging
★ Discusses the assessment and treatment of emergencies commonly seen in the elderly

Chapter 4 **Abuse and Assault 204**

★ Provides information about detecting abusive or dangerous situations
★ Discusses the special needs of victims of abuse or assault

Chapter 5 **The Challenged Patient 224**

★ Addresses the special needs of patients with physical, mental, or cultural challenges
★ Emphasizes strategies that can be used to reduce challenged patient stress
★ Describes methods to conduct a thorough and accurate assessment of a challenged patient

Chapter 6 **Acute Interventions for the Chronic Care Patient 248**

★ Discusses the role of EMS personnel in treating home care patients and patients with chronic medical conditions
★ Provides an overview of equipment commonly found in a home care setting
★ Examines strategies for working with the family and caregivers encountered in most home care situations

Chapter 7 **Assessment-Based Management 292**

★ Discusses the diagnostic skills involved in assessment-based management
★ Provides scenarios that illustrate comprehensive patient assessment

Chapter 8 **Ambulance Operations 320**

★ Reviews the medical equipment aboard most ambulances and stresses the need for safe driving procedures
★ Emphasizes the need for a constant state of readiness for every call

Content Overview
Volume 5 Special Considerations/Operations

Detailed Contents

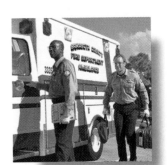

Chapter 1   Introduction to Advanced Prehospital Care 2

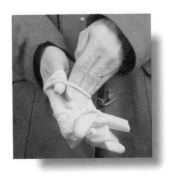

Chapter 2   The Well-Being of the Paramedic 14

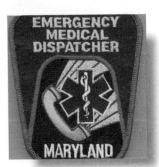

Chapter 3   EMS Systems 44

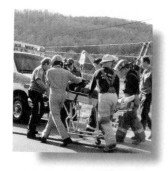

Chapter 4   Roles and Responsibilities of the Paramedic 76

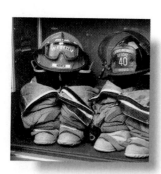

Chapter 5   Illness and Injury Prevention 96

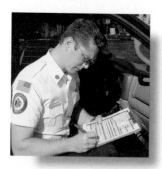

Chapter 6   Medical/Legal Aspects of Advanced Prehospital Care 110

Chapter 7 — Ethics in Advanced Prehospital Care 142

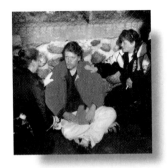

Chapter 8 — General Principles of Pathophysiology 162

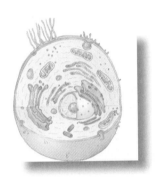

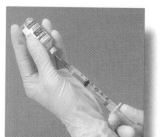

Chapter 9   General Principles of Pharmacology 274

Chapter 10   Intravenous Access and Medication Administration 368

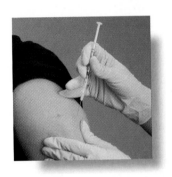

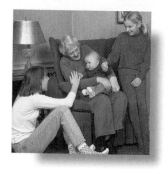

Chapter 11   Therapeutic Communications 464

Chapter 12   Life-Span Development 482

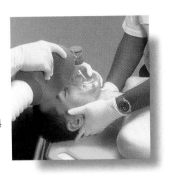

Chapter 13 Airway Management and Ventilation 504

Photo Scans/Procedures

It's Your Profession

Dear Student:

Thank you for using Brady's *Paramedic Care: Principles & Practice* series. These five volumes, based on the widely used *Paramedic Emergency Care* text we developed more than 15 years ago, will provide the core foundation for your paramedic education. Coupled with quality classroom instruction and clinical rotations, you are assured of receiving the knowledge and skills required of a quality paramedic. We know you want to pass your certification exam, and you also want to be prepared for the challenges you'll encounter on the street. *Paramedic Care: Principles & Practice* is the textbook series that will help you accomplish both goals.

We are proud to tell you that Brady has made a top-down commitment to quality, a commitment that is evident in the book you now hold. William A. Foster once wrote, "Quality is never an accident; it is always the result of high intention, sincere effort, intelligent direction, and skilled execution; it represents the wise choice of many alternatives." Every person at Brady involved in the preparation of this text has made a sincere commitment to quality, beginning with our efforts as authors. We know you have made a significant investment in your program, and we have gone to great effort to ensure that our paramedic program is accurate, current, and complete. The second edition has been extensively reviewed and revised to reflect changes in EMS that have occurred since the first edition was published. The three of us, as well as contributors to this series, have made a tremendous effort to ensure that the material accurately reflects the current state of and best practices in EMS.

Brady makes a considerable investment in "development editing," and its development team is among the most dedicated and skilled in the publishing industry. Development editing ensures that content is reviewed appropriately for accuracy and currency, explanations are consistent, and the material remains at the appropriate level for the paramedic student. Brady's editors have worked hard toward these goals. Another of Brady's strongest assets is its production team. These publishing experts have many years of experience in the business and an undeniable commitment to producing books with distinctive designs and clear formatting. Working together, Brady's development and production teams help to ensure that our books are the best on the market. Brady's commitment to a standard of excellence continues with the customer service and feedback system provided by the sales team, the most experienced group in EMS publishing.

In summary, EMS is about quality. Welcome. Be safe. Have fun. We wish you all the best in your education and in the practice of EMS.

Sincerely,

Bryan Bledsoe   Robert Porter   Richard Cherry

Series Preface

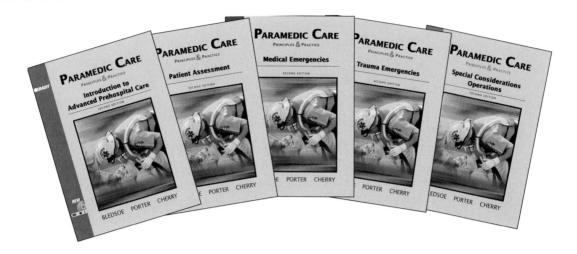

Congratulations on your decision to further your EMS career by undertaking the course of education required for certification as an Emergency Medical Technician–Paramedic! The world of paramedic emergency care is one that you will find both challenging and rewarding. Whether you will be working as a volunteer or a paid paramedic, you will find the field of advanced prehospital care very interesting.

This textbook, **the 2nd edition of *Paramedic Care: Principles & Practice,*** will serve as your guide and reference to advanced prehospital care. It is based on the 1998 U.S. Department of Transportation's *Emergency Medical Technician–Paramedic National Standard Curriculum* and is divided into five volumes:

Volume 1 *Introduction to Advanced Prehospital Care*
Volume 2 *Patient Assessment*
Volume 3 *Medical Emergencies*
Volume 4 *Trauma Emergencies*
Volume 5 *Special Considerations/Operations.*

Volume 1, *Introduction to Advanced Prehospital Care,* presents the foundations of paramedic practice as well as an introduction to pathophysiology, pharmacology, medication administration, and airway management and ventilation. **Volume 2, *Patient Assessment,*** adds the cognitive and psychomotor skills of patient assessment, communications, and documentation. This knowledge base expands as the series applies it to the medical patient in **Volume 3, *Medical Emergencies,*** and to the trauma patient in **Volume 4, *Trauma Emergencies.*** **Volume 5, *Special Considerations/Operations***, enriches these general patient care concepts and principles with applications to special patients and circumstances we commonly see as paramedics. The product of this complete and integrated series is a set of principles of care you will be required to practice as a twenty-first-century paramedic.

Your paramedic education program should include ample classroom, practical laboratory, in-hospital clinical, and prehospital field experience. These educational experiences must be guided by instructors and preceptors with special training and experience in their areas of participation in your program.

DEVELOPING ADVANCED SKILLS

The psychomotor skills of fluid and medication administration, advanced airway care, ECG monitoring and defibrillation, and advanced medical and trauma patient care are best learned first in the classroom and the skills laboratory and then in the clinical and field settings. Commonly required advanced prehospital skills are discussed in the text as well as outlined in the accompanying procedure sheets. Review these before and while practicing each skill.

It is important to underscore that neither this nor any other text can teach skills. Care skills are learned only under the watchful eye of a paramedic instructor and perfected during your clinical and field internship.

CONTENT OF THE FIVE VOLUMES

It is intended that your program coordinator will assign reading from *Paramedic Care: Principles & Practice* in preparation for each classroom lecture and discussion section. The knowledge gained from reading this text will form the foundation of the information you will need in order to function effectively as a paramedic in your EMS system. Your instructors will build on this information to strengthen your knowledge and understanding of advanced prehospital care so that you may apply it in your practice.

The content of each volume of *Paramedic Care: Principles & Practice* is summarized below, with an emphasis on "what's new" in this 2nd edition.

VOLUME 1: INTRODUCTION TO ADVANCED PREHOSPITAL CARE

Volume 1 addresses the fundamentals of paramedic practice, including paramedic roles and responsibilities, pathophysiology, pharmacology, medication administration, and advanced airway management.

What's New in Volume 1?

★ In Chapter 2, "The Well-Being of the Paramedic," former discussions of critical incident stress management (a technique that is no longer recommended) have been replaced with new sections on specific **EMS stresses** and on **general mental health services** and **disaster mental health services** available to EMS personnel.

★ Chapter 6, "Medical/Legal Aspects of Advanced Prehospital Care," contains a new section on the **Health Insurance Portability and Accountability Act (HIPAA) privacy rules.**

★ Chapter 8, "General Principles of Pathophysiology," and Chapter 10, "Medication Administration," include new sections on **HBOCs (hemoglobin-based oxygen-carrying substances),** which are considered to have significant advantages over standard crystalloids and colloids for fluid resuscitation.

★ Chapter 9, "General Principles of Pharmacology," includes updated information on **insulin preparations,** an updated **immunization schedule,** and discussion of **new drugs for erectile dysfunction.**

★ Chapter 13, "Airway Management and Ventilation," includes a new section on **capnography,** particularly its uses in monitoring tube placement during endotracheal intubation. New sections are also included on the **Intubating LMA (laryngeal mask airway),** the **Cobra Perilaryngeal Airway,** and the **Ambu Laryngeal Mask.** For assistance in intubation, the **bougie** device is newly discussed and illustrated as are techniques for **nasotracheal auscultation.**

VOLUME 2: PATIENT ASSESSMENT

Volume 2 builds on the assessment skills taught in the basic EMT course, emphasizing advanced-level patient assessment and clinical decision-making at the scene.

What's New in Volume 2?

★ Chapter 2, "Physical Exam Techniques," includes much-expanded information and photos to illustrate the **ophthalmic (eye) exam** and the **otoscopic (ear) exam.**

★ Chapter 2, "Physical Exam Techniques," and Chapter 3, "Patient Assessment in the Field," feature new sections on **capnography** as an assessment tool.

★ Chapter 5, "Communications," includes new information on **wireless phones and 911 calls** (new technology for identifying locations and call-back numbers). There is a section on the promising new technology of **automatic collision notification (ACN)** and also a discussion of the importance of **speaking to medical direction on a recorded line** (which will help in the event of a lawsuit).

VOLUME 3: MEDICAL EMERGENCIES

Volume 3 addresses the paramedic level of care in medical emergencies. Particular emphasis is placed on respiratory and cardiovascular emergencies, which are the most common EMS medical calls.

What's New in Volume 3?

★ Chapter 1, "Pulmonology," features new information on **capnography** as a prehospital diagnostic tool and means of monitoring the patient's respiratory status, specifically in upper airway obstruction and asthma emergencies. New material on **severe acute respiratory syndrome (SARS)** is included.

★ Chapter 2, "Cardiology," introduces the use of the **15-lead and 18-lead ECGs in right ventricular and left ventricular posterior wall infarctions.**

★ Chapter 3, "Neurology," has added information on the **pediatric Glasgow Coma Scale.**

★ Chapter 7, "Urology and Nephrology," has a new section on **priapism.**

★ Chapter 11, "Infectious Disease"—like Chapter 1—includes new information on **SARS.**

★ Chapter 12, "Psychiatric and Behavior Disorders," features completely revised text and photos regarding **restraint of violent patients** to emphasize supine placement and monitoring the airway and breathing of the restrained patient.

VOLUME 4: TRAUMA EMERGENCIES

Volume 4 discusses advanced prehospital care of the trauma patient, from mechanism-of-injury analysis to care of specific types of trauma to general principles of shock/trauma resuscitation.

What's New in Volume 4?

★ Chapter 2, "Blunt Trauma," includes new information on **side air bags** and on **deactivation of undeployed air bags.** Notes are included regarding **terrorist use of explosives** that contain nails, screws, and other materials intended to cause maximum injury and destruction.

★ Chapter 4, "Hemorrhage and Shock," includes a new section on the use of **capnography** as a guide to ventilation rates and volumes as well as for ensuring proper tube placement. A new section has been added on the use of two techniques to improve ventilatory efficiency: **positive end-expiratory pressure (PEEP)** and **continuous positive airway pressure (CPAP).**

- In Chapter 5, "Soft-Tissue Trauma," **fentanyl** is introduced as a drug for pain control.
- Chapter 6, "Burns," includes new information on **keratitis**, an eye injury welders may suffer; on the unreliability of **pulse oximetry** to measure oxygen saturation in the burn patient and the patient who has inhaled carbon monoxide; and on **fentanyl** as a pain management drug. Illustrations and text on factors affecting **radiation exposure** have been revised to provide greater detail.
- In Chapter 7, "Musculoskeletal Trauma," discussions and illustrations of the **vacuum splint** and the **pelvic sling** have been added. The Hare splint has been deleted from the section on traction splinting and the **Fernotrac splint** has been added. Under pain control medications, **fentanyl** has been added and nalbuphine has been deemphasized.
- Chapter 8, "Head, Facial, and Neck Trauma," has an added discussion of **capnography** as an assessment tool with the head injury patient and as a tool for confirmation of tube placement. A section on **recognition of herniation** is newly included. Both **adult and pediatric Glasgow coma scales** are now included. The importance of obtaining **blood glucose readings** in the head injury patient is newly emphasized. In the directed intubation section, the **bougie** device is introduced. Recommended **ventilation rates and volumes for the head injury patient** have been updated, as has information on **maintenance of blood pressure in the head injury patient.** Caveats regarding the use of **rapid sequence intubation** in the prehospital setting have been included. In the discussion of medications, mannitol has been deleted as a diuretic, **atracurium** has been added as a paralytic, and **etomidate** and **fentanyl** have been added as sedatives.
- In Chapter 9, "Spinal Trauma," extensive discussions of **spinal clearance** and a spinal clearance protocol have been added. A term that is gaining acceptance, **spinal motion restriction,** is discussed. **Capnography** is now included, along with pulse oximetry, as an aid in ensuring adequate oxygenation. An explanation is included as to why routine use of **steroids in spine injury is no longer recommended.**
- Chapter 12, "Shock Trauma Resuscitation," now includes **pediatric trauma scoring** in addition to adult trauma scoring.

VOLUME 5: SPECIAL CONSIDERATIONS/OPERATIONS

Volume 5 addresses such topics as neonatal, pediatric, and geriatric care; home health care and challenged patients; and incident command, ambulance service, rescue, hazardous material, crime scene operations, and responding to terrorist acts.

What's New in Volume 5?

- Chapter 1, "Neonatology," includes expanded text regarding congenital anomalies and, in particular, more information on **congenital heart problems.**
- Chapter 2, "Pediatrics," has a new section on **verification of tube placement in the pediatric patient.**
- Chapter 4, "Abuse and Assault," features a new section on **date rape drugs.**
- In Chapter 8, "Ambulance Operations," the **criteria for air medical dispatch** have been updated.
- Chapter 9, "Medical Incident Management," makes reference to the new **U.S. Department of Homeland Security National Incident Management System (NIMS).** The former emphasis on critical incident stress debriefings has been deleted and replaced by new sections on **mental health support** and **disaster mental health services.**
- Chapter 14, "Responding to Terrorist Acts," is an entirely new chapter that did not appear in the first (pre-September 11, 2001) edition of *Paramedic Care.* It includes information on **explosive, nuclear, chemical, and biological agents** as well as **scene safety, recognizing a terrorist attack,** and **responding to a terrorist attack.**

Preface

Modern EMS is based on sound principles and practice. The paramedic of the twenty-first century must be knowledgeable in all aspects of EMS. This begins with a fundamental understanding of EMS operations and basic medical science. The paramedic curriculum follows the medical model. Students are first educated in the basic sciences. They are then introduced to the clinical sciences, reinforcing the basic science knowledge attained earlier. The 1998 U.S. DOT *EMT-Paramedic: National Standard Curriculum* that is now in use markedly expanded both the basic science and clinical science knowledge base of paramedics. With ***Paramedic Care: Principles & Practice***, we have followed the DOT curriculum and provided the preparatory material *Volume 1, Introduction to Advanced Prehospital Care.*

This volume provides paramedic students with the principles of advanced prehospital care and EMS operations. The first five chapters detail EMS operations and paramedic roles and responsibilities. There is an added emphasis on personal wellness and injury and illness prevention. The next two chapters deal with the medical-legal aspects of emergency care and ethics. Both are increasingly important in EMS. As a part of the current curriculum, there is significant emphasis on pathophysiology and the disease process. This volume presents this material in detail so that the paramedic student will have insight into the various disease and injury concepts presented in the clinical portions of this and the later volumes. The last four chapters of this volume are comprehensive discussions of pharmacology, airway management, and other essential advanced prehospital skills. This volume provides the paramedic student with the basic science knowledge necessary to delve into the clinical portions of the curriculum, including patient assessment, medical emergencies, trauma emergencies, and special situations.

OVERVIEW OF THE CHAPTERS

Chapter 1 "Introduction to Advanced Prehospital Care" introduces the paramedic student to the world of paramedicine and the current DOT curriculum. It summarizes the expanding roles of the paramedic as well as the importance of professionalism.

Chapter 2 "The Well-Being of the Paramedic" presents material crucial to the survival of the paramedic in EMS. It addresses such important issues as physical fitness, nutrition, and personal protection from disease. It details the role of stress in EMS and presents important coping strategies.

Chapter 3 "EMS Systems" reviews the history of EMS and provides an overview of EMS today. It details the various, integrated aspects of EMS system design and operation. It emphasizes the importance of medical direction in all aspects of prehospital care.

Chapter 4 "Roles and Responsibilities of the Paramedic" is a detailed discussion of the expectations and responsibilities of the modern paramedic. It emphasizes the importance of ethical behavior, appearance, and patient advocacy in a field that is becoming more technical and more impersonal.

Chapter 5 "Illness and Injury Prevention" addresses the importance of preventing illness and injury among the public as well as in EMS. It emphasizes the importance of scene safety and the role the paramedic has in assuring the safety of all rescuers. It also emphasizes the importance of paramedics participating in community illness and injury prevention programs.

Chapter 6 "Medical/Legal Aspects of Advanced Prehospital Care" is a detailed treatise of law and emergency care. In addition to an overview of the law and the legal system, this chapter discusses how the legal system can impact the paramedic. It also provides important tips on how the paramedic can avoid exposure in a malpractice action.

Chapter 7 "Ethics in Advanced Prehospital Care" presents the fundamentals of medical ethics. As EMS becomes more sophisticated, the paramedic will be faced with an ever-increasing number of ethical dilemmas. This chapter provides the paramedic student with an overview of medical ethics so as to be able to make sound decisions when confronted with ethical problems.

Chapter 8 "General Principles of Pathophysiology" provides a detailed description of basic pathophysiology. The first part of the chapter describes the cell and the cellular environment, including a detailed look at such important concepts as acid-base balance and fluid and electrolyte therapy. The second part of the chapter discusses the causes and pathophysiology of disease. The final part of the chapter details the body's response to disease and injury.

Chapter 9 "General Principles of Pharmacology" is a comprehensive chapter covering the various medications used in medical practice. It initially presents an overview of pharmacology. This is followed by a discussion of drug classifications.

Chapter 10 "Medication Administration" details the fundamental paramedic skills of medication administration by various routes as well as an overview of medical mathematics including dosage calculations.

Chapter 11 "Therapeutic Communications" addresses an important but often overlooked aspect of prehospital care. Communications among the paramedic and the patient and the paramedic and other health care providers is discussed.

Chapter 12 "Life Span Development" provides an overview of physiological and psychosocial developmental and age-related changes from infancy to late adulthood.

Chapter 13 "Airway Management and Ventilation" is a core chapter that presents the crucial prehospital skill of airway management. It addresses both basic manual and advanced airway management techniques. In addition, this chapter details ventilation techniques, suctioning, rapid sequence intubation, and surgical airways.

Appendix "Research in EMS" introduces the student to the understanding that, as EMS evolves, research will be the driving force. To function effectively during a career in EMS, the paramedic must have a basic understanding of research and its role in EMS development.

SUMMARY OF VOLUME 1

This volume, *Introduction to Advanced Prehospital Care*, details the basic knowledge and skills expected of twenty-first century paramedics. The material should be mastered before undertaking the clinical aspects of paramedic education set forth in the subsequent volumes of this text. The best paramedics are those who have a working understanding of the basic science and underlying pathophysiology of every emergency they are called upon to treat.

Note: Please refer to the Brady supplement *Drug Guide for Paramedics.*

▼Acknowledgments

CHAPTER CONTRIBUTORS

We wish to acknowledge the remarkable talents and efforts of the following people who contributed to this volume of *Paramedic Care: Principles & Practice.* Individually, they worked with extraordinary commitment on this new program. Together, they form a team of highly dedicated professionals who have upheld the highest standards of EMS instruction.

Chapter 1   Introduction to Advanced Prehospital Care
Bryan E. Bledsoe, D.O., F.A.C.E.P., EMT-P, Emergency Physician, Midlothian, Texas; Adjunct Associate Professor of Emergency Medicine, The George Washington University Medical Center, Washington, DC

Chapter 2   The Well-Being of the Paramedic
Kate Dernocoeur, BS, EMT-P, Lowell, Michigan

Chapter 3   EMS Systems
Eric C. Chaney, NREMT-P, Administrator, Office of the State EMS Medical Director, Maryland Institute for Emergency Medical Services Systems, Baltimore, Maryland

Chapter 4   Roles and Responsibilities of the Paramedic
Eric C. Chaney, MS, NREMT-P, Administrator, Office of the State EMS Medical Director, Maryland Institute for Emergency Medical Services Systems, Baltimore, Maryland

Chapter 5   Illness and Injury Prevention
Eric W. Heckerson, RN, MA, NREMT-P, EMS Coordinator, Mesa Fire Department, Mesa, Arizona
Sandra Hultz, BS, NREMT-P, EMS Instructor, University of Mississippi Medical Center, Jackson, Mississippi

Chapter 6   Medical/Legal Aspects of Advanced Prehospital Care
Emily Vacher, Esq., MPA, EMT-CC, Associate Director of Judicial Affairs, Syracuse University, Syracuse, New York
W. E. (Gene) Gandy, JD, LP, Hill-Gandy Associates, Albany, Texas

Chapter 7   Ethics in Advanced Prehospital Care
J. Nile Barnes, BS, NREMT-P, Associate Professor of EMS Professions, Austin Community College, Austin, Texas and Paramedic, Williamson County (Texas) EMS Department
Michael F. O'Keefe, MS, NREMT-P, EMS Training Coordinator, Vermont Department of Health

Chapter 8 General Principles of Pathophysiology

John S. Saito, MPH, EMT-P, Director, EMS/Paramedic Education, Assistant Professor, Oregon Health Sciences University, School of Medicine, Department of Emergency Medicine, Portland, Oregon

Matthew S. Zavarella, BSAS, REMT-P, CCTEMT-P, Instructor, Department of Emergency Medical Technology, School of Health Related Professions, University of Mississippi Medical Center, Jackson, Mississippi

Chapter 9 General Principles of Pharmacology

Jeffrey L. Jarvis, MS, LP, Medical Student, The University of Texas Medical Branch, Galveston, Texas

Chapter 10 Medication Administration

James W. Drake, MS, NREMT-P, EMS Coordinator, Jameson Memorial Hospital, New Castle, Pennsylvania

Chapter 11 Therapeutic Communications

Kate Dernocoeur, BS, EMT-P, Lowell, Michigan

Chapter 12 Life Span Development

Jo Anne Schultz, BA, NREMT-P, Paramedic, Lifestar Ambulance, Inc., Salisbury, Maryland; Level II Emergency Medical Services Instructor, Maryland Fire and Rescue Institute, University of Maryland; Paramedic Instructor, Maryland Institute of Emergency Medical Services Systems, University of Maryland; ACLS, BTLS, and PALS instructor

Chapter 13 Airway Management and Ventilation

Joseph P. Funk, MD, FACEP, Peachtree Emergency Associates, Piedmont Hospital, Atlanta, Georgia

Kathleen G. Funk, MD, FACEP, Emergency Medicine Physician, Atlanta, Georgia

Appendix Research in EMS

Michael F. O'Keefe, MS, REMT-P, EMS Training Coordinator, Vermont Department of Health

REVIEW BOARDS

Our special thanks to Dr. Edward T. Dickinson, Assistant Professor and Director of EMS Field Operations in the Department of Emergency Medicine, University of Pennsylvania School of Medicine in Philadelphia. Dr. Dickinson's reviews of first edition material were carefully prepared, and we appreciate the thoughtful advice and keen insight he shared with us.

INSTRUCTOR REVIEWERS

The reviewers of *Paramedic Care: Principles & Practice* have provided many excellent suggestions and ideas for improving the text. The quality of the reviews has been outstanding, and the reviews have been a major aid in the preparation and revision of the manuscript. The assistance provided by these EMS experts is deeply appreciated.

Brenda M. Beasley, RN, BS, EMT-P
Department Chair, Allied Health
Calhoun College
Decatur, AL

Jeff Fritz, BS, NREMT-P
Temple College
Temple, TX

Frank J. Gilligan, EMT-P, CECM
Lackawanna College
Scranton, PA

David M. LaCombe, NREMT-P
National EMS Academy
Lafayette, LA

Andrew Lewis, EMT-P
American Aviation Management
Fort Pierce, FL

Lawrence Linder, BA, NREMT-P
EMS Faculty
St. Petersburg College
Pinellas Park, FL

Keith A. Monosky, MPM, EMT-P
Assistant Professor
The George Washington University
Washington, DC

Douglas A. Paris, BS NREMT-P
Faculty, Dept. of Emergency Medical
  Technology
Greenville Technical College
Greenville, SC

Allen O. Patterson
Holmes Community College
Ridgeland, MS

Randy Perkins, CEP
Paramedic Program Director
Scottsdale Community College
Scottsdale, AZ

Richard Peterson, EMT-P
Paramedic Program Director
Rochester Community and Technical
  College
Rochester, MN

Gina Riggs, EMT-P, I/C
Kiamichi Technology Center
Poteau, OK

Judith A. Ruple, PhD, RN, NREMT-P
Associate Professor
Director
The University of Toledo
College of Health and Human Services
Emergency Medical Health Services
Toledo, OH

Christopher T. Ryther, MS, NREMT-P
Emergency Services and Mobile
  Healthcare Associates
Sacramento, CA

Janet L. Schulte, BS, AS, NR-CDEMT-P
IHM Health Studies Center
St. Louis, MO

Andrew R. Turcotte, NREMT-P, EMS
  I/C
Old Orchard Beach Fire Department
Old Orchard Beach, ME

We also wish to express appreciation to the following EMS professionals who reviewed the 1st edition of *Paramedic Care: Principles & Practice.* Their suggestions and perspectives helped to make this program a successful teaching tool.

Brenda Beasley, RN, BS, EMT-P
EMS Program Director
Calhoun College
Decatur, AL

Tom Blake, MS, EMT-P
Director, Paramedic Associates Degree
  Program
Southern Maine Technical College
South Portland, ME

Alan Brower, RN, NREMT-P
Ricks College Paramedic Program
Rexbury, ID

Kerry Campbell, NREMT-P
Lakeshore Technical College
Cleveland, WI

Albert Dimmitt, Jr.
Penn Valley Community College
Kansas City, MO

Robert Dotterer, BSEd, MEd, NREMT-P
Phoenix Fire Department
Phoenix College
Phoenix, AZ

Bill Gentry, MICP
Paramedic Program Coordinator
Northern California Training Institute
Sacramento, CA

Blaine Griffiths, BS, NREMT-P
Youngstown State University
Youngstown, OH

Jeffrey Grunow, MSN, NREMT-P
Director, Prehospital Education
Carolinas Medical Center
Charlotte, NC

Samuel D. Marciano, MS, EMT-I
Assistant Professor
Erie Community College
Lancaster, NY

Larry W. Masterman, MICP, CEM
Northern California EMS Agency
Redding, CA

Michael E. Murphy, RN, EMT-P
Deputy Chief
Rockland Paramedic Services
Orangeburg, NY

Gerard Oncale, RN, BSN, CEN, REMT-P
EMS Faculty
University of South Alabama
Mobile, AL

Judith Ruple, PhD, RN
Associate Professor
The University of Toledo
Toledo, OH

Larry Ryland
Director of Emergency Medical Services
L.B. Wallace College
Andalusia Rescue Squad
Andalusia, AL

John Saito, EMT-P, MPH
EMS/Paramedic Education
Oregon Health Sciences University
Portland, OR

Brad L. Sparks
Paramedic Program Coordinator
St. Francis Hospital and Health Centers
Indianapolis, IN

Andrew W. Stern, NREMT-P, MPA, MA
Senior Paramedic/Flightmedic
Town of Colonie Emergency Medical
  Services
Colonie, NY

Regina M. Twisdale, AS, MICP
Director, School of Paramedic Sciences
Virtua Health/Camden County College
Camden County, NJ

Michael D. Zemany
Director of Education
Mt. Lakes Regional EMS Program
Saranac Lake, NY

PHOTO ACKNOWLEDGMENTS

All photographs not credited adjacent to the photograph or in the photo credit section below were photographed on assignment for Brady/Prentice Hall Pearson Education.

Organizations

We wish to thank the following people and organizations for their valuable assistance in creating the photo program for the paramedic volumes:

Marshall Eiss, REMT
Special Events Coordinator
Indian Rocks Volunteer Firemen's Association
Indian Rocks Beach, FL

Steve Fravel, NREMT-P
Pinellas County EMS & Fire Administration
Largo, FL

C.T. "Chuck" Kearns, MBA, EMT-P
Director, Pinellas County EMS/Sunstar
Largo, FL

Chief John R. Leahy, Jr.
Pinellas Suncoast Fire & Rescue
Indian Rocks Beach, FL

Darryl Quigley
TLC Ambulance Service
Dallas, TX

Rural/Metro Medical Services,
   Syracuse, NY
North Area Volunteer Ambulance
   Corps (NAVAC)
North Syracuse, NY

Chief David Schrodt
Midlothian Fire Department
Midlothian, TX

Rev. Robert A. Wagenseil, Jr.
Chaplain—Pinellas Suncoast Fire &
   Rescue
Rector—Cavalry Episcopal Church
Indian Rocks Beach, FL

Robert A. Walley, REMT
District Chief
Pinellas Suncoast Fire & Rescue
Indian Rocks Beach, FL

Special thanks to Jeff Goethe of Philips Medical Systems for provision of electronic monitors.

Technical Advisors

Thanks to the following people for providing valuable technical support during the photo shoots:

Richard A. Cherry, MS, NREMT-P
Clinical Assistant Professor of Emergency
   Medicine
Assistant Residency Director
Upstate Medical University
Syracuse, NY

Michael Cox, Instructor
Division of State Fire Marshal
Florida Bureau of Fire Standards
   and Training
Florida State Fire College
Ocala, FL

Richard T. Walker, EMT-P
District Chief
Pinellas Suncoast Fire & Rescue
Indian Rocks Beach, FL

Digital postproduction:
   Richard Carter, Tampa, FL

About the Authors

BRYAN E. BLEDSOE, D.O., F.A.C.E.P., EMT-P

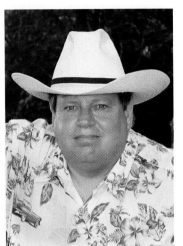

Dr. Bryan Bledsoe is an emergency physician with a special interest in prehospital care. He received his B.S. degree from the University of Texas at Arlington and his medical degree from the University of North Texas Health Sciences Center/Texas College of Osteopathic Medicine. He completed his internship at Texas Tech University and residency training at Scott and White Memorial Hospital/Texas A&M College of Medicine. Dr. Bledsoe is board certified in emergency medicine. Dr. Bledsoe is an Adjunct Associate Professor of Emergency Medicine at The George Washington University Medical Center in Washington, DC.

Prior to attending medical school, Dr. Bledsoe worked as an EMT, a paramedic, and a paramedic instructor. He completed EMT training in 1974 and paramedic training in 1976 and worked for 6 years as a field paramedic in Fort Worth, Texas. In 1979, he joined the faculty of the University of North Texas Health Sciences Center and served as coordinator of EMT and paramedic education programs at the university. Dr. Bledsoe is active in emergency medicine and EMS research. He is a popular speaker at state, national, and international seminars and writes regularly for numerous EMS journals.

Dr. Bledsoe has authored several EMS books published by Brady including *Paramedic Care: Principles & Practice, Essentials of Paramedic Care, Intermediate Emergency Care: Principles & Practice, Anatomy & Physiology for Emergency Care, Prehospital Emergency Pharmacology,* and *Pocket Reference for EMTs and Paramedics.* He is married to Emma Bledsoe. They have two children, Bryan and Andrea, and a grandson, Andrew, and live on a ranch south of Dallas, Texas. He enjoys saltwater fishing and warm latitudes.

ROBERT S. PORTER, M.A., NREMT-P

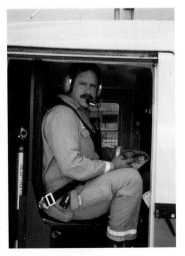

Robert Porter has been teaching in emergency medical services for 30 years and currently serves as the Senior Advanced Life Support Educator for Madison County, New York, and as a Flight Paramedic with the Onondaga, New York, County Sheriff's Department helicopter service, AirOne. Mr. Porter is a Wisconsin native and received his bachelor's degree in education from the University of Wisconsin. He completed his paramedic training at Northeast Wisconsin Technical Institute in 1978 and earned a master's degree in health education at Central Michigan University in 1990.

Mr. Porter has been an EMT and EMS educator and administrator since 1973 and obtained his national registration as an EMT-Paramedic in 1978. He has taught both basic and advanced EMS courses in the states of Wisconsin, Michigan, Louisiana, Pennsylvania, and New York. Mr. Porter served for more than 10 years as a paramedic program accreditation-site evaluator for the American Medical Association and is a past chair of the National Society of EMT Instructor/Coordinators. He has authored Brady's

Paramedic Care: Principles & Practice, Essentials of Paramedic Care, Intermediate Emergency Care: Principles & Practice, Tactical Emergency Care, and *Weapons of Mass Destruction: Emergency Care,* as well as the workbooks accompanying this text, *Paramedic Emergency Care,* and *Intermediate Emergency Care.* When not writing or teaching, Mr. Porter enjoys offshore sailboat racing and historic home restoration.

RICHARD A. CHERRY, M.S., NREMT-P

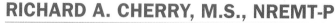

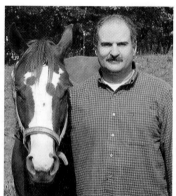

Richard Cherry is Clinical Assistant Professor of Emergency Medicine and Assistant Residency Director at Upstate Medical University in Syracuse, New York. His experience includes years of classroom teaching and emergency fieldwork. A native of Buffalo, Mr. Cherry earned his bachelor's degree at nearby St. Bonaventure University in 1972. He taught high school for the next 10 years while he earned his master's degree in education from Oswego State University in 1977. He holds a permanent teaching license in New York State.

Mr. Cherry entered the emergency medical services field in 1974 with the DeWitt Volunteer Fire Department, where he served his community as a firefighter and EMS provider for more than 15 years. He took his first EMT course in 1977 and became an ALS provider 2 years later. He earned his paramedic certificate in 1985 as a member of the area's first paramedic class.

Mr. Cherry has authored several books for Brady. Most notable are *Paramedic Care: Principles & Practice, Essentials of Paramedic Care, Intermediate Emergency Care: Principles & Practice,* and *EMT Teaching: A Common Sense Approach.* He has made presentations at many state, national, and international EMS conferences on a variety of teaching topics. He regularly teaches in the paramedic program he helped establish and is Regional Faculty for ACLS and PALS. As Assistant Residency Director he is responsible for implementing the 3-year emergency medicine core curriculum through weekly conferences. He and his wife Sue run a horse-riding camp for children with cancer and other life-threatening diseases on their property in West Monroe, New York. He also plays guitar in a Christian band.

Welcome to Paramedic Care

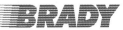

Brady
Prentice Hall Health
Upper Saddle River, NJ 07458

Dear Instructor:

Brady, your partner in education, is pleased to present the 2nd edition of our best-selling *Paramedic Care: Principles & Practice*. This revision is one of the most important we've published to date. Since we published the 1st edition, changes in education, publishing, technology, and the EMS profession have been occurring at a greater rate than ever. Indeed, the world is a different place today. Responding to these changes in a meaningful way required us to look at this series from several perspectives—its history, its quality, its experience, and its commitment. Getting to the next edition meant taking a close look at the past and discovering the things that make us a unique choice.

PCPP has a rich and long history. Since the advent of the EMS profession, several things have happened in the Advanced Life Support arena: a curriculum emerged; care is more widely available; care is more consistent; and it's now beginning to benefit from research. Our authors have been associated with this product all along the way, taking care to ensure that the latest and safest practices are taught. This edition is an extension of that care.

When the 1st edition of *PCPP* was published, two unique things happened: 1) the series went to the #1 position in the market; and 2) there were very few errors. This is an exceptional success story in the publishing world. What made this happen? In a word, quality. The authoring, developmental, and production acumen on this series is second to none. They take no shortcuts, and they never compromise the needs of their customers. This new edition has the same individuals at work together to create an even better solution.

Quality also comes from experience. Our authors have been known for their clear, comprehensive, and accurate style of presentation for more than 25 years. They are active, accessible teachers, writers, and practitioners who enjoy respect among their peers. At Brady, our combined editorial experience is 70 years, with more than 20 years focused on EMS exclusively. Our production and design experience totals more than 70 years. Finally, our EMS-exclusive sales and marketing experience is over 100 years! This means that we're specialists; we have in-depth product knowledge; and we can truly understand what we can offer our customers based on their individual needs.

Last is our commitment. The people—inside and outside Brady—affiliated with this series can't think of anything they'd rather be doing. This dedication comes through, every step of the way, in our writing, reviewing, photography, marketing, and selling. We truly believe we have an obligation to provide the best possible product, so that you can teach students to provide the best possible care. In the world of educational publishing, there are few equals to this combination. We believe it translates into what you'll see as you take a look inside this series. We also believe it represents the work of professionals and hope that our work enables your students to become the same—professionals.

We know you have many choices when it comes to choosing a textbook and appreciate the support you've given us over the years. This support has enabled us to continue to bring you up-to-date, accurate, consistent, comprehensive, and relevant products for EMS education. We're committed to helping students learn to become the best professionals possible. After all, it's they who may help us in an emergency some day. This new edition is an extension of our promise to you and to them.

Sincerely,

Julie Levin Alexander
VP/Publisher

Katrin Beacom
Senior Marketing Manager

Marlene McHugh Pratt
Executive Editor

Thomas Kennally
National Sales Manager

Lois Berlowitz
Senior Managing Editor

▼Emphasizing Principles

Objectives

Part 1: Cardiovascular Anatomy and Physiology, ECG Monitoring, and Dysrhythmia Analysis (begins on p. 73)

After reading Part 1 of this chapter, you should be able to:

1. Describe the incidence, morbidity, and mortality of cardiovascular disease. (pp. 71, 241)
2. Discuss prevention strategies that may reduce the morbidity and mortality of cardiovascular disease. (pp. 71–72)
3. Identify the risk factors most predisposing to coronary artery disease. (pp. 71–72)

◄ **Chapter Objectives with Page References.** List the objectives that form the basis of each chapter, in addition to the page on which each objective is covered.

One of your most important skills as a paramedic will be obtaining and interpreting ECG rhythm strips.

▲ **Key Points.** Help students identify and learn fundamental points.

cardiovascular disease (CVD) *disease affecting the heart, peripheral blood vessels, or both.*

▲ **Key Terms.** Located in margins near the paragraphs in which they first appear, these help students master new terminology.

✓ Review

Content

Factors Affecting Stroke Volume

- Preload
- Cardiac contractility
- Afterload

▲ **Content Review.** Summarizes important content, giving students a format for quick review.

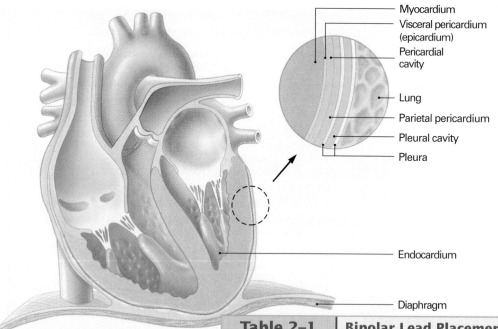

Figure 2-2 Layers of the heart.

Myocardium
Visceral pericardium (epicardium)
Pericardial cavity
Lung
Parietal pericardium
Pleural cavity
Pleura
Endocardium
Diaphragm

◄▼ **Tables and Illustrations.** Provide visual support to enhance understanding.

Table 2–1	Bipolar Lead Placement Sites	
Lead	Positive Electrode	Negative Electrode
I	Left arm	Right arm
II	Left leg	Right arm
III	Left leg	Left arm

Emphasizing Principles ▼

Summary

▶ **Summary.** Provides students with a concise review of important chapter information.

Cardiovascular disease is the number-one cause of death in the United States and Canada. Many deaths from heart attack occur within the first 24 hours—frequently within the first hour. With the advent of fibrinolytic therapy, time is of the essence when managing the patient with suspected ischemic heart disease. EMS plays an ever-increasing role in the early recognition of patients suffering coronary ischemia. In certain areas, EMS provides definitive care by initiating fibrinolytic therapy in the field. This is especially important in cases where transport times can be long. With cardiovascular disease, EMS can truly mean the difference between life and death.

Review Questions

1. The _____ is a protective sac surrounding the heart and consists of two layers, visceral and parietal.
   a. myocardium
   b. pericardium
   c. mesocardium
   d. endocardium
2. The outermost lining of the walls of arteries and veins is the _____ _____, a fibrous tissue covering that gives the vessel strength to withstand the pressures generated by the heart's contractions.
   a. tunica media
   b. tunica intima
   c. tunica adventitia
   d. visceral media

◀ **NEW Review Questions.** Ask students to recall information and to apply the principles they've just learned.

Further Reading

Beasley, B. M. *Understanding 12-Lead EKGs: A Practical Approach.* 2nd ed. Upper Saddle River, N.J.: Pearson/Prentice Hall, 2001.

Beasley, B. M. *Understanding EKGs: A Practical Approach.* 2nd ed. Upper Saddle River, N.J.: Pearson/Prentice Hall, 2003.

Bledsoe, B. E., and D. E. Clayden. *Prehospital Emergency Pharmacology.* 6th ed. Upper Saddle River, N.J.: Pearson/Prentice Hall, 2005.

▶ **Further Reading.** Recommendations for books and journal articles.

On the Web

Visit Brady's Paramedic Website at **www.bradybooks.com/paramedic.**

◀ **On the Web.** www.bradybooks.com/paramedic refers students to a Companion Website, where additional activities and information can be found on the chapter's topics. Also, links to other topic-specific website are listed.

Case Study

The crew of Paramedic Unit 112 is called to a local nursing home to evaluate Mr. Evan Henry, an 80-year-old male with chest pain. It is Sunday afternoon, and Mr. Henry's family has been visiting from out of town. Not used to all the attention and excitement, Mr. Henry has developed substernal chest pain that radiates to his left arm. He has a history of this type of pain, but it usually resolves after one or two sublingual nitroglycerin tablets. This time, however, the nitroglycerin tablets have failed to alleviate his pain. Because of this, the nursing home staff has activated the EMS system.

◀ **Case Study.** Draws students into the reading and creates a link between the text content and real-life situations and experiences.

You Make the Call

▶ **You Make the Call.** Promotes critical thinking by requiring students to apply principles to actual practice.

You and your partner on Medic 3 are dispatched to a well-kept residence about three blocks from the station. The dispatch information relates the nature of the call as a medical emergency. On your arrival at the residence, the patient's wife meets you and shows you to a back room. The patient is a male who appears to be in his late 60s. He is complaining of severe back pain that began approximately 30 minutes ago. He thinks it may be due to some light yard work he did earlier in the day. The patient appears in severe distress, however, and is sweaty and diaphoretic.

| Procedure 2–5 | **12-Lead Prehospital ECG Monitoring** |

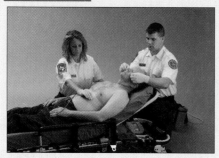

2-5a   Prep the skin.

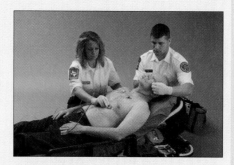

2-5b   Place the four limb leads according to the manufacturer's recommendations.

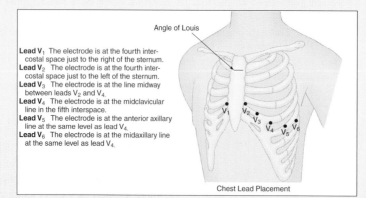

Angle of Louis

Lead V₁ The electrode is at the fourth intercostal space just to the right of the sternum.
Lead V₂ The electrode is at the fourth intercostal space just to the left of the sternum.
Lead V₃ The electrode is at the line midway between leads V₂ and V₄.
Lead V₄ The electrode is at the midclavicular line in the fifth interspace.
Lead V₅ The electrode is at the anterior axillary line at the same level as lead V₄.
Lead V₆ The electrode is at the midaxillary line at the same level as lead V₄.

Chest Lead Placement

◀ **Procedure Scans.** Provide step-by-step visual support on how to perform skills.

2-5c   Proper placement of the precordial leads.

Emphasizing Practice ▼

▶ **Patient Care Algorithms.**
Provide graphic "pathways" that
integrate assessment and care
procedures.

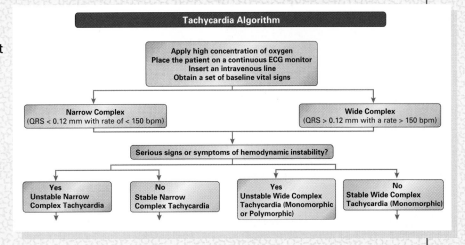

Patho Pearls

The Best Treatment for Stroke Despite the great strides in medicine, there is
still very little that can be provided to help minimize the effects of a stroke. Stroke therapy usually involves medically stabilizing the patient after the stroke and then getting
him into a physical rehabilitation program where he can regain as much motor function as possible.

◀ **NEW Patho Pearls.** Offer a
snapshot of pathological
considerations students will
encounter in the field.

▶ **NEW Legal Notes.**
Present instances in
which legal or ethical
considerations should
be evaluated.

Legal Notes

Reporting Contagious Diseases All states have provisions for reporting contagious diseases without fear of violating the patient's privacy or confidentiality issues.
Even the Health Insurance Portability and Accountability Act (HIPAA) has provisions in
place for reporting contagious disease without violating provisions of the act. There
are over 60 diseases in the United States that are reportable at a national level. In addition, there are state-reportable diseases which vary from state to state. Some illnesses, including anthrax, brucellosis, diphtheria, pertussis, plague, and others, must
be immediately reported. Others, including AIDS, gonorrhea, leprosy, and syphilis,
must be reported within 1 week. Some require reporting of individual cases and others require reporting of numbers only.

Cultural Considerations

Culture and Cardiovascular Disease Cardiovascuar disease remains the
number-one cause of death in the United States and Canada. The incidence of cardiovascular disease increased steadily during the twentieth century although it has
stabilized somewhat over the last decade or so.

◀ **NEW Cultural Considerations.**
Provide an awareness of beliefs
that might affect patient care.

Student CD

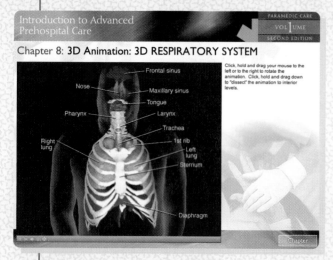

Chapter 8: 3D Animation: 3D RESPIRATORY SYSTEM

◀ **3D Animation.** Interactive 3D models encourage a deeper understanding of the body and its processes. 360° rotation and virtual dissection reinforce the concepts presented in each volume.

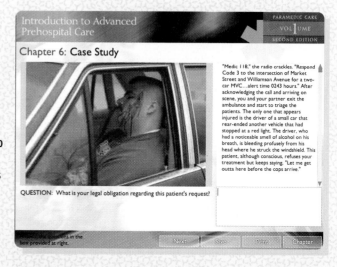

Chapter 6: Case Study

"Medic 11B," the radio crackles. "Respond Code 3 to the intersection of Market Street and Williamson Avenue for a two-car MVC...alert time 0243 hours." After acknowledging the call and arriving on scene, you and your partner exit the ambulance and start to triage the patients. The only one that appears injured is the driver of a small car that rear-ended another vehicle that had stopped at a red light. The driver, who had a noticeable smell of alcohol on his breath, is bleeding profusely from his head where he struck the windshield. This patient, although conscious, refuses your treatment but keeps saying, "Let me get outta here before the cops arrive."

QUESTION: What is your legal obligation regarding this patient's request?

▶ **Case Study.** Designed to develop critical thinking skills, each case study offers questions and rationales that help to hone the student's assessment skills.

Drug Guide

Select a drug from the list below and click. To return to this page, press the 'Home' button on your computer keyboard.

Activated Charcoal
Adenosine
Albuterol
Aminophylline
Amiodarone
Aspirin
Atenolol
Atropine
Calcium Chloride
Dextrose 50%
Diazepam
Digoxin
Dobutamine
Dopamine
Epinephrine
Etomidate
Fentanyl Citrate
Furosemide
Glucagon
Hydralazine
Ipratropium

Magnesium Sulfate
Mannitol
Metaproterenol
Methylprednisolone
Midazolam
Morphine
Naloxone
Nitroglycerin
Nitrous Oxide
Norepinephrine
Oxygen
Oxytocin
Pancuronium Bromide
Phenytoin
Procainamide
Propranolol
Sodium Bicarbonate
Sodium Nitroprusside
Succinylcholine
Thiamine
Vasopressin

◀ **Drug Guide.** A valuable reference tool, this hotlinked PDF allows quick access to important information regarding the drugs most commonly used by today's paramedic.

Focused History and Physical Exam: Trauma

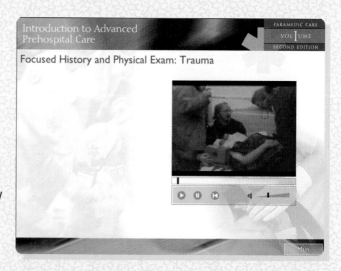

▶ **EMS Scenes.** Video clips of real-life situations put you in the action. See what you might encounter at an actual emergency scene.

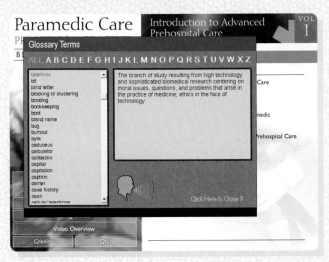

◀ **Glossary.** This interactive, indexed glossary contains the definitions and audio pronunciations of the key terms presented in each volume.

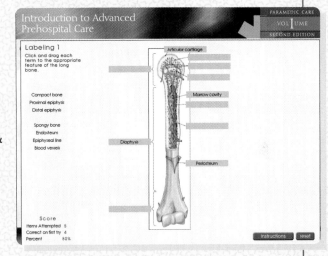

▶ **Interactives.** From Bone Structure to Body Cavities, drag & drop interactive exercises make learning both engaging and fun.

◀ **Multiple Choice.** Each chapter offers self-testing in a multiple-choice format. Upon completion, a score and feedback are provided for post-assessment.

▶ **Virtual Tours.** Including the airway, cardiovascular system, muscle-skeletal system, nervous system and heart, these narrated tours guide you through the intricate workings of the body systems in an easy-to-understand presentation.

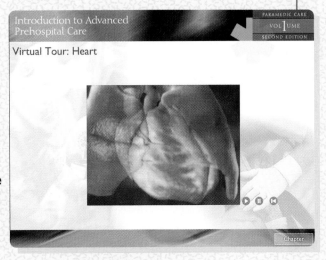

Student Workbook

A student workbook with review and practice activities accompanies each volume of the Paramedic Care series. The workbooks include multiple-choice questions, other exercises, case studies, and special projects, along with an answer key with text page references. National Registry Practical Evaluation forms and Flash Cards are also provided in each volume.

▶ **Review of Chapter Objectives. Reviews important content elements addressed by chapter objectives.**

Review of Chapter Objectives

After reading this part of the chapter, you should be able to:

1. Describe the incidence, morbidity, and mortality of cardiovascular disease.   **pp. 71, 241**

Cardiovascular disease (CVD) is serious and extremely common, with more than 60 million Americans affected. Morbidity is considerable: An American has a nonfatal heart attack (myocardial infarction, MI) roughly every 29 seconds. Coronary heart disease (CHD), one type of CVD, is the single largest killer of Americans and Canadians. Roughly 466,000 Americans die annually from CHD, half of them before reaching a hospital. Many deaths from CHD are sudden and involve lethal cardiac dysrhythmias. Many deaths from MI occur within the first 24 hours, frequently within the first hour.

Case Study Review

Reread the case study in Chapter 2 of Paramedic Care: Medical Emergencies *before reading the discussion below.*

    This case study demonstrates how paramedics react to a typical medical emergency involving chest pain. In addition to observing how the team conducts the patient's initial assessment, note how they respond as the situation quickly changes into a more complex and urgent one.

◀ **Case Study Review. Reviews and points out essential information and applied principles.**

▶▼ **Content Self-Evaluation. Multiple-choice, matching, and short-answer questions to test reading comprehension.**

Content Self-Evaluation

MULTIPLE CHOICE

_____ 1. From innermost to outermost, the three tissue layers of the heart are:
    A. the endocardium, the pericardium, and the myocardium.
    B. the endocardium, the myocardium, and the syncytium.
    C. the endocardium, the myocardium, and the pericardium.
    D. the myocardium, the epicardium, and the pericardium.
    E. the epicardium, the myocardium, and the endocardium.

MATCHING

Write the letter of the ECG leads in the space provided next to the type of leads they are.

A. I, II, III

B. V_1, V_2, V_3, V_4, V_5, V_6

C. aVR, aVL, aVF

_____ 9. unipolar (augmented)

_____ 10. bipolar

_____ 11. precordial

Fill-in-the-Blanks

56. The _____ valves lie between the atria and ventricles, whereas the _____ valves lie between the ventricles and the arteries into which they open.

57. The four properties of cells in the cardiac conductive system are _____ , _____ , _____ , and _____ .

Student Workbook ▼

Special Project

Assessing Respiratory Emergencies

Read the assessment written for each of three patients evaluated in a prehospital setting and identify the probable cause for each emergency. Check the Assessment section of the textbook for each disorder to refamiliarize yourself with characteristic findings on history and physical examination.

Scenario 1: You are called to an elementary school where a student has become "suddenly ill" during a class birthday party. You find a distressed seven-year-old child who is breathing rapidly and shallowly and whose skin tone is becoming dusky. The use of accessory muscles to breathe is evident. The school nurse offers you a box containing an inhaler that she says the child uses on an "as needed" basis and states she isn't sure what ingredients were in the cupcakes brought for the party. She adds that the boy has several severe food allergies.

Probable cause: _____

Scenario 2: You are called to a home where an elderly man is "short of breath." On arrival, you find a thin, elderly man with a broad chest whose breathing is labored despite use of a home supplemental oxygen setup. His daughter tells you that he has had a cold recently, and he suddenly became "shorter of breath" this morning. On exam, the man has a fever of

◄ **Special Projects.** Experiences designed to help students remember information and principles.

EMT-Paramedic Form

National Registry of Emergency Medical Technicians
Advanced Level Practical Examination

PATIENT ASSESSMENT - TRAUMA

Candidate: _____ Examiner: _____
Date: _____ Signature: _____

Scenario # _____

► **National Registry Practical Evaluation Forms.** Gives a clearer picture of what is expected during the practical exam.

Time Start: NOTE: Areas denoted by "*" may be integrated within sequence of Initial Assessment	Possible Points	Points Awarded
Takes or verbalizes body substance isolation precautions	1	
SCENE SIZE-UP		
Determines the scene/situation is safe	1	
Determines the mechanism of injury/nature of illness	1	
Determines the number of patients	1	
Requests additional help if necessary	1	
Considers stabilization of spine	1	

CARD 1 PATIENT HISTORY

Dispatch Information: Responding to a residence for a patient complaining of chest pain.

Scene Size-Up: Small but clean home with the patient seated on the couch, in obvious pain, and clutching his chest; no hazards noted.

Medical History
A—anesthetic at the dentist's office ("caine" family)
M—nitroglycerin and calcium supplements
P—sees his doctor yearly but doesn't have any medical problems
L—breakfast an hour ago, 2 eggs, toast, and coffee
E—watching television, nothing unusual

◄ **Patient Scenario Flash Cards.** Present scenarios with signs and symptoms and information to make field diagnoses.

Teaching and Learning Package

FOR THE INSTRUCTOR

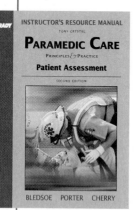

Instructor's Resource Manual. The Instructor's Resource Manual for each volume contains everything needed to teach the 1998 U.S. DOT National Standard Curriculum for Paramedics. It fully covers the DOT curriculum with:

- Time estimates for various topics
- Listing of additional resources
- Lecture outlines
- Student activities handouts
- Answers to student review questions
- Case study discussion questions
- Transition guides from current edition and competing text

This manual is also available on disk in Word and PDF format so instructors can customize resources to their individual needs.

 TestGen. Thoroughly updated and reviewed. Contains more than 2,000 exam-style questions, including DOT objectives and book page references.

PowerPoints. Updated to include additional illustrations, photos, animations, video clips, and sound. Includes all images from the textbooks.

FOR THE STUDENT

NEW Student CD. In-text CD contains quizzes, a virtual airway tour, animations, case study exercises, video skills clips, on-scene video footage, and audio glossary.

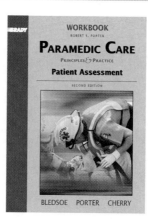

Workbook. Contains review of chapter objectives with summary information; case study review; content self-evaluation that includes multiple-choice, matching, and short-answer questions; special projects; content review; practical evaluation forms; and patient scenario flash cards.

ONLINE RESOURCES

Companion Website. Contains quizzes, labeling exercises, state EMS directories, *New York Times* link, weblinks, and trauma gallery.

 OneKey. A distance learning program to support the series, offered on one of three platforms: Course Compass, Blackboard, or WebCT. Includes the IRM, PowerPoints, Test Manager, and Companion Website for instruction. Features include:

- Course outline
- Online gradebook, which automatically keeps track of students' performance on quizzes, class participation, and attendance
- Ability to upload questions authored offline and to randomize question order for each student
- Ability to add your own URLs and course links, set up discussion boards, modify navigation features
- A virtual classroom for real-time sessions and communication with students
- Weblinks
- Ability to include your teaching assistants into course creation/management

Other Titles of Interest

SKILLS

Brady Skills Series: Advanced Life Support (0-13-119307-4—video; 0-13-119326-0—CD)
26 skills presented in step-by-step format with introduction, equipment, overview, and close-up, including assessment.

Advanced Life Support Skills (0-13-093874-2)
26 skills presented in full color, with step-by-step photos and rationales.

ALS Skills Review (0-13-193637-9)
Close-ups for 26 skills, for student review.

REVIEW & REFERENCE

Beasley, Mistovich, *EMT Achieve: Paramedic Test Preparation* (0-13-119269-8)
Online test preparation, with full-length exams and quizzes, with rationales and supporting text, artwork, and video.

Cherry, Mistovich, *EMT-Paramedic Self-Assessment Exam Review*, 3rd edition (0-13-112869-8)
Best-selling review, containing test questions with DOT and text page references and rationales.

Miller, *Paramedic National Standards Self-Test*, 4th edition (0-13-110500-0)
Based on the 1998 DOT curriculum, uses self-test format to target areas students need to study further. Includes multiple-choice and scenario-based questions.

Bledsoe, Clayden, *Pocket Reference for ALS Providers*, 3rd edition (0-13-170728-0)
Drugs, dosages, algorithms, tables and charts, pediatric emergencies, advanced skills, and home medications provided in an easy-to-use field guide.

Cherry, Bledsoe, *Drug Guide for Paramedics* (0-13-028798-9)
Handy field resource for accurate, easily accessed information about patient medication.

Cherry, *Patient Assessment Handbook* (0-13-061578-1)
Concise, illustrated, step-by-step procedures for assessment techniques.

ANATOMY & PHYSIOLOGY

Martini, Bartholemew, Bledsoe, *Anatomy & Physiology for Emergency Care* (0-13-042298-3)
EMS-specific applications at the end of every chapter provide an emergency care focus to A&P discussions.

CARDIAC/EKG

Walraven, *Basic Arrhythmias*, 6th edition (0-13-117591-2)
Classic best-seller covers all the basics of EKG and includes a new student CD. Also contains appendices on clinical implications, cardiac anatomy & physiology, 12-lead EKG, basic 12-lead interpretation, and pacemakers.

Beasley, *Understanding EKGs: A Practical Approach*, 2nd edition (0-13-045215-7)
A direct approach to EKG interpretation that presents all the essential concepts for mastering the basics of this challenging field, while assuming no prior knowledge of EKGs.

Page, *12-Lead ECG for Acute and Critical Care Providers* (0-13-022460-X)
This full-color text presents ECG interpretation in a practical, easy-to-understand, and user-friendly manner.

Beasley, *Understanding 12-Lead EKGs: A Practical Approach*, 2nd edition (0-13-170789-2)
This comprehensive, reader-friendly text teaches beginning students basic 12-lead EKG interpretation.

Mistovich, et al., *Prehospital Advanced Cardiac Life Support*, 2nd edition (0-13-110143-9)
Straightforward and easy to follow, this text offers clear explanations, a colorful design, and covers all of the core concepts covered in an advanced cardiac life support course.

MEDICAL

Dalton, et al., *Advanced Medical Life Support*, 2nd edition (0-13-098632-1)
This groundbreaking text offers a practical approach to adult medical emergencies. Each chapter discusses realistic methods that a seasoned EMS practitioner would use.

Other Titles of Interest

MEDICAL TERMINOLOGY

Rice, *Medical Terminology with Human Anatomy*, 5th edition (0-13-048706-6)
Providing comprehensive coverage of all aspects of medical terminology, along with overviews of anatomy and physiology, this popular text is arranged by body systems and specialty areas.

PEDIATRICS

Markenson, et al., *Pediatric Prehospital Care* (0-13-022618-1)
Written for all levels of EMS providers, this text presents a physiological approach to rapid and accurate pediatric assessment, identification of potential problems, establishing treatment priorities with effective on-going assessment, and rapid and safe transport.

PHARMACOLOGY

Bledsoe, Clayden, *Prehospital Emergency Pharmacology*, 6th edition (0-13-150711-7)
This text and handy reference is a complete guide to the most common medications used in prehospital care.

TRAUMA

Campbell, *Basic Trauma Life Support for Paramedics and Advanced Providers*, 5th edition (0-13-112351-3)
Best-selling BTLS text provides a complete course that covers all the skills necessary for rapid assessment, resuscitation, stabilization, and transportation of the trauma patient.

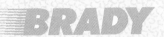

Paramedic Care

Principles & Practice

INTRODUCTION TO ADVANCED PREHOSPITAL CARE

SECOND EDITION

Introduction to Advanced Prehospital Care

Objectives

After reading this chapter, you should be able to:

1. Describe the relationship between the paramedic and other members of the allied health professions. (pp. 5–6)
2. Identify the attributes and characteristics of the paramedic. (pp. 6–7)
3. Explain the elements of paramedic education and practice that support its stature as a profession. (pp. 7–8)
4. Define and give examples of the expanded scope of practice for the paramedic. (pp. 7–8, 10)

Case Study

Stephen Fletcher retired earlier this year after a 30-year career as a computer systems analyst with a Fortune 500 company. He is approaching retirement with the same vigor in which he approached his former job. Stephen and his wife, Karen, are planning to fulfill a longtime dream by visiting every national park in the continental United States. They recently arrived at Big Bend National Park in remote west Texas and expect to spend a week exploring this massive park.

Stephen, as usual, awakens at the crack of dawn. He and Karen are planning a hike through the Chisos Mountains, taking a trail that is not far from the lodge and is well traveled. Shortly after setting off, Stephen develops a dull, pressure-like sensation in his chest. At the same time, he becomes slightly nauseated. His wife notices that he is pale and sweaty. Stephen attributes these symptoms to last night's dinner. He decides to sit down and wait until the symptoms resolve before going on with the hike.

After a 15-minute rest, however, Stephen's chest pressure and nausea persist and he is still pale and sweaty. He is becoming increasingly anxious and finally tells his wife what he's thinking: "You know, Karen, I'm afraid I could be having a heart attack." They agree that Karen should go and look for help. The Park Service has a ranger station near the lodge.

Karen makes Stephen as comfortable as she can and then starts back down the trail. Fortunately, within a quarter of a mile, she runs into a park ranger guiding a group of tourists. She tells him about Stephen and gives an approximate location. The ranger immediately uses his radio to summon EMS and First Responders. He asks the tour group to return to the lodge and goes with Karen to assist Stephen.

Medic-2 of Brewster County EMS is dispatched along with Park Service First Responders. The First Responders reach Stephen's side within 5 minutes of dispatch and perform a brief assessment. Stephen is still having chest pressure and is now also having some shortness of breath. In addition, he has vomited twice. The First Responders administer oxygen via a nonrebreather mask. They make Stephen comfortable and open a canvas tarp to keep off the hot west Texas sun.

Medic-2 is a specially staffed and equipped EMS unit assigned to Big Bend National Park during the peak season. The park covers 801,163 acres of rugged mountains and high desert. It is the least visited U.S. National Park in the lower 48 states. The closest major medical center is over 200 miles away, which is generally too far for helicopter transport. The paramedics who staff Medic-2 are in a unique situation. Because of problems accessing patients and long transport times, they often must provide patient care for periods exceeding 3 hours.

The crew of Medic-2, Keith Bundick and Dudley Wilcoxson, arrive at the scene approximately 15 minutes after dispatch. Park Service personnel have carried the patient to the trailhead where he is immediately moved into the air-conditioned ambulance. Keith and Dudley begin their assessment. While Keith continues with the assessment, Dudley starts an IV with a heparin lock. In addition, he attaches the electrodes for the 12 lead ECG.

The patient's initial vital signs reveal a blood pressure of 142/98 mmHg, a pulse rate of 56 beats per minute, and respirations of 22 breaths per minute. The SpO$_2$ is 98 percent with the nonrebreather mask. The 12 lead ECG reveals a sinus bradycardia with an elevation of the ST segments in Leads II, III, and aVF. Based on the ECG and physical exam findings, Keith and Dudley conclude that the patient is suffering an acute inferior wall myocardial infarction. By now, approximately 1 hour has passed since the onset of symptoms. The paramedics contact medical direction and fax the ECG via the radio.

The medical direction physician agrees with their assessment. Because of the location and transport time, he feels that the patient may benefit from prehospital fibrinolytic therapy. The paramedics screen the patient for possible fibrinolytic therapy and determine that he has no contraindications. His only chronic health problems are mild hypertension that is being treated with atenolol (Tenormin) and prostate problems.

The paramedics explain their findings and treatment plan to Stephen and Karen. The Fletchers understand and agree to fibrinolytic therapy. An additional heparin lock is placed and the patient is given an aspirin tablet by mouth. Keith also administers 4 milligrams of morphine sulfate and 12.5 milligrams of promethazine (Phenergan) intravenously. This decreases the patient's pain from a score of 5/10 to 1/10 or better. Keith prepares the tissue-plasminogen activator (tPA) for administration. Per their standing orders, 15 milligrams of tPA are administered over 2 minutes as a bolus. This is followed by an infusion of 50 mg over 30 minutes with the remaining 35 milligrams being administered over an hour.

Following the tPA bolus and initiation of tPA infusion therapy, they depart for the airport at Lajitas. While en route, approximately 25 minutes into the tPA protocol, Stephen develops several runs of ventricular tachycardia and exhibits frequent multifocal premature ventricular contractions (PVCs). Keith administers 100 milligrams of lidocaine intravenously and the PVCs disappear. Per protocol, he begins a lidocaine infusion at 2 milligrams per minute. About the same time the dysrhythmias begin, the patient becomes pain-free. His skin color improves and his shortness of breath completely resolves. Keith notes also that the patient's ST segments in Leads II, III, and aVF have returned to normal.

Medic-2 arrives at the rural airstrip where a Beech King Air 350 is waiting. Since Big Bend is too far from a major medical center to allow for helicopter transport, fixed-wing aircraft are dispatched from Odessa, Midland, or El Paso when transport is needed. Stephen is moved from the ambulance to the aircraft. Keith and Dudley turn care over to the two Critical Care Paramedics who staff the aircraft. They provide the patient report, and the handoff is smooth. Keith and Dudley return to the ambulance and watch as the King Air lifts off for the 30-minute flight to Odessa.

Upon arrival at the medical center, Stephen is admitted directly to the Coronary Care Unit (CCU). He remains pain-free. Upon completion of tPA therapy, a heparin infusion is started. The next day, he is taken to the cardiac lab and a cardiac catheterization is completed. The cath reveals a 95 percent blockage in the right coronary artery. Balloon angioplasty is performed, which results in marked improvement in the blockage. Fortunately, Stephen only has mild coronary artery disease and will not require coronary artery bypass surgery. Overall, his prognosis is very good.

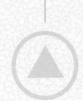

The best news is that the tPA administered by the paramedics was successful in breaking down the clot in the right coronary artery that was causing the myocardial ischemia. Stephen did not sustain any permanent damage to his myocardium. In fact, he did not even have any elevation of cardiac enzymes. He is released the next day and returns home to Missouri for some rest before he and Karen resume their quest to visit every national park in the continental United States.

INTRODUCTION

Congratulations on your decision to become an EMT-Paramedic. Before you begin this long but rewarding endeavor, it is important to understand what the job of an EMT-Paramedic in the twenty-first century entails.

Emergency Medical Services (EMS) has made significant advances over the last 30 years. Understandably, the roles and responsibilities of the paramedic have advanced accordingly. Not that long ago, the ambulance was simply a vehicle that provided rapid, horizontal transportation to the hospital. Today, equipped with the latest in equipment and technology, the modern ambulance is truly a mobile emergency room. The paramedic of the twenty-first century is a highly trained health care professional who provides comprehensive, compassionate, and efficient prehospital emergency medical care.

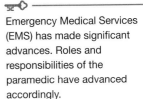

Emergency Medical Services (EMS) has made significant advances. Roles and responsibilities of the paramedic have advanced accordingly.

DESCRIPTION OF THE PROFESSION

The paramedic is the highest level of prehospital care provider and the leader of the prehospital care team. As a member of the allied health professions (ancillary health care professions, apart from physicians and nurses), the paramedic is highly regarded by society (Figure 1-1 ■).

The primary task of the paramedic is to provide emergency medical care in an out-of-hospital setting. As a paramedic, you will use your advanced training and equipment to extend the care of the emergency physician to the patient in the field. However, you must also be able to make accurate independent judgments. The ability to do this in a timely manner is essential, as it can mean the difference between life and death for the patient.

In order to function as a paramedic—to practice the art and science of out-of-hospital medicine in conjunction with medical direction—you must have fulfilled the prescribed requirements of the appropriate licensing or credentialing body. Licensing

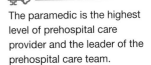

The paramedic is the highest level of prehospital care provider and the leader of the prehospital care team.

The ability to make independent judgments in a timely manner can mean the difference between life and death for the patient.

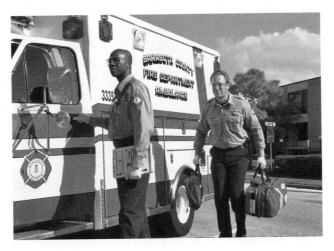

■ Figure 1-1   The paramedic of the twenty-first century is a highly trained health care professional.

or credentialing is typically provided by a state or provincial agency. All paramedics must be licensed, registered, or otherwise credentialed by the appropriate agency in the area where they work.

Paramedics may only function under the direction and license of the EMS system's medical director. Because of this, in addition to being appropriately licensed or credentialed, the paramedic must also be approved by the system's medical director before being permitted to practice advanced prehospital care. Paramedics must possess knowledge, skills, and attitudes consistent with the expectations of the public and the profession.

As a paramedic, you must recognize that you are an essential component in the continuum of care. Furthermore, paramedics often serve as a link between various health resources. In the future, there will be a continuing demand to control or cut health care costs. As a consequence, paramedics may find themselves in the role of a gatekeeper to the health care system. For example, you may be charged with the responsibility of assuring that your patient gets to the appropriate health care facility in a timely manner, even though the appropriate health care facility may not be a hospital emergency department.

Paramedics must always strive toward maintaining high quality health care at a reasonable cost. Nevertheless, you must always be an advocate for your patient and assure that the patient receives the best possible care—without regard to the patient's ability to pay or insurance status (Figure 1-2 ■).

While paramedics of the twenty-first century will continue to fill the well-defined and traditional role of 911 response, they will also find themselves taking on a wide variety of additional responsibilities. The emerging roles and responsibilities of the paramedic include public education, health promotion, and participation in injury and illness prevention programs. As the scope of paramedic service continues to expand, the paramedic will function as a facilitator of access to care as well as an individual treatment provider.

Paramedics are responsible and accountable to the system medical director, their employer, the public, and their peers. Although this may seem like a difficult standard to meet, if you always act in the best interest of the patient, you will seldom run into problems.

PARAMEDIC CHARACTERISTICS

There are many different types of EMS system designs and operations. As a paramedic, you may work for a fire department, private ambulance service, third city service, hospital, police department, or other operation. Regardless of the type of service provider you work for, you must be flexible in order to meet the demands of the ever-changing emergency scene.

You must always be an advocate for your patient and assure that the patient receives the best possible care—without regard to the patient's ability to pay.

The emerging roles and responsibilities of the paramedic include public education, health promotion, and participation in injury and illness prevention programs.

Paramedics are accountable to their medical director, their employer, the public, and peers. However, if you always act in the best interest of the patient, you will seldom have problems.

■ Figure 1-2   The paramedic must always be an advocate for the patient. (© *Craig Jackson/ In the Dark Photography*)

Which Hat Are You Wearing? The modern paramedic must wear several hats. Many paramedics are also cross-trained as firefighters or police officers. The role of each of these professions is different, but there is often significant overlapping of duties. Paramedics may participate in rescue operations, directing traffic, firefighting, and other tasks on an emergency scene. However, it is essential that, when functioning in the role of paramedic, you remember that your primary responsibility is the patient and patient care. You must also be an advocate for the patient.

If you are cross-trained, this can cause a certain degree of confusion and conflict. For example, if you are a cross-trained police officer/paramedic who is treating an intoxicated driver, you may have conflicting responsibilities. However, as noted above, when you are functioning as a paramedic your priority should be the patient. Legal issues and other tasks normally addressed by police officers must be handled by other police officers on scene or dealt with after the patient has been treated and transported. Similarly, paramedics who are cross-trained may learn information about a patient that is protected from disclosure by the Health Insurance Portability and Accountability Act (HIPAA) and other medical privacy laws and regulations. In a case like this, you may not be able to disclose certain information to your law enforcement colleagues despite the fact that you are also a police officer.

Laws regarding responsibilities of cross-trained individuals vary from state to state. You must be familiar with the laws of the state where you are employed. Remember: When you function as a paramedic, you must put care of the patient above all other tasks—and always remember which hat you are wearing.

As a paramedic, you must be a confident leader who can accept the challenge and responsibility of the position. You must have excellent judgment and be able to prioritize decisions so as to act quickly in the best interest of the patient. You must be able to develop rapport with a wide variety of patients so that, for example, you can safely interview hostile patients and communicate with members of diverse cultural groups and the various ages within those groups. Overall, you must be able to function independently at an optimum level in a nonstructured, constantly changing environment. The job is never easy and always challenging.

You must be a confident leader—able to function independently at an optimum level in a nonstructured, constantly changing environment. The job is never easy and always challenging.

THE PARAMEDIC: A TRUE HEALTH PROFESSIONAL

Despite its relative youth as a profession, the field of emergency medical services is now recognized as an important part of the health care system. With this, paramedics are now highly respected members of the health care team. As a paramedic, you must never take this status for granted. Instead, you must always strive to earn your acceptance as a health care professional.

You must always strive to earn your status as a health care professional.

You should consider the completion of your initial paramedic course to be the start of your professional education, not the end. You should participate in various continuing education programs when they become available. Skills that are infrequently used should be frequently reviewed and practiced to assure competency when the skill is needed. As a rule, the less a skill or procedure is used, the more frequent should be the review of that skill or procedure. Most quality continuing education programs acknowledge this by scheduling periodic review and practice of infrequently used skills or procedures. Professional development should be a never-ending, career-long pursuit. Additionally, you should participate in routine peer-evaluation and assume an active role in professional and community organizations (Figure 1-3 ■).

Professional development should be a never-ending, career-long pursuit.

A major step toward the development of EMS as a true health care profession has been to raise the standards of education for prehospital personnel. A significant advance

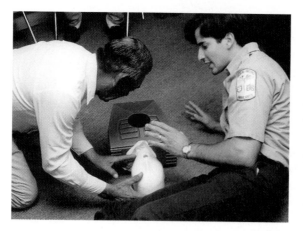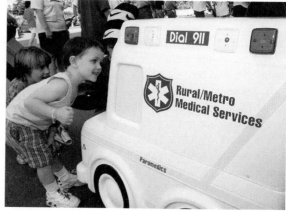

■ Figure 1-3 Public education is an important part of the paramedic's job. *(Both © Craig Jackson/In the Dark Photography)*

was the 1998 publication by the U.S. Department of Transportation of the revised *EMT-Paramedic: National Standard Curriculum*. This curriculum has taken paramedic education to a much higher level. An anatomy and physiology course is now a prerequisite to the paramedic course. The paramedic course itself requires a far more extensive foundation of medical knowledge to underlie the required skills. In particular, the curriculum provides for a much improved understanding of the pathophysiology of the various illness and injury processes paramedics encounter in their work. The 1998 DOT paramedic curriculum (Figure 1-4 ■) is the guideline for this textbook.

As a paramedic, you must actively participate in the design, development, evaluation, and publication of research on topics relevant to your profession. For years, paramedic practice was based on anecdotal data and tradition. Only during the 1990s did we truly begin applying the scientific method to various aspects of prehospital practice. Surprisingly, we found that there were little or no scientific data to support many of our prehospital practices. As a result of research, many traditional EMS treatments have been abandoned or refined. There are still many unanswered questions about paramedic practice, and these can only be answered by sound scientific research.

An essential aspect of a health professional is acceptance and adherence to a code of professional ethics and etiquette. Ethics are standards of right or honorable behavior, while etiquette refers to good manners. Both can apply to all human relationships. However, you will find that questions of ethics most often arise in relationships with patients and the public, while etiquette more often relates to behavior between health professionals.

The public must feel confident that, for the paramedic, the patient's and public's interests are always placed above personal, corporate, or financial interests. You must never forget that the emergency patient is your primary concern. Emergency patients are vulnerable and in need. Always keep this in mind and serve as their advocate until you turn patient care over to another health care professional.

EXPANDED SCOPE OF PRACTICE

Paramedics have a very bright future. New technologies and therapies can literally bring the emergency department to the patient. Paramedics must be willing to step up to these expanding roles, or persons from other health care disciplines will fill them. There are many aspects of out-of-hospital care that can provide you with the opportunity to work in an environment other than the typical 911 response vehicle. These include:

★ Critical care transport
★ Primary care

EMT-PARAMEDIC: NATIONAL STANDARD CURRICULUM
EDUCATIONAL MODEL

COMPETENCIES
Mathematics, reading, and writing

PRE- or CO-REQUISITE
EMT or EMT-Basic Human Anatomy and Physiology

Clinical/Field	**PREPARATORY** EMS Systems/The Roles and Responsibilities of the Paramedic The Well-Being of the Paramedic Illness and Injury Prevention Medical/Legal Issues Ethics General Principles of Pathophysiology Pharmacology Venous Access and Medication Administration Therapeutic Communications Life Span Development	Clinical/Field
	AIRWAY MANAGEMENT AND VENTILATION	
MEDICAL Pulmonary Cardiology Neurology Endocrinology Allergies and Anaphylaxis Gastroenterology Renal/Urology Toxicology Hematology Environmental Conditions Infectious and Communicable Diseases Behavioral and Psychiatric Disorders Gynecology Obstetrics	**PATIENT ASSESSMENT** History Taking Techniques of Physical Examination Patient Assessment Clinical Decision Making Communications Documentation	**TRAUMA** Trauma Systems/Mechanism of Injury Hemorrhage and Shock Soft Tissue Trauma Burns Head and Facial Trauma Spinal Trauma Thoracic Trauma Abdominal Trauma Musculoskeletal Trauma
Clinical/Field	**SPECIAL CONSIDERATIONS** Neonatology Pediatrics Geriatrics Abuse and Assault Patients with Special Challenges Acute Interventions for the Chronic Care Patient	Clinical/Field
	ASSESSMENT BASED MANAGEMENT	
	OPERATIONS Ambulance Operations Medical Incident Command Rescue Awareness and Operations Hazardous Materials Incidents Crime Scene Awareness	

LIFELONG LEARNING
Continuing education

Figure 1-4 The 1998 EMT-Paramedic Curriculum.

* Industrial medicine
* Sports medicine

Paramedics are now stepping into nontraditional roles such as these because of their unique education and ability to think and work independently.

CRITICAL CARE TRANSPORT

As a result of the specialization of health care facilities that began to occur in the 1990s, an increasing number of patients are being moved from one health care facility to another for specialized care. Many of these patients are critically ill and require equipment and care more sophisticated than that available on standard ambulances. Because of this, many EMS systems have developed specialized critical care transport vehicles to move these patients between facilities.

These vehicles include specialized ground ambulances, fixed-wing aircraft, and helicopters. Many services have elected to utilize large vehicles mounted on a truck chassis to provide the added space needed for critical care transport (Figure 1-5 ■). To staff these vehicles, paramedics have been educated in various aspects of critical care medicine. These include advanced airway management, ventilator management, fluid and electrolyte therapy, advanced pharmacology, specialized monitoring, operation of intraaortic balloon pumps, and other techniques usually found in an intensive care setting. This provides a safe and efficient way to move critical patients between facilities without compromising hospital staffing (Figure 1-6 ■).

PRIMARY CARE

Today, many patients can receive primary care outside the hospital at far less cost, for example, in physicians' offices and minor-care or outpatient clinics. Additionally, many patients can be cared for at home. In certain cases, paramedics, in close contact with medical direction, can provide care at the scene without transport to the hospital, for example, to treat simple lacerations or to change dressings or gastrostomy tubes.

INDUSTRIAL MEDICINE

Paramedics have long been the principal health care providers on oil rigs, movie sets, and similar industrial operations. Paramedics are specially trained for the industry in question and often assume additional responsibilities, including safety inspection, accident prevention, medical screening of employees, and vaccinations and immunizations. Many industries use paramedics to assist with sick calls and minor medical care. Having paramedics on site allows for increased employee safety and decreased time lost from work (Figure 1-7 ■).

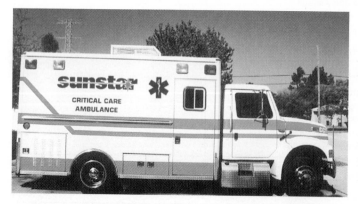

■ Figure 1-5 The modern critical care transport vehicle provides virtually all of the capabilities of the hospital intensive care unit.

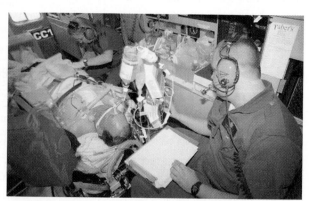

■ Figure 1-6 Critical care transport provides for the safe transfer of critically ill or injured patients between health care facilities. (© *Eddie Sperling*)

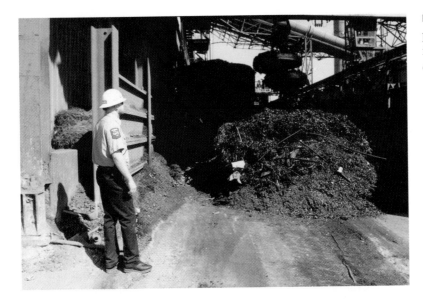

SPORTS MEDICINE

Another area in the expanded scope of paramedic practice is sports medicine. Many teams, including those in professional sports, have found that paramedics complement their athletic trainers. In this role, paramedics assume considerably more responsibility for injury prevention. They are also trained to deal with injuries specific to the sport in question. For example, paramedics working with a football team will assist in pregame preparation of players. During the game, they provide any needed emergency medical care. They can also advise the staff whether an injured or ill player may return to the game. Paramedics working with hockey teams often learn to perform simple laceration repairs and provide care for orthopedic injuries so as to safely return the players to action as soon as possible.

Summary

It is an exciting time for EMS and prehospital medicine. The paramedic of the twenty-first century can provide a significant impact on health care. You will often be the first member of the health care system with whom the patient interacts. At the very least, the results of patients' interaction with you and other EMS personnel will affect their opinion of the health care system in general. EMS is a profession where you can make a difference. Every call and every patient interaction can literally mean the difference between life and death for the patient. Few professions carry such awesome responsibility.

You Make the Call

Finally, after two straight years of urban EMS work without a vacation, you and two of your best paramedic friends, Eileen and Dee Dee, are taking the trip you've been planning for some time. The small airplane grinds to a bumpy halt as you land on a tiny speck of land in the midst of a bright turquoise sea. The ride from the mainland was rough and Eileen has thrown up. To make matters worse, two of your bags didn't make it aboard the plane. You question the ticket agent who says, "Maybe a plane come Monday. No plane Sunday." Your dream vacation is quickly turning into a nightmare.

After standing in the sun for 45 minutes waiting for a taxi, a 1963 Chevrolet shows up. The driver tells you that your hotel is about 45 minutes away. He throws your bags into the trunk, ties the trunk shut with a piece of manila rope, and takes off like a dragster from the starting line. You and your friends hang on for dear life as the cab speeds through the winding streets. You try to remember whether people on this island drive on the left side or the right. You certainly cannot tell based upon your driver's actions. The driver seems to know everybody and honks accordingly. Loud island music crackles through the small speakers in the cab. Dee Dee, the friend who managed not to vomit on the plane, leans over to you and tells you that she thinks she needs to vomit now.

Suddenly, you see a plume of smoke billowing up on the road ahead. As the cab slows, you spot what appears to be an accident. On closer inspection, you see that another cab has plowed into a station wagon at an intersection. Several people are lying on the ground and there is the general appearance of pandemonium. Dee Dee throws up.

The three of you, experienced paramedics, get out of the cab to take a look. The scene appears safe to approach. Unfortunately, the accident looks severe with several persons suffering serious injuries. Bystanders begin to reach inside the station wagon and drag the occupants out to a nearby shade tree. You try to offer some advice on providing cervical spine precautions, but they aren't paying any attention to you. You cringe as you see a patient's head fall back and strike the ground.

Before long, all six victims are spread out under a large magnolia tree. A woman is crying loudly and reciting a prayer. A dog walks among the victims. One of the bystanders says that the police should be there "pretty soon." You ask if anyone has called the fire department. The bystander responds with a confused look on his face. "Why do we call the fire department?" he asks. "I do not see a fire."

One victim is obviously dead of a massive head injury. The others are alive but with various injuries. You and your friends try to provide what care you can with absolutely no medical equipment available. Before long, you hear the shrill siren of an approaching police car. The police officers get out of their vehicle and take a significant amount of time putting their hats on. One officer goes to the vehicles. The other goes to the magnolia tree where he proceeds to get into a heated argument with one of the bystanders. Nobody is paying much attention to the victims except you and your friends.

Before long, there is some excitement as another vehicle pulls up. It seems to be some sort of ambulance. It is an old delivery van painted white with a large orange cross on the side. There are two attendants dressed in white smocks. They carry a canvas litter and, again with no spinal precautions and in no particular order, they begin to load up the victims. You and your friends try to relay the results of your assessment and care. The attendants continue with their tasks, both disinterested and unimpressed with your work. From what you can tell, absolutely no medical care is being provided.

When the last victim is loaded with the other five in the van, both attendants take their seats in the front of the van and leave for the hospital. The shrill sound of the siren slowly fades into the distance and you and your friends go on to the hotel. You look at the local paper each day, hoping to find out something about the crash victims, but you never find a story about the accident.

Although you are still upset about the accident and the unsophisticated level of medical care you witnessed—and after your bags finally arrive—you, Dee Dee, and Eileen have a nice vacation with no further adverse events.

1. Discuss the vast differences between EMS and paramedic care in the United States, Canada, and other economically developed nations compared with those that exist in some less developed countries of the world. How should awareness of such differences affect your attitude about your work?

See Suggested Responses at the back of this book.

Review Questions

1. Paramedics may only function under the direction and license of the EMS system's:
   a. town council.
   b. company owner.
   c. medical director.
   d. Board of Directors.

2. The emerging roles and responsibilities of the paramedic include:
   a. public education.
   b. health promotion.
   c. participation in injury and illness prevention programs.
   d. all of the above.

3. The rules, standards, and expected actions governing the activities of a group or profession are called:
   a. ethics.
   b. morals.
   c. manners.
   d. etiquette.

4. Which of the following is an aspect of professionalism?
   a. being well groomed
   b. maintaining patient confidentiality
   c. attending continuing education sessions
   d. all of the above

5. All of the following are considered new, nontraditional roles for the paramedic except:
   a. primary care.
   b. sports medicine.
   c. family practitioner.
   d. industrial medicine.

See answers to Review Questions at the back of this book.

Further Reading

Bledsoe, B. E. "EMS Needs a Few More Cowboys." *Journal of Emergency Medical Services (JEMS)* 28(12) (2003):112–113.

Bledsoe, B. E. "Where Are the Wise Men?" *Emergency Medical Services (EMS)* 31(10) (2002):172.

EMT-Paramedic: National Standard Curriculum. Washington, D.C.: U.S. Department of Transportation, National Highway Traffic Safety Administration, 1998.

Page, J. O. *The Paramedics.* Morristown, N.J.: Backdraft Publications, 1979. [No longer available for purchase except as a used book. Entire book can be viewed online at *www.JEMS.com/Paramedics.*]

Rogan, Dennis. *For Love of Life.* Sydney, NSW, Australia: NSW Ambulance Publishing Services, 1986.

On the Web

Visit Brady's Paramedic Website at **www.bradybooks.com/paramedic**.

The Well-Being of the Paramedic

Objectives

After reading this chapter, you should be able to:

1. Discuss the concept of wellness and its benefits. (pp. 16–17)
2. Define the components of wellness. (pp. 17–23)
3. Describe the role of the paramedic in promoting wellness. (pp. 16–17)
4. Discuss how cardiovascular endurance, weight control, muscle strength, and flexibility contribute to physical fitness. (pp. 17–20)
5. Describe the impact of shift work on circadian rhythms. (p. 35)
6. Discuss the contributions that periodic risk assessments and warning sign recognition make to cancer and cardiovascular disease prevention. (p. 20)
7. Differentiate proper from improper body mechanics for lifting and moving patients in emergency and nonemergency situations. (pp. 21–23)
8. Describe the problems that a paramedic might encounter in a hostile situation and the techniques used to manage the situation. (p. 40)
9. Describe the considerations that should be given to using escorts, dealing with adverse environmental conditions, using lights and siren, proceeding through intersections, and parking at an emergency scene. (pp. 39–40)
10. Discuss the concept of "due regard for the safety of all others" while operating an emergency vehicle. (p. 40)
11. Describe the equipment available in a variety of adverse situations for self-protection. (pp. 24–25, 39–40)
12. Describe the benefits and methods of smoking cessation. (p. 21)
13. Describe the three phases of the stress response. (p. 34)

14. List factors that trigger the stress response. (p. 33)
15. Differentiate between normal/healthy and detrimental physiological and psychological reactions to anxiety and stress. (pp. 35–37)
16. Identify causes of stress in EMS. (p. 37)
17. Describe behavior that is a manifestation of stress in patients and those close to them, and describe how that behavior relates to paramedic stress. (p. 33)
18. Identify and describe the defense mechanisms and management techniques commonly used to deal with stress. (pp. 35–38)
19. Describe the research about possible problems in the use of critical incident stress management (CISM) and the appropriate mental health services that should be available to EMS personnel. (p. 38)
20. Describe the stages of the grieving process (Kübler-Ross). (p. 30)
21. Describe the unique challenges for paramedics in dealing with themselves, adults, children, and special populations related to their understanding or experience of death and dying. (pp. 29–33)
22. Describe the body substance isolation steps to take for personal protection from airborne and bloodborne pathogens. (pp. 24–26)
23. Given a scenario where equipment and supplies have been exposed to body substances, plan for the proper cleaning, disinfection, and disposal of the items. (pp. 27–28)
24. Given photos of various motor-vehicle collisions, assess scene safety and propose ways to make the scene safer. (pp. 39–40)
25. Given a scenario involving a stressful situation, formulate a strategy to help adapt to the stress. (pp. 33–38)

Key Terms

anchor time, p. 35
body substance isolation (BSI), p. 24
burnout, p. 35
circadian rhythms, p. 35
cleaning, p. 27

disinfecting, p. 27
exposure, p. 28
incubation period, p. 23
infectious disease, p. 23
isometric exercise, p. 17
isotonic exercise, p. 17

pathogens, p. 23
personal protective equipment (PPE), p. 24
sterilizing, p. 27
stress, p. 33
stressor, p. 33

Case Study

Howard is a 15-year veteran of a high-volume, inner-city EMS service. When he first started his career, Howard thought he knew what he was getting into, but the years have taught him differently.

Right now, Howard is in the spotlight for saving the life of a police officer who was shot. "That call forced me to reflect on a few important things," he says. "Two years ago, I had a minor heart problem, and it was a good wake-up call. Since then I've been lifting weights and running, so I was able to get to the officer with enough strength to carry him to safety.

"Another thing is that I always use personal protective equipment. I never go to work without steel-toe boots and a pair of disposable gloves. Can you believe there are still paramedics who knock the concept of infection control? If any one of my partners sticks a needle into the squad bench in my ambulance, they know I'll speak up."

Howard, a mild mannered, nondescript man, doesn't realize that his young colleagues regard him as a role model. They've seen him handle himself at chaotic scenes as well as when a situation demands sensitivity, patience, and gentleness. "Howard is the man I'd want to tell bad news to my mother," one of his partners says. "He can handle people involved in just about any circumstance—death situations, panicked parents, lonely elderly people, and even hostile drunks. I've never seen anyone treat others with such dignity and respect. He's the best partner anyone could want, especially when we have to manage patients who are thrashing around. But that was not always so, was it, Howard?"

"No, it wasn't," Howard replies. "There was a time when no one wanted to work with me. I was a cowboy, and I figured there was only one way to do things: my way. But an incident that occurred a few years ago changed all that. It's a long story. But the upshot is that when I recovered from the stress, my outlook had been altered. I realized that though I couldn't save the world, I could save myself. That's when I learned how to deal with the effects of a stressful job. I started eating right, lost a bunch of weight, and adopted a new attitude. Anyway, if I can maintain my own well-being, I can do a lot more to help others. Right? Isn't that what we're about?"

INTRODUCTION

Well-being is a fundamental aspect of top-notch performance.

Eat well, work to stay physically fit, and avoid potentially addictive and harmful substances so you have the strength and stamina to do the job.

Well-being is a fundamental aspect of top-notch performance in EMS. It includes your physical well-being as well as your mental and emotional well-being. If your body is fed well and kept fit, if you use the principles of safe lifting, and if you avoid potentially addictive and harmful substances, you stand a chance of having the physical strength and stamina to do the job.

If you seize the information about safe practice and apply it to your life, you will be better able to avoid harm from violent people, roadway hazards, and insidious infections. If you let your spirit appreciate the fear and sadness on other faces, you will find ways to combat your prejudices and treat people with dignity and respect. By doing all these things, you will also be able to promote the benefits of well-being to your EMS colleagues.

Death, dying, stress, infection, fear—all threaten your wellness and conspire to interfere with your good intentions. But you can do something about them. Each person has choices about how to live. Every choice has outcomes and consequences. Many patients in nursing homes are living with their choices, paying for lifestyle decisions made decades ago when they were about your age. Is that what you want for yourself?

Most paramedic injuries are due to lifting and being in and around motor vehicles. Those who train to be physically fit for their jobs as paramedics stand a better chance of avoiding early, forced retirement due to injured backs or knees. Those who train themselves to be mentally alert in the ambulance and at roadway scenes stand a better chance of staying alive and uninjured. Those who can inspire their colleagues to work towards a state of well-being are role models of the highest order.

This chapter introduces the many elements of well-being. If you listen now and enhance your knowledge later, you stand a good chance of enjoying a long and rewarding career of helping others—all because you helped yourself.

BASIC PHYSICAL FITNESS

The benefits of achieving acceptable physical fitness are well known. They include a decreased resting heart rate and blood pressure, increased oxygen-carrying capacity, increased muscle mass and metabolism, and increased resistance to illness and injury. Quality of life is enhanced, too, because of the ability to do more, and there is a positive correlation between fitness, personal appearance, and self-image. Other benefits of physical fitness are improved mental outlook and reduced anxiety levels. Finally, a physically fit body enhances a person's ability to maintain sound motor skills throughout life.

CORE ELEMENTS

Core elements of physical fitness are muscular strength, cardiovascular endurance (aerobic capacity), and flexibility. Like a three-legged stool, if any one of the three is deficient, the whole becomes unstable. Each is equally important.

Be careful about plunging into a well-intended effort to get in shape. For example, before starting an exercise or stretching regimen, it can be helpful to measure your current state of fitness. There are various methods of assessing the three core elements of fitness. Many EMS agencies have access to facilities where precise assessment methods—with trained personnel—are available. Take advantage of any information available to you.

Muscular strength is achieved with regular exercise that trains muscles to exert force and build endurance. Exercise may be isometric or isotonic. **Isometric exercise** is active exercise performed against stable resistance, where muscles are exercised in a motionless manner. **Isotonic exercise** is active exercise during which muscles are worked through their range of motion. Take time to get in-depth information about the best approach from a trainer or other knowledgeable person.

Weight lifting is an obvious way to achieve muscular strength, and it is excellent all-around training for the body. You can vary the amount of weight lifted, the number of times it is lifted, and the frequency of the demands on the muscle. Whatever type of strength-building exercise is best for you, consider rotating between training the muscles of your upper body and shoulders, chest and back, and lower body. Do abdominal exercises daily.

Cardiovascular endurance is a result of exercising at least three days a week vigorously enough to raise your pulse to its target heart rate (Table 2–1). Many people shy away from aerobic exercise, thinking the effort will be too great or the results will take too long. However, there is no need to become a marathon runner to gain aerobic capacity. Try a brisk walk, or ride a stationary bike while watching TV. Make it a daily habit.

Even modest exercise programs, which can be done most days of the week, will improve cardiovascular endurance and muscular strength. Walking briskly from the outer reaches of the employee parking lot, using stairs whenever possible, and playing actively with your children can all "count" toward physical fitness.

Flexibility seems to be the forgotten element of fitness. Without an adequate range of motion, your joints and muscles cannot be used efficiently or safely. A body builder with tight hamstrings may be as much at risk for back injury as anyone else. To achieve

 Review

Basics of Physical Fitness

Cardiovascular endurance
Strength and flexibility
Nutrition and weight control
Freedom from addictions
Back safety

isometric exercise *active exercise performed against stable resistance, where muscles are exercised in a motionless manner.*

isotonic exercise *active exercise during which muscles are worked through their range of motion.*

Table 2-1	Finding Your Target Heart Rate

1. Measure your resting heart rate. (You will use this total later.)

2. Subtract your age from 220. This total is your estimated maximum heart rate.

3. Subtract your resting heart rate from your maximum heart rate, and multiply that figure by 0.7.

4. Add the figure you just calculated to your resting heart rate.

EXAMPLE: In a 44-year-old woman whose resting heart rate is 52, her maximum heart rate would be 176 (220–44). Her maximum heart rate minus resting heart rate is 124 (176–52). Multiply 124 by 0.7 for a value of 86.8. Resting heart rate plus the calculated figure is 138.8 (52 + 86.8). Rounded up, this person's target heart rate is 140 beats per minute.

(or regain) flexibility, stretch the main muscle groups regularly. Try to stretch daily. Never bounce when stretching; this causes microtears in muscle and connective tissues. Hold a stretch for at least 60 seconds. A side benefit of good flexibility is prevention or reduction of back pain. Stretching is an excellent TV-time activity. If you are interested, consider studying yoga for improved flexibility.

NUTRITION

It is a myth that people in EMS cannot maintain an adequate diet. Even so, the "hit-and-run" nature of emergency care requires planning and awareness of your options. The most difficult part of improving nutrition is altering established bad habits. A change in your behavior requires some commitment and self-discipline, understanding the change process, and patience with what will become long-term

Patho Pearls

Obesity Obesity has become a major problem in the United States and other industrialized countries. EMS personnel are not immune to this trend. In fact, EMS personnel are becoming, on the average, progressively more overweight. There are several factors inherent in EMS that can contribute to obesity. First, much of EMS work is sedentary. A great deal of time is spent seated in an ambulance or in a station. Second, physical activity on the job is usually limited to short periods of sometimes intense effort. While these periods of work can be strenuous, they seldom last long enough to provide any significant degree of exercise. Third, the duties of the job require EMS personnel to "eat on the run," which often means relying on fast food or processed food. These meals provide plenty of "empty calories" and significantly contribute to obesity.

Obesity can lead to numerous health problems, such as back pain, and can place paramedics at increased risk of sustaining a back injury. Obesity can also lead to cardiovascular disease, diabetes, and other long-term chronic problems. As an EMS professional, you must recognize that, in order to provide the best care for your patient—and to provide a good role model for your patients and the public—you must first care for yourself. This includes watching your weight, finding ways to eat a reasonable diet, and obtaining an adequate amount of exercise. More and more EMS employers are recognizing the obesity epidemic and are developing employee assistance and physical fitness programs designed to minimize the chances of obesity cutting an EMS career short.

self-improvement. Set realistic goals, and understand that backsliding happens. Whatever your goals may be, such as reducing excess weight, gaining weight, or regularly eating more wholesome foods, it is helpful to be able to analyze your progress by using charts or daily intake tallies.

Excercise and good nutrition are fundamental to your well-being. The following are exercise and diet guidelines published as "My Pyramid" by the U.S. Department of Agriculture.

★ *Physical activity.* Be physically active at least 30 minutes most days.

★ *Whole grains.* Eat at least 3 ounces of whole grain bread, cereal, crackers, rice, or pasta per day.

★ *Fruits and vegetables.* Eat 2 cups of fruit and 2-1/2 cups of vegetables each day. Eat more dark green and orange vegetables. Eat a variety of fresh, frozen, canned or dried fruit (go easy on fruit juices).

★ *Fats.* Get most of your fats from fish, nuts, and vegetable oils. Limit solid fats like butter, stick margarine, shortening, and lard.

★ *Milk.* Drink 3 cups per day of fat free or low fat milk.

★ *Meat and beans.* Choose broiled, baked, or grilled lean meats and poultry. Vary it with fish, beans, peas, nuts, and seeds.

In short, exercise and eat (in moderation) a balanced variety of wholesome foods. (The USDA website MyPyramid.gov provides details about how you can tailor the guidelines to meet your own needs.)

Food labels contain abundant information about nutritional content. Learn to read them. Standardization of food labels has reduced much of the confusion. Be sure to check the serving size to avoid misinterpreting the food's overall nutritional value (Figure 2-2).

⊘ **Review**

Major Food Groups

Whole grains
Fruits and vegetables
Fats and oils
Milk and dairy products
Meat, fish, and beans

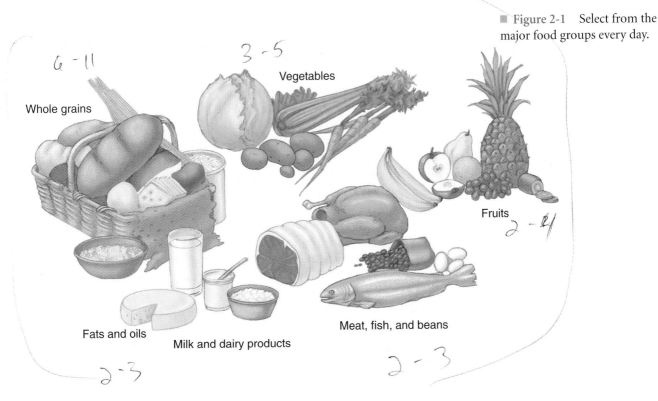

■ Figure 2-1 Select from the major food groups every day.

Whole grains

Vegetables

Fruits

Fats and oils

Milk and dairy products

Meat, fish, and beans

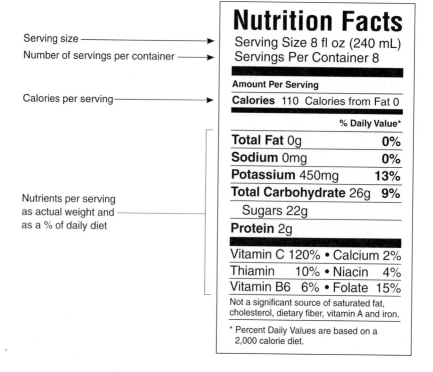

■ Figure 2-2 Example of a standardized food label.

Serving size

Number of servings per container

Calories per serving

Nutrients per serving as actual weight and as a % of daily diet

Nutrition Facts

Serving Size 8 fl oz (240 mL)
Servings Per Container 8

Amount Per Serving

Calories 110 Calories from Fat 0

% Daily Value*

Total Fat 0g	**0%**
Sodium 0mg	**0%**
Potassium 450mg	**13%**
Total Carbohydrate 26g	**9%**
Sugars 22g	
Protein 2g	

Vitamin C 120% • Calcium 2%

Thiamin 10% • Niacin 4%

Vitamin B6 6% • Folate 15%

Not a significant source of saturated fat, cholesterol, dietary fiber, vitamin A and iron.

* Percent Daily Values are based on a 2,000 calorie diet.

Eating on the run, as EMS providers must often do, can be less detrimental if you plan ahead and carry a small cooler filled with whole-grain sandwiches, cut vegetables, fruit, and other wholesome foods. If you must, stop at a local market instead of the fast-food place next door. Buy fresh fruit, yogurt, and sensible deli selections. They are more nutritious and much cheaper than "fast foods."

Finally, monitor your fluid intake. Your body needs plenty of fluids to flush food through your system and eliminate toxins. Pay attention to what you are drinking. Fill a "go-cup" with fresh ice water when you stop by the emergency department instead of spending your money on soft drinks. Water is more thirst-quenching, cheaper, and much better for you.

Exercising and eating well can help you prevent both cancer and cardiovascular disease. Although for the typically youthful EMS provider, the likelihood of being hit by either of these diseases seems remote, it happens. You can do a lot to prevent it. Minimizing stress through healthy stress management practices, for example, can work wonders. In addition, assess yourself and your family history.

Exercise will improve cardiovascular endurance, help lower blood pressure, and tip the balance of your body composition favorably—all good measures against cardiovascular disease. Know your cholesterol and triglyceride levels, and keep them in check. For women who are menopausal, be informed about the risks and benefits of using hormone replacement therapy (particularly estrogen).

Diet can also do much to minimize the chances of getting certain cancers. Certain foods, such as broccoli and high-fiber foods, can help reduce the incidence of cancer; others, such as charcoal-cooked foods, can increase it. The connection between sun exposure and skin cancer is well known. So, take the precaution of using sunblocks and wear sunglasses and a hat when you can. Watch out for the warning signs of cancer, such as blood in the stools (even in young people, especially men), a changing mole, unexplained weight loss, unexplained chronic fatigue, and lumps.

Be sure to include appropriate periodic risk-assessment screening and self-examination habits in your personal well-being program. That includes tests like mammograms and prostate exams as you gain in years.

HABITS AND ADDICTIONS

Many people who work high-stress jobs overuse and abuse substances such as caffeine and nicotine. These bad habits are rampant in EMS. Each can contribute to long-term diseases such as cancer and cardiovascular disease. Choose a healthier life, and avoid overindulging in these and other harmful substances such as alcohol. For example, smoking cessation programs are usually easily accessed in local areas or on the Internet.

There are abundant approaches to this common addiction, including behavior modification, nicotine replacement therapy ("patches"), aversion therapy, hypnotism, and "cold turkey." Part of understanding your addiction is knowing whether it is a psychological dependency, sociocultural dependency, or a true physical addiction. Whatever it takes, the message is clear: get free of addictions, particularly those that threaten your well-being. Substance abuse programs, nicotine patches, 12-step groups—all exist to help you help yourself. But the first step has to be yours.

BACK SAFETY

EMS is a physically demanding endeavor. Of the host of movements needed (scrambling down embankments, climbing ladders or trees, squeezing into narrow spaces, and so on), none will be more frequent than lifting and carrying equipment and patients. To avoid back injury, you must keep your back fit for the work you do. You also must use proper lifting techniques each time you pick up a load, whether the load is heavy or light.

Back fitness begins with conditioning the muscles that support the spinal column. These are the "guy wires" that stabilize the spine, much the way cables help keep telephone poles upright. Note that the muscles of the abdomen are also crucial to overall spinal-column strength and safe lifting. Never perform old-fashioned sit-ups. They can seriously strain your lumbar spine. Instead, use abdominal crunches, which target only the stomach muscles. Consult an exercise coach or trainer for specifics.

Correct posture will minimize the risk of back injury (Figure 2-3). Good nutrition helps to maintain healthy connective tissue and intervertebral discs. Excess weight contributes to disc deterioration. So does smoking. Thus, proper weight management and smoking cessation are relevant to back health. Finally, adequate rest gives the spine non-weight-bearing time to nourish discs and repair itself.

Proper lifting techniques should ideally be taught by and practiced with a trainer who understands the variety of challenges faced by EMS providers. Important principles of lifting are as follows:

★ Move a load only if you can safely handle it.

★ Ask for help when you need it—for *any* reason.

★ Position the load as close to your body and center of gravity as possible.

★ Keep your palms up whenever possible.

★ Do not hurry. Take the time you need to establish good footing and balance. Keep a wide base of support with one foot ahead of the other.

Pay particular attention to keeping your back fit for the work you do. Always use the proper techniques for lifting and moving patients and equipment.

Legal Notes

Back Injuries Back injuries are one of the greatest risks to EMS providers and account for a significant monetary expenditure in worker compensation claims. Programs to help reduce the incidence of such injuries should be an ongoing aspect of any EMS system.

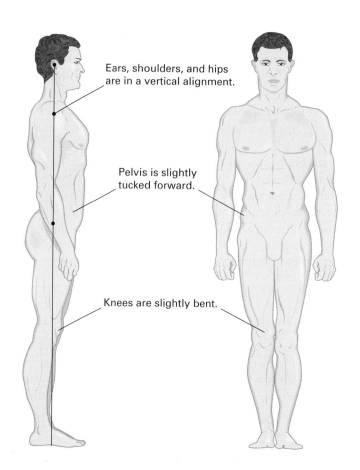

Figure 2-3a   Correct standing posture. Note the straight line from ear through shoulder, hip, knee, to arch of foot.

Ears, shoulders, and hips are in a vertical alignment.

Pelvis is slightly tucked forward.

Knees are slightly bent.

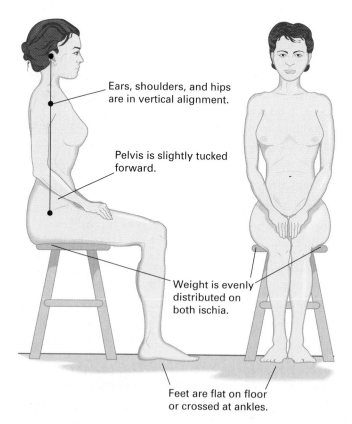

Figure 2-3b   Correct sitting posture.

Ears, shoulders, and hips are in vertical alignment.

Pelvis is slightly tucked forward.

Weight is evenly distributed on both ischia.

Feet are flat on floor or crossed at ankles.

- ★ Bend your knees, lower your buttocks, and keep your chin up. If your knees are bad, do not bend them more than 90 degrees.
- ★ "Lock in" the spine with a slight extension curve, and tighten the abdominal muscles to support spinal positioning.
- ★ Always avoid twisting and turning.
- ★ Let the large leg muscles do the work of lifting, not your back.
- ★ Exhale during the lift. Do not hold your breath.
- ★ Given a choice, push. Do not pull.
- ★ Look where you are walking or crawling. Take only short steps, if you are walking. Move forward rather than backward whenever possible.
- ★ When rescuers are working together as a team to lift a load, only one person should be in charge of verbal commands.

Heed your own body's signals. You are stronger some days than others. Know when you are physically depleted due to exhaustion, lack of food, or minor illness. Use volunteers wisely, and be sure to ask if their backs are strong enough for the job.

Never reach for an item and twist at the same time. Most back injuries occur because of the cumulative effect of such low-level everyday stresses. Everything you do on behalf of back safety adds up to choices that can mean the difference between a long and rewarding career in EMS, or one shortened by an injury. Be careful!

PERSONAL PROTECTION FROM DISEASE

In recent years the emphasis on infection control has focused on the most devastating diseases, such as HIV/AIDS, hepatitis B, and tuberculosis—and rightly so. There is enough risk in EMS without having to worry about dying of a disease you caught while caring for others. Fortunately, there is a lot you can do to minimize your risk of infection. A good first step is to develop a habit of doing the things promoted in this chapter. Eating well, getting adequate rest, and managing stress are among the building blocks of a good defense against infection. In addition, it is a good idea to periodically assess your risk for infection, such as noticing when you are run down or when your hands are dangerously chapped.

INFECTIOUS DISEASES

Infectious diseases are caused by **pathogens** such as bacteria and viruses, which may be spread from person to person. For example, infection by way of bloodborne pathogens can occur when the blood of an infected person comes in contact with another person's broken skin (cuts, sores, chapped hands) or by way of parenteral contact (stick by a needle or other sharp object). Infection by airborne pathogens can occur when an infected person sneezes or coughs, causing body fluids in the form of tiny droplets to be inhaled or to come in contact with the mucous membranes of another person's eyes, nose, or mouth.

HIV/AIDS, hepatitis B, and tuberculosis are diseases of great concern because they are life threatening. However, one may be exposed to many different infectious diseases. See Table 2–2 for some common ones, their modes of transmission, and **incubation periods.**

Even when someone is carrying pathogens for disease, signs of an illness may not be apparent. For this reason, *you must consider the blood and body fluids of every patient you treat as infectious.* Safeguards against infection are mandatory for all medical personnel. They involve a form of infection control called "body substance isolation (BSI)."

infectious disease *any disease caused by the growth of pathogenic microorganisms, which may be spread from person to person.*

pathogens *microorganisms capable of producing disease, such as bacteria and viruses.*

incubation period *the time between contact with a disease organism and the appearance of the first symptoms.*

Treat all blood and body fluids as if they are infectious, and take appropriate body substance isolation (BSI) precautions whenever you treat a patient.

Table 2-2 | Common Infectious Diseases

Disease	Mode of Transmission	Incubation Period
AIDS (Acquired Immune Deficiency Syndrome)	AIDS- or HIV-infected blood via intravenous drug use, semen and vaginal fluids, blood transfusions, or (rarely) needle sticks. Mothers also may pass HIV to their unborn children.	Several months or years
Hepatitis B, C	Blood, stool, or other body fluids, or contaminated objects.	Weeks or months
Tuberculosis	Respiratory secretions, airborne or on contaminated objects.	2 to 6 weeks
Meningitis, bacterial	Oral and nasal secretions.	2 to 10 days
Pneumonia, bacterial and viral	Oral and nasal droplets and secretions.	Several days
Influenza	Airborne droplets, or direct contact with body fluids.	1 to 3 days
Staphylococcal skin infections	Contact with open wounds or sores or contaminated objects.	Several days
Chicken pox (varicella)	Airborne droplets, or contact with open sores.	11 to 21 days
German measles (rubella)	Airborne droplets. Mothers may pass it to unborn children.	10 to 12 days
Whooping cough (pertussis)	Respiratory secretions or airborne droplets.	6 to 20 days
SARS (severe acute respiratory syndrome)	Airborne droplets and personal contact.	4 to 6 days

INFECTION CONTROL PRACTICES

Body Substance Isolation (BSI)

body substance isolation (BSI) *a strict form of infection control that is based on the assumption that all blood and other body fluids are infectious.*

personal protective equipment (PPE) *equipment used by EMS personnel to protect against injury and the spread of infectious disease.*

Body substance isolation (BSI) is a strategy that is based on the assumption that all blood and body fluids are infectious. It dictates that all EMS personnel take BSI precautions with every patient. To achieve this, appropriate **personal protective equipment** (PPE) should be available in every emergency vehicle. The minimum recommended PPE includes the following:

★ *Protective gloves.* Wear disposable protective gloves before initiating any emergency care. When an emergency involves more than one patient, change gloves between patients. When gloves have been contaminated, remove and dispose of them properly as soon as possible (Figure 2-4 ■).

★ *Masks and protective eyewear* (Figure 2-5 ■). These should be worn together whenever blood spatter is likely to occur, such as with arterial bleeding, childbirth, endotracheal intubation and other invasive procedures, oral suctioning, and clean-up of equipment that requires heavy scrubbing or brushing. Both you and your patient should wear masks whenever the potential for airborne transmission of disease exists.

★ *HEPA and N-95 respirators* (Figure 2-6 ■). Due to the resurgence of tuberculosis (TB), you must protect yourself from infection through the use of a high-efficiency particulate air (HEPA) or N-95 respirator. Wear one whenever you care for a patient with confirmed or suspected TB. This is especially true during procedures that involve the airway, such as the administration of nebulized medications, endotracheal intubation, or suctioning.

★ *Gowns.* Disposable gowns protect your clothing from splashes. If large splashes of blood are expected, such as with childbirth, wear an impervious gown.

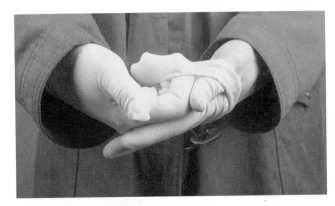

Figure 2-4a To remove gloves, first hook the gloved fingers of one hand under the cuff of the other glove. Then pull that glove off without letting your gloved fingers come in contact with bare skin.

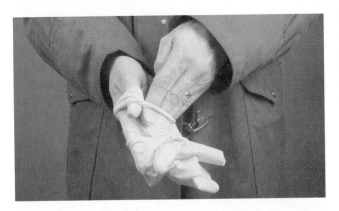

Figure 2-4b Then slide the fingers of the ungloved hand under the remaining glove's cuff. Push that glove off, being careful not to touch the glove's exterior with your bare hand.

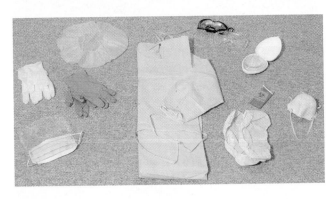

Figure 2-5 Proper gloves, eyewear, and mask prevent a patient's blood and body fluids from contacting a break in your skin or spraying into your eyes, nose, and mouth.

★ *Resuscitation equipment.* Use disposable resuscitation equipment as your primary means of artificial ventilation in emergency care. Such items should be used once, then disposed of properly.

The garments and equipment previously described are intended to serve the paramedic by protecting against infection through contact with both potentially contaminated body substances, such as blood, vomit, and urine, as well as other agents, such as airborne droplets. These garments and equipment will assist you in achieving, to the extent possible, the universal precautions recommended by the Centers for Disease Control, which help to protect against bloodborne infection.

Infectious diseases also are minimized through the use of appropriate work practices and equipment especially engineered to minimize risk. For example, most invasive equipment is now used on a one-time, disposable basis. Of course, it is important to launder reusable clothing with infection control in mind.

General cleanliness and appropriate personal hygiene will do much to prevent infection. Probably the most important infection control practice is handwashing

Perhaps the most important infection control practice is handwashing.

■ Figure 2-6a A high-efficiency particulate air (HEPA) respirator.

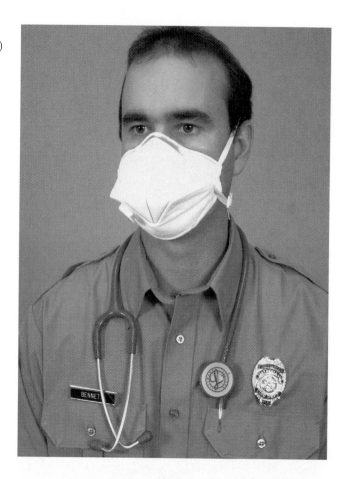

■ Figure 2-6b An N-95 respirator.

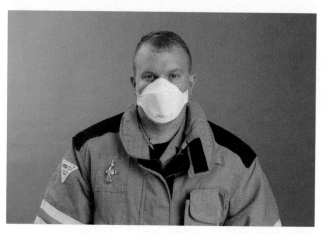

(Figure 2-7 ■). As soon as possible after every patient contact and decontamination procedure, thoroughly wash your hands. To do so, first remove any rings or jewelry from your hands and arms. Then use soap and water. Lather your hands vigorously front and back for at least 15 seconds up to 2 or 3 inches above the wrist. Be sure to lather and rub between your fingers and in the creases and cracks of your knuckles. Scrub under and around the fingernails with a brush. Rinse your hands well under running water, holding your hands downward so that the water drains off your fingertips. Dry your hands on a clean towel.

Plain soap works perfectly well for handwashing. At those times when soap is not available, you might use an antimicrobial handwashing solution or an alcohol-based foam or towelette.

✓ **Review**

Handwashing

Lather with soap and water
Scrub for at least
15 seconds
Rinse under running water
Dry on a clean towel

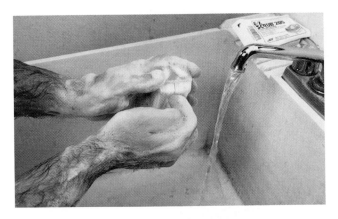

■ Figure 2-7a To wash your hands properly, lather up well and be sure to scrub under your nails.

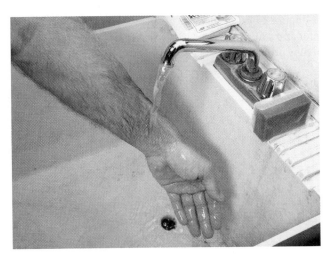

■ Figure 2-7b When you rinse off your hands, point them downward so that soap and water run off away from your body.

Vaccinations and Screening Tests

Immunizations against many illnesses are available. Get them. Even "nuisance" illnesses can be avoided if you get vaccinated. Immunizations that are available include those for rubella (German measles), measles, mumps, chicken pox, and other childhood diseases, as well as for tetanus/diphtheria, polio, influenza, hepatitis B, and Lyme disease. Some, such as tetanus, may require booster shots periodically, so monitor your personal medical history well. Also arrange for routine tuberculosis (TB) screenings and record the results.

Monitor your personal medical history accurately, and be sure to get all appropriate vaccinations, boosters, and screenings on a regular basis.

Decontamination of Equipment

Any personal protective equipment (PPE) designed for a single use should be properly disposed of after use. The same is true of contaminated medical devices designed for a single use. Such materials should be discarded in a red bag marked with a biohazard seal (Figure 2-8 ■). Needles and other sharp objects should be discarded in properly labeled, puncture-proof containers. Once an item is placed in the appropriate container, the container should be disposed of according to local guidelines.

Nondisposable equipment that has been contaminated must be cleaned, disinfected, or sterilized:

Infection control includes properly cleaning, disinfecting, sterilizing, or discarding all equipment after contact with a patient.

★ **Cleaning** refers to washing an object with soap and water. After caring for a patient, wash your work areas down with approved soaps. Throw away single-use cleaning supplies in a proper biohazard container.

cleaning washing an object with cleaners such as soap and water.

★ **Disinfecting** includes cleaning with a disinfecting agent, which should kill many microorganisms on the surface of an object. Disinfect equipment that had direct contact with the intact skin of a patient, such as backboards and splints. Use a commercial disinfectant or bleach diluted in water (one part bleach to 10 parts water), or follow local guidelines.

disinfecting cleaning with an agent that can kill some microorganisms on the surface of an object.

★ **Sterilizing** is the use of a chemical, or a physical method such as pressurized steam, to kill all microorganisms on an object. Items that were inserted into the patient's body (a laryngoscope blade, for example) should be sterilized by heat, steam, or radiation. There are also EPA-approved solutions for sterilization.

sterilizing use of a chemical or physical method such as pressurized steam to kill all microorganisms on an object.

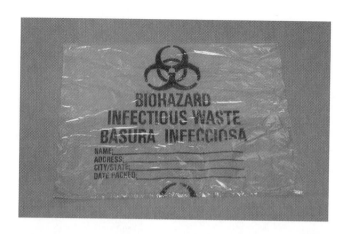

■ Figure 2-8a   Dispose of biohazardous wastes in a bag that is properly marked.

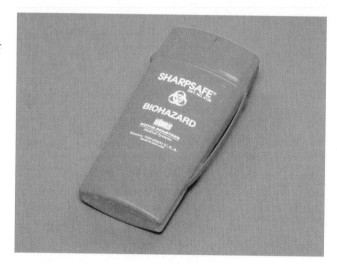

■ Figure 2-8b   Discard needles and other sharp objects in a properly labeled, puncture-proof container.

If your equipment needs more extensive cleaning, bag it and remove it to an area designated for this purpose. Disposable work gloves worn during cleaning and decontamination should be properly discarded. If your clothing has become contaminated, bag the items and wash them in accordance with local guidelines. After removing contaminated clothing, take a shower before dressing again.

Post-Exposure Procedures

exposure   *any occurrence of blood or body fluids coming in contact with nonintact skin, mucous membranes, or parenteral contact (needle stick).*

By definition, an **exposure** is any occurrence of blood or body fluids coming in contact with nonintact skin, the eyes or other mucous membranes, or parenteral contact (needle stick). In most areas, an EMS provider who has had an exposure should (Figure 2-9 ■):

Follow your EMS system guidelines on all management and documentation of any exposure to a patient's blood or body fluids.

★ Immediately wash the affected area with soap and water.

★ Get a medical evaluation.

★ Take the proper immunization boosters.

★ Notify the agency's infection control liaison.

★ Document the circumstances surrounding the exposure, including the actions taken to reduce chances of infection.

In general, the EMS provider should cooperate with the incident investigation and comply with all required reporting responsibilities and time frames.

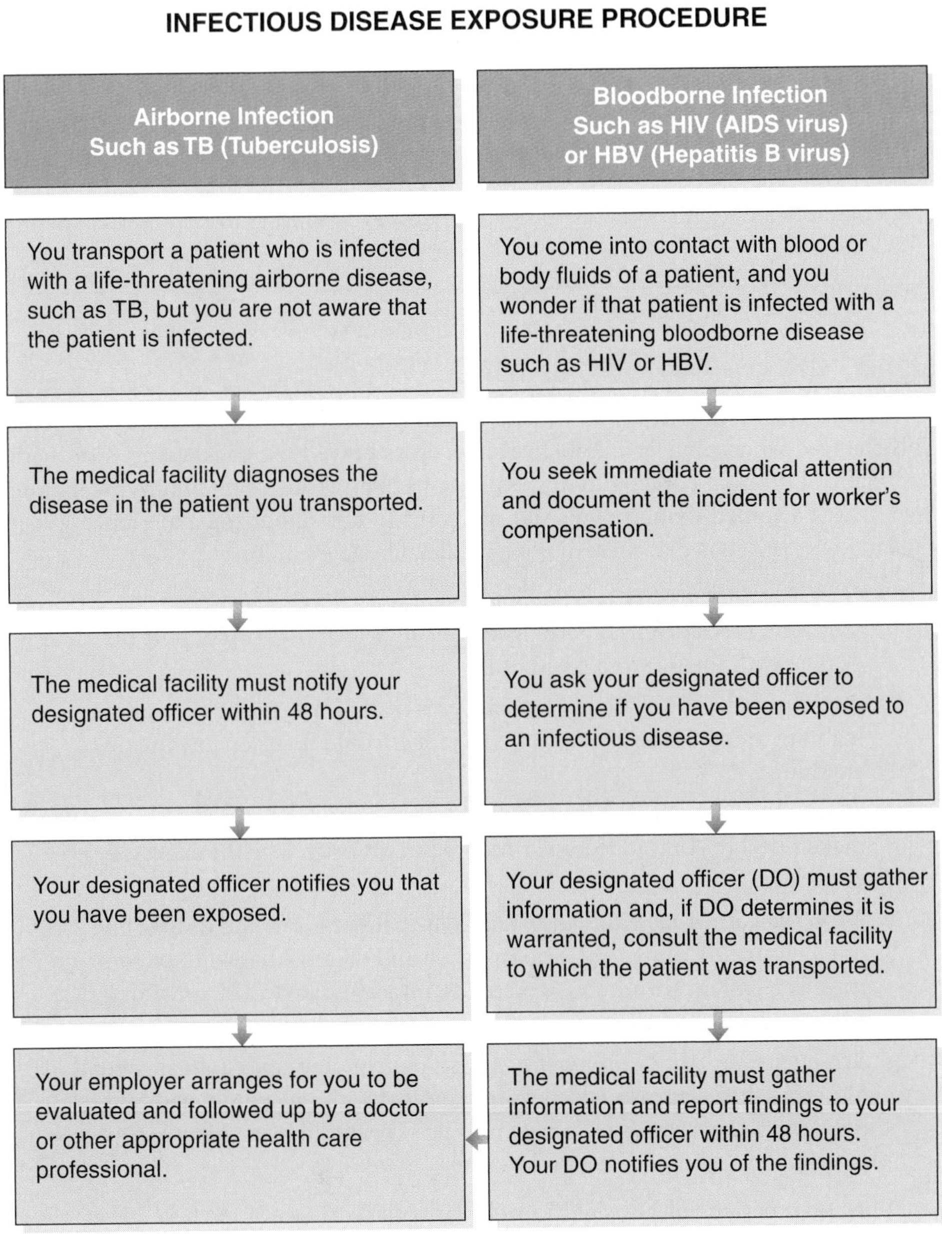

INFECTIOUS DISEASE EXPOSURE PROCEDURE

Airborne Infection Such as TB (Tuberculosis)	Bloodborne Infection Such as HIV (AIDS virus) or HBV (Hepatitis B virus)
You transport a patient who is infected with a life-threatening airborne disease, such as TB, but you are not aware that the patient is infected.	You come into contact with blood or body fluids of a patient, and you wonder if that patient is infected with a life-threatening bloodborne disease such as HIV or HBV.
The medical facility diagnoses the disease in the patient you transported.	You seek immediate medical attention and document the incident for worker's compensation.
The medical facility must notify your designated officer within 48 hours.	You ask your designated officer to determine if you have been exposed to an infectious disease.
Your designated officer notifies you that you have been exposed.	Your designated officer (DO) must gather information and, if DO determines it is warranted, consult the medical facility to which the patient was transported.
Your employer arranges for you to be evaluated and followed up by a doctor or other appropriate health care professional.	The medical facility must gather information and report findings to your designated officer within 48 hours. Your DO notifies you of the findings.

■ Figure 2-9   A federal regulation called the Ryan White Comprehensive AIDS Resources Emergency (CARE) Act outlines procedures to follow after an occupational exposure to human immunodeficiency virus (HIV), hepatitis B, diphtheria, meningitis, plague, hemorrhagic fever, rabies, and tuberculosis (TB).

DEATH AND DYING

Most paramedics agree that of all prehospital situations, those involving death or dying are among the most personally uncomfortable and challenging. There are many reasons for this. A death is regarded as a sad event of loss. There is an air of unalterable finality. Each person carries into a death situation formative impressions based on prior experiences of loss, coping skills, religious convictions, and other personal background. Paramedics encounter death much more frequently than other people do. They often see it as it happens. This can lead to a sense of cumulative overload, which the smart paramedic recognizes and deals with in a healthy manner through appropriate grief work and stress management.

Cultural Considerations

Responses to Death The emotional response to the death of a friend or family member varies significantly among cultures as well as among individuals. Some people will accept the news quietly while others will react with an emotional outburst. Use simple terms and avoid euphemisms. Realize that grieving is a cultural as well as a personal phenomenon, and that it is normal for people to respond to bad news in different ways.

LOSS, GRIEF, AND MOURNING

 Review

Stages of Loss

Denial
Anger
Bargaining
Depression
Acceptance

For decades, discussing death and dying openly was difficult due to cultural taboos. This changed when pioneer Elisabeth Kübler-Ross braved the backlash to meet with terminally ill hospital patients to discuss their feelings about death and dying. Before then, it was assumed dying people did not want to talk about the experience. What Kübler-Ross learned is that there are five predictable stages of loss:

★ *Denial, or "not me."* This is the inability or refusal to believe the reality of the event. It is a defense mechanism, during which the patient puts off dealing with the inevitable end of life.

★ *Anger, or "why me?"* The patient's anger is really frustration related to his inability to control the situation. That anger could focus on anyone or anything.

★ *Bargaining, or "okay, but first let me . . ."* In the patient's mind, he tries to make a deal to "buy additional time" to put off or change the expected outcome.

★ *Depression, or "okay, but I haven't . . ."* The patient is sad and despairing, often mourning things not accomplished and dreams that will not come true. The patient withdraws, or retreats, into a private world, unwilling to communicate with others.

★ *Acceptance, or "okay, I'm not afraid."* The patient may come to realize his fate and achieve a reasonable level of comfort with the anticipated outcome. At this stage, the family may need more support than the patient.

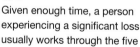

Given enough time, a person experiencing a significant loss usually works through the five predictable stages: denial, anger, bargaining, depression, and acceptance.

A person experiencing any significant loss usually works through these stages, given enough time. Although there is a tendency to progress from one stage to the next in order, both dying patients and their loved ones experience the stages in their own unique ways. They may jump around among the stages, they may go back and forth, or they may never finish them. It is important for you to remain flexible, so you can decide how best to help, if asked.

Because paramedics encounter death and dying often, there is a mistaken belief that they handle it better. However, paramedics are human, too. Let yourself deal with death and dying when it occurs. Do not shirk the support of friends and family. Do not try to "tough it out." Use every opportunity to process a specific incident in a healthy manner, through appropriately grieving losses that have an impact on you.

Grief is a feeling. Mourning is a process. A grieving person feels mostly sadness or distress. A person in mourning is immersed in the process of displaying and ultimately dissipating the feelings of grief. The sense of loss is predictably most intense immediately after the news is received. Although numerous models for the mourning process exist, a good rule of thumb is that after the loss of a close friend or relative, a period of 1 year of mourning is normal.

Upon initially hearing the news of a death, a person experiences a "paralyzing, totally incapacitating surge of grief that is exactly comparable to the incapacitating pain of an acute blow to an eye or testicle—in that the whole world shrinks down to that acute pain." Typically, the feeling lasts for 5 to 15 minutes. When you deliver the news of a death, remember that a survivor cannot function during this grief spike. After delivering the news, wait until it is past and the survivor is ready and able to receive information and make decisions.

A period of intense feelings that continues for around 4 to 6 weeks follows the grief spike. Feelings may include loss, anger, resentment, sadness, and even guilt, depending on the relationship and the circumstances surrounding the death. Gradually, the intensity and immediacy of the loss fade into a phase dominated by a sense of loneliness, which lasts about 6 months. Finally, a period of recovery ensues. The survivor begins to view the loss more objectively and rediscovers an interest in living. Key to the process of mourning is the passage of significant dates and anniversaries, such as birthdays, holidays, and the monthly (then annual) date when the loss occurred.

How different people cope with difficult moments, such as death, varies. If you are dealing with a child, understand that children's perceptions are different from an adult's. (See Table 2–3 for a summary.) This is true of all the special populations you will encounter, such as the elderly and people with mental disabilities. The elderly, for example, may be particularly concerned about the effects of the loss on other family members, about further loss of their own independence, and about the costs of a funeral and burial. There is a wide variety of responses to death among different peoples and cultures as well. Be flexible, and be ready for anything.

WHAT TO SAY

As "Do Not Resuscitate" orders and other out-of-hospital death situations increase, EMS personnel are more often placed in the position of telling people that someone has died. It would be nice to have a script for those difficult moments, but the reality is that you have to assess the scene and the people in each situation to determine the safest and most compassionate way to deliver the sad news.

In terms of safety, you never know how people will respond, even if you know them. Most people accept the news quietly. However, some allow their grief to flood out of them in very physical ways, such as throwing things, kicking walls, or screaming and running in circles. Before speaking, consciously position yourself between them and the door or other escape route. Remember, initially the grief spike has its grip on the survivors. There is little you can do but give them a safe, private place to get through it. Also, for safety, do not deliver the news to a large group. Ask the primary people (no more than four or five) to step aside with you to a private place. Let them tell the others in their own way.

Find out who is who among the survivors. Do not make assumptions. Then address the closest survivor, preferably in a way that shows compassion. That is, avoid standing above the survivor. Instead, sit or squat so that your eyes are at the same level. If the survivor is alone, call for a friend, neighbor, clergy member, or relative. Wait to tell the survivor the news until that person has arrived.

Introduce yourself by name and function ("My name is Kate. I'm a paramedic with West End Ambulance.") A careful choice of words is helpful. Although it may seem blunt, use the words "dead" and "died," rather than euphemisms that may be misinterpreted or misunderstood. Use gentle eye contact and, if appropriate, the power of touching an arm or holding a hand. Basic elements of your message should include:

★ A loved one has died.

★ There is nothing more anyone could have done.

	Table 2–3	Needs and Expectations of Children Regarding Death

Age Range	Characteristics	Suggestions
Newborn to age 3	Senses that something has happened in family, and notices that there is much activity in the household. Realizes that people are crying and sad. Watch for irritability and changes in eating, sleeping, or other behavioral patterns.	Be sensitive to the child's needs. Try to maintain consistency in routines. Maintain consistency with significant people in child's life.
Ages 3 to 6	Believes death is a temporary state, and may ask continually when the person will return. Believes in magical thinking, and may feel responsible for the death or that it is punishment for own behavior. May be fearful of catching the same illness and die, or may believe that everyone else he loves will die also. Watch for changes in behavior patterns with friends and at school, difficulty sleeping, and changes in eating habits.	Emphasize that the child was not responsible for the death. Reinforce that when people are sad, they cry, and that crying is normal and natural. Encourage the child to talk about and/or draw pictures of his feelings, or to cry.
Ages 6 to 9	May prefer to hide or disguise feelings to avoid looking babyish. Is afraid significant others will die. Seeks out detailed explanations for death, and differences between fatal illness and "just being sick." Has an understanding that death is real, but may believe that those who die are too slow, weak, or stupid. Fantasizes in an effort to make everything the way it was. Denial is the most helpful coping skill.	Talk about the normal feelings of anger, sadness, and guilt. Share your own feelings about death. Do not be afraid to cry in front of the child. This and other expressions of loss help to give the child permission to express his feelings.
Ages 9 to 12	Begins to understand the irreversibility of death. May seek details and specifics of the situation, and may need repeated, explicit explanations. Hard-won sense of independence becomes fragile, and may show concern about the practical matters of his lifestyle. May try to act "adult," but then regress to earlier stage of emotional response. When threatened, expresses anger toward the ill/deceased, himself, or other survivors.	Set aside time to talk about feelings. Encourage sharing of memories to facilitate grief response.
Ages 12 to 18	Demanding developmental processes are an awkward fit with the need to take on different family roles. Retreats to safety of childhood. Feels pressure to act as an adult, while still coping with skills of a child. Suppresses feelings in order to "fit in," leaving teen isolated and vulnerable.	Encourage talking, but respect need for privacy. See if a trusted, reliable friend or adult can provide appropriate support. Locate support group for teens.

★ Your EMS service is available to assist the survivors if needed. (Sometimes, medical emergencies occur in survivors in the wake of such stressful news.)

★ Information about local procedures for out-of-hospital death, such as the inspection of the scene by the medical examiner or coroner, and so on.

Do not include statements about God's will or relief from pain or any subjective assumption. You do not know the people well enough to know the details about their relationship or their religious preferences.

WHEN IT IS SOMEONE YOU KNOW

Many paramedics are called to serve in small communities, where calls often involve people they know. Elements of this are both rewarding and heart-wrenching. People may be greatly relieved to see a familiar, trusted face arriving in the ambulance. There also is a lot of support for paramedics in small communities because you are there to help others during their most fearful moments. However, being involved when the life of someone you know is threatened—or lost—can have a powerful impact upon your own emotions. If it is too much, you must find a way to manage the stress. Oftentimes, you must grieve as well. Your well-being demands it.

STRESS AND STRESS MANAGEMENT

Many aspects of EMS are stressful. A time-honored definition of stress, according to stress researcher Hans Selye, is "the nonspecific response of the body to any demand." The word **stress** also refers to a hardship or strain, or a physical or emotional response to a stimulus. Stress results from the interaction of events and the capabilities of each individual to adjust to that stress. A person's reactions to stress are individual. They are affected by previous exposure to the stressor, perception of the event, general life experience, and personal coping skills.

stress *a hardship or strain; a physical or emotional response to a stimulus.*

A stimulus that causes stress is known as a **stressor.** Stress is usually understood to generate a negative effect, or *distress*, in an individual. There is also "good" stress, which is called *eustress* (for example, seeing a lost loved one for the first time in years). However, even eustress generates physiological and psychological signs and symptoms.

stressor *a stimulus that causes stress.*

Adapting to stress is a dynamic, evolving process. As a person adapts, he develops:

★ *Defensive strategies.* While sometimes helpful for the short term, these strategies deny and distort the reality of a stressful situation.

★ *Coping.* This is an active process during which a person confronts the stressful situation. By acknowledging the existence of stressors, the patient is able to gather information about them and then change or adjust as necessary. Coping may not serve as the best strategy for the long term.

★ *Problem-solving skills.* These skills are regarded as the healthiest approach to everyday concerns. They involve problem analysis, which generates options for action, and determination of a course of action. Reflected in the ability to recognize multiple options and potential solutions for stressful situations, mastery generally comes only as a result of extensive experience with similar situations.

EMS has abundant stressors, which provide ample opportunities for the development of problem-solving skills. There are administrative stressors, such as waiting for calls, shift work, loud pagers, and inadequate pay. There are scene-related stressors, such as violent and abusive people, flying debris, vomit, loud noises, and chaos. There are emotional and physical stressors, such as fear, demanding bystanders, abusive patients, frustration, exhaustion, hunger or thirst, and lifting heavy objects.

Environmental stress may be in the form of siren noise, inclement weather, confined work spaces, and the frequent urgency of rapid scene responses and life-or-death decisions. In addition, the often difficult world of EMS can strain a paramedic's family relationships and possibly lead to conflicts with supervisors and co-workers. Add this to the common personality traits of paramedics, which include a strong need to be liked and often unrealistically high self-expectations, and the combination can lead to disturbing feelings of guilt or anxiety. All these stressors take a toll on the paramedic.

To manage stress, identify your own personal stressors, the amount of stress you can take before it becomes a problem, and what specific stress-management techniques work for you.

Your job in managing stress is to learn these things:

★ *Your personal stressors.* Each person has an individual list. What is stressful to you may be enjoyable to someone else. What was stressful to you last year may be replaced by new stressors this year.

★ *Amount of stress you can take before it becomes a problem.* Stress occurs in a tornado-like continuum. It starts with a few breezes, but it can increase in force until it is whirling out of control. Stopping the "storm" early is key to your well-being. You need to know which stress responses are early indicators for you, so you can deal with them at that point.

★ *Stress management strategies that work for you.* Again, this is totally individual. Those who seek personal well-being must become well-versed about personally appropriate options.

Adapting to stressors is a dynamic process of receiving, processing, and dissipating stressors and their effects. You bring your life experience, temperament, emotional maturity, spiritual convictions, habits (good and bad), interpersonal skills, ability to be self-aware, gender, and recent activity to each moment of adapting to the world. If a person piles on stressor after stressor without regard for the consequences, the results are likely to be bad. In fact, the U.S. Surgeon General once estimated that stress-related diseases kill 80 percent of people who die of nontraumatic causes. Stress-related disease is avoidable if you make a habit of doing what is necessary to preserve your personal well-being.

There are three phases of a stress response: *alarm*, *resistance*, and *exhaustion*. At the end comes a period of rest and recovery (Figure 2-10 ■).

★ *Stage I: Alarm.* The alarm phase is the "fight-or-flight" phenomenon. It occurs when the body physically and rapidly prepares to defend itself against a perceived threat. The pituitary gland begins by releasing adrenocorticotropic (stress) hormones. Hormones continue to flood the body via the autonomic nervous system, coordinated by the hypothalamus. Epinephrine and norepinephrine from the adrenal glands increase heart rate and blood pressure, dilate pupils, increase blood sugar and slow digestion, and relax the bronchial tree. This reaction ends when the event is recognized as not dangerous.

★ *Stage II: Resistance.* This stage starts when the individual begins to cope with the stress. Over time, an individual may become desensitized or adapted to stressors. Physiological parameters, such as pulse and blood pressure, may return to normal.

★ *Stage III: Exhaustion.* Prolonged exposure to the same stressors leads to exhaustion of an individual's ability to resist and adapt. Resistance to all stressors declines. Susceptibility to physical and psychological ailments increases. A period of rest and recovery is necessary for a healthy outcome.

It would be great if we could manage each stressor to the point of recovery before the next one hits, but that is not how it works. Typically, people are still dealing with one stress (or the same ongoing one, such as the chronic stress of shift work) when additional stressors pile on, resulting in cumulative stress. If stress accumulates without intervention, the consequences can be serious.

Content

■ Figure 2-10   Phases of a stress response. [*Adapted from J. Mitchell and G. Bray's* Emergency Services Stress *(Englewood Cliffs, N.J.: Prentice Hall, 1990), p. 11.*]

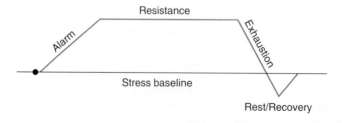

SHIFT WORK

There will always be shift work in EMS. Because EMS is a 24-hour, 7-days-a-week endeavor, someone has to be functional at all times. This is inherently stressful because of disruptions in the biorhythms of the body, known as **circadian rhythms,** and sleep deprivation.

Circadian rhythms are biological cycles that occur at approximately 24-hour intervals. These include hormonal and body temperature fluctuations, appetite and sleepiness cycles, and other bodily processes. When life patterns disrupt the circadian rhythms, such as with extensive time-zone travel, there are biological effects that can be stressful. Sleep deprivation is also common among people who work at night. The inherent dangers to paramedics are clear. Indeed, one study shows a conservative estimate of 56,000 motor-vehicle crashes annually between 1989 and 1993 due to driver drowsiness and fatigue.

If you have to sleep in the daytime, there are some tips to minimize the stress:

★ Sleep in a cool, dark place that mimics the nighttime environment.

★ Stick to sleeping at your **anchor time** (times you can rest without interruption), even on days off. Do not try to revert to a daytime lifestyle on days off. For example, if you work 9 P.M. to 5 A.M. and your anchor time is 8 A.M. to 12 noon, then go to bed "early" on days off and on workdays sleep from 8 A.M. to 3 P.M.

★ Unwind appropriately after a shift in order to rest well. Do not eat a heavy meal or exercise right before bedtime.

★ Post a "day sleeper" sign on your front door, turn off the phone's ringer, and lower the volume of the answering machine.

circadian rhythms physiological phenomena that occur at approximately 24-hour intervals.

anchor time set of hours when a night-shift worker can reliably expect to rest without interruption.

SIGNS OF STRESS

A variety of factors can trigger a stress response. They include the loss of something valuable, injury or the threat of injury, poor health or nutrition, general frustration, and ineffective coping mechanisms. Remember, each individual is susceptible to different stressors and therefore has a different constellation of signs and symptoms.

These signs and symptoms are a blessing in a way, because they are the body's way of warning that corrective stress management is needed. The warnings typically are mild at first, but left uncorrected they will build in intensity until you are forced to rest. If it means having a heart attack or collapsing, that is what the body will do. So, pay attention early.

The signs and symptoms of excessive stress can occur physically, emotionally, cognitively, or behaviorally (Table 2–4). They are unique to each person. Once again, an individual must perform a self-assessment. If you catch a warning sign of excessive stress early and manage it, there is no need to reach the extreme endpoint commonly referred to as **burnout.**

burnout occurs when coping mechanisms no longer buffer job stressors, which can compromise personal health and well-being.

COMMON TECHNIQUES FOR MANAGING STRESS

There are two main groups of defense mechanisms and techniques for managing stress: beneficial and detrimental. Detrimental techniques may provide a temporary sense of relief, but they will not cure the problem. They only make things worse. They include substance abuse (alcohol, nicotine, illegal and prescription drugs), overeating or other compulsive behaviors, chronic complaining, freezing out or cutting off others and the support they could give you, avoidance behaviors, and dishonesty about your actual state of well-being ("I'm just fine!").

Table 2–4	Warning Signs of Excessive Stress

Physical

Nausea/vomiting

Upset stomach

Tremors (lips, hands)

Feeling uncoordinated

Diaphoresis (profuse sweating), flushed skin

Chills

Diarrhea

Aching muscles and joints

Sleep disturbances

Fatigue

Dry mouth

Shakes

Headache

Vision problems

Difficult, rapid breathing

Chest tightness or pain, heart palpitations, cardiac rhythm disturbances

Cognitive

Confusion

Lowered attention span

Calculation difficulties

Memory problems

Poor concentration

Difficulty making decisions

Disruption in logical thinking

Disorientation, decreased level of awareness

Seeing an event over and over

Distressing dreams

Blaming someone

Emotional

Anticipatory anxiety

Denial

Fearfulness

Panic

Survivor guilt

Uncertainty of feelings

Depression

Grief

Hopelessness

Feeling overwhelmed

Feeling lost

Feeling abandoned

Feeling worried

Wishing to hide

Wishing to die

Anger

Feeling numb

Identifying with victim

Behavioral

Change in activity

Hyperactivity, hypoactivity

Withdrawal

Suspiciousness

Change in communications

Change in interactions with others

Change in eating habits

Increased or decreased food intake

Increased smoking

Increased alcohol intake

Increased intake of other drugs

Being overly vigilant to environment

Excessive humor

Excessive silence

Unusual behavior

Crying spells

It is far better for you to spend your energy on beneficial, or healthy, techniques that serve to dissipate the accumulation of stress and promote actual recovery. In situations where your stress response threatens your ability to handle the moment, you can:

★ *Use controlled breathing.* Focus attention on your breathing. Take in a deep breath through your nose. Then exhale forcefully but steadily through your mouth, so that you can hear the air rush out. Press all the air out of your lungs with your abdomen. Do this two or more times, until you feel steadier. This technique helps to reduce your adrenaline levels and slow your heart rate, so you can do your job appropriately.

★ *Reframe.* Mentally reframe interfering thoughts, such as "I can't do this" or "I'm scared." Be sure to deal with the thoughts later, or they will continue to interfere with the performance of your duties.

★ *Attend to the medical needs of the patient.* Even if you know the people involved, do not let those relationships interfere with your responsibilities as an EMS provider. Later, when it is appropriate to do so, address your stress about the call.

For long-term well-being, one of the best stress management techniques is to take care of yourself—physically, emotionally, and mentally. Remember that regular exercise does not have to be extreme. Do something that you enjoy and find relaxing. At stressful times, pay especially close attention to your diet. If you smoke, make it a goal to quit.

Create a non-EMS circle of friends, and renew old friendships or activities. Take a vacation or a few days off. Say "no!" to the next offer of an overtime shift. Listen to music, meditate, and learn positive thinking. Try the soothing techniques of guided imagery and progressive relaxation. Some paramedics have even quit EMS for a while. In general, you can make many choices. The key principle is to generate positive options for yourself, and keep choosing them until you have recovered.

For long-term well-being, the best stress-management technique is to take care of yourself; that is, eat properly, exercise regularly, and take time off!

SPECIFIC EMS STRESSES

There are three types of clearly defined EMS stresses:

★ *Daily stress.* Most EMS stress is unrelated to critical incidents and disasters. Instead, it is related to such things as pay, working conditions, dealing with the public, administrative matters, and other hassles of day-to-day living. To help deal with daily stress, all emergency personnel should develop personal stress management strategies such as a personal support system made up of co-workers, family, clergy, and others.

★ *Small incidents.* Incidents involving only one or two patients, including incidents that result in injuries or deaths of emergency workers, are best handled by competent mental health personnel in individual or small group settings. Mental health professionals should be familiar with EMS and be ready to respond when needed. They should then continue to screen affected emergency workers for signs and symptoms of abnormal response to stress and, if these are detected, refer these workers, as appropriate, to other competent mental health professionals who use accepted treatment methods.

★ *Large incidents and disasters.* Most EMS personnel will never encounter a disaster situation. However, all must be ready in case such a catastrophe occurs. The stress of large-scale disasters can be mitigated by a well-coordinated and organized response. Use of the Incident Management System (IMS) or Incident Command System (ICS) in large incidents and disasters serves to appropriately direct responding personnel. It also provides for rotating personnel through rehabilitation and surveillance stations. Those who are showing signs of stress or fatigue are removed from duty, at least temporarily. Here, too, there is a role for competent mental health professionals, who should be readily available to provide psychological first aid.

MENTAL HEALTH SERVICES

Mental health professionals can provide the information and education needed for rescuers to understand trauma, what to expect, and where to get help if needed. In addition, competent mental health personnel should be available at all major incidents to provide psychological first aid to rescuers and victims. Psychological first aid includes:

- ★ Listening
- ★ Conveying compassion
- ★ Assessing needs
- ★ Ensuring that basic physical needs are met
- ★ Not forcing personnel to talk
- ★ Providing or mobilizing family or significant others
- ★ Encouraging, but not forcing, social support
- ★ Protecting rescuers and victims from additional harm

Psychological first aid is not a treatment or packaged proprietary intervention technique. It is an attempt to provide practical palliative care and contact while respecting the wishes of those who may not be ready to deal with the possible onslaught of emotional responses in the early days following an incident. It entails providing comfort and information and meeting people's immediate practical and emotional needs.

DISASTER MENTAL HEALTH SERVICES

The emotional well-being of both rescuers and victims is an important concern in any multiple-casualty incident. In the past, Critical Incident Stress Management (CISM) was recommended for use in emergency services. However, recent evidence has clearly shown that CISM and Critical Incident Stress Debriefing (CISD) do not appear to mitigate the effects of traumatic stress and, in fact, may interfere with the normal grieving and healing process and should not be used.

However, there remains an important role for competent mental health professionals in any multiple-casualty incident. Mental health personnel should be available on scene to provide psychological first aid to all those affected by an incident—including EMS personnel. At the same time, they can survey rescuers and victims for the development of abnormal stress-related symptoms. In addition, mental health professionals should be available during the 2 months following a critical incident to screen and assist anyone who may be developing stress-related symptoms. Persons so affected may be referred for additional counseling or mental health care.

GENERAL SAFETY CONSIDERATIONS

The topic of scene safety is vast and requires career-long attention. Considering the many problems that can occur, it is impressive how few injuries there are. Your risks include violent people, environmental hazards, structural collapse, motor vehicles, and infectious disease. Many of these hazards can be minimized with protective equipment, such as helmets, body armor, reflective tape for night visibility, footwear with ankle support, and BSI precautions against infectious disease. Whatever protective equipment you have should be used.

INTERPERSONAL RELATIONS

Safety issues that arise in out-of-hospital care often stem from poor interpersonal relations. Paramedics are public ambassadors of health care. Interpersonal safety begins with effective communication. If you can build a rapport with the strangers you have been sent to serve, you will gain their trust. Suspicious, angry, and upset people are far more likely to be defensive and inflict harm than those who see a reason to trust what you are doing.

Building rapport depends on the ability to put your personal prejudices aside. Everyone has prejudices. But as a representative of an institution far greater than yourself, you must never allow them to interfere with appropriate patient and bystander management. In fact, go beyond curbing prejudice, and challenge yourself to treat every person you meet with dignity and respect.

Treat every person you meet with dignity and respect, no matter what their race, sex, age, religion, economic background, or present condition.

You can begin by taking time to pay attention to the rich array of cultural diversity and learning to see those differences as valuable and positive. In particular, learn about the different cultural backgrounds of people in your area and how to work with them effectively. For example, although you may like a lot of eye contact, understand that it is regarded as more polite in several cultures to avoid eye contact. Therefore, someone showing you esteem might avoid eye contact with you. This is not wrong. It is just different. Listen well to the stories of other people and see what you can learn. When a person can accept differences easily, it becomes easier to work toward win-win situations on the streets.

ROADWAY SAFETY

One of the greatest hazards in EMS is the motor vehicle. Roadways are unsafe places. There are good books, classes, and mentors to help you become aware of the various roadway hazards. For all related emergency situations, acquire the necessary training for emergency rescue and for the safe use of emergency rescue equipment. Learn the principles of:

One of the greatest hazards in EMS is the motor vehicle. Be sure to obey roadway laws and follow all driving safety guidelines.

★ Safely following an emergency escort vehicle.

★ Intersection management, when traffic is moving in several directions.

★ Noting hazardous conditions, such as spilled hazardous materials (gasoline, industrial chemicals, and so on), downed power lines, and proximity to moving traffic. Also notice adverse environmental conditions.

★ Evaluating the safest parking place when arriving at a roadway incident.

★ Safely approaching a vehicle in which someone is slumped over the wheel.

★ Patient compartment safety—in particular, bracing yourself against sudden deceleration or swerving to avoid roadway hazards; and making a habit of hanging on consistently, especially when changing positions.

★ Safely using emergency lights and siren.

An ambulance escort can create additional hazards. Inexperienced ambulance operators often follow the escort vehicle too closely and are unable to stop when the escort does. Inexperienced operators also may assume that other drivers know the ambulance is following an escort. In fact, other drivers do not know another emergency vehicle is coming and often pull out in front of the ambulance just after the escort vehicle passes.

Multiple-vehicle responses can be just as dangerous, especially when responding vehicles travel in the same direction close together. When two vehicles approach the same intersection at the same time, not only may they fail to yield to each other, but other drivers may yield for the first vehicle only, not the second one. Extreme caution must be taken when approaching intersections.

Certain equipment is intended to promote your safety on roadways. For example, to be visible to oncoming drivers, who may have dirty, smeared, pitted windshields and may not be sober, wear reflective tape and orange or lime-green safety vests. In fact, you also may be issued other protective gear, especially if you are in the fire service. Using respiratory protection, gloves, boots, turnout coat and pants (or coveralls), and other specialty safety equipment is the mark of an aware, professional paramedic. Ask non-medical personnel to set out flares or cones, if needed. Leave some emergency lights flashing, although you should be careful not to blind oncoming drivers.

To park safely at a roadway incident, make it a habit to scan each individual setting. Notice curves, hilltops, volume, and the speed of surrounding traffic. Ideally, park in the front of a crash site on the same side of the street. This facilitates access to the patient compartment and equipment, and it protects you from traffic coming from behind. However, when responding to an incident such as "person slumped behind wheel," maintain the defensive advantage by staying behind the vehicle, and use spotlights to "blind" the person until you know there are no hostile intentions. Walk to the vehicle with cautious alertness until you are sure it is not a trap.

The use of seat belts in the front of an ambulance should be an obvious habit, both for safety and for role modeling. Less obvious is the use of safety restraints in the patient compartment. An improper assumption is that the paramedic is too busy attending to the patient and passengers to wear a seat belt. However, buckling into a seat belt for a safer ride is, in fact, possible during much or most of ambulance transport times. Death and major disability is common when someone is in the patient compartment during a crash. For your well-being, wear a seat belt whenever possible, even "in back."

Because ambulances represent help and hope, it is doubly tragic when a paramedic crew is involved in a motor-vehicle crash caused by the misuse of lights and siren. Lights and siren are tools, not toys. They are the paramedic's means for gaining quick access to people in dire need. Those who misuse the mandate to operate them chip away at the public's trust in EMS. Whether using lights and siren or not, the paramedic has a responsibility to drive with due regard for the safety of others. As a professional, you are obligated to study and use safe driving practices at all times.

Summary

The paramedic has the training and responsibility to manage the most complicated health problems posed by out-of-hospital citizens. This makes the paramedic a leader within the prehospital care community. Paramedics who attend to their own well-being are not only helping themselves, but they are also providing a positive role model for other EMS providers and the community at large.

Continuous assessment of personal lifestyle includes practices that affect the immediate future to practices that affect the paramedic in old age. They range from wearing personal protective equipment (PPE) and parking safely at a crash site, to managing stress daily, eating right, and exercising.

There are numerous elements to the topic of well-being, and the paramedic must strive continually to address each one. Take your knowledge beyond the introduction offered in this chapter. Be a lifelong student of well-being, and you are more likely to have a healthy long life. Your biggest challenge is this: be well, so that you can help others be well, too.

Always use the proper personal protective equipment (PPE) to keep yourself safe from injury at the scene of an emergency.

You Make the Call

It's been a tough year for you on the paramedic squad. Lately, it just seems as if everything that can go wrong does. Arguing (again) with your spouse about paying the mortgage is not helping your irritation one bit. It is 2300 hours. You are tired, and all you ate all day was glazed doughnuts and fast food. Suddenly, the tone alert sounds: "Ambulance 44, respond to the corner of Fero and Bailey on a two-vehicle crash. Number of victims unknown."

You are the second EMS crew to arrive. You prefer the job of triage, and the paramedic who is doing it is too new to know much. Anyway, he has already triaged four patients. As you walk up to the scene, you notice the bumper sticker on one crash vehicle, and realize it is your neighbor's daughter's car. You do not see her in the group of patients, and your heart leaps into your throat when you see the DOA covered with a sheet.

You are assigned two patients, one an unconscious teen with a crushed leg, and the other an adult with a broken arm.

You take pride in your medical abilities, so handling the immobilization and other medical care is smooth. On the way to the hospital, the teen wakes up and presses you to tell him, "Is Debbie okay? Is she? Please! Tell me, is she all right?" Thus you find out that, indeed, the other person in your neighbor's car was Debbie, their daughter.

After delivering the patients to the hospital, you pop an antacid for your sour stomach and chew out your partner for his bumpy driving.

A couple of days later, you take on yet another overtime shift. Your mortgage payment is due and, besides, you can't face going to the funeral of your neighbor's daughter. You've seen enough death. Who needs another funeral anyway?

1. Are your stress levels inappropriately high? What are the indications?
2. Might it be a good idea for you to go to the funeral? Why or why not?
3. How can you improve stress management in the future?

See Suggested Responses at the back of this book.

Review Questions

1. Most paramedic injuries are due to _____ and being in and around motor vehicles.
   a. falls
   b. stress
   c. lifting
   d. violence

2. Which of the following is not a benefit of achieving acceptable physical fitness?
   a. increased muscle mass and metabolism
   b. increased oxygen-carrying capacity
   c. increased resting heart rate and blood pressure
   d. increased resistance to illness and injury

3. Based on the major food groups list, the paramedic should consume _____ servings of vegetables per day, for fiber, iron, vitamins A and C, and folate.
   a. 2–3
   b. 2–4
   c. 3–5
   d. 6–11

4. Which of the following is not an important principle of lifting?
   a. always avoid twisting and turning
   b. keep your palms up whenever possible
   c. move a load only if you can safely handle it
   d. position the load far away from your body and center of gravity

5. A strict form of infection control that is based on the assumption that all blood and other body fluids are infectious is termed:
   a. personal protective equipment.
   b. mode of transmission.
   c. incubation period.
   d. body substance isolation.

6. _____ is the use of a chemical, or a physical method such as pressurized steam, to kill all microorganisms on an object.
   a. cleaning
   b. disinfecting
   c. sterilizing
   d. decontaminating

7. How many stages are identified in the grief process?
   a. 3
   b. 5
   c. 7
   d. 8

8. The first step in the grieving process is:
   a. anger.
   b. denial.
   c. depression.
   d. bargaining.

9. This is an active process during which a person confronts the stressful situation.
   a. coping
   b. resistance
   c. defensive strategies
   d. problem-solving skills

10. For safety at a roadway incident it is appropriate to do all of the following except:
    a. ask non-medical personnel to set out flares or cones.
    b. wear reflective tape and an orange or lime-green vest.
    c. blind a slumped-over passenger with a spotlight as you approach.
    d. park on the opposite side of the street from the crashed vehicle.

See Answers to Review Questions at the back of this book.

Further Reading

Becknell, J. *Medic Life*. St. Louis: Mosby Lifeline, 1996.

Bledsoe, B. E. "Critical Incident Stress Management (CISM): Benefit or Rise for Emergency Services." *Prehospital Emergency Care* 7(2) (2003):272–329.

Dernocoeur, K. B. *Streetsense: Communication, Safety, and Control*. 3rd ed. Redmond, WA: Laing Research Services, 1996.

"Effects of Partial and Total Sleep Deprivation on Driving Performance." #FHWA-RD-94-046. McLean, VA: Federal Highway Administration, 1994.

"EMS Safety: Techniques and Applications," FA-144. Washington: Federal Emergency Management Agency (FEMA), April 1994.

"Fitting Fitness in Even When You're Pressed for Time." Chicago: National Cattlemen's Beef Association, 1996. (Reviewed favorably by American Heart Association and others.)

Krebs, D. R., et al. *When Violence Erupts*. St. Louis: C.V. Mosby, 1990.

Kübler-Ross, E. *On Death and Dying*. (Originally published 1969.) Scribner Classics reprint edition. New York: Simon & Schuster, 1997.

Markiwitz, E. "Eating on the Run: Finding Fast Food That Feeds Your Health." *JEMS* 18 (January, 1993).

McNally, R. J., R. A. Bryant, and A. Ehlers. "Does Early Psychological Intervention Promote Recovery from Posttraumatic Stress?" *Psychological Science in the Public Interest* 4(2)(2003):45–79 [available at *http://www.psychologicalscience.org/journals/pspi/index.html*].

Mitchell, J., and G. Bray. *Emergency Services Stress: Guidelines for Preserving the Health and Careers of Emergency Services Personnel*. Upper Saddle River, N.J.: Pearson/Prentice Hall, 1990.

On the Web

Visit Brady's Paramedic Website at **www.bradybooks.com/paramedic**.

EMS Systems

Objectives

After reading this chapter, you should be able to:

1. Describe key historical events that influenced the national development of Emergency Medical Services (EMS) systems. (pp. 47–52)
2. Define the following terms:
    a. EMS systems (p. 46)
    b. Licensure (p. 59)
    c. Certification (p. 59)
    d. Registration (p. 59)
    e. Profession (p. 59)
    f. Professionalism (p. 69)
    g. Health care professional (p. 61)
    h. Ethics (p. 69)
    i. Peer review (p. 69)
    j. Medical direction (p. 54)
    k. Protocols (p. 55)
3. Identify national groups important to the development, education, and implementation of EMS. (pp. 62–63)
4. Discuss the role of national associations, the National Registry of EMTs, and the roles of various EMS standard-setting agencies. (pp. 62–63)
5. Identify the standards (components) of an EMS system as defined by the National Highway Traffic Safety Administration. (pp. 51–52)
6. Differentiate among EMS provider levels: First Responder, Emergency Medical Technician-Basic, Emergency Medical Technician-Intermediate, and Emergency Medical Technician-Paramedic. (pp. 59–60)

7. Describe what is meant by "citizen involvement in the EMS system." (pp. 55–56)

8. Describe the role of the EMS physician in providing medical direction. (pp. 54–55)

9. Discuss prehospital and out-of-hospital care as an extension of the physician. (pp. 54–55)

10. Describe the benefits of both on-line and off-line medical direction. (pp. 54–55)

11. Describe the process for the development of local policies and protocols. (pp. 54–55)

12. Describe the relationship between a physician on the scene, the paramedic on the scene, and the EMS physician providing on-line medical direction. (p. 55)

13. Describe the components of continuous quality improvement and analyze its contribution to system improvement, continuing medical education, and research. (pp. 67–70)

14. Describe the importance, basic principles, process of evaluating and interpreting, and benefits of research. (pp. 70–71; Appendix)

Key Terms

advanced life support
  (ALS), p. 47
basic life support (BLS),
  p. 47
certification, p. 59
continuous quality
  improvement (CQI),
  p. 68
emergency medical
  dispatcher (EMD), p. 57
emergency medical
  services (EMS) system,
  p. 46

ethics, p. 69
health care professionals,
  p. 61
intervener physician, p. 55
licensure, p. 59
medical direction, p. 51
medical director, p. 54
off-line medical direction,
  p. 55
on-line medical direction,
  p. 54
peer review, p. 69
profession, p. 59

professionalism, p. 69
protocols, p. 55
quality assurance (QA),
  p. 68
quality improvement (QI),
  p. 52
reciprocity, p. 59
registration, p. 59
rules of evidence, p. 69
standing orders, p. 55
trauma, p. 49
trauma center, p. 52
triage, p. 49

Case Study

It is a beautiful Fourth of July. You and your family are traveling down the interstate on your way to a concert and fireworks show. Just an hour from your destination, a tire blows out on the BMW ahead of you, and you see it skid into the median and crash into some pine trees. You pull onto the shoulder. As an experienced paramedic, you assure scene safety before approaching the mangled car. You see no movement inside the passenger compartment.

Your daughter grabs her cellular phone and calls 911. The dispatcher asks for the location of the crash and transfers your call to the 911 center for that area. The emergency medical dispatcher gathers the appropriate information and dispatches the local volunteer fire service and an advanced life support (ALS) ambulance. While you attempt to gain access to the patients, your daughter continues to provide the dispatcher with information that he, in turn, relays to the responding units.

The local volunteer fire and rescue team arrives on scene in about 7 minutes. You provide a verbal report to the arriving rescuers. They do their own scene safety check, approach the car, and determine that there are four patients. Two are priority-1 patients (one of these is a 2-year-old child), and two are priority-3 patients. Based on the initial assessment, Rescuer Lt. C. J. Greenlee requests an aeromedical helicopter and a second ALS unit. Approximately 2 minutes later, a fire truck crew arrives. They reroute traffic and establish a landing zone for the helicopter.

When all EMS personnel summoned are on scene, they decide that the 2-year-old patient will be flown to Children's Hospital, a pediatric specialty center. The other priority-1 patient will be transported by ground to the closest level-one trauma center. The priority-3 patients will be taken to the local hospital by ground transport. Working as a team, the fire and ambulance personnel extricate the patients and package them for transport.

Approximately 22 minutes after the arrival of the first ALS unit, all patients are extricated and en route to a receiving facility capable of providing the level of care they need. Within 15 minutes of arrival at the pediatric trauma center and just 31 minutes after the crash, the 2-year-old is moved to surgery for the repair of a ruptured liver and spleen. The other patients are being treated at their destinations as well.

INTRODUCTION

emergency medical services (EMS) system *a comprehensive network of personnel, equipment, and resources established for the purpose of delivering aid and emergency medical care to the community.*

An **emergency medical services (EMS) system** is a comprehensive network of personnel, equipment, and resources established to deliver aid and emergency medical care to the community. To meet the needs of the community it serves, an EMS system must function as a unified whole. In general, an EMS system is comprised of both out-of-hospital and in-hospital components. The out-of-hospital component includes:

★ Members of the community who are trained in first aid and CPR
★ A communications system that allows public access to emergency services dispatch and allows EMS providers to communicate with each other
★ EMS providers, including paramedics
★ Fire/rescue and hazardous-materials services
★ Public utilities, such as power and gas companies
★ Resource centers, such as regional poison control centers

The in-hospital component includes:

★ Emergency nurses
★ Emergency physicians and specialty physicians
★ Ancillary services, such as radiology and respiratory therapy
★ Specialty physicians, such as trauma surgeons and cardiologists
★ Rehabilitation services

Every EMS system must rely on the strength of its components. A weakness in one will diminish the overall quality of patient care. For example, a typical EMS operation begins with citizen activation. That is, a bystander—a family member, friend, or a stranger to the patient—initiates contact with a 911 dispatch center. EMS dispatch is then responsible for collecting essential information and sending out the closest appropriately staffed and equipped unit. In many EMS systems, the dispatcher also provides prearrival instructions to the patient or caller so that care may begin immediately.

Usually, the first EMS provider to respond to the scene of an emergency is a police officer, firefighter, lifeguard, teacher, or other community member who has received basic medical training in an approved First Responder program. His role is to stabilize the patient until more advanced EMS personnel arrive.

The next EMS provider likely to arrive on scene depends on the type of EMS system involved. In most areas, the dispatcher will send a **basic life support (BLS)** or **advanced life support (ALS)** ambulance. In other areas of the country, EMS uses a "tiered response," sending multiple levels of emergency care personnel to the same incident. In still other areas of the country, ALS personnel may respond to every incident regardless of the level of care needed to treat a patient (Figure 3-1 ■).

Once emergency care has been initiated, EMS providers must quickly decide on the medical facility to which the patient should be transported. This decision is based on the type of care needed, transport time, and local protocols. In a comprehensive EMS system where specialty centers have been designated (such as pediatric, trauma, and burn centers), it may be necessary to transport the patient to a facility other than the closest hospital.

Upon arrival at the receiving medical facility, where an emergency nurse or physician assumes responsibility for the patient, the patient is assigned a priority of care. If needed, a surgeon or other specialist will be summoned.

basic life support (BLS) *refers to basic life-saving procedures such as artificial ventilation and cardiopulmonary resuscitation (CPR).*

advanced life support (ALS) *refers to advanced life-saving procedures such as intravenous therapy, drug therapy, intubation, and defibrillation.*

HISTORY OF EMS

The Emergency Medical Services (EMS) system developed from the traditional and scientific beliefs of many cultures.

ANCIENT TIMES

There is evidence that emergency medicine has a very long history. It may be traced back to biblical times when it was recorded that a "good Samaritan" provided care to a wounded traveler by the side of a road. In fact, about 4,000 to 5,000 years ago, scribes in Sumer, a civilization in Mesopotamia (southwest Asia), inscribed clay tablets with some of our earliest medical records.

Similar to protocols that EMS uses today, the ancient tablets provided healers with step-by-step instructions for patient care based on the patient's description of symptoms. The tablets also included instructions on how to create the medications needed to cure the patient and explained how and when to administer them. The most striking difference between these first "protocols" and EMS today is the absence of a physical exam.

In 1862, the Egyptologist Edwin Smith purchased a papyrus scroll dating back to about 1500 B.C.E. It contained 48 medical case histories with data arranged in head-to-toe order and in order of severity, an arrangement very similar to today's patient assessment. Each case also had a particular format, including a title, specific instructions to the healer, and a projection of possible outcomes. One section, called the "Book of Wounds," explains the treatment of injuries such as fractures and dislocations. It includes descriptions of the materials needed for making bandages and splints, as well as information about sutures and solutions that may be used to clean wounds.

At about the same time in another civilization in the Mesopotamian region, King Hammurabi of Babylon commissioned a large painting of 282 case laws known today as the "Code of Hammurabi." That code governed criminal and civil matters, and it established strict penalties for violations, a concept called *lex talionis* or "law of the claw" (very similar to the idea of "an eye for an eye").

TIERED RESPONSE

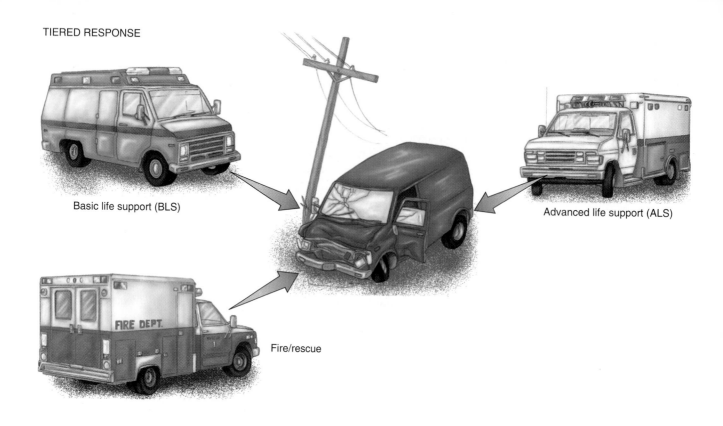

Basic life support (BLS)

Advanced life support (ALS)

FIRE DEPT.

Fire/rescue

ALTERNATIVE RESPONSE

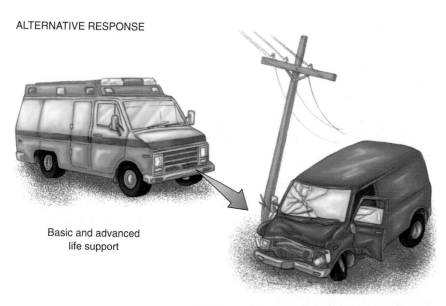

Basic and advanced
life support

■ Figure 3-1   In a tiered response, BLS providers arrive on scene first and then, if required, ALS care arrives later. Other systems dispatch an ALS team to all calls.

One particular section of the code was devoted to the regulation of medical fees and penalties, which were based on the social class of the patient. For example, if a surgeon operated successfully on a commoner, he would be paid only half of what his fee would be if he had operated on a rich man. Social class was also the basis for penalties. If a surgeon caused the death of a rich man, the surgeon's hand would be cut off. But if a slave died under his care, he only had to replace the slave.

EIGHTEENTH AND NINETEENTH CENTURIES

In the more recent times of the Napoleonic Wars (Table 3–1), one of Napoleon's chief surgeons, Jean Larrey, recognized the importance of reducing the time from injury to definitive surgery. In response, Larrey formed the *ambulance volante*, or "flying ambulance," which focused efforts on providing emergency surgery as close to the battlefield as possible. Though the *ambulance volante* was little more than a covered horse-drawn cart, Larrey is credited with the development of the first prehospital system that used **triage** and transport.

triage *a method of sorting patients by the severity of their injuries.*

Between 1861 and 1865 during the U.S. Civil War, a nurse named Clara Barton coordinated care for the sick and injured at battlefield sites along the East Coast. Defying army leaders, she persisted in going to the front where wounded men suffered and often died from lack of the simplest medical attention. She continued the concept of the *ambulance volante* by organizing the triage and transport of injured soldiers to improvised hospitals in nearby houses, barns, and churches away from the battlefield.

The first civilian ambulance service was formed about the same time (1865) in Cincinnati, Ohio. Four years later, in 1869, the New York City Health Department Ambulance Service began operating out of Bellevue Hospital. The ambulances of both services were specially designed horse-drawn carts, which were staffed with physician interns from the various hospital wards.

TWENTIETH CENTURY

During World War I, a high mortality rate of soldiers was associated with an average evacuation time of 18 hours. As a result, in World War II a system of transportation to echelons (levels) of care was created. Battlefield ambulance corps transported wounded soldiers from the front lines to the echelons of care. However, many of the echelons were so far from the battlefield and each other that there were huge delays in patient care. In many cases, it was often days from the injury itself to definitive surgery.

During the Korean and Vietnam conflicts, there were great advances in the patient care delivery system. At last, the wounded soldier was treated in the battlefield when the injury occurred and was evacuated by helicopter to a field hospital where he would receive definitive surgery. In Vietnam, in many cases, this occurred within 10 to 20 minutes. Once stabilized and able to be moved (generally within 24 to 48 hours), the patient would be flown by jet to Clark Air Force Base in the Philippines, where he would receive any necessary further treatment. The decrease in the amount of time to definitive care plus the advances in medical procedures significantly reduced mortality rates.

Throughout history, significant advances in **trauma** care occurred during wartime. However, until the late 1960s, few areas of the United States provided adequate civilian prehospital emergency care. The prevailing thought was that medical care began in the hospital emergency department. Rescue techniques were crude, ambulance attendants poorly educated, and equipment minimal. Police, fire, and EMS personnel had no radio communication. Proper medical direction was not available, and the only interaction between physicians and EMS personnel was at the receiving facility.

trauma *a physical injury or wound caused by external force or violence.*

Eventually, as costs and demand for additional services forced many rural mortician-operated ambulances to withdraw, local police and fire departments found that they had to provide the ambulance service. In many areas, volunteer ambulance services made up of local, independent EMS provider agencies proliferated. In the urban setting, the increased demand on hospital-based EMS systems resulted in the development of municipal services, which were operated on city, county, or regional levels. However, because they could not communicate with each other, it was impossible to coordinate a response to any but the simplest local calls.

In 1966 the publication of *Accidental Death and Disability: The Neglected Disease of Modern Society* by the National Academy of Sciences, National Resource Council,

Table 3-1 | An EMS Timeline

1797	Napoleon's chief physician implements a prehospital system designed to triage and transport the injured from the field to aid stations.
1855	Florence Nightingale introduces hygienic standards into military hospitals during Crimean War.
1860s	First civilian ambulance services begin in Cincinnati and New York City.
	Clara Barton coordinates medical care at U.S. Civil War battlefield sites.
1915	First known air medical transport occurs during the retreat of the Serbian army from Albania.
1920s	First volunteer rescue squads organize in Roanoke, Virginia, and along the New Jersey coast.
1958	Dr. Peter Safar demonstrates the efficacy of mouth-to-mouth ventilation.
1960	Cardiopulmonary resuscitation (CPR) is shown to be efficacious.
1966	Highway Safety Act of 1966 establishes the Emergency Medical Services Program in the Department of Transportation.
	Accidental Death and Disability: The Neglected Disease of Modern Society is published.
1969	DOT publishes first EMT-Ambulance Curriculum.
1970	Military Assistance to Safety and Traffic (MAST) program tests use of helicopters and paramedics in civilian emergencies.
	National Registry of EMTs founded.
1971	White House funds demonstration of model EMS system development.
1972	Department of Health, Education, and Welfare allocates $16 million to EMS demonstration programs in five states.
1973	The Robert Wood Johnson Foundation appropriates $15 million to fund 44 regional EMS projects in 32 states and Puerto Rico.
	The Emergency Medical Services Systems (EMSS) Act provides additional federal guidelines and funding for the development of regional EMS systems; the law establishes 15 components of EMS systems.
1974	"KKK-A-1822 Federal Specifications for Ambulances" is the first attempt to standardize ambulance design.
1977	DOT publishes first EMT-Paramedic Curriculum.
1980	"KKK-A-1822A" replaces ambulance light bars and beacons with low-amp lighting system.
1981	Omnibus Budget Reconciliation Act consolidates EMS funding into state preventive-health and health-services block grants, and eliminates funding under the EMSS Act.
1983	Standard equipment for BLS services identified by American College of Surgeons Committee on Trauma.
1984	EMS for Children program, under the Public Health Act, provides funds for enhancing the EMS system to better serve pediatric patients. Since its inception, over 40 states have received funding.
1985	National Research Council publishes *Injury in America: A Continuing Public Health Problem*, which describes deficiencies in the progress of addressing accidental death and disability; renewed focus on developing regional trauma care systems.
	"KKK-A-1822B" upgrades standards for ambulances, including reduced internal siren noise and venting systems for oxygen compartments.
1988	NHTSA initiates the Statewide EMS Technical Assessment Program based on 10 key components of EMS systems.
	Standard equipment for ALS services recommended by American College of Emergency Physicians.
1990	The Trauma Care Systems and Development Act encourages development of inclusive trauma systems and provides funding to states for trauma system planning, implementation, and evaluation.
1993	The Institute of Medicine publishes *Emergency Medical Services for Children*, which points out deficiencies in our health-care system's ability to address the emergency medical needs of pediatric patients.
1995	Congress does not reauthorize funding under the Trauma Care Systems and Development Act.
1996	*EMS Agenda for the Future* is published.
1997	NHTSA publishes *A Leadership Guide to Quality Improvement for Emergency Medical Services Systems*.
1998	DOT publishes revised EMT-Paramedic Curriculum.
2002	"KKK-A-1822E" guidelines are released, designed to markedly increase the safety of ambulances.
2003	Health Insurance Portability and Accountability Act (HIPAA) becomes effective, strictly regulating the flow of confidential patient information.

focused attention on the problem. "The White Paper," as the report was called, spelled out the deficiencies in prehospital emergency care. It suggested guidelines for the development of EMS systems, the training of prehospital emergency medical providers, and the upgrading of ambulances and their equipment. This landmark publication set off a series of federal and private initiatives, including these:

* *1966.* Congress passed the National Highway Safety Act, which established the U.S. Department of Transportation (DOT), a cabinet-level department. It provided matching grants to states for emergency medical services and forced them to develop effective EMS systems or risk losing federal highway construction funds. The Highway Safety Act distributed more than $142 million between 1968 and 1979. Funds were also provided for the development of educational programs for emergency services and for early advanced life support (ALS) pilot programs. In 1969 the Emergency Medical Technician–Ambulance program was made public. The first paramedic curriculum followed in 1977.
* *1971.* The White House gave nearly $9 million to EMS demonstration projects, which were designed to be models for subsequent system development.
* *1972.* The Department of Health, Education, and Welfare funded a $16 million five-state initiative for the development of regional EMS systems. The next year, the Robert Wood Johnson Foundation provided approximately $15 million in grants for establishing regional EMS projects and communication systems.

Then, in 1973 Congress passed the Emergency Medical Services Systems Act, which provided additional funding for a series of projects related to the delivery of trauma care. As a result, the development of regional EMS systems continued from 1974 through 1981. A total of $300 million was allocated to study the feasibility of EMS planning, operations, expansion, and research.

In order to be eligible for this funding, an EMS system had to include the following 15 components: manpower, training, communications, transportation, emergency facilities, critical care units, public safety agencies, consumer participation, access to care, patient transfer, standardized record keeping, public information and education, system review and evaluation, disaster management plans, and mutual aid. Unfortunately, the designers of this legislation omitted two major components: system financing and **medical direction.**

When federal funding was significantly reduced in the early 1980s, many systems faced economic disaster. Even worse, many were operating without medical direction. So, the Emergency Medical Services Systems Act was amended in 1976 and again in 1979, and a total of $215 million was appropriated over a 7-year period toward the establishment of regional EMS systems.

In 1981, the passage of the Consolidated Omnibus Budget Reconciliation Act (COBRA) essentially wiped out federal funding for EMS. The small amount of funding that remained was placed into state preventive-health and health-services block grants. The National Highway Traffic Safety Administration (NHTSA) attempted to sustain the efforts of the Department of Health and Human Services, but with its other EMS responsibilities and no additional funding, the momentum for continued development was lost.

In 1988, the Statewide EMS Technical Assessment Program was established by the NHTSA. It defines elements necessary to all EMS systems. Briefly, they are:

* *Regulation and policy.* Each state must have laws, regulations, policies, and procedures that govern its EMS system. It also is required to provide leadership to local jurisdictions.

Content

Review

**1973 EMSS Act:
15 Components
of EMS Systems**

Manpower
Training
Communications
Transportation
Emergency facilities
Critical care units
Public safety agencies
Consumer participation
Access to care
Patient transfer
Standardized record keeping
Public information and education
System review and evaluation
Disaster management plans
Mutual aid

medical direction *medical policies, procedures, and practices that are available to providers either on-line or off-line.*

Review

Content

1988 NHTSA: "10 System Elements"

Regulation and policy
Resources management
Human resources and training
Transportation
Facilities
Communications
Trauma systems
Public information and education
Medical direction
Evaluation

trauma center *medical facility that has the capability of caring for the acutely injured patient. Trauma centers must meet strict criteria to use this designation.*

quality improvement (QI) *an evaluation program that emphasizes service and uses customer satisfaction as the ultimate indicator of system performance.*

★ *Resources management.* Each state must have central control of EMS resources so all patients have equal access to acceptable emergency care.

★ *Human resources and training.* A standardized EMS curriculum should be taught by qualified instructors, and all personnel who transport patients in the prehospital setting should be adequately trained.

★ *Transportation.* Patients must be safely and reliably transported by ground or air ambulance.

★ *Facilities.* Every seriously ill or injured patient must be delivered in a timely manner to an appropriate medical facility.

★ *Communications.* A system for public access to the EMS system must be in place. Communication among dispatchers, the ambulance crew, and hospital personnel must also be possible.

★ *Trauma systems.* Each state should develop a system of specialized care for trauma patients, including one or more **trauma centers** and rehabilitation programs. It also must develop systems for assigning and transporting patients to those facilities.

★ *Public information and education.* EMS personnel should participate in programs designed to educate the public. The programs are to focus on the prevention of injuries and how to properly access the EMS system.

★ *Medical direction.* Each EMS system must have a physician as its medical director. This physician delegates medical practice to nonphysician caregivers and oversees all aspects of patient care.

★ *Evaluation.* Each state must have a **quality improvement** (**QI**) system in place for continuing evaluation and upgrading of its EMS system.

Many EMS providers today fail to realize that each component of the EMS system has gone through many stages of development. Nevertheless, in this technologically advanced country, there are still startling regional differences in the quality of prehospital care.

THE EMS AGENDA FOR THE FUTURE

The EMS Agenda for the Future was published in 1996 as an opportunity to examine what has been learned during the prior three decades and to create a vision for the future for EMS in the United States. This opporunity came at an important time, when those agencies, organizations, and individuals that affect EMS were evaluating its role in the context of a rapidly evolving health care system—a process of evaluation that is ongoing.

The EMS Agenda for the Future project was supported by the National Highway Traffic Safety Administration and the Health Resources and Services Administration, Maternal and Child Health Bureau. This document focuses on aspects of EMS related to emergency care outside of traditional health care facilities. It recognizes the changes occurring in the health care system of which EMS is a part. EMS of the future will be a community-based health management system that is fully integrated with the overall health care system. EMS of the future will have the ability to identify and modify illness and injury risks, provide acute illness and injury care and follow-up, and contribute to the treatment of chronic conditions and to community health monitoring. EMS will be integrated with other health care providers and public health and public safety agencies in the effort to improve community health, which will result in more appropriate use of acute health care resources. EMS will remain the public's emergency medical safety net.

To realize this vision, *The EMS Agenda for the Future* proposes continued development of 14 EMS attributes. They are:

- ★ Integration of health services
- ★ EMS research
- ★ Legislation and regulation
- ★ System finance
- ★ Human resources
- ★ Medical direction
- ★ Education systems
- ★ Public education
- ★ Prevention
- ★ Public access
- ★ Communication systems
- ★ Clinical care
- ★ Information systems
- ★ Evaluation

This document serves as guidance for EMS providers, health care organizations and institutions, governmental agencies, and policy makers who must be committed to improving the health of their communities and to ensuring that EMS efficiently contributes to that goal. They must invest the resources necessary to provide the nation's population with emergency health care that is reliably accessible, effective, subject to continuous evaluation, and integrated with the remainder of the health system.

The EMS Agenda for the Future provides a vision for out-of-facility EMS. Achieving such a vision requires deliberate action and application of the knowledge gained during the past decades of EMS experience. If pursued conscientiously, it will be an achievement that greatly benefits all of society.

TODAY'S EMS SYSTEMS

The efficient delivery of emergency medical care requires a systematic approach and team effort to make the best use of existing resources. That means each community must develop an EMS system that best meets its needs. Though EMS systems across the country and the world will vary, certain elements are essential to ensure the best possible patient care.

Each community must develop an EMS system that best meets its needs.

LOCAL AND STATE-LEVEL AGENCIES

At the municipal and regional levels, the first step in developing a comprehensive EMS system is to establish an administrative agency. This agency is responsible for managing the local system's resources, developing operational protocols, and establishing standards and guidelines. Within the agency, a planning board is formed. The planning board should be composed of community representatives, including emergency physicians, the emergency nurse association, the firefighter association, state and local police, and "consumers." It develops a budget and selects a qualified administrative staff capable of managing an EMS agency.

Once established, the agency designates who may function within the system and develops policies consistent with existing state requirements. It also creates a quality assurance or quality improvement program to evaluate the system's effectiveness and to ensure that the best interests of the patient are always a top priority. State EMS agencies are typically responsible for allocating funds to local systems, enacting legislation concerning the prehospital practice of medicine, licensing and certification of field providers, enforcing all state EMS regulations, and appointing regional advisory councils.

In essence, EMS is made up of a series of systems within a system. The integration of these systems and the cooperation of all participants help to result in the best quality of emergency care.

MEDICAL DIRECTION

medical director *a physician who is legally responsible for all of the clinical and patient-care aspects of an EMS system. Also referred to as medical direction.*

An EMS system must retain a **medical director**—a physician who is legally responsible for all clinical and patient-care aspects of the system. Prehospital medical care provided by nonphysicians is considered an extension of the medical director's license; that is, prehospital care providers are the medical director's designated agents, regardless of who their employers may be.

The medical director's role in an EMS system is to:

All prehospital care providers are the medical director's designated agents, regardless of who their employer may be.

* Educate and train personnel
* Participate in personnel and equipment selection
* Develop clinical protocols in cooperation with expert EMS personnel
* Participate in quality improvement and problem resolution
* Provide direct input into patient care
* Interface between the EMS system and other health care agencies
* Advocate within the medical community
* Serve as the "medical conscience" of the EMS system, including advocating for quality patient care

In addition to the responsibilities previously listed, the medical director is the ultimate authority for all on-line (direct) and off-line (indirect) medical direction.

On-Line Medical Direction

on-line medical direction *occurs when a qualified physician gives direct orders to a prehospital care provider by either radio or telephone.*

On-line medical direction occurs when a qualified physician gives direct orders to a prehospital care provider by either radio or telephone (Figure 3-2 ■). Medical direction may be delegated to a mobile intensive care nurse (MICN), a physician assistant (PA),

■ Figure 3-2   The medical director can provide on-line guidance to EMS personnel in the field. (© Ken Kerr)

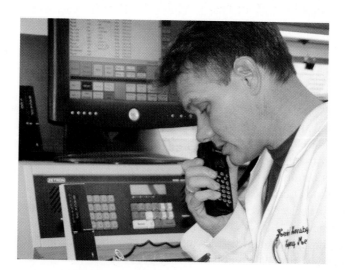

or a paramedic. In all circumstances, ultimate on-line responsibility remains with the medical director.

On-line medical direction offers several benefits to the patient. It gives the EMS provider direct and immediate access to medical consultation for patient-specific care. It also allows the use of telemetry, which provides the on-line medical director with diagnostic information that can be used to make critical decisions while the patient is still on scene or en route. Most EMS systems have the equipment to record on-line consultations. Those recordings can then be used for peer review and other continuous quality improvement activities.

When at the scene of an emergency, the health care provider with the most knowledge and experience in the delivery of prehospital emergency care should be in charge. When a nonaffiliated physician, or **intervener physician** is on scene and on-line medical direction does not exist, the paramedic should relinquish responsibility to the physician. However, the intervener physician must first identify himself, demonstrate a willingness to accept responsibility, and document the intervention as required by the local EMS system. If his treatment differs from established protocol, the intervener physician must accompany the patient in the ambulance to the hospital.

If an intervener physician is on scene and on-line medical direction does exist, the on-line physician is ultimately responsible. In case of a disagreement, the paramedic must take orders from the on-line physician.

Off-Line Medical Direction

Off-line medical direction refers to medical policies, procedures, and practices that a system physician has set up in advance of a call. It includes "prospective medical direction," such as guidelines on the selection of personnel and supplies, training and education, and protocol development. It also includes "retrospective medical direction," such as auditing, peer review, and other quality assurance processes.

Protocols are the policies and procedures of all components of an EMS system. They provide a standardized approach to common patient problems and a consistent level of medical care, as well as a standard for accountability. When treatment is based on such protocols, the on-line physician can assist prehospital personnel in interpreting the patient's complaint, understanding the findings of their evaluations, and providing the appropriate treatment. Protocols are designed around the four "Ts" of emergency care:

- ★ *Triage.* Guidelines that address patient flow through an EMS system, including how system resources are allocated to meet the needs of patients.
- ★ *Treatment.* Guidelines that identify procedures to be performed upon direct order from medical direction and procedures that are preauthorized protocols called **standing orders.**
- ★ *Transport.* Guidelines that address the mode of travel (air vs. ground) based on the nature of the patient's injury or illness, the condition of the patient, the level of care required, and estimated transport time.
- ★ *Transfer.* Guidelines that address receiving facilities to ensure that the patient is admitted to the one most appropriate for definitive care.

Protocols also are established for special circumstances, such as the proper handling of "Do Not Resuscitate" orders, patients who refuse treatment, sexual abuse, abuse of children or elderly people, termination of CPR, and intervener physicians. Although protocols standardize field procedures, they should allow the paramedic the flexibility necessary to improvise and adapt to special circumstances.

intervener physician *a licensed physician, professionally unrelated to patients on scene, who attempts to assist EMS providers with patient care.*

off-line medical direction *refers to medical policies, procedures, and practices that medical direction has set up in advance of a call.*

protocols *the policies and procedures for all components of an EMS system.*

 Review

Content

Four "Ts" of Emergency Care

Triage
Treatment
Transport
Transfer

standing orders *preauthorized treatment procedures; a type of treatment protocol.*

PUBLIC INFORMATION AND EDUCATION

The public is an essential, yet often overlooked, component of an EMS system. EMS should have a plan to educate the public on recognizing an emergency, accessing the system, and initiating basic life support procedures.

Recognizing an emergency can save lives. For example, the American Heart Association (AHA) estimates that over 300,000 cardiac arrests per year occur before the patient reaches the hospital. Such arrests are called "sudden death" because most happen within 2 hours of the onset of cardiac symptoms. Many patients delay calling for help when symptoms occur. If the patient and bystanders are taught to recognize the emergency and call for help in time, many cases of sudden death could be prevented.

The second aspect of public education is system access. Citizens must know how to activate EMS in an emergency to avoid life-threatening delays. Whether access is by way of 911 or a local seven-digit phone number, the number should be well publicized, and citizens should be taught how to give the necessary information to the emergency medical dispatcher.

Finally, after recognizing an emergency and activating EMS, citizens must know how to provide basic life support assistance, such as cardiopulmonary resuscitation (CPR) and bleeding control after major trauma. Abundant research indicates that a relationship exists between EMS response times and mortality (death) rates of patients. Communities have proven that when many citizens are trained in basic life support—and there is a rapid advanced life support (ALS) response—a larger number of patients can be successfully resuscitated. The American Heart Association (AHA) estimates that thousands of lives could be saved each year with implementation of bystander CPR programs and rapid ALS response.

Note that future public involvement may include bystander defibrillation (the application of an electric shock to the chest of a nonbreathing, pulseless patient). Research shows increasing numbers of successful programs. With the development of automated external defibrillator (AED) technology, it is now possible to place affordable, portable AEDs in the homes of cardiac patients as well as in all public places.

COMMUNICATIONS

The communications network is the heart of a regional EMS system. Coordinating the components into an organized response to urgent medical situations requires a comprehensive, flexible communications plan. Such a plan should include:

★ *Citizen access.* A well-publicized universal number, such as 911, provides direct citizen access to emergency services. Multiple community numbers only add life-threatening minutes to emergency response times. Enhanced 911, or E-911, gives automatic location of the caller, instant routing of the call to the appropriate emergency service (fire, police, or EMS), and instant callback capability.

★ *Single control center.* One control center that can communicate with and direct all emergency vehicles within a large geographical area is best. Ideally, all public service agencies should be dispatched from the same communications center in order to ensure the best use of resources in an emergency response.

★ *Operational communications capabilities.* With these, EMS dispatch can manage all aspects of system response and assess the system's readiness for the next response. Emergency units can communicate with each other and with other agencies during mutual aid and disaster operations. Hospitals also can communicate with other hospitals in the region to assess specialty capabilities.

★ *Medical communications capabilities.* EMS providers can communicate with the receiving facility and, in many areas, transmit ECG telemetry signals to the on-line physician. Hospitals also can communicate with each other, usually by a landline or microwave network, to facilitate patient transfer.

★ *Communications hardware.* Radios, consoles, pagers, cellular phone transmission towers, repeaters, telephone landlines, and other telecommunications equipment are required to operate a system.

★ *Communications software.* This includes the radio frequencies needed for in-system communication and, in many systems, the satellite and high-tech computer programs that track ambulances. Radio procedures, policies consistent with FCC standards and local protocols, and back-up communication plans for disaster operations are essential.

An EMS system must have an effective and efficient communications network in place. Because no single design will meet the needs of all communities, each system should design a network that is simple, flexible, and practical.

Emergency Medical Dispatcher (EMD)

The activities of the **emergency medical dispatcher (EMD)** are crucial to the efficient operation of EMS (Figure 3-3 ■). EMDs not only send ambulances to the scene, but they also make sure that system resources are in constant readiness to respond. EMDs must be both medically and technically trained. Their training should cover basic telecommunication skills, medical interrogation (questioning), giving prearrival instructions, and dispatch prioritization. The course should be standardized, and it should include certification by a government agency.

emergency medical dispatcher (EMD) *EMS person responsible for assignment of emergency medical resources to a medical emergency.*

EMS Dispatch

Emergency medical dispatching is the nerve center of an EMS system. It is the means of assigning and directing appropriate medical care to patients and should be under the

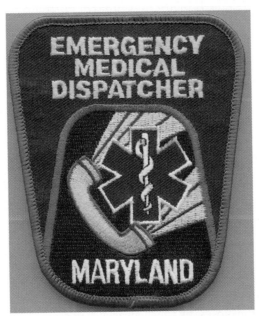

■ Figure 3-3   An emergency medical dispatcher patch.

full control of the medical director and the EMS agency. An emergency medical dispatch plan should include interrogation protocols, response configurations, system status management, and prearrival caller instructions.

In general, EMS system status management relies on projected call volumes and locations to make strategic placement of ambulances and crews. This method helps to reduce response times. Another management method is called "priority dispatching," which was first used by the Salt Lake City Fire Department. Using a set of medically approved protocols, EMDs are trained to medically interrogate a distressed caller, prioritize symptoms, select an appropriate response, and give life-saving prearrival instructions.

In 1974, the Phoenix Fire Department introduced a prearrival instruction program developed by medically trained dispatchers. In that program, callers initiate life-saving first aid with the dispatcher's help while they wait for emergency units to arrive on scene. In 1985, the Seattle EMS system initiated a successful program of instructing callers in CPR. Critics point out that prearrival instruction programs may result in increased liability. Even so, the increased liability of *not* providing such a service may far outweigh the risk of providing it.

An effective EMS dispatching system places the first responding units on scene within 4 minutes of the onset of the emergency. The American Heart Association (AHA) reports that brain resuscitation will not be successful if response time exceeds 4 minutes unless there was proper BLS intervention (CPR). Many studies also suggest that defibrillation within 8 minutes can reverse sudden-death mortality. So, the goal of emergency response is: BLS care in less than 4 minutes and ALS care in less than 8 minutes after the event. High-performance systems meet this standard more than 90 percent of the time.

> An effective EMS dispatching system places BLS care on scene within 4 minutes of onset and ALS care in less than 8 minutes.

EDUCATION AND CERTIFICATION

The two kinds of EMS education programs for EMS personnel are initial education and continuing education. *Initial education* programs are the original training courses for prehospital providers. They involve the completion of a standardized course that meets or exceeds the U.S. Department of Transportation's national curriculum. *Continuing education* programs include refresher courses for recertification and periodic in-service training sessions. All education programs should have a medical director who is involved in the EMS system. The EMS agency is responsible for assuring funding.

Initial Education

A paramedic's initial education is accomplished by successfully completing a course following the most recent *EMT-Paramedic: National Standard Curriculum* published by the U.S. DOT. It establishes the minimum content for the course and sets a standard for paramedic programs across the country. It also offers criteria for the minimum number of lecture, laboratory, and clinical hours a program should require. The National Standard Curriculum is divided into three specific learning domains:

- ★ *Cognitive,* which consists of facts, or information knowledge
- ★ *Affective,* which requires students to assign emotions, values, and attitudes to that information
- ★ *Psychomotor,* which consists of hands-on skills students learn while in laboratory and clinical settings

> certification   *the process by which an agency or association grants recognition to an individual who has met its qualifications.*

Once initial education is completed, the paramedic will become either certified or licensed, depending on the laws governing EMS in the particular state. **Certification** is the process by which an agency or association grants recognition to an individual who has met its qualifications. Many states certify paramedics. After attaining state certification, paramedics are permitted to work within an established EMS system under the direct supervision of a physician medical director.

Licensure is a process of occupational regulation. Through licensure, a governmental agency (usually a state agency) grants permission to engage in a given trade or **profession** to an applicant who has attained the degree of competency required to ensure the public's protection. Some states choose to license paramedics instead of certifying them. (Note that there is an unfounded general belief that a licensed professional has greater status than one who is certified or registered. However, a certification granted by a state, conferring a right to engage in a trade or profession, is in fact a license.)

Registration is accomplished by entering your name and essential information within a particular record. Paramedics are registered so that the state can verify the provider's initial certification and monitor recertification. Almost every state has an EMS office that tracks the registration of emergency care providers. While some states track only ALS providers, others maintain registers on the certifications of First Responders, EMT-Basics, EMT-Intermediates, and EMT-Paramedics.

Reciprocity is the process by which an agency grants automatic certification or licensure to an individual who has comparable certification or licensure from another agency. For example, some states grant reciprocity to paramedics who are certified in another state.

Certification Levels

There are a variety of prehospital certification levels for communities to choose from. In 1983, because of variations in state and regional EMS terminology, there were as many as 30 levels of prehospital care providers. Since then, the National Registry of EMTs has recognized—and the DOT has developed curricula for—four different levels of providers. They are:

★ *First Responder* (Figure 3-4). Usually the first EMS-trained provider to arrive on scene, the First Responder's role is to stabilize the patient until more advanced EMS personnel arrive. He is trained to perform a general patient assessment and to provide emergency care such as bleeding control, spinal stabilization, and CPR. He also may assist in emergency childbirth. In some areas, he is trained in the administration of oxygen and in the use of an automated external defibrillator (AED).

licensure *the process by which a governmental agency grants permission to engage in a given occupation to an applicant who has attained the degree of competency required to ensure the public's protection.*

profession *refers to the existence of a specialized body of knowledge or skills.*

registration *the process of entering your name and essential information within a particular record. In EMS this is done in order for the state to verify the provider's initial certification and to monitor recertification.*

reciprocity *the process by which an agency grants automatic certification or licensure to an individual who has comparable certification or licensure from another agency.*

✓ **Review**

EMS Certification Levels

First Responder
EMT-Basic
EMT-Intermediate
EMT-Paramedic

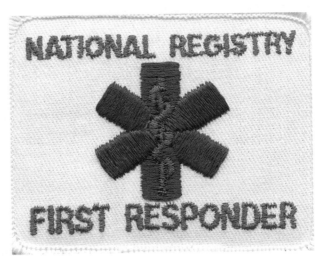

■ Figure 3-4   A First Responder patch.

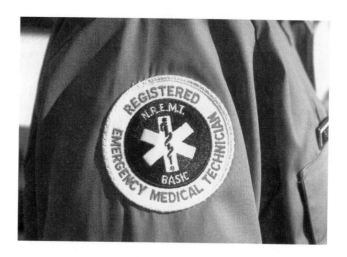

★ *Emergency Medical Technician-Basic (EMT-B)* (Figure 3-5 ■). This EMS
provider is trained to do all that a First Responder can do, plus perform
complex immobilization procedures, restrain patients, and drive and staff
ambulances. The EMT-B also may assist in the administration of certain
medications and, in some areas, perform an endotracheal intubation.

★ *Emergency Medical Technician-Intermediate (EMT-I)* (Figure 3-6 ■). The
EMT-I should possess all EMT-B skills and be competent in advanced
airway management, intravenous fluid therapy, and certain other
advanced skills. In some states, the EMT-I may be trained as a cardiac
technician and authorized to administer additional medications.

★ *Emergency Medical Technician-Paramedic (EMT-P)* (Figure 3-7 ■). As the
most advanced EMS provider, the paramedic is trained in all EMT-I skills,
plus advanced patient assessment, trauma management, pharmacology,
cardiology, and other medical skills. He should successfully complete
advanced cardiac life support (ACLS) and pediatric advanced life support
(PALS) courses offered by the American Heart Association. Basic trauma
life support (BTLS) or prehospital trauma life support (PHTLS) course
completion is also desirable.

■ Figure 3-6   An EMT-
Intermediate patch.

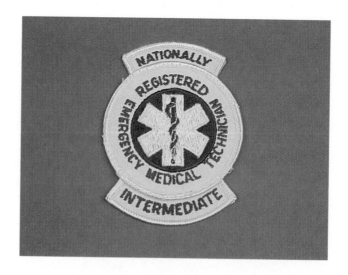

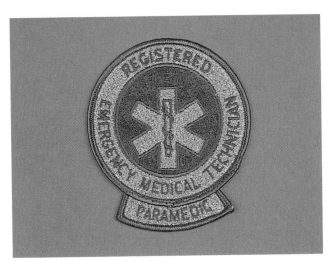

■ Figure 3-7 An EMT-Paramedic patch.

The training of prehospital personnel is a critical phase of EMS system design. In addition to gaining the knowledge and skills necessary to perform their jobs well, paramedics should graduate with the high regard for human dignity and passion for excellence expected of all **health care professionals.**

Expanding Roles

The success of EMS is now widely accepted. Because of this, EMS personnel are filling a growing number of nontraditional roles. They include:

★ *Critical care transport.* Paramedics manage complicated interhospital transports—typically from one intensive care unit to another—in specially equipped ambulances or aircraft designed to provide a higher level of care.

★ *Industrial or occupational EMS.* Paramedics specially trained in occupational health are used to staff construction sites, oil rigs, and other facilities where unique skills are required. These personnel may also serve as safety officers and inspectors.

★ *Tactical EMS.* Paramedics accompany specially trained law enforcement officers on tactical operations such as hostage rescue, drug raids, and similar high-risk emergencies. The tactical paramedic is a member of the operations team but is also trained to provide sophisticated, prolonged, definitive patient care.

★ *Primary care.* In the era of managed care, one goal is to keep patients with nonemergency problems out of the hospital emergency department. As a result, the EMS system has been involved in triaging and directing patients to the proper nonhospital facilities. In many cases, cost-effective, convenient medical care can be provided in the field by paramedics with additional skills.

National Registry of EMTs

The National Registry of Emergency Medical Technicians (NREMT) prepares and administers standardized tests for the First Responder, EMT-Basic, EMT-Intermediate, and EMT-Paramedic. It establishes the qualifications for registration and biennial

In addition to knowledge and skills necessary to perform their jobs well, EMS personnel should have a high regard for human dignity and a passion for excellence.

health care professionals
properly trained and licensed or certified providers of health care.

re-registration and serves as a vehicle for establishing a national minimum standard of competency. Through these services, the National Registry serves as a major tool for reciprocity by providing a process for EMTs to become certified when moving from one state to another. The National Registry also develops and evaluates EMT training programs with the goal of developing nationwide professional standards for EMS providers.

Currently, in the majority of states, National Registry examinations are being used at some level by EMS regulators. Several states offer locally developed examinations because their levels of certification or licensure differ from those recognized by the National Registry. The states that do use the National Registry examinations benefit from savings that result from spreading exam development costs over a large user base as well as from the assurance that the examinations are widely recognized as providing a national standard.

Professional Organizations

Belonging to a professional organization is a good way to keep informed about the latest technology. Communicating with members from other parts of the country also provides an excellent opportunity to share ideas. National EMS organizations include the following:

- ★ National Association of Emergency Medical Technicians (NAEMT)
- ★ National Association of Search and Rescue (NASAR)
- ★ National Association of EMS Educators (NAEMSE)
- ★ National Association of EMS Physicians (NAEMSP)
- ★ International Flight Paramedics Association (IFPA)
- ★ National Council of State EMS Training Coordinators (NCSEMSTC)

These are just some examples of organizations through which paramedics, emergency physicians, and nurses can enrich themselves and pursue their particular interests. Such organizations assist in the development of educational programs, operational policies and procedures, and the implementation of EMS. They establish guidelines with input from the public and the profession, which ensure that the public interest is served in the delivery of emergency medical services. They also provide a means to promote and enhance the status of EMS within the health care community, and their efforts help to create a unified voice for EMS providers.

The Joint Review Committee on Educational Programs for the EMT-Paramedic is an example of a standard-setting organization. It is responsible for establishing national standardization within the didactic and clinical portion of paramedic education programs. The standards applied by the Joint Review Committee are developed with input from national professional groups such as the NAEMT.

Professional Journals

A variety of journals are available to keep the paramedic aware of the latest changes in this ever-changing industry. These journals provide an abundant source of continuing-education material, as well as an excellent opportunity for EMS professionals to write and publish articles. The following is just a partial list of journals that routinely publish articles relating to the medical care of patients in EMS:

- ★ *Annals of Emergency Medicine*
- ★ *Emergency Medical Services*
- ★ *Journal of Emergency Medical Services*
- ★ *Academic Emergency Medicine*

★ *Journal of Pediatric Emergency Medicine*
★ *Journal of Trauma*
★ *Prehospital Emergency Care*

PATIENT TRANSPORTATION

Patients who are transported under the direction of an EMS system should be taken to the nearest appropriate medical facility whenever possible. Medical direction should designate that facility, based on the needs of the patient and the availability of services. In some cases, the patient's need for special services (such as care for burns) means designating a facility that is not nearby. At other times, the closest facility will be designated for stabilization of the patient while transfer is arranged. The ultimate authority for this decision remains with on-line medical direction.

Patients may be transported by ground or air (Figure 3-8 ■). The use of helicopters for medical transport was introduced during the Korean War and expanded in Vietnam. The success of military evacuation procedures led to their use in civilian ambulance systems. In 1970, the Military Assistance to Safety and Traffic (MAST) program was established. This demonstration project set up 35 aeromedical transportation programs nationwide to test the feasibility of using military helicopters and paramedics in civilian medical emergencies.

Today, trauma care systems use law enforcement, municipal, hospital-based, private, and military helicopter transport services to transfer patients (Figure 3-9 ■). Fixed-wing aircraft also are used when patients must be transported long distances, usually more than 200 miles.

All transport vehicles must be licensed and meet local and state EMS requirements. Equipment lists should be consistent with systemwide standards. In 1983, the

Legal Notes

Emergency Department Closures Numerous factors have resulted in emergency department closures and ambulance diversions. This can significantly impact the EMS system. All systems must address this situation so that patient care does not suffer.

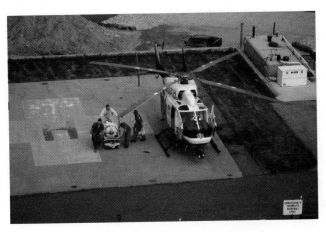

■ Figure 3-8 The helicopter has become an integral part of prehospital care. (*© Mark C. Ide*)

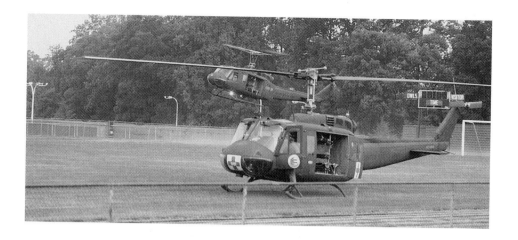

■ Figure 3-9   Military helicopters frequently assist civilian EMS systems.

American College of Surgeons Committee on Trauma recommended a standard set of equipment to be carried by providers of BLS services. In 1988, the American College of Emergency Physicians (ACEP) recommended a list of ALS supplies and equipment. Both sets of recommendations serve as guidelines for all prehospital EMS systems. Regional standardization of equipment and supplies is most effective in facilitating interagency efforts during disaster operations.

In 1974, in response to a request from the DOT, the General Services Administration developed the "KKK-A-1822 Federal Specifications for Ambulances." This was the first attempt at standardizing ambulance design to permit intensive life support for patients en route to a definitive care facility. The act defined the following basic types of ambulances:

★ *Type I* (Figure 3-10 ■). This is a conventional cab and chassis on which a module ambulance body is mounted, with no passageway between the driver's and patient's compartments.

★ *Type II* (Figure 3-11 ■). A standard van, body, and cab form an integral unit. Most have a raised roof.

★ *Type III* (Figure 3-12 ■). This is a specialty van with forward cab and integral body. It has a passageway from the driver's compartment to the patient's compartment.

■ Figure 3-10   Type I ambulance. *(© Jeff Forster)*

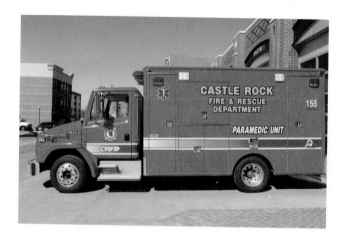

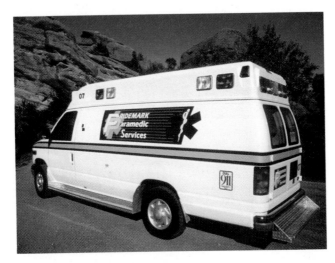

Figure 3-11 Type II ambulance. (© Jeff Forster)

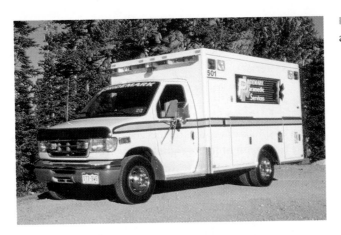

Figure 3-12 Type III ambulance. (© Jeff Forster)

Only these certified ambulances may display the registered "Star of Life" symbol as defined by the National Highway Traffic Safety Administration (NHTSA). The word "ambulance" should appear in mirror image on the front of the vehicle so that other drivers can identify the ambulance in their rear-view mirrors.

Many services now place a variety of specialized equipment on board ambulances, including specialty rescue, HAZMAT, and additional advanced life support equipment. This has often meant exceeding the gross vehicle weight and has resulted in introduction of a medium-duty truck chassis built for rugged durability and large storage and work areas. Another newer type of ambulance, developed for fuel economy, is the diesel hybrid ambulance (Figure 3-13 ■). Ambulance standards will continue to evolve.

In 1980, the revision "KKK-A-1822A" aimed at improving ambulance electrical systems by designing a low-amp lighting system to replace antiquated light bars and beacons. This standard helped to reduce electrical system overloads. In 1985, another revision "KKK-A-1822B" specified changes based on the National Institute for Occupational Safety and Health (NIOSH) standards. These include reduced internal siren noise, high engine temperatures, and exhaust emissions; safer cot-retention systems; wider axles; handheld spotlights; battery conditioners for longer life; and venting systems for oxygen compartments. In 2002, revision "KKK-A-1822E" provided guidelines to improve occupant protection in the patient compartment including additional occupant restraints, more rounded interior corners, and more secure locations of the sharps container for needles and other potentially dangerous items.

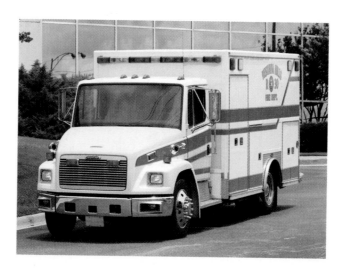

■ Figure 3-13 Diesel hybrid ambulance. *(© Ken Kerr)*

All ambulances purchased with federal funds during the 1970s were required to comply with the KKK criteria. Since then, however, some states have adopted their own stricter criteria.

RECEIVING FACILITIES

Not all hospitals are equal in emergency and support service capabilities. So how do you get the right patient to the right facility in an appropriate amount of time? EMS systems organize hospitals into categories that identify the readiness and capability of each hospital and its staff to receive and effectively treat emergency patients. EMS coordinators can use these categories to quickly recognize the most appropriate medical facility for definitive treatment or life-saving stabilization.

Once categorization has been established, regionalizing available services helps give all patients reasonable access to the appropriate facility. Burn, trauma, pediatric, psychiatric, perinatal, cardiac, spinal, and poison centers are examples of specialty service facilities that offer high-level care for specific groups of patients (Figure 3-14 ■). Large EMS systems should designate a resource hospital that will coordinate specialty resources and ensure appropriate patient distribution.

Ideally, all receiving facilities should have the following capabilities: an emergency department with an emergency physician on duty at all times, surgical facilities, a lab and blood bank, x-ray capabilities available around the clock, and critical and intensive care units. They should have a documented commitment to participate in the EMS system, a willingness to receive all emergency patients in transport regardless of their ability to pay, and medical audit procedures to ensure quality care and medical accountability. Finally, receiving facilities should exhibit a desire to participate in multiple-casualty preparedness plans.

MUTUAL AID AND MASS-CASUALTY PREPARATION

The resources of any one EMS system can be overwhelmed. A mutual-aid agreement ensures that help is available when needed. Such agreements may be between neighboring departments, municipalities, systems, or states. Cooperation among EMS agencies must transcend geographical, political, and historical boundaries.

Each EMS system should put a disaster plan in place for catastrophes that can overwhelm available resources. There should be a coordinated central management

An EMS system should have a disaster plan that is practiced frequently.

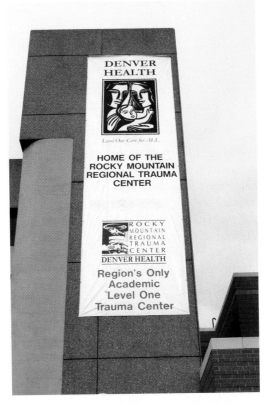

Legal Notes

9/11/01 and Beyond Since the attacks on the United States on September 11, 2001, disaster response and EMS have taken on significantly more and different responsibilities. All EMS personnel must be prepared for disasters, regardless of the cause. Biological and chemical agents pose significant risks to EMS personnel. Preparation and education are the keys to survival if such events are encountered.

agency that identifies commanders within the framework of the incident command system and an existing mutual-aid agreement. The plan should integrate all EMS system components and have a flexible communications system. Frequent drills should test the plan's effectiveness and practicality. The communications and control systems should be capable of coordinating a systemwide response to a major medical incident without a major change in personnel, equipment, or operating protocol.

QUALITY ASSURANCE AND IMPROVEMENT

An EMS system must be designed to meet the needs of the patient. Therefore, the only acceptable quality is excellence. For quality assurance and improvement programs to be effective, they must be dynamic and comprehensive. The EMS system must also be willing to cooperate with other systems and adjust its practices and procedures accordingly.

In 1997, the National Highway Traffic Safety Administration (NHTSA) released a manual called *A Leadership Guide to Quality Improvement for Emergency Medical Services Systems.* Its guidelines are based on the following components:

An EMS system must be designed to meet the needs of the patient. Therefore, the only acceptable quality of an EMS system is excellence.

 Review

Guidelines for Quality Improvement

Leadership
Information and analysis
Strategic quality planning
Human resources development and management
EMS process management
EMS system results
Satisfaction of patients and other stakeholders

* Leadership
* Information and analysis
* Strategic quality planning
* Human resources development and management
* EMS process management
* EMS system results
* Satisfaction of patients and other stakeholders

quality assurance (QA) *a program designed to maintain continuous monitoring and measurement of the quality of clinical care delivered to patients.*

Many EMS systems have developed ongoing quality assurance programs, while others have gone a step further with quality improvement programs. A **quality assurance (QA)** program is primarily designed to maintain continuous monitoring and measurement of the quality of clinical care delivered to patients. QA programs emphasize evaluation of objective data such as response times, adherence to protocols, patient survival, and other key indicators of system performance.

QA programs document the effectiveness of the care provided. They also help to identify problems and selected areas that need improvement. A common complaint about QA programs is that they tend to identify only the problems and therefore focus only on punitive corrective action. Thus, prehospital personnel often view QA programs negatively.

continuous quality improvement (CQI) *a program designed to refine and improve an EMS system, emphasizing customer satisfaction.*

As a result, many EMS systems have taken QA a step further with a **continuous quality improvement (CQI)** program. This is an ongoing effort to refine and improve the system in order to provide the highest level of service possible. A CQI program emphasizes customer satisfaction and includes evaluations of such aspects as billing and maintenance. In contrast to QA programs, CQI focuses on recognizing, rewarding, and reinforcing good performance. The dynamic process of CQI includes six basic steps: researching and identifying systemwide problems; elaborating on the probable causes; listing possible solutions; outlining a plan of corrective action; providing the resources and support needed to ensure the plan's success; and reevaluating results continuously.

In general, EMS quality can be divided into two categories: "take-it-for-granted" quality and service quality.

Legal Notes

QI: A Risk Management Strategy A good EMS Quality Improvement (QI) program is also an excellent risk management strategy. Problems in the system or with individual EMS providers can often be identified early through the QI program and remedied before patient care is harmed. Experience has shown that EMS services with an ongoing QI program have a decreased incidence of being sued. A good QI program should continuously monitor all high-risk cases and high-risk procedures.

High-risk cases in EMS include cardiac arrest patients, patients who must be restrained, patients who refuse EMS care, those who later file a complaint about care, and others. High-risk procedures include endotracheal intubation, medication administration, and others. A good QI program will continuously monitor high-risk cases and procedures such as these at both a system and provider level. If a provider is determined not to be managing these cases appropriately, that provider can be referred for additional education. Similarly, if it is learned that the system is not managing these cases appropriately, then changes must be made in the system to assure that the problems are corrected.

So never look at an EMS QI program as punishment. If properly utilized, it will make you a better paramedic and your system a better EMS system.

"Take-It-for-Granted" Quality

People take it for granted that EMS will respond quickly to a 911 call. Because patients do not usually have medical training, they must assume that we are always acting in their best interests and at the highest level of **professionalism.** Thus, they also take it for granted that the care they receive from us is safe, appropriate, and the best that is available.

Quality improvement in this area is accomplished through continuous evaluation. Such clinical evaluation and improvement should be subject to rigorous examination prior to implementation and periodically thereafter. When considering a new medication, process, or procedure, for example, we must follow set rules before permitting its use in EMS. These rules are often called **rules of evidence.** Joseph P. Ornato, M.D., Ph.D., developed them. They include the following guidelines:

★ *There must be a theoretical basis for the change.* That is, the change must make sense based on relevant anatomy, physiology, biochemistry, and other basic medical sciences.

★ *There must be ample scientific human research to support the idea.* Any device or medication used in patient care must have adequate scientific human research to justify its use.

★ *It must be clinically important.* The device, medication, or procedure must make a significant clinical difference to the patient. For example, a device such as an automated external defibrillator (AED) may mean the difference between living and dying for some patients, while color-coordinated stretcher linen has little clinical significance.

★ *It must be practical, affordable, and teachable.* Some medical devices remain too expensive and too impractical for use in routine prehospital emergency care.

If a clinical innovation or improvement meets all these guidelines, then the change should be made. Only devices, medications, and procedures that pass these rigorous tests should be implemented.

Another way to accomplish "take-it-for-granted" quality improvement is through the ongoing education of personnel. Paramedics can improve their skills by reading, taking classes, soliciting feedback on clinical performance from receiving hospitals, and following up on patients. **Peer review**—the process of EMS personnel reviewing each other's patient reports, emergency care, and interactions with patients and families—is another way for paramedics to improve their knowledge and skills.

Ethics are the rules or standards that govern the conduct of members of a particular group or profession. Prehospital providers at all levels have an ethical responsibility to their patients and to the public. (See Chapter 7 for a detailed discussion of professional ethics.) The public expects excellence from the EMS system, and we should accept no less than excellence from ourselves.

Service Quality

In the business world, service quality is called "customer satisfaction." This is the kind of quality that individual customers get excited about, feel good about, and tell stories about. These are the little extras that exceed a customer's expectations and elicit thank-you letters. Prime examples of customer satisfaction include patient statements such as: "You fed my cat before we left." "You remembered my name and introduced me to the nurse." "You held my hand." "You seemed like a friend when I needed one."

Customer satisfaction can be created or destroyed with a simple word or deed. A significant part of the way we communicate with one another is through body language and tone of voice. Paramedics who genuinely care about their patients communicate it

professionalism *refers to the conduct or qualities that characterize a practitioner in a particular field or occupation.*

rules of evidence *guidelines for permitting a new medication, process, or procedure to be used in EMS.*

peer review *an evaluation of the quality of emergency care administered by an individual, which is conducted by that individual's peers (others of equal rank). Also, an evaluation of articles submitted for publication.*

ethics *the rules or standards that govern the conduct of members of a particular group or profession.*

Customer satisfaction can be created or destroyed with a simple word or deed.

The ultimate reason for the existence of EMS: to serve the patient by providing the highest quality service and care available.

A formal, ongoing research program is an essential component of the EMS system for moral, educational, medical, financial, and practical reasons.

in many subtle ways. From the patient's perspective this is much more important than IVs, backboards, and ECGs. It is essential to remember the ultimate reason for our existence: to serve the patient by providing the highest quality service and care available.

RESEARCH

A formal, ongoing research program is an essential component of the EMS system for moral, educational, medical, financial, and practical reasons. The future enhancement of EMS is strongly dependent on the availability of quality research. Future changes in EMS procedures, techniques, and equipment must be evaluated to prove they make a positive difference prior to implementation. The current trend of introducing "new and improved" ideas or new "high tech" equipment to existing procedures must be evaluated scientifically. Unfortunately, many EMS protocols and procedures in use today have evolved without clinical evidence of usefulness, safety, or benefit to the patient.

One particular area that will rely heavily on research is funding. As managed care increases its influence on the delivery of emergency care, EMS systems will be forced to scientifically validate their effectiveness and necessity. The restrictions on reimbursement by managed care organizations and governmental agencies will drive the need for quality EMS research. Outcome studies will also be required to justify funding and assure the future of EMS.

Future EMS research must address the following issues: Which prehospital interventions actually reduce morbidity and mortality? Are the benefits of certain field procedures worth the potential risks? What is the cost-benefit ratio of sophisticated prehospital equipment and procedures? Is field stabilization possible, or should paramedics begin immediate transport in every case?

Paramedics can play a valuable role in data collection, evaluation, and interpretation of research. The components of a research project include the following:

★ Identify a problem, explain the reason for the proposed study, and state the hypothesis or a precise question.

★ Identify the body of published knowledge on the subject.

★ Select the best design for the study, clearly outline all logistics, examine all patient-consent issues, and get them approved through the appropriate investigational review process.

★ Begin the study, and collect raw data.

★ Analyze and correlate your data in a statistical application.

★ Assess and evaluate the results against the original hypothesis or question.

★ Write a concise, comprehensive description of the study for publication in a medical journal.

Current EMS practice must be justified by hard clinical data derived from an objective, valid program of ongoing research. EMS providers at all levels share the responsibility for identifying research opportunities, conducting peer review programs, and publishing the results of their projects. As leaders in the prehospital care environment, paramedics should set an example in the development of and participation in research projects.

For a more detailed discussion of research in EMS, see the Appendix.

Evidence-Based Medicine

A movement has been building in the house of medicine called *evidence-based medicine (EBM)*. This movement has been widely embraced by those in emergency medicine. It is only logical that the principles of EBM be applied to EMS. After all, EMS is an extension of the practice of emergency medicine. There is really nothing all that new about EBM. Its roots can be traced back to the mid-nineteenth century and beyond. The current resurgence of EBM began in Great Britain and has spread throughout the medical world.

EBM is the conscientious, explicit, and judicious use of the current best evidence in making decisions about the care of individual patients. It requires combining clinical expertise with the best available clinical evidence from systematic research. Thus, to practice effective EBM, EMS personnel must first be proficient in prehospital care and exercise sound clinical judgment. These traits can only be developed following a comprehensive initial education program, followed by clinical experience and practice.

To move to the next level, prehospital personnel must be familiar with the current and past research pertinent to prehospital care and be able to integrate that knowledge into the care of individual patients. An essential skill is knowing how to read and interpret the scientific literature and to determine whether the information is sound. (Again, refer to the Appendix, Research in EMS, which discusses how to read and evaluate research.)

External clinical evidence can invalidate previously accepted treatments and procedures and replace them with new ones that are more powerful, more effective, and safer. Good paramedics can become excellent paramedics by using both their clinical expertise and the best available external evidence. In today's medical setting, neither clincial experience nor external evidence alone is enough; there must always be a balance between the two.

Some might say that EBM is simply "cookbook" medicine. This is simply not true. As previously noted, EBM requires paramedics to be, first, clinically proficient. Anybody can follow simple "cookbook" directions and provide some level of patient care. But to achieve excellent patient care, external evidence can inform but never replace the individual paramedic's clinical expertise. Clinical expertise is required to form the best determination of the optimum treatment for each individual patient.

There has been a trend in EMS over the last decade or so to study the various practices and procedures of prehospital care. When studied, some treatments, such as pneumatic anti-shock garments (PASG), did not stand up to the test. Likewise, some treatments, such as early defibrillation, were found to have significant positive impact on survival following out-of-hospital cardiac arrest. Looking at this from a different perspective, by using the best research data available, we were able to abandon a practice (PASG) that helped few if any patients. Later, we were able to embrace a practice (early defibrillation) that has saved countless lives through diverse programs that include bystander defibrillation.

Practicing EBM helps to assure that we are providing our patients the best possible care at the lowest possible price.

For many years, EMS practice has been based on anecdotes and unproven theories. Today, EMS personnel must base their practice on sound scientific evidence. Because of this, all paramedics must fundamentally understand EMS research.

SYSTEM FINANCING

At present in the United States, there is a wide variety of EMS system designs. EMS can be hospital-based, fire- or police-department based, a municipal service, a private commercial business, a volunteer service, or some combination. Major differences exist in methods of EMS system finance, too. They range from fully tax-subsidized municipal systems to all-volunteer squads supported solely by contributions.

EMS funding can come from many sources. However, the most common is fee-for-service revenue, which may be generated from Medicare, Medicaid, private insurance companies, specialty service contracts, or private paying patients. Most of these sources of revenue are referred to as "third-party payers," because payment comes from someone other than the patient. To date, almost all third-party payers require the patient to be transported or the EMS service will not be compensated for a response. Reimbursement may also be based on the level of care the patient receives during transport.

Because of the high costs of health care and complex billing and reimbursement systems, the "Public Utility Model" and the "Failsafe Franchise" are becoming increasingly popular. In these systems, a municipality establishes the design and standards for the contract bid, then periodically—usually every 3 or 4 years—holds a wholesale competition open to the market. The provider firm that wins the contract must manage services properly and efficiently throughout the contract term or face severe penalties, usually in the form of fines. The use of models such as these shifts the financial burden of operating an EMS system from the local community to the service franchise.

Summary

The evolution of EMS has occurred over thousands of years. Many of its innovations are the result of lessons learned from military conflicts. EMS today is also largely the result of federal legislation and investment from private foundations.

A comprehensive EMS system has many components. EMS provides a continuum of care that extends from the EMT who conducts public education classes to the mechanic who keeps the ambulance fleet running; from the emergency medical dispatcher who calms a distressed caller to the emergency department physician, surgeon, and physical therapist who see the patient through to definitive care and rehabilitation. No one component, no one person, is more important than another. EMS is a total team effort.

EMS systems are designed with the patient as the highest priority. Each system has an administrative agency, which structures the system around the community's needs and grants the medical director ultimate authority in all issues of patient care.

Most EMS systems may be activated by way of a single, universal number (911). They rely on a centralized communications center, which handles all medical emergencies in the area and coordinates all levels of communication—operational and medical—within a region. The goal of an emergency response is: BLS care in less than 4 minutes, and ALS care in less than 8 minutes after the onset of an event. Coordination of ground and air transport follows established protocols at the communications center.

Mutual-aid agreements ensure a continuum of care during multiple-casualty incidents. Disaster plans are formalized, rehearsed regularly, continuously evaluated, and revised when necessary. Hospitals are categorized according to their readiness to provide essential and specialty services within a region. EMS providers are trained according to U.S. DOT national standard curricula. Continuing education programs encourage providers to achieve excellence.

A continuous quality improvement program documents the EMS system's performance. Ongoing research validates the actions of prehospital providers through scientific evaluation. Finally, EMS systems flourish because of strong, stable financial plans that ensure consistent development on a regional, state, and national basis.

You Make the Call

While you and your family are watching the fireworks display, one of the rockets tips over, shoots into the air, and explodes just above the crowd. There is a mad rush of people, and moments later everyone has scattered, leaving 11 injured people lying on the ground. You and your family are unhurt and move to a safe distance from the scene.

Luckily, the local fire and ambulance service has units on stand-by at the show. The crews immediately call dispatch and request additional ground and air transport units. The 911 dispatcher puts the region's mass-casualty plan into effect and dispatches the appropriate law enforcement and fire personnel.

Meanwhile, the EMS crews on scene are triaging the patients. Five minutes after the incident, a breakdown of patients is reported to the incident commander. There are seven injured adults: one priority-1, three priority-2, and three priority-3. There are four injured children: one priority-1 and three priority-3.

It isn't long before the top-priority patient is transported by helicopter to a regional burn center, which is 80 miles from the scene. As the ambulances arrive on scene, the remaining patients are loaded and transported to appropriate receiving facilities. During transport, EMS providers follow local protocols for patient care. One EMS provider radios medical direction for guidance in the care of the youngest injured child. All units radio the receiving facility to provide updated patient information and an estimated time of arrival.

1. Which of the "10 system elements" identified by NHTSA are mentioned in this scenario?
2. For what possible reason was the top-priority patient sent so far from the scene?
3. How important was the role played by the emergency medical dispatcher in this scenario? Explain.
4. How might the EMS system benefit from an evaluation of this incident?

See Suggested Responses at the back of this book.

Review Questions

1. Which of the following is not an out-of-hospital component of an EMS system?
   a. EMS providers, including paramedics
   b. fire/rescue and hazardous-materials services
   c. ancillary services, such as radiology and respiratory therapy
   d. public utilities, such as power and gas companies

2. The first civilian ambulance service was formed in:
   a. New York City.
   b. Cincinnati, Ohio.
   c. Miami, Florida.
   d. Pittsburgh, Pennsylvania.

3. The _____ was published in 1996 as an opportunity to examine what had been learned during the prior three decades and to create a vision for the future for EMS in the United States.
   a. *EMS Agenda for the Future*
   b. Statewide EMS Technical Assessment Program
   c. Consolidated Omnibus Budget Reconciliation Act
   d. Emergency Medical Services Systems Act

4. Verbal orders regarding patient management guidelines are examples of:
   a. direct medical direction.
   b. indirect medical direction.
   c. intermittent medical direction.
   d. reciprocal medical agreements.

5. Medical direction can best be described as:
   a. paramedic development of patient care protocols.
   b. on-scene physician's direction of all patient care.
   c. delegated practice involving physicians on scene in the field.
   d. physician direction of actions of his designated agents.

6. Retrospective medical direction includes all of the following except:
   a. auditing.
   b. peer review.
   c. quality improvement.
   d. training and education.

7. An effective EMS dispatching system places BLS care on scene within _____ minutes of onset and ALS care in less than _____ minutes.
   a. 3, 9
   b. 4, 9
   c. 4, 8
   d. 5, 7

8. In 1985, the Seattle EMS initiated a successful program of instructing callers in:
   a. childbirth assistance.
   b. defibrillation.
   c. orotracheal intubation.
   d. CPR.

9. The process by which an agency or association grants recognition to an individual who has met its qualifications is called:
   a. profession.
   b. licensure.
   c. registration.
   d. certification.

10. _____ is the conscientious, explicit, and judicious use of the current best evidence in making decisions about the care of individual patients.
    a. QI
    b. QA
    c. CQI
    d. EBM

See Answers to Review Questions at the back of this book.

Further Reading

Alonzo-Sierra, H., D. Blanton, and R. E. O'Connor. "Physician Medical Direction in EMS." *Prehospital Emergency Care* 2(2)(1998):153–157.

Bledsoe, B. E. "The Golden Hour: Fact or Fiction?" *Emergency Medical Services (EMS)* 31(6)(2002):105.

Bledose, B. E. "Searching for the Evidence behind EMS." *Emergency Medical Services (EMS)* 31(1)(2003):63–67.

Koenig, K. L., A. A. Salvucci, B. S. Zachariah, and R. E. O'Conner. "Systems and Managed Care Integration." *Prehospital Emergency Care* 2(1)(1998):67–69.

Kuehl, A. E. *Prehospital Systems and Medical Oversight.* 3rd ed. Dubuque, IA: Kendall-Hunt Publishing, 2002.

National Academies of Emergency Dispatch. *Emergency Telecommunicator Course Manual.* Sudbury, MA: Jones and Bartlett Publishers, 2001.

National Highway Traffic Safety Administration. *Emergency Medical Dispatch National Standard Curriculum, Instructor's Guide.* Washington, D.C.: National Highway Traffic Safety Adminstration, 1996.

National Highway Traffic Safety Administration. *The EMS Agenda for the Future.* Washington, D.C.: National Highway Traffic Safety Administration, 1996. [available at *http://www.nhtsa.dot.gov/people/injury/ems/agenda/emsman.html*]

Walz, B. J. *Introduction to EMS Systems.* Albany, NY: Delmar/Thomson Learning, 2002.

On the Web

Visit Brady's Paramedic Website at **www.bradybooks.com/paramedic.**

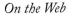

Roles and Responsibilities of the Paramedic

Objectives

After reading this chapter, you should be able to:

1. Describe the attributes of a paramedic as a health care professional. (pp. 86–92)
2. Describe the benefits of paramedic continuing education and the importance of maintaining one's paramedic license/certification. (pp. 86, 92)
3. List the primary and additional responsibilities of paramedics. (pp. 78–86)
4. Define the role of the paramedic relative to the safety of the crew, the patient, and bystanders. (pp. 79–80)
5. Describe the role of the paramedic in health education activities related to illness and injury prevention. (p. 85)
6. Describe examples of professional behaviors in the following areas: integrity, empathy, self-motivation, appearance and personal hygiene, self-confidence, communications, time management, teamwork and diplomacy, respect, patient advocacy, and careful delivery of service. (pp. 87–92)
7. Identify the benefits of paramedics teaching in their community. (p. 85)
8. Analyze how the paramedic can benefit the health care system by supporting primary care for patients in the out-of-hospital setting. (pp. 83, 85)
9. Describe how professionalism applies to the paramedic while on and off duty. (p. 87)

Key Terms

Case Study

The central dispatch center for your city receives a call for a medical emergency. The patient's name, address, and street number appear on the computer monitor, so the dispatcher clicks a mouse and a map of the city appears on screen. In this EMS system, satellites are used continuously to track and monitor the location and availability of emergency vehicles. The dispatcher selects Medic 49, the unit closest to the scene, and, by way of the computer-aided dispatch (CAD) system, gives them specific directions and patient information.

While the ambulance is responding, the dispatcher talks to the caller and provides him with emotional support and prearrival instructions for immediate patient care.

Upon arrival, the ambulance personnel find a 66-year-old female patient lying in bed, unable to speak clearly or move the right side of her body. An initial assessment reveals her to be disoriented. It also finds that she has an open airway, a normal rate of breathing, and strong radial and carotid pulses.

Paramedic Bobby Moore directs his partner to place the patient on oxygen and prepare for transport. Then he performs a rapid stroke assessment, after which he determines that the patient has had a stroke. She is immediately moved to the stretcher and placed into the ambulance.

In the ambulance, the paramedics complete a more detailed assessment and determine that the patient requires transport to a hospital with fibrinolytic capabilities. During transport, they radio the hospital and report the patient's condition and estimated time of arrival. Vital signs and pulse oximetry are continuously monitored and an ECG is performed.

After approximately 18 minutes en route, the patient is delivered to the emergency department where the stroke team—the emergency physician, a neurologist, and a radiologist—is waiting for her. One hour later, after an emergency CT scan of the brain, the patient is receiving fibrinolytic therapy to help minimize the size of the infarct in her brain. One week later, the patient is discharged to her home with a schedule of appointments for rehabilitation. A home health nurse is also scheduled to perform follow-up assessments twice each week.

INTRODUCTION

In the past 10 years, the United States has seen dramatic changes in the health care delivery system. EMS has not been immune to these changes. Driving forces such as technology, cost, and trends in patient population are forcing change. One such change involves the EMT-Paramedic, whose roles and responsibilities are dramatically different than they were 10 years ago.

Today, paramedic emergency care is an enormous responsibility for which you must be mentally, physically, and emotionally prepared. You will be required to have a strong knowledge of **pathophysiology** and of the most current medical technology. You will have to be capable of maintaining a professional attitude while making medical and ethical decisions about severely injured and critically ill patients. You will be required to provide not only competent emergency care but also emotional support to your patients and their families.

As a paramedic, the most highly trained prehospital emergency care provider in the EMS system, you will often serve people who are unaware of your knowledge and skills. However, if self-satisfaction and pride in a job well done are rewards enough—and if you have a genuine desire to help people in need—then being a paramedic will be a very fulfilling career.

PRIMARY RESPONSIBILITIES

A paramedic's responsibilities are diverse. They include emergency medical care for the patient (Figure 4-1 ■) and a variety of other responsibilities that are attended to before, during, and after a call.

pathophysiology *the study of how disease affects normal body processes.*

 Review

Content

Primary Responsibilities

- Preparation
- Response
- Scene size-up
- Patient assessment
- Treatment and management
- Disposition and transfer
- Documentation
- Clean-up, maintenance, and review

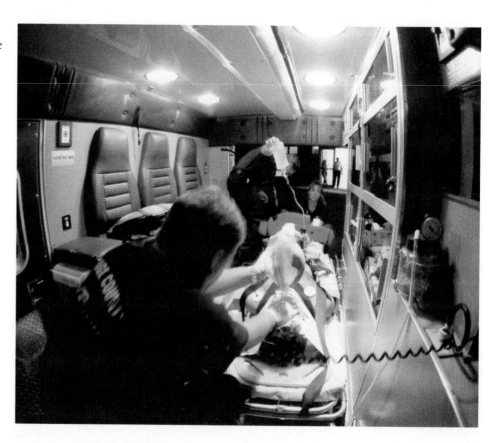

■ Figure 4-1   A paramedic provides emergency medical care to ill and injured patients. (© *Craig Jackson/In the Dark Photography*)

PREPARATION

Prior to responding to a call, you must be mentally, physically, and emotionally able to meet the demands of the patient, his family, and other health care providers. Your on-going training should include aerobics for cardiovascular fitness, exercises for muscle strength and endurance, stretching for increased flexibility, and an understanding of the biomechanics of lifting for prevention of lower-back injuries. Other keys to a successful career are recognizing the effects of stress and practicing ways to alleviate it.

You must be prepared. This means making sure that inspection and routine maintenance have been completed on your emergency vehicle and on all equipment. It means restocking medications and intravenous solutions and checking their expiration dates. In addition, you must be very familiar with:

★ All local EMS protocols, policies, and procedures

★ Communications system hardware (radios) and software (frequency utilization and communication protocols)

★ Local geography, including populations during peak utilization times, and alternative routes during rush hours

★ Support agencies, including services available from neighboring EMS systems, and the methods by which efforts and resources are coordinated

Prior to responding to a call, a paramedic must be mentally, physically, and emotionally able to meet the demands of the job.

RESPONSE

During an emergency response, remember that personal safety is your number one priority. If your ambulance crashes en route to an incident because of speeding or running red traffic lights, you will be of no benefit to the patient. Responding safely to an emergency will reduce the risk to you, your partners, and other agencies responding to the same incident. Always follow basic safety precautions en route to an incident. Wear a seat belt, obey posted speed limits, and monitor the road for potential hazards.

Just as important as getting to the scene safely is getting to the scene in a timely manner. Make certain you know the correct location of the incident and that the appropriate equipment is en route. Also while you are en route, request any additional personnel or services that you think may be needed. Waiting to ask for such assistance until you get to a chaotic scene can only delay the appropriate response. Learn to anticipate potential high-risk situations based on dispatch information and experience. For example, if any of the following is reported, you may need to call for assistance:

★ Multiple patients

★ Motor-vehicle collisions

★ Hazardous materials

★ Rescue situations

★ Violent individuals (patients or bystanders)

★ Use of a weapon

★ Knowledge of previous violence

SCENE SIZE-UP

Your primary concern during scene size-up is the safety of your crew, the patient, and bystanders. Identify all potential hazards such as fire, smoke, traffic, bystanders, angry or distraught family members, unstable structures or vehicles, and hazardous materials (Figure 4-2). Never enter an unsafe scene until the hazards have been dealt with.

A paramedic's primary concern at the scene of an emergency is safety.

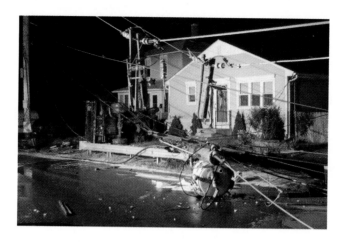

■ Figure 4-2 Assess for potential hazards when you size up the scene. (© *Mark C. Ide*)

mechanism of injury (MOI)
the force or forces that caused an injury.

nature of the illness (NOI)
a patient's general medical condition or complaint.

Remember that any scene has the potential to deteriorate, so learn to anticipate problems and be prepared for anything.

When the scene is safe to enter, determine the number of patients. In medical emergencies, there usually is only one. However, in some cases—such as carbon monoxide poisoning or exposure to other toxic substances—it may be necessary to search the entire area for patients. Once the number of patients and the severity of their illnesses or injuries are determined, quickly request any additional or specialized services required to manage the incident.

The **mechanism of injury (MOI)** or the **nature of the illness (NOI)** also must be identified. For a trauma patient, some mechanisms of injury are a cause for alarm. For example, a child struck by a fast-moving car is likely to have serious, multiple injuries. Knife and gunshot wounds suggest severe injury to internal organs and life-threatening internal bleeding. How far a patient is found from a collision or explosion, or how far a patient fell from a height, will also indicate how severe an injury may be. For a medical patient, clues identified at the scene can provide important insights into the nature of the illness. Identifying medications, such as insulin, or devices, such as an inhaler, may prevent misdiagnosis and speed the proper treatment of the patient.

PATIENT ASSESSMENT

One of the most critical skills you will learn is patient assessment. Though the order of the steps may vary for trauma and medical patients, the basic components are the same: initial assessment, physical examination, patient history, and ongoing assessment. (Volume 2 deals with patient assessment in detail.)

The initial assessment of a patient is usually performed in a scant minute or so. During this assessment, you must note your general impression of the patient's appearance. Then assess the patient's responsiveness; that is, determine if the patient is alert, responding to verbal or painful stimuli, or not responding at all. Finally, you will assess the patient's airway, breathing, and circulation (Figure 4-3 ■). If you discover any life threats, you will treat them immediately.

As part of the initial assessment, you will decide whether to continue the assessment on scene or immediately transport the patient to a medical facility. The next step of assessment is performing a physical examination of the patient and gathering the facts of the patient's medical history from the patient and/or bystanders, with all information recorded and reported to the hospital. It is also the paramedic's responsibility to continuously monitor the patient and provide any additional emergency care needed until the patient is transferred to the care of the hospital's emergency department staff.

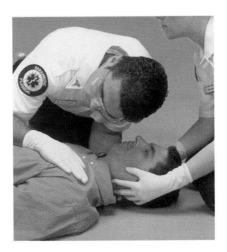

■ Figure 4-3 During the initial assessment of your patient, you will look for and immediately treat any life-threatening conditions.

RECOGNITION OF ILLNESS OR INJURY

Recognizing the nature of the illness or severity of injury, accomplished during the scene size-up and the initial assessment, is the first aspect of patient prioritization. Most commonly, patient priority is based on the urgency for transport. For example, a priority-1 patient would be transported as soon as the initial assessment and the rapid physical exam are completed. A priority-3 patient may have a full assessment and treatment completed before transport. Trauma patients are generally categorized, or triaged, by severity of injury. Priority-1 trauma patients are the most critical. Priority-4 trauma patients have very minor injuries and can wait for treatment, or they are dead and no treatment is necessary.

No matter what method of prioritization your EMS system uses, it is essential that you learn and practice it. Note that the method should be standardized so that all health care professionals within your system understand each other and can respond appropriately.

PATIENT MANAGEMENT

Almost all EMS systems have a set of protocols that providers follow. As a paramedic, you must always follow your system's protocols. They ensure that various personnel, when presented with the same emergency, will respond in the same manner. Protocols related to patient care also specify when it is necessary for you to communicate with medical direction. In response, medical direction will give you instructions on how to proceed with emergency care, permission to perform certain procedures, or alternatives to the standard care.

Patient management includes the task of moving the patient from one location to another. In order to do so, you must make sure that the proper equipment is used and the proper number of personnel are available. Remember, back injury is the number one career injury in EMS. Assure your own safety, and call dispatch for any additional assistance needed whenever you must lift or move a patient.

APPROPRIATE DISPOSITION

Transportation

A critical decision to be made is the mode of transportation for your patient. Time and distance are key. For example, if an unstable patient needs to be taken to a facility that is far from the scene, an aeromedical service—helicopter or fixed-wing aircraft—rather than ground transport may be the best choice. However, there may be only a single receiving facility option if you practice in a rural setting. Know the resources available in your EMS system. Follow all local protocols on their use.

Gatekeeper to the Health Care System The EMS system is often the initial point of contact for a person entering the health care system. Thus, to a certain extent, a paramedic frequently functions as a sort of gatekeeper to the health care system as a whole.

Part of a paramedic's responsibility is to ensure that a patient is taken to a facility that can appropriately care for the patient's condition. Today, hospitals have become more specialized. That is, some hospitals have chosen to provide certain services and not provide others. For example, one hospital may elect to specialize in cardiac care, another in stroke care, another in burn care, and so on. This is especially true in communities with multiple hospitals. Because of this, it is essential that paramedics understand the capabilities of the hospitals in the system where they work. Also, with overcrowding in modern emergency departments, diversion of ambulances by hospitals whose emergency departments are full has become commonplace.

For all these reasons, local EMS system protocols must be available to guide prehospital personnel in ensuring that each patient is delivered to a facility that can adequately care for the patient's condition.

Receiving Facilities

Selecting the appropriate receiving facility for your patient is your responsibility. In order to do so, it is important for you to know which medical facilities in your area offer the following services:

★ Fully staffed and equipped emergency department

★ Trauma care capabilities

★ Operating suites available 24 hours a day and 7 days a week

★ Critical care units, such as post-anesthesia recovery rooms and surgical intensive care units

★ Cardiac facilities with on-staff cardiologists

★ Neurology department that provides a "stroke team"

★ Acute hemodialysis capability

★ Pediatric capabilities, including pediatric and neonatal intensive care units

★ Obstetric capabilities, including facilities for high-risk delivery

★ Radiological specialty capabilities, such as computerized tomography (CT) and magnetic resonance imaging (MRI)

★ Burn specialization for infants, children, and adults

★ Acute spinal-cord and head-injury management capability

★ Rehabilitation staff and facilities

★ Clinical laboratory services

★ Toxicology, including HAZMAT decontamination facilities

★ Hyperbaric oxygen therapy capability

★ Microvascular surgical capabilities for replants

★ Psychiatric facilities

Receiving facilities are categorized by the level of care they can provide. For example, the American College of Surgeons categorizes trauma centers by levels:

* *Level I*—provides the highest level of trauma care.
* *Level II*—may not have specialty pediatrics or a neurosurgeon on site.
* *Level III*—generally does not have immediate surgical facilities available.

A fourth designation may be given to specialty referral centers, which offer unique services. They include burn, pediatric, psychiatric, perinatal, cardiac, spinal, and poison centers.

Knowing the capabilities of the hospitals in your area will allow you to decide on the one best able to care for your patient. Most patients request transportation to the nearest medical facility. However, patients enrolled in managed-care programs, such as health maintenance organizations (HMOs) or designated provider groups, may request transport to a facility approved by their group, which may be a facility other than the nearest hospital. Other patients may ask you to transport them to a facility outside of your run area. Even though the requested facility may be appropriate for the patient, there may be an equally appropriate hospital that is closer. Remember, you are responsible for patient care and, therefore, ultimately responsible for selecting the transport destination. When in doubt, contact on-line medical direction for advice and support.

Other Types of Disposition

In some areas, paramedics provide **primary care.** They have well-defined protocols that allow them to treat patients at the scene and transfer them to facilities other than a hospital. For example, consider a child who cuts his arm on a rusty nail. The father activates EMS by calling 911. When the paramedics arrive, they control the bleeding and perform a patient assessment. They find a simple 2-inch laceration on the child's forearm. Instead of transporting the patient to the hospital and using resources that are not needed for the treatment of this patient, the paramedics contact medical direction and request permission to transport the child to a local outpatient center for treatment. This decision saves the family from paying a costly emergency department fee, and it keeps the emergency department available for a more serious emergency.

primary care *basic health care provided at the patient's first contact with the health care system.*

Another type of disposition is called "treat and release." In this type of program, paramedics arrive on scene, assess the patient, and provide emergency care. If they determine that there is no need for further medical attention, they contact medical direction and request orders not to transport. In some systems, paramedics may then contact a specialized dispatch center where an office appointment is made with a physician in the patient's area.

While disposition systems such as these are not widely accepted, the increasing numbers of people in managed-care programs (which generally attempt to achieve optimum care while finding ways to control costs) may change that. Innovative programs such as these are setting standards for the future of EMS.

PATIENT TRANSFER

The managed-care environment has caused many people—both laypersons and health care providers—to occasionally question whether certain actions that are intended to reduce the cost of medical care are actually in the patient's best interest. For example, to avoid the cost of duplicating equipment and services in a number of facilities that serve the same geographic area, managed-care systems have encouraged facilities to specialize and, often, to transfer patients to a facility that can provide the specific care needed.

Occasionally, there may be a question as to whether the transfer of a patient from one facility to another has been approved for cost reasons but may not actually be in the patient's best interest. When you are assigned to transport a patient, you share responsibility—with the receiving and accepting physician—for the treatment and care of the patient. When you are in doubt about the patient's stability for the duration of transport, or about the capabilities of the receiving facility, contact medical direction.

Prior to removing the patient from a hospital, request a verbal report from the primary-care provider (usually a registered nurse or a physician). Also request a copy of essential parts of the patient's chart, including a summary of the patient's past and present medical history. However, if the results of diagnostic tests taken at the facility are not ready when you are prepared to leave, do not delay patient transport. The data can be sent by fax, e-mailed, or telephoned to the receiving facility.

Your first priority during transport is the patient. While en route, contact the receiving facility and provide them with an estimated time of arrival (ETA) and an update on the patient's condition. Upon arrival at your destination, seek out the contact person (usually a registered nurse or physician). Provide that person with an updated patient report, including any treatment or changes in status while en route. All documents provided by the sending facility should be turned over to the receiving care provider along with a copy of your run report. If required by your service, obtain appropriate billing/insurance information at this time.

DOCUMENTATION

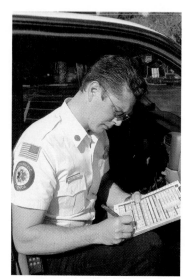

Maintaining a complete and accurate written patient care report is essential to the flow of patient information, to research efforts, and to the quality improvement of your EMS system. The patient care report should be completed in its entirety as soon as emergency care has been completed—no later. Any brief notes that were taken during patient assessment—vital signs, for example—should be copied into the report.

The importance of accurate and complete documentation cannot be overemphasized. Proper record keeping helps to ensure continuity of patient care from the emergency scene to the hospital setting. To avoid potential legal problems and embarrassing court situations, record only your observations, not your opinions. For example, do record "patient has an odor of alcohol on his breath." Do not record "patient is drunk." The former cannot be disputed, and the latter cannot be proved. Your final report should be complete, neat in appearance, and written legibly with no spelling errors. This assures that other health care providers can readily understand your assessment and interventions as well as the patient's responses to your treatment. It is important to note that your patient care report will be a reflection of the emergency care you provided if a lawsuit is filed in the future.

■ Figure 4-4 A paramedic's responsibility does not end with delivering the patient to the emergency department. Documentation, restocking, and a run critique are as important as the call itself.

RETURNING TO SERVICE

Once you have completed patient care, turned the patient over to the hospital staff, and completed all documentation, immediately prepare to return to service (Figure 4-4 ■). Clean and decontaminate the unit, properly discard disposable materials, restock supplies, and replace and stow away equipment. If necessary, refuel the unit on the way back to your station or post. Review the call with crew members, including any problems that may have occurred. Such a dialogue can lead to solutions that enhance the delivery of quality patient care. Finally, the paramedic team leader should check crewmembers for signs of critical incident stress and assist anyone who needs help.

Review

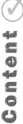

Additional Responsibilities

- Community involvement
- Support for primary care
- Citizen involvement
- Personal and professional development

ADDITIONAL RESPONSIBILITIES

The role of the paramedic involves duties in addition to those associated with emergency response. They may include training civilians in CPR, EMS demonstrations and seminars, teaching first aid classes, organizing prevention programs, and engaging in professional development activities. All involve taking an active role in promoting positive health practices in your community.

COMMUNITY INVOLVEMENT

Prehospital providers should take the lead in helping the public learn how to recognize an emergency, how to provide basic life support (BLS), and how to properly access the EMS system. A successful effort can save lives. Providing educational programs can also encourage positive health practices in the community, such as the American Heart Association's "prudent heart living" campaign. EMS injury prevention projects, such as seat belt awareness and the proper use of child safety seats, are essential to the reduction of long-term disability and accidental death.

In order to decide what injury prevention projects need to be developed in a community, EMS systems often conduct illness and injury risk surveys, both formally and informally. For example, consider an EMS service that reviews run reports for a 6-month period. They might find that for a single county they responded to 10 different vehicle collisions at various railroad crossings. A public safety campaign directed at the safe crossing of railroad tracks may be appropriate. Once an EMS service has identified a problem and the target audience, EMS personnel should seek out community agencies—including the local political structure—to assist in the development, promotion, and delivery of the campaign.

Among the benefits of community involvement are the following: It enhances the visibility of EMS, promotes a positive image, and puts forth EMS personnel as positive role models. It also creates opportunities to improve the integration of EMS with other health care and public safety agencies through cooperative programs.

SUPPORT FOR PRIMARY CARE

Promoting wellness and preventing illness and injury will be important components of EMS in the future. Some systems have already begun to direct resources toward the development of prevention and wellness programs that decrease the need for emergency services. The theory is to reduce the cost of the services provided to the community by decreasing the burden on the system.

One strategy is to establish protocols that specify the mode of transportation for nonemergency patients. Some systems already operate vans rather than ambulances to transport such patients to and from nursing facilities or from their residences to a doctor's office. Though an additional expense to the system, this service reduces emergency equipment costs and the demand for emergency personnel. The result is a decrease in the overall operating expense, which results in an increase in revenue.

Another strategy being used in many areas of the country is having EMS and hospitals team up to provide an alternative to the emergency department. They transport patients to freestanding outpatient centers or clinics, which ultimately reduces the cost of care to the patient and the system. The development of such alliances will undoubtedly continue. However, caution should be taken to ensure that the patient always receives the appropriate emergency care based on need, not cost.

CITIZEN INVOLVEMENT IN EMS

Citizen involvement in EMS helps to give "insiders" an outside, objective view of quality improvement and problem resolution. Whenever possible, members of the community should be used in the development, evaluation, and regulation of the EMS system. When considering the addition of a new service or the enhancement of an existing one, community members should help to establish what is needed. After all, they are your "customers," and their needs are your priority.

PERSONAL AND PROFESSIONAL DEVELOPMENT

Only through continuing education and recertification can the public be assured that quality patient care is being delivered consistently. Therefore, after you are certified and/or licensed, you have an important responsibility to continue your personal and professional development. Remember, everyone is subject to the decay of knowledge and skills over time. Use this as a rule of thumb: As the volume of calls decreases, training should correspondingly increase. Refresher requirements and courses vary from state to state, but the goal is the same: to review previously learned materials and to receive new information.

Since EMS is a relatively young industry, new technology and data emerge rapidly. Make a conscious effort to keep up. A variety of journals, seminars, computer news groups, and learning experiences are available to help. So are professional EMS organizations, which exist at the local, state, and national levels.

There are other options for keeping up your interest and staying informed, too. By participating in activities designed to address work-related issues—such as case reviews and other quality improvement activities, mentoring programs, research projects, multiple-casualty incident drills, in-hospital rotations, equipment in-services, refresher courses, and self-study exercises—you can expect substantial career growth.

Alternative career paths may be open to you as well. For example, a career paramedic may decide to explore management by applying for a supervisory position or may take a critical care class to prepare for a job on a transport unit. Nontraditional careers for paramedics include working in the primary care setting, providing emergency care on off-shore oil rigs, and taking on the occupational-safety role in an industrial setting.

PROFESSIONALISM

The paramedic is a health care professional.

A paramedic is a member of the health care professions. Note that the word *profession* refers to the existence of a specialized body of knowledge or skills. Generally self-regulating, a profession will have recognized standards, including requirements for initial and ongoing education. When you have satisfied the initial education requirements for your training as a paramedic, you may then be either certified or licensed. The EMS profession has regulations that ensure that members maintain standards. For the paramedic, these regulations come in the form of periodic recertification with a specified amount of continuing education time.

In addition, the term *professionalism* refers to the conduct or qualities that characterize a practitioner in a particular field or occupation. Health care professionals promote quality patient care and generate pride in their profession. They set and strive for the highest standards. They earn the respect and confidence of team members and the public by performing their duties to the best of their ability. Attaining professionalism is not easy. It requires an understanding of what distinguishes the professional from the nonprofessional.

PROFESSIONAL ETHICS

allied health professions
term used to describe members of ancillary health care professions, apart from physicians and nurses, such as paramedics, respiratory therapists, and physical therapists.

Ethics are the rules or standards that govern the conduct of members of a particular group or profession. Physicians have long subscribed to a body of ethical standards developed primarily for the benefit of the patient. These standards cover the **allied health professions,** such as paramedic, respiratory therapist, and physical therapist. Ethics are not laws, but they are standards for honorable behavior. Conformity to ethical standards is expected. As members of an allied health profession, paramedics must recog-

OATH OF GENEVA

I solemnly pledge myself to consecrate my life to the service of humanity; I will give to my teachers the respect and gratitude which is their due; I will practice my profession with conscience and dignity; the health of my patient will be my first consideration; I will respect the secrets which are confided in me; I will maintain by all the means in my power the honor and noble traditions of the medical profession; my colleagues will be my brothers; I will not permit considerations of religion, nationality, race, party, politics, or social standing to intervene between my duty and my patient; I will maintain the utmost respect for human life from the time of conception; even under threat, I will not make use of my medical knowledge contrary to the laws of humanity. I make these promises solemnly, freely and upon my honor.

■ Figure 4-5   The Oath of Geneva.

nize a responsibility not only to patients, but also to society, to other health professionals, and to themselves.

In 1948, the World Medical Association adopted the "Oath of Geneva" (Figure 4-5 ■). In 1978, the National Association of Emergency Medical Technicians adopted the "EMT Code of Ethics" (Figure 4-6 ■). These documents detail the guiding principles for professional EMT service.

PROFESSIONAL ATTITUDES

A commitment to excellence is a daily activity. While on duty, health care professionals place their patients first; nonprofessionals place their egos first. True professionals establish excellence as their goal and never allow themselves to become complacent about their performance. They practice their skills to the point of mastery and then keep practicing them to stay sharp and improve. They also take refresher courses seriously, because they know they have forgotten a lot and because they are eager for new information. Nonprofessionals believe their skills will never fade.

Professionals set high standards for themselves, their crew, their agency, and their system. Nonprofessionals aim for the minimum standard and can be counted on to take the path of least resistance. Professionals critically review their performance, always seeking ways to improve. Nonprofessionals look to protect themselves, hide their inadequacies, and place blame on others. Professionals check out all equipment prior to the emergency response. Nonprofessionals hope that everything will work, supplies will be in place, batteries will be charged, and oxygen levels will be adequate.

A professional paramedic is responsible for acting in a professional manner both on and off duty. Remember, the community you serve will judge other EMS providers, the service you work for, and the EMS profession as a whole by your actions.

Professionalism is an attitude, not a matter of pay. It cannot be bought, rented, or faked. Although it is a young industry, EMS has achieved recognition as a bona fide allied health profession. Gaining professional stature is the result of many hard-working, caring individuals who refused to compromise their standards. Always strive to maintain that level of performance and commitment.

PROFESSIONAL ATTRIBUTES

Leadership

Leadership is an important but often forgotten aspect of paramedic training. Paramedics are the prehospital team leaders (Figure 4-7 ■). They must develop a leadership

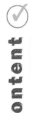

✓ **Review**

Professional Attributes

- Leadership
- Integrity
- Empathy
- Self-motivation
- Professional appearance and hygiene
- Self-confidence
- Communication skills
- Time-management skills
- Diplomacy in teamwork
- Respect
- Patient advocacy
- Careful delivery of service

Figure 4-6 EMT Code of Ethics.

EMT CODE OF ETHICS

Professional status as an Emergency Medical Technician-Paramedic is maintained and enriched by the willingness of the individual practitioner to accept and fulfill obligations to society, other medical professionals, and the profession of Emergency Medical Technician. As an Emergency Medical Technician at the basic level or an Emergency Medical Technician-Paramedic, I solemnly pledge myself to the following code of professional ethics: A fundamental responsibility to the Emergency Medical Technician is to conserve life, to alleviate suffering, to promote health, to do no harm, and to encourage the quality and equal availability of emergency medical care. The Emergency Medical Technician provides services based on human need, with respect for human dignity, unrestricted by consideration of nationality, race, creed, color, or status. The Emergency Medical Technician does not use professional knowledge and skills in any enterprise detrimental to the public well being. The Emergency Medical Technician respects and holds in confidence all information of a confidential nature obtained in the course of professional work unless required by law to divulge such information. The Emergency Medical Technician, as a citizen, understands and upholds the law and performs the duties of citizenship; as a professional, the Emergency Medical Technician has the never-ending responsibility to work with concerned citizens and other health care professionals in promoting a high standard of emergency medical care to all people. The Emergency Medical Technician shall maintain professional competence and demonstrate concern for the competence of other members of the Emergency Medical Services health care team. An Emergency Medical Technician assumes responsibility in defining and upholding standards of professional practice and education. The Emergency Medical Technician assumes responsibility for individual professional actions and judgement, both in dependent and independent emergency functions, and knows and upholds the laws which affect the practice of the Emergency Medical Technician. The Emergency Medical Technician has the responsibility to be aware of and participate in matters of legislation affecting the Emergency Medical Technician and the Emergency Medical Services System. The Emergency Medical Technician adheres to standards of personal ethics which reflect credit upon the profession. Emergency Medical Technicians, or groups of Emergency Medical Technicians, who advertise professional services, do so in conformity with the dignity of the profession. The Emergency Medical Technician has an obligation to protect the public by not delegating to a person less qualified, any service which requires the professional competence of an Emergency Medical Technician. The Emergency Medical Technician will work harmoniously with and sustain confidence in Emergency Medical Technician associates, the nurse, the physician, and other members of the Emergency Medical Services health care team. The Emergency Medical Technician refuses to participate in unethical procedures, and assumes the responsibility to expose incompetence or unethical conduct of others to the appropriate authority in a proper and professional manner. *National Association of Emergency Medical Technicians*

The paramedic is the prehospital team leader.

style that suits their personalities and gets the job done. Although there are many successful styles of leadership, certain characteristics are common to all great leaders. They include:

★ Self-confidence

★ Established credibility

★ Inner strength

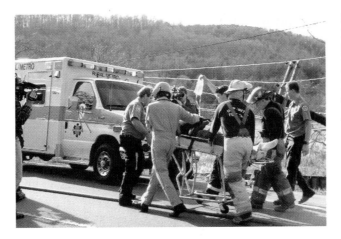

■ Figure 4-7 As leader of the EMS team, the paramedic must interact with patients, bystanders, and other rescue personnel in a professional and efficient manner. (© *Glen Jackson*)

- ★ Ability to remain in control
- ★ Ability to communicate
- ★ Willingness to make a decision
- ★ Willingness to accept responsibility for the consequences of the team's actions

The successful team leader knows the members of the crew, including each one's capabilities and limitations. Ask crew members to do something beyond their capabilities and they will question your ability to lead, not their ability to perform.

Integrity

Paramedics assume the leadership role for patient care in the prehospital setting. As a paramedic, you represent the EMS service and the health care system. The patient and other members of the health care team assume you are sincere and trustworthy. The single most important behavior that you will be judged by is honesty. The environment you work in will often put you in the patient's home or in charge of the patient's wallet and other personal possessions, such as jewelry and items left in a vehicle. You must be trustworthy. The easiest way for a paramedic to lose respect is to be dishonest.

A paramedic functions as an extension of the system's medical director, with authority delegated by the medical director. Because you may be practicing in an area that is remote from your medical director, you will be depended upon to follow protocols and accurately document all patient care.

Empathy

Successfully interacting with a patient and family is a challenging skill to master. One of the most important components is empathy. To have empathy is to identify with and understand the circumstances, feelings, and motives of others. To be considered a professional, you will often have to place your own feelings aside to deal with others, even when you are having a bad day. Paramedics who act in a professional manner can show empathy by:

- ★ Being supportive and reassuring
- ★ Demonstrating an understanding of the patient's feelings and the feelings of the family
- ★ Demonstrating respect for others
- ★ Having a calm, compassionate, and helpful demeanor

Self-Motivation

The environment in which you work is often unsupervised, so it is up to you to be able to motivate yourself and establish a positive work ethic. Examples of a positive work ethic are:

★ Completing assigned duties without being asked or told to do so
★ Completing all duties and assignments without the need for direct supervision
★ Correctly completing all paperwork in a timely manner
★ Demonstrating a commitment to continuous quality improvement
★ Accepting constructive feedback in a positive manner
★ Taking advantage of learning opportunities

Self-motivation is an internal drive for excellence. Remember, providing adequate patient care is not enough. You must strive for excellence in the care that you provide.

Appearance and Personal Hygiene

Society has high expectations for everyone in the allied health professions. From the moment you arrive at the scene of an emergency, you are being judged by the way you present yourself. Good appearance and personal hygiene are critical. If you do not look like a health care provider, then your patient may feel you must not be one. If you have a sloppy appearance, your patient may suspect that your medical care will be sloppy, too. Using slang, foul, abusive, or off-color language is not acceptable and will alienate you from your patients. Your appearance, as well as your behavior, are vital to establishing credibility and instilling confidence.

A paramedic should always wear a clean, pressed uniform. Multiple pagers and holsters with tape hanging from them, or rubber gloves pulled through a belt loop, simply do not give you a professional appearance. Also, avoid wearing an abundance of patches and pins on your uniform. Remember that it is the care you provide, not the patches and pins you wear, that will impress the patient.

The paramedic should always be well groomed. Hair should be kept off the collar. If facial hair is allowed, it should be kept neat and trimmed. A light-colored tee shirt may be worn under your uniform shirt, which should be buttoned up, with only the top collar button open. Jewelry, other than a wedding ring, a watch, or small plain earrings, is unprofessional. Long fingernails that have the potential to puncture protective gloves also should be avoided.

Self-Confidence

Having confidence in yourself and your abilities is very important. The patient and family will not trust you if they sense you do not trust yourself. A lack of self-confidence shows and is the basis of many lawsuits. The easiest way to gain self-confidence is to accurately assess your strengths and limitations, and then seek every opportunity to improve any weaknesses. Also, keep in mind that self-confidence does not equal cockiness. When a self-confident paramedic is presented with a complex situation, he will ask for assistance.

Communication

Communication is the process of exchanging thoughts, messages, and information. It is a skill often underestimated in EMS services. Providing emergency care in the prehospital environment requires constant communication with the patient, family, and bystanders, as well as with other EMS providers and rescuers from other public agencies.

To be an effective communicator, the paramedic should remember to gather all patient information and present it in a clear and concise format. Speaking clearly, listening actively, and writing legibly are obviously very important skills. Remember, too, to speak in a way that is appropriate for your audience. For example, just as you would not refer to a laceration as a "booboo" when consulting with a physician, you should not use complicated medical terminology to explain a procedure to an injured child.

Being able to adjust your communication strategies to various situations is also an important skill. For example, learning a manual alphabet (sign language) or learning simple medical questions in foreign languages common in your area are just two ways to prepare yourself.

Time Management

Good time-management skills are important to the paramedic. The experienced paramedic who plans ahead, prioritizes tasks, and organizes them to make maximum use of time will generally be more effective in the field. A paramedic with good time-management skills is punctual for shifts and meetings and completes tasks such as paperwork and maintenance duties on or ahead of schedule.

Some simple time-management techniques that you can use are: making lists, prioritizing tasks, arriving at meetings or appointments early, and keeping a personal calendar. By implementing just one or two of these techniques, you may find your schedule to be more manageable and less stressful.

Teamwork and Diplomacy

The paramedic is a leader. Leadership implies the ability to work with other people—to foster teamwork. Teamwork requires diplomacy, or tact and skill, in dealing with people, even when you are under siege from the patient or family.

Diplomacy requires the paramedic to place the interest of the patient or team ahead of his own interests. It means listening to others, respecting their opinions, and being open-minded and flexible when it comes to change. A strong leader of any team realizes that he will be successful only if he has the support of all team members. A confident leader will:

★ Place the success of the team ahead of personal self-interests

★ Never undermine the role or opinion of another team member

★ Provide support for members of the team, both on and off duty

★ Remain open to suggestions from team members and be willing to change for the benefit of the patient

★ Openly communicate with everyone

★ Above all, respect the patient, other care providers, and the community you serve

Respect

To respect others is to show—and feel—deferential regard, consideration, and appreciation for others. A paramedic respects all patients, and provides the best possible care to each and every one of them, no matter what their race, religion, sex, age, or economic condition. Showing that you care for a patient's or family member's feelings, being polite, and avoiding the use of demeaning or derogatory language toward even the most difficult patients are simple ways to demonstrate respect. By demonstrating respect, you will earn credit for yourself, your service, and the EMS profession.

Patient Advocacy

The paramedic should always be an advocate for the patient.

A paramedic is also an advocate for patients, defending them, protecting them, and acting in their best interests. For example, as a paramedic you should not allow your personal biases (religious, ethical, political, social, or legal) to interfere with proper emergency care of your patients. Except when your safety is threatened, you should always place the needs of your patient above your own self-interests. In addition, always keep a patient's health care information confidential. (Refer to Chapter 6 for details about patient confidentiality.)

Careful Delivery of Service

Professionalism requires the paramedic to deliver the highest quality of patient care with very close attention to detail. Examples of behaviors that demonstrate a careful delivery of service include:

* ★ Mastering and refreshing skills
* ★ Performing complete equipment checks
* ★ Careful and safe ambulance operations
* ★ Following policies, procedures, and protocols

Review of individual performance—and attitude—is also important in ensuring that all patients are receiving the proper care in the proper setting. Most EMS agencies have adopted or developed continuous quality improvement (CQI) programs to identify and correct substandard patient care.

CONTINUING EDUCATION

Maintaining certification is the responsibility of the paramedic. Most paramedics utilize continuing education programs to develop further knowledge or skills in a particular area of emergency health services. This type of education is most often acquired by attending lectures, seminars, conferences, and demonstrations. Each state, region, and local system may have its own policies, regulations, and procedures for recertification. Paramedics cannot work without satisfying those requirements.

There are many benefits to participating in as much continuing education as possible. The most obvious is the expansion of the paramedic's own personal knowledge and skills. Another important reason is to keep up with an emergency health care delivery system that is constantly being updated with more technologically advanced equipment and procedures.

The paramedic must continually strive to stay abreast of changes in EMS.

Finally, the skills you learn in this course will need to be practiced. Continuing education programs provide the opportunity to review material and address weak points in patient care.

Summary

To become a paramedic, you must be willing to accept the responsibility of being a leader in the prehospital phase of emergency medical care. Your responsibilities include on-call emergency duties and off-duty preparation. When the emergency call comes in, you must already be prepared to respond. If not, you are likely to be too late.

Most of your time as a paramedic will be spent on preparing yourself to do the job properly—not providing emergency care. If you can accept this reality, and if you are willing to undertake the responsibility of preparing for this dynamic occupation, then you are ready to proceed with your education. Remember: the best paramedics are those who make a commitment to excellence.

The best paramedics are those who make a commitment to excellence.

You Make the Call

The First Response Ambulance Service receives a call for a patient experiencing chest pain and difficulty breathing. You, as a paramedic, and your EMT-Basic partner are immediately dispatched to the scene. While en route, the dispatcher tells you that the patient is a 55-year-old male who has had a sudden onset of chest pain shoveling snow in his driveway and has audible labored breathing. The dispatcher also informs you that the patient has a history of heart disease and routinely takes multiple medications.

Approximately 7 minutes later, your ambulance arrives on scene. You observe that your patient, Mr. Yates, is sitting on his porch holding his chest. His wife and son are sitting beside him. As soon as you and your partner get out of the unit, the son runs to you and starts yelling "Hurry!" and "Just get him to the hospital!"

While you are performing an initial assessment of the patient, the son continuously exclaims, "Just load my father and get him to the hospital!" In 2 minutes, the initial assessment is complete. Due to the cold weather, you decide to move the patient into the unit. Once inside the ambulance, you quickly complete the history and physical exam and begin to treat the patient. Meanwhile, the patient's wife and son are outside the ambulance yelling at your partner, "Leave immediately, or we'll sue you!" He attempts to calm them but is unsuccessful.

After placing the patient on oxygen and connecting him to the monitor, you open the door and ask the family if they are going to ride in the ambulance to the hospital. Mrs. Yates tells you that she will, and she attempts to enter the unit. She is stopped by your partner, who explains that if she is going to ride with the ambulance, she must ride up front in the passenger seat. She immediately and loudly protests. At this point, you ask your partner to sit with the patient. You exit the unit as your partner enters, and you close the unit door. You quickly but calmly explain to Mrs. Yates that First Response Ambulance Service has a policy that requires her to ride in a seat with a seat belt in place, and that the passenger seat is the only seat available. After you explain that during the transport you will keep her updated on her husband's condition, she reluctantly gets into the front seat.

While en route to the hospital, you establish an IV, administer nitroglycerin and aspirin, run numerous ECG strips, and maintain a close watch on the patient's vital signs. Every few minutes you stick your head up front to inform Mrs. Yates about her husband's condition. About 10 minutes from the hospital, you consult with the emergency department physician, providing him with an estimated time of arrival, the patient's medical history, and the patient's current status.

Upon arrival, your partner assists you in unloading the patient. After allowing her to talk with her husband, your partner escorts Mrs. Yates to the hospital waiting area. In the emergency department, you provide the hospital staff with a verbal report and assist them in moving the patient to a stretcher. Then you give a copy of the run report to the unit clerk who is responsible for placing it on the patient's chart. You then walk to the waiting area where you find Mrs. Yates and her son. You take a minute to tell them that Mr. Yates is now in the care of Dr. Zimmer, and that he or one of the staff members will be out to speak with them as soon as an assessment is completed.

You and your partner meet outside the hospital and prepare the unit for the next call. The stretcher is made up and the unit is cleaned and restocked. While driving back to the station, you discuss the difficulty you both had dealing with Mrs. Yates and her son.

1. What were your key responsibilities in the previously detailed scenario?
2. How should you have prepared yourself mentally and physically for this call?
3. Did you and your partner act professionally? If so, explain how.

See Suggested Responses at the back of this book.

Review Questions

1. During an emergency response, remember that _____ _____ is your number one priority.
   a. patient care
   b. personal safety
   c. documentation
   d. medical direction

2. The force or forces that caused an injury define the:
   a. nature of illness.
   b. chief complaint.
   c. mechanism of injury.
   d. primary illness.

3. _____ trauma patients have very minor injuries and can wait for treatment, or they are dead and no treatment is necessary.
   a. priority-1
   b. priority-2
   c. priority-3
   d. priority-4

4. A _____ trauma center provides the highest level of trauma care.
   a. level I
   b. level II
   c. level III
   d. specialty referral

5. Maintaining a complete and accurate written patient care report is essential to:
   a. research efforts.
   b. the flow of patient information.
   c. the quality improvement of EMS systems.
   d. all of the above.

6. Nontraditional careers for paramedics include:
   a. working in the primary care setting.
   b. providing emergency care on off-shore rigs.
   c. taking on the occupational-safety role in an industrial setting.
   d. all of the above.

7. The term _____ refers to the conduct or qualities that characterize a practitioner in a particular field or occupation.
   a. licensure
   b. registration
   c. professionalism
   d. certification

8. _____ are the rules or standards that govern the conduct of members of a particular group or profession.
   a. ethics
   b. morals
   c. etiquette
   d. protocols

See Answers to Review Questions at the back of this book.

Further Reading

Bailey, E. D., and T. Sweeney. "Considerations in Establishing Emergency Medical Services Response Time Goals." *Prehospital Emergency Care* 7(3) (2003):397–399.

Bledsoe, B. E. "EMS Needs a Few More Cowboys." *Journal of Emergency Medical Services (JEMS)* 28(12)(2003):112–113.

Bledsoe, B. E. "Searching for the Evidence behind EMS." *Emergency Medical Services (EMS)* 31(1)(2003):63–67.

Heightman, A. J. "EMS Workforce. A Comprehensive Listing of Certified EMS Providers by State and How the Workforce Has Changed Since 1993." *Journal of Emergency Medical Services (JEMS)* 25(2)(2000):108–112.

Jaslow, D., J. Ufberg, and R. Marsh. "Primary Injury Prevention in an Urban EMS System." *Journal of Emergency Medicine* 25(2)(2003):167–170.

National Academy of Sciences, National Research Council. *Accidental Death and Disability: The Neglected Disease of Modern Society.* Washington, DC: U.S. Department of Health, Education, and Welfare, 1966.

Page, J. O. *The Magic of 3 AM.* San Diego, CA: JEMS Publishing, 2002.

Page, J. O. *The Paramedics.* Morristown, N.J.: Backdraft Publications, 1979. [No longer available for purchase except as a used book. Entire book can be viewed online at *www.JEMS.com/Paramedics.*]

Page, J. O. *Simple Advice.* San Diego, CA: JEMS Publishing, 2002.

Persse, D. E., C. B. Key, R. N. Bradley, C. C. Miller, and A. Dhingra. "Cardiac Arrest Survival as a Function of Ambulance Deployment Strategy in a Large Urban Emergency Medical Services System." *Resuscitation* 59(1)(2003):97–104.

Streger, M. "Professionalism." *Emergency Medical Services (EMS)* 23(1)(2003):35.

On the Web

Visit Brady's Paramedic Website at **www.bradybooks.com/paramedic**.

Illness and Injury Prevention

Objectives

After reading this chapter, you should be able to:

1. Describe the incidence, morbidity and mortality, and the human, environmental, and socioeconomic impact of unintentional and alleged unintentional injuries. (p. 98)

2. Identify health hazards and potential crime areas within the community. (pp. 99, 103–105)

3. Identify local municipal and community resources available for physical, socioeconomic crises. (pp. 99–101, 106–107)

4. List the general and specific environmental parameters that should be inspected to assess a patient's need for preventive information and direction. (pp. 103–105)

5. Identify the role of EMS in local municipal and community prevention programs. (pp. 97–98, 99–101, 103–107)

6. Identify the injury and illness prevention programs that promote safety for all age populations. (pp. 103–104)

7. Identify patient situations where the paramedic can intervene in a preventive manner. (pp. 99, 101, 103–107)

8. Document primary and secondary injury prevention data. (pp. 99–107)

Key Terms

Case Study

It's a hot July day, and Timmy is spending it with John, whose family has an in-ground pool. At approximately 9:00 A.M., John's mom receives a phone call. The two boys, who had been watching cartoons in the living room, run out to the patio, grab the large inflatable alligator raft, and head for the water. Timmy pronounces himself "king of the alligator killers" as he jumps on the raft. John says he is the "true king" and plops himself down on top of Timmy. In the resulting tussle, Timmy rolls off the raft and into the water. He tries but is unable to get a good enough grasp on the edge of the concrete pool. John watches his friend struggle and, terrified, runs to the side of the house to hide. All this takes about 7 minutes.

At approximately 9:10 A.M., John's mom hangs up the phone. As she steps out onto the patio, she sees Timmy's small form floating face down in the pool. She races to the pool, jumps in, and pulls Timmy out. She checks to see if he is breathing, but he is not. She starts for the phone, but stops short. Where is John? It takes her another minute to find him and another 30 seconds to get to the phone to dial 911.

It takes you and your partner 6 minutes to respond. While waiting, John's mother stays with Timmy, turning him on his side to let the water drain from his mouth and lungs and pleads with him softly to "hang in there." When you arrive on scene, you perform a scene size-up and an initial assessment and start CPR. Timmy begins to breathe in about a minute, but he does not regain consciousness. You rush him to the hospital emergency department. There the staff praises your actions and tells you, "You did the best you could."

Almost a year later, Timmy has still not regained consciousness. The costs for Timmy's care so far have reached more than $650,000. It is difficult to predict the total cost. With good medical care, Timmy could live for many years.

INTRODUCTION

Many EMS providers are first drawn to emergency medical services because of the opportunity to make a dramatic contribution to a person in need. They respond to countless scenes of crisis and tragedy and feel genuine excitement when the critically ill patient improves after receiving emergency medical care. But beyond the excitement of the moment is a sobering reality. How often do EMS crews respond to incidents that could easily have been prevented? How often have you thought to yourself "What a shame" or "I wish there was something I could have done" in the wake of senseless circumstances surrounding an accidental injury or illness?

Such thoughts are all too common after an incident, but what if EMS providers, leaders, and administrators asked these questions *before* an incident occurred? How many injuries could be prevented? How many lives could be saved? This chapter focuses on these questions and discusses illness and injury prevention as a paramedic's crucial duty and responsibility.

EPIDEMIOLOGY

Injury is one of our nation's most important health problems. Consider the following facts offered by the U.S. Department of Transportation:

★ Injury surpassed stroke as the third leading cause of death in the United States, and it is the leading cause of death in people ages 1 to 44.

★ Injuries that are unintentional result in nearly 70,000 deaths and millions of nonfatal injuries each year. The leading causes of death from unintentional injuries are motor-vehicle collisions, fires, burns, falls, drownings, and poisonings.

★ The estimated lifetime cost of injuries will exceed $114 billion.

★ For every one death caused by injury, there are an estimated 19 hospitalizations and 254 emergency department visits.

Though many people believe that injuries "just happen," evidence shows that injuries result from interaction with potential hazards in the environment. Thus, it has been suggested that "MVAs" (motor-vehicle accidents) should be called "MVCs" (motor-vehicle collisions), since driving drunk or at 80 mph and crashing is no accident. In other words, many injuries may be predictable and preventable. The study of the factors that influence the frequency, distribution, and causes of injury, disease, and other health-related events in a population is called **epidemiology.**

Concepts related to epidemiology that you should know include **years of productive life,** a calculation made by subtracting the age at death from 65. (For example, in a liability suit concerning the death of a 45-year-old, a jury might assess damages based on the deceased's loss of 20 years as a wage-earner.) Another concept is **injury,** which refers to the intentional or unintentional damage to a person resulting from acute exposure to thermal, mechanical, electrical, or chemical energy or from the absence of such essentials as heat and oxygen. An accident is an *unintentional injury,* but an injury that is purposefully inflicted either on oneself (e.g., suicide) or on another person (e.g., homicide) is an *intentional injury.* Intentional injuries make up about a third of all injury deaths. Other categories of intentional injury include rape, assault, and domestic, elder, and child abuse.

Other concepts related to epidemiology include **injury risk,** which is a real or potentially hazardous situation that puts people in danger of sustaining injury. As medical professionals, EMS providers should assess every scene and situation for injury risk and maintain statistics as part of an **injury-surveillance program,** or the ongoing systematic collection, analysis, and interpretation of injury data essential to the planning, implementation, and evaluation of public health practice.

An injury-surveillance program must also include a component for the timely dissemination of data to those who need to know. The final link in the injury-surveillance chain is the application of these data to prevention and control. **Teachable moments** occur shortly after an injury when the patient and observers remain acutely aware of what has happened and may be more receptive to learning about how similar injury or illness could be prevented in the future.

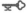

Injury is one of our nation's most important health problems.

Injuries result from interaction with potential hazards in the environment, which means that they may be predictable and preventable.

epidemiology *the study of factors that influence the frequency, distribution, and causes of injury, disease, and other health-related events in a population.*

years of productive life *a calculation made by subtracting the age at death from 65.*

injury *intentional or unintentional damage to a person resulting from acute exposure to thermal, mechanical, electrical, or chemical energy or from the absence of such essentials as heat and oxygen.*

injury risk *a real or potentially hazardous situation that puts people in danger of sustaining injury.*

injury-surveillance program *the ongoing systematic collection, analysis, and interpretation of injury data essential to the planning, implementation, and evaluation of public health practice.*

teachable moments *these occur shortly after an injury, when the patient and observers remain acutely aware of what has happened and may be more receptive to teaching about how similar injury or illness could be prevented in the future.*

By becoming involved in injury prevention, EMS providers can focus on **primary prevention,** or keeping an injury from ever occurring. Medical care and rehabilitation activities that help to prevent further problems from occurring are referred to, respectively, as **secondary prevention** and **tertiary prevention.**

PREVENTION WITHIN EMS

Other than the survivors and their families, no one experiences the aftermath of trauma more directly than EMS providers. Every day, paramedics witness the tragic effects of preventable injuries. Even armed with the best equipment and technology, they cannot save every life. However, by being first on the scene of emergencies, EMS personnel have become prime candidates to be advocates of injury prevention.

EMS providers perform CPR and other life-saving procedures as part of an everyday routine. As partners in public health and safety, members of the EMS community must go beyond their normal daily routine and work cooperatively with members of the public to prevent avoidable illness and injury.

EMS providers are widely distributed in the population, often reflecting the composition of their communities. They are often considered to be champions of the health care consumer and are welcome in schools and other community institutions. Medical personnel are high-profile role models and, as such, can have a significant impact on the reduction of injury rates in this country. In rural areas, EMS providers may be the most medically educated individuals, and are often looked to for advice and direction. Essentially, the more than 600,000 EMS providers in the United States comprise a great arsenal in the war to prevent injury and disease.

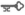

The more than 600,000 EMS providers in the United States comprise a great arsenal in the war to prevent injury and disease.

ORGANIZATIONAL COMMITMENT

EMS organizational commitment is vital to the development of any prevention activities. As a member of the EMS community, you should become familiar with available resources and your responsibilities in preventing illness and injury:

EMS organizational commitment is vital to the development of any prevention activities.

★ *Protection of EMS providers.* The leadership of EMS agencies must assure that policies are in place to promote response, scene, and transport safety. The appropriate body substance isolation (BSI) and personal protective equipment (PPE) should be issued to protect against exposure to bloodborne and airborne pathogens, as well as environmental hazards. An overall commitment to safety and wellness should be emphasized and supported.

★ *Education of EMS providers.* EMS personnel must understand the need for involvement in prevention activities. A "buy-in" from employees at every level is key to the success of any prevention program. EMS managers have the responsibility of instructing them in the fundamentals of primary prevention during initial training and in continuing education courses. Public and private sector specialty groups may be called upon for specific EMS education and training (Figure 5-1 ■). EMS providers should also have the skills and training necessary to defend against violent patients or other hostile attackers. Classes in on-scene survival techniques should be commonplace in every EMS agency.

★ *Data collection.* Monitoring and maintaining records of patient illnesses and injuries is essential in determining trends and in developing and measuring the success of prevention programs. Each agency should contribute data to local, regional, state, and national systems that track such information.

 Review

Organizational Commitment

- Assure the protection of EMS providers
- Provide initial and continuing education
- Collect and distribute illness and injury data
- Provide financial support
- Empower EMS personnel

Content

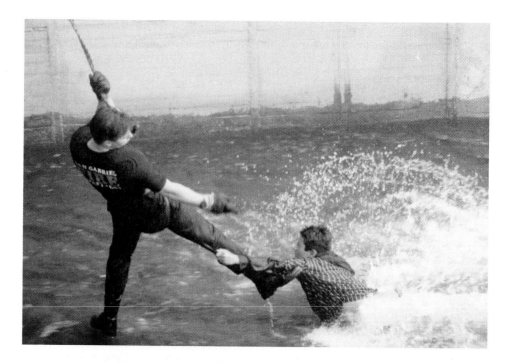

■ Figure 5-1 When appropriate, specific EMS education and training in specialized safety procedures should be available to you. (© Jonathan Alcorn/ ZUMA/Corbis)

■ Figure 5-2 Funding for illness and injury prevention campaigns may be contributed by corporations and advertising agencies, as well as nonprofit organizations.

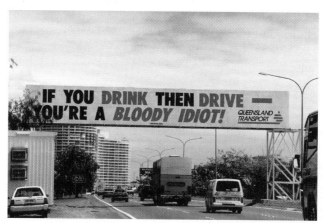

★ *Financial support.* An agency's internal budget should reflect support for prevention strategies as a priority. If necessary, support must be sought from outside the organization. Large corporations are often willing to donate funds in exchange for stand-by coverage at an event or company function. State highway safety offices can offer funding for traffic-related projects, such as those involving child safety seats, seat belts, and drunk driving. Advertising agencies may contribute billboards for safety messages and public service announcements (Figure 5-2 ■). Partnerships with local hospitals can result in advertising safety messages in newsletters and flyers. Community groups such as Mothers Against Drunk Driving (MADD) and junior auxiliaries also are great resources for initiating community and school programs.

★ *Empowerment of EMS providers.* The ultimate factor in achieving success in a prevention program lies in the hands of the frontline personnel. Managers should identify, encourage, and foster employee interest, support, and involvement. Likewise, such involvement should be recognized and rewarded from top management. In addition, it is also recommended that managers rotate assignment to prevention programs and provide salary for off-duty injury prevention activities.

EMS PROVIDER COMMITMENT

Illness and injury prevention should begin at home and be carried over into the workplace. The priority for EMS providers is to protect themselves from harm. Employers have an obligation to provide a safe environment. Written guidelines and policies should promote wellness and safety among employees. (See Chapter 2 for more information on the points discussed in the following sections.)

Body Substance Isolation (BSI) Precautions

Under the guidelines of the Occupational Safety and Health Administration (OSHA), employers and employees share responsibility for body substance isolation (BSI) precautions. Following BSI guidelines assists in preventing contamination from blood and other bodily fluids. BSI equipment, such as gloves and eyewear, plays a major role in EMS operations and is one of the provider's basic lines of defense (Figure 5-3 ■).

Physical Fitness

The often hectic and chaotic lifestyle of a paramedic does not always permit you to follow your normal, healthy daily routine. Therefore, you must consistently incorporate exercise, fitness, and a health-minded attitude into your life to minimize the risk of injury and to improve your overall quality of life. Encourage your partner, crew members, and other co-workers to do the same. A wellness program that includes a proper diet, cardiovascular fitness, and strength training can increase energy levels, boost immune systems, and help fend off disease and injury.

Note that though lifting and moving techniques and back safety programs have become routine for prehospital staff, back injuries remain a leading cause of disability among EMS workers. Make a solid effort to follow proper lifting techniques in order to prevent bodily injury, strain, and pain.

Stress Management

Members of today's workforce, particularly EMS providers, must learn to control, or at least handle, the stress in their lives. It is often difficult for even the healthiest individual to balance their personal, family, and work life. Know your limits and take time out when necessary. Take time to relax; pick a pastime or hobby that alleviates stress. If work becomes too stressful, speak with a supervisor in order to avoid burnout or future conflicts. Balance your life with exercise, good nutrition, and healthy activities to keep stress in check.

✓ **Review**

EMS Provider Commitment

- Take BSI precautions
- Maintain physical fitness
- Use proper lifting and moving techniques
- Manage stress in personal, family, and work life
- Seek professional care when needed
- Drive safely
- Assess and maintain scene safety

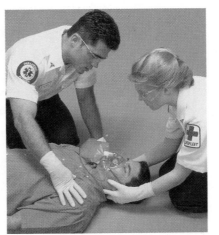

■ Figure 5-3 BSI equipment, such as protective gloves and eyewear, is one of a provider's basic lines of defense.

Seeking Professional Care

EMS providers should not be ashamed of needing or asking for professional counseling. Paramedics are called in to assess and treat people during the worst times of their lives. Facing tragedy, disease, death, and despair are part of the daily routine for EMS personnel. Do not forget that paramedics are vulnerable to the same stressors, emotions, illnesses, and injuries as everyone else. If your job or life becomes overwhelming, you may choose to consider counseling from a trained professional.

Many employers will offer employee assistance programs that include counseling, stress management, nutrition, healthy lifestyle inventories, and general wellness. It is often a great benefit for employees to take advantage of these opportunities to help themselves through a crisis or stressful time.

Driving Safety

Safe driving is an essential part of EMS response. As an emergency vehicle operator, be familiar with traffic laws and obey them. Never drink and drive. In addition, you must be able to understand the capabilities and limitations of your emergency vehicle, handle weather and road conditions with precision, and accurately respond to all traffic conditions quickly. Safe emergency operation of EMS vehicles can only be achieved when proper use of warning devices is coupled with sound emergency and defensive driving practices.

Scene Safety

Safety is always your first priority. Once your unit is dispatched to a call, evaluate the dispatch information prior to arrival. Focus your attention on response and equipment needed (Figure 5-4 ■). Upon arrival, park the unit in the safest and most convenient place to load the patient as well as to leave the scene. Consider traffic, road conditions, and all other possible hazards. Directing traffic is primarily the responsibility of local law enforcement agencies. The safest method for traffic control at serious vehicle collisions is to stop all traffic and re-route it to different roads. This is for the safety of patients, bystanders, and rescue personnel.

Note that if you are called to an area with potential health hazards, such as an industrial park of a chemical plant, or an area with high crime rates, approach the scene with caution. Be sure to protect yourself appropriately. If you do not have adequate protection or are not specifically trained to control specific hazards, never enter a hazardous scene. Call in specialized teams, such as a hazardous materials crew, if necessary. Law enforcement agencies should be contacted for any violent, potentially violent, or dangerous scene, including those involving domestic abuse or other crimes.

Do not forget that paramedics are vulnerable to the same stressors, emotions, illnesses, and injuries as everyone else.

Safety is always your first priority.

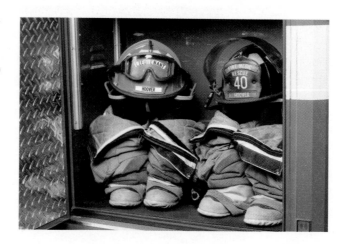

■ Figure 5-4   Keep your safety equipment in good condition and readily available in your emergency vehicle. (© Ken Kerr)

If the scene is safe to enter, be sure to wear reflective clothing to provide added protection on the scene. With BSI precautions in place, approach patients with your safety in mind. Determine the mechanisms of injury (forces that caused injury) or the nature of illness. Treat the patient according to protocol.

After patient care is addressed and a transport decision is made, make sure your unit is secure before departure. Have your partner check the outside of the unit to make certain that all doors are secured. The patient should be secured on an ambulance stretcher with at least three straps, as well as shoulder straps if available. If a family member is allowed to accompany the patient, that person should be placed in the passenger seat in the front compartment with vehicle restraints in place.

PREVENTION IN THE COMMUNITY

As a component of health care, EMS has a responsibility to not only prevent injury and illness among EMS workers, but also to promote prevention among the members of the public. EMS providers can be an appropriate and effective means of prevention in several situations.

AREAS OF NEED
Infants and Children

Each year, nearly 290,000 infants are born weighing less than 5.5 pounds (2,500 grams), often as a result of inadequate prenatal care. Low birth weight is a key indicator of poor health at the time of birth. Babies born too small or too soon are far more likely to die in the first year of life. Annually, over 4,000 die of low birth weight and prematurity. Among those who survive, an estimated 2 to 5 percent have a disability, and one quarter of the smallest survivors (born weighing less than 1,500 grams) have serious disabilities such as mental retardation, cerebral palsy, seizure disorders, or blindness.

One of every three deaths among children in the United States results from an injury. The number of injuries, of course, far exceeds the number of deaths. The most common causes of fatal injuries in children include motor-vehicle collisions, pedestrian or bicycle injuries, burns, falls, and firearms. Injuries generally can be classified into intentional events (such as shootings and assaults), unintentional events (such as motor-vehicle collisions), and alleged unintentional events (such as suspicious injury patterns that suggest possible abuse).

In motor-vehicle collisions, young children are easily thrown on impact. Because a young child's head is large in proportion to the body, unrestrained children tend to fly head first into the windshield or out of the car when a collision occurs. The back seat is the best seat for children 12-years-old or younger. In this location, the properly restrained child is least likely to sustain injuries in a crash. Car safety seats and seat belts can prevent most severe injuries to passengers of all ages if they are used correctly. Air bags are designed to save people's lives when used with seat belts, and they can protect drivers and passengers who are correctly buckled.

Infants and toddlers are commonly injured by cars backing up in driveways or parking lots. Children between the ages of 5 and 9 who are struck by cars typically dart out in front of traffic. Children riding bicycles can be injured when they collide with cars or other fixed objects or when they are thrown from the bicycle. The most serious bicycle-related injuries are head injuries, which can cause death or permanent brain damage.

Falls are the most frequent cause of injury to children younger than 6 years old. About 200 children die from falls each year. Fire and burn injuries occur in the highest

EMS has a responsibility to not only prevent injury and illness among EMS workers, but also to promote prevention among the members of the public.

Review

Content

Areas in Need of Prevention Activities

- Low birth weight in newborns
- Unrestrained children in motor vehicles
- Bicycle-related injuries
- Household fire and burn injuries
- Unintentional firearm-related deaths
- Alcohol-related motor-vehicle collisions
- Fall injuries in the elderly
- Workplace injuries
- Sports and recreation injuries
- Misuse or mishandling of medications
- Early discharge of patients

numbers in the very young. Most are caused by scalding from a hot liquid such as when children grab pot handles and spill the contents.

In this modern age of media and the Internet, children and young adults are bombarded with an incredible amount of information and are often faced with some of the same stressors as adults. Sometimes those stressors become overwhelming.

One of the most troubling recent trends is the increased number of violent acts among young people, occurring in the form of self-destructive behavior, gang violence, and assaults. In addition, firearm injury is becoming more common as a result of the accessibility of hand guns to children. An increasing number of injuries and deaths occur when children and adolescents take guns to school. The number of firearm deaths has doubled since 1953. About 15 percent of all firearm-related deaths are unintentional, often resulting from improper handling and lack of safety mechanisms.

Motor-Vehicle Collisions

For years, the EMS industry and law enforcement have referred to collisions among trucks and automobiles as motor-vehicle accidents (MVAs). However, that term does not accurately reflect the circumstances of the incident. The term motor-vehicle collision (MVC) more accurately reflects the fact that no collision is an accident: something caused the crash to occur. Such crashes are responsible for over half of all deaths from unintentional injuries. Alcohol use is a factor in about half of all motor-vehicle fatalities.

Geriatric Patients

Falls account for the largest number of preventable injuries for persons over 75 years of age. As a result of slower reflexes, failing eyesight and hearing, and arthritis, the elderly are at increased risk of injury from falls. Falls frequently result in fractures since the bones become weaker and more brittle with age.

The aging process also places the elderly at greater risk for serious head injury as well as other injuries. Although many geriatric patients are completely coherent, many others suffer from some degree of dementia. Alzheimer's disease is merely one example of the conditions that can affect the elderly. The associated confusion can contribute to dangerous behaviors such as wandering away from home or into a roadway, which places these patients at greater risk of injury.

Work and Recreation Hazards

In the workplace, back injuries account for 22 percent of all disabling injuries. Injuries to the eyes, hands, and fingers are responsible for another 22 percent. Even the quietest office setting can be a hazardous area. Never underestimate the potential dangers in an area that appears to be safe. Many areas and aspects of the work environment are potentially dangerous, including copy machines, electrical cords, faulty wiring, and shoddy building construction, among others.

Sports injuries are commonly seen in persons of all ages due to the increased popularity and participation in outdoor recreational activities. Football, soccer, and baseball, as well as running, hiking, and biking, are among popular sports that can result in fractures, dislocations, sprains, and strains.

Cultural Considerations

Elderly and Impoverished Populations Studies have shown that the incidence of EMS calls is higher in areas where there is poverty and many elderly. EMS personnel must recognize that this will be a significant part of the job.

Medications

When an illness or injury occurs and treatment is sought, medications are often part of the treatment regimen. These medications are occasionally taken improperly (too much or not enough), or they are taken by others, sometimes causing serious medical problems. Medications of any kind should be taken only by those for whom they are prescribed. They should be stored according to label directions. They should also be continued until the prescription is completed. Following the physician's, the pharmacist's, and the label directions is imperative.

Early Discharge

Managed-care organizations such as HMOs and insurance companies often mandate shorter hospital stays and early discharges from the hospital, urgent care centers, and other outpatient facilities. Such policies often result in more patients being at home sooner with illnesses that are less completely treated. These patients may call upon 911 for supportive care and intervention.

IMPLEMENTATION OF PREVENTION STRATEGIES

The following is a list of prevention strategies which you should be able to implement:

* ★ *Preserve the safety of the response team.* Always remember that your first priority is your safety and the safety of your fellow crew members. The next priorities are the patient and, finally, bystanders. Do what you can and what is within your training to maintain a safe and secure working area. If there is a chance of risk or further danger on scene, act quickly and appropriately to correct the situation. Do not hesitate to contact back-up units and law enforcement personnel, if necessary.

* ★ *Recognize scene hazards.* To prevent illness or injury to EMS personnel and further illness or injury to patients, size up the scene for potential risks or dangers before entering. Be aware of your surroundings. Is there anyone or anything that could cause harm to you, your crew, or the patient? Does the mechanism that injured the patient still pose a threat to the rescuers?

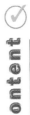

Review

Content

Prevention Strategies

- Preserve the safety of the response team
- Recognize scene hazards
- Document findings
- Engage in on-scene education
- Know community resources
- Conduct a community needs assessment

Cultural Considerations

Immunizing At-Risk Populations Many illnesses can be prevented through immunization of at-risk populations. The Centers for Disease Control and Prevention and other organizations frequently update and publish a list of recommended immunizations for children and persons at increased risk of contracting a preventable disease. However, for various reasons, some patients are hesitant to obtain these life-saving immunizations. This is especially true in communities with a large number of illegal immigrants. People who are in the country illegally often will not seek health care for fear their presence in the country will be revealed to immigration authorities and they will be deported. As a result, this population is at increased risk of developing diseases that could be prevented through proper immunization.

In several areas, paramedics have been called upon to provide immunizations as a community service. In these situations, it has been demonstrated that persons unlikely to go to a standard health clinic for immunizations are more likely to attend an immunization session provided by EMS. Thus, by using the trustworthy image of EMS, paramedics can help target populations for preventative immunizations who might not obtain them by traditional means.

It is important to remember that, for many conditions, the best treatment is prevention.

Are there any hazardous materials in the area? Has any crime been committed? Are there structural risks? Are there temperature extremes for which you are unprepared? If the scene is not safe and there is an immediate and imminent danger, retreat immediately and call for the appropriate assistance.

★ *Document findings.* Document your patient-care findings at the end of every call. Note that EMS patient forms often can be designed to include specific data on injury prevention in order to benefit researchers and implement future prevention programs. Such a form should include scene conditions at the time of EMS arrival, which play a major role in determining intentional and unintentional injuries, and the mechanism of injury, which is the best determinant of patient care on scene. It should also include a place where you can describe any risks that were overcome. If protective devices were used (or not used) during the emergency, these should be documented, too. (See Figure 5-5 ■ for an example.)

★ *Engage in on-scene education.* Taking advantage of a teachable moment is a chance to decrease future emergency responses. Remember that, to communicate effectively, you must gain your listeners' trust. Remain objective, nonjudgmental, and nonthreatening. Inform them of how they can prevent the recurrence of a similar emergency and, if needed, instruct them on the use of protective devices.

★ *Know your community resources.* Treating the medical needs of a patient is often not enough. You must also seek to identify and meet the

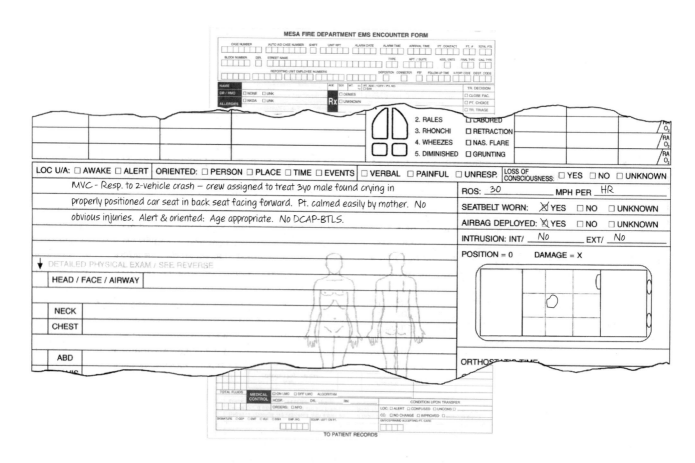

■ Figure 5-5   Example of documentation of primary and secondary injury prevention data.

psychosocial needs of your patient. At times, you may find it appropriate to consider your patient a "customer." Determine what his needs are and how you may assist him. Your patient may require a referral to an outside agency such as a prenatal clinic, a social service organization that offers food, shelter, clothing, mental health resources or counseling, or other services. Your system may also allow for referral or transportation to a clinic, urgent care, or alternative form of health care. Be aware of the presence of both licensed and unlicensed child care centers in your area. Encourage parents to provide preexisting consent for treatment and transport in case of illness or injury at a child care facility. Be sure to follow local protocols and report suspected abuse situations to the appropriate child protective agency. Consider developing a social service resource guide for your organization to determine solutions and ideas for these and other situations.

★ *Conduct a community needs assessment.* Each community should determine its own specific approaches to prevention. Conducting a formal needs assessment will assist in identifying priorities. Consider the following:

–Childhood and flu immunizations

–Prenatal and well-baby clinics

–Elder-care clinics

–Defensive driving classes

–Workplace safety courses

–Health clinics (co-sponsored by local hospitals or health care organizations)

–Prevention information on your agency's Internet website

These are just a few of the ideas that may be appropriate for your organization. The population served and its ethnic, cultural, and religious makeup may affect the needs and approaches that are most appropriate. Also consider community members who are learning disabled or physically challenged.

Summary

Each member of EMS shares the responsibility of promoting wellness and preventing illness and injury among co-workers and the community. Consider offering programs to the public such as first aid and CPR classes, infectious disease prevention classes, safe driving classes, and swimming lessons. Partner with members of your community in new and innovative ways to make everyone more aware of how to prevent avoidable illness and injury. If we can prevent one injury, one disabling disease, or one avoidable death, it will have been more than worth the effort.

You Make the Call

As you walk into work on a sunny, warm Saturday morning, your supervisor greets you at the door. He is beaming with excitement as he tells you, "The boss just approved our budget for EMS week. And he and I agree that you are just the person to coordinate this year's effort." He continues by insisting that the organization must become "more active" in injury and illness prevention, and EMS week is the perfect platform to begin such a campaign. You agree to the concept and accept the assignment. The supervisor responds, "Here is the budget overview and the planning kit for this year and last. I would like a preliminary plan from you by the end of today's shift" and wanders back into his office. You briefly scan the packet and proceed to prepare for your shift.

Later, during an hour or so of down time, you and your partner decide to brainstorm ideas on how best to prepare for the event. Your partner mentions that he thinks, "This whole idea of us doing prevention is hokey and ridiculous." He continues by saying, "That stuff is for the public health people. I'm a paramedic. I don't have time to be working on prevention." Another paramedic, fresh out of medic school, joins in on the conversation and adds, "Yeah. If we prevented all of the injuries and illnesses, we would be out of a job. I don't want that after all I went through to get my certification." You slump slightly into your chair as you begin to discover how difficult this task might become.

1. How will you counter the arguments the two paramedics made?
2. Why is prevention an important responsibility of being a paramedic?
3. List 10 ideas for an illness and injury prevention program that may be appropriate in your area.

See Suggested Responses at the back of this book.

Review Questions

1. The study of the factors that influence the frequency, distribution, and causes of injury, disease, and other health-related events in a population is called:
   a. logistics.
   b. census gathering.
   c. epidemiology.
   d. pathophysiology.

2. Intentional injuries make up about _____ of all injury deaths.
   a. 1/4
   b. 1/3
   c. 2/3
   d. 1/2

3. Rehabilitation after an injury or illness that helps to prevent further problems from occurring is referred to as:
   a. primary prevention.
   b. tertiary prevention.
   c. secondary prevention.
   d. teachable moments.

4. Under the guidelines of _____, employers and employees share responsibility for body substance isolation precautions.
   a. DOT
   b. FEMA
   c. OSHA
   d. HIPAA

5. It should be noted that, though lifting and moving techniques and back safety programs have become routine for prehospital staff, _____ injuries remain a leading cause of disability among EMS workers.
   a. fall
   b. back
   c. head
   d. chest

6. _____ account for the largest number of preventable injuries for persons over 75 years of age.
   a. burns
   b. falls
   c. MVCs
   d. head injuries

See Answers to Review Questions at the back of this book.

Further Reading

Greenwood, M. D. "Community Cooperatives Combat Sexual Assault and Domestic Violence." *Emergency Medical Services (EMS)* 32(2)(2003):60–61.

Jaslow, D., J. Ufberg, and R. Marsh. "Primary Injury Prevention in an Urban EMS System." *Journal of Emergency Medicine* 25(2)(2003):167–170.

Mosesso, V. N., Jr., C. R. Packer, J. McMahon, T. E. Auble, and P. M. Paris. "Influenza Immunizations Provided by EMS Agencies: The MEDICVAX Project." *Prehospital Emergency Care* 7(1)(2003):74–78.

Streger, M. "Keeping Kids Safe: Injury Prevention Programs in EMS." *Emergency Medical Services (EMS)* 31(6)(2002):24.

Weiss, S. J., R. Chong, M. Ong, A. A. Ernst, and M. Balash. "Emergency Medical Services Screening of Elderly Falls in the Home." *Prehospital Emergency Care* 7(1) (2003):79–84.

Yancey, A. H. 2nd, R. Martinez, and A. L. Kellermann. "Injury Prevention and Emergency Medical Services: The 'Accendents Aren't' Program." *Prehospital Emergency Care* 6(2)(2002):204–209.

On the Web

Visit Brady's Paramedic Website at **www.bradybooks.com/paramedic.**

Medical/Legal Aspects of Advanced Prehospital Care

Objectives

After reading this chapter, you should be able to:

1. Differentiate among legal, ethical, and moral responsibilities of the paramedic. (pp. 113–114)
2. Describe the basic structure of the legal system and differentiate between civil and criminal law. (pp. 114–115)
3. Differentiate between licensure and certification as they apply to the paramedic. (p. 117)
4. List the specific reportable problems or conditions encountered while providing care and identify to whom the reports are to be made. (p. 117)
5. Define the following terms:
   a. Abandonment (p. 130)
   b. Advance directives (pp. 132–135)
   c. Assault (p. 130)
   d. Battery (p. 130)
   e. Breach of duty (p. 119)
   f. Confidentiality (pp. 123–124)
   g. Consent (expressed, implied, informed, involuntary) (pp. 125–127)
   h. Do Not Resuscitate (DNR) orders (pp. 132, 134–135)
   i. Duty to act (p. 119)

   j. Emancipated minor (p. 126)

   k. False imprisonment (p. 130)

   l. Immunity (pp. 118, 121)

   m. Liability (p. 113)

   n. Libel (p. 124)

   o. Minor (p. 126)

   p. Negligence (pp. 118–121)

   q. Proximate cause (p. 120)

   r. Scope of practice (pp. 116–117)

   s. Slander (p. 124)

   t. Standard of care (p. 119)

   u. Tort (p. 115)

6. Discuss the legal implications of medical direction, including off-line medical direction and on-line medical direction, and its relationship to the paramedic's standard of care. (pp. 116–117, 119)

7. Describe the four elements that must be present in order to prove negligence. (pp. 119–120)

8. Explain liability as it applies to emergency medical services, including the physicians providing medical direction and the paramedic's supervision of other care providers. (pp. 113, 116–117, 119)

9. Discuss immunity, including Good Samaritan statutes and governmental immunity, as it applies to the paramedic. (pp. 118, 121)

10. Explain the importance and necessity of patient confidentiality and the standards for maintaining patient confidentiality that apply to the paramedic. (pp. 123–124)

11. Differentiate among the types of consent: expressed, informed, implied, and involuntary. (pp. 125–126)

12. Given various scenarios with a patient in need of care, describe the process used to obtain informed or implied consent. (pp. 125–126)

13. Given several refusal-of-care scenarios, demonstrate appropriate patient interaction and documentation techniques. (pp. 127–128)

14. Identify the legal issues involved in the decision not to transport a patient, or to reduce the level of care being provided. (pp. 126–128)

15. Describe how hospitals are selected to receive patients based on patient need and hospital capability and the role of the paramedic in such selection. (p. 131)

16. Differentiate between assault and battery and describe how to avoid committing each. (pp. 130–131)

17. Describe the conditions under which the use of force, including restraint, is acceptable. (pp. 130–131)

18. Explain the purpose of advance directives and how they impact your patient care. (pp. 132–135)

19. Discuss the paramedic's responsibilities relative to resuscitation efforts for patients who are potential organ donors. (p. 135)

20. Describe how a paramedic may preserve evidence at a crime or accident scene. (pp. 135–136)
21. Describe the importance of providing accurate documentation (oral and written) in substantiating an emergency medical services response. (pp. 136–137)
22. Describe the characteristics of a patient care report required to make it an effective legal document. (pp. 136–137)
23. Review several patient care reports and evaluate the content from a legal and liability perspective. (pp. 136–137)
24. Given several scenarios in which a patient is injured while a paramedic is providing care, determine whether the four components of negligence are present. (pp. 119–120)
25. Given several scenarios, describe patient care behaviors that would protect the paramedic from claims of negligence. (p. 121)

Key Terms

Case Study

A police officer has pulled a 27-year-old female driver off to the side of the road at the intersection of Quincy Place and Route 122. Because of the dangerous driving he witnessed and the driver's erratic behavior, unsteady gait, and slurred speech, the officer suspects that the driver is intoxicated. To be safe, the officer requests immediate EMS backup.

EMS 117 paramedics arrive on scene in 2 minutes and find a young woman arguing with the police officer. As the paramedics are assessing scene safety, they see the patient turn and lunge at the officer. The officer subdues the patient, who thrashes around briefly before losing consciousness.

At the officer's signal, the paramedics run in to do their jobs. They perform an initial assessment, quickly determining that the patient's airway is clear and breathing and circulation are adequate. They do not detect any immediate life threats, and they begin to review possible causes of the altered mental status. To rule out hypoglycemia, they perform a rapid glucose determination using a glucometer. Then, while one paramedic conducts a physical exam of the patient, the other notes that her blood sugar is 22 mg/dL. Per approved standing orders, an IV is established and 50 mL of 50 percent dextrose is administered. The patient quickly responds, becomes fully oriented, and thanks the paramedics for their help. She then mentions that she has been ill for a few days and has not been eating well.

The paramedics urge the patient to go to the hospital for additional evaluation. She declines, stating that she has recently scheduled a physician's appointment and that she is late for a meeting. The paramedics advise the patient of the risks of refusing care. Nevertheless, she continues to refuse assistance. The paramedics assure themselves that the patient is fully conscious, oriented, and capable of refusing consent. They instruct the patient to go immediately to the mini-mart across the street to get something to eat, and she agrees. They then aseptically discontinue the IV and have the patient sign a "release-from-liability" form, which is witnessed by the police officer. They return their equipment to the ambulance, and notify the dispatcher that they are back in service.

INTRODUCTION

To practice competent prehospital care today, paramedics must become familiar with the legal issues they are likely to encounter in the field. As a paramedic, you must be prepared to make the best medical decisions and the most appropriate legal decisions. This chapter addresses general legal principles in addition to specific laws and legal concepts that affect the paramedic's daily practice.

Note that since laws vary from state to state, and protocols can vary from county to county, the information contained in this chapter cannot be used as a substitute for competent legal advice. Just like the practice of medicine, the practice of law involves some art, some science, and is always heavily dependent on the unique facts present in each situation. If you are faced with a specific legal question, you must rely on the advice of your attorney.

LEGAL DUTIES AND ETHICAL RESPONSIBILITIES

As a paramedic, you have specific legal duties to your patient, crew, medical director, and the public (Figure 6-1 ■). These duties are based on generally accepted standards and are often set by statutes and regulations. The failure of a paramedic to perform his or her job appropriately can result in civil or criminal liability. Your best protection from **liability** (legal responsibility) is to perform a systematic patient assessment, provide the appropriate medical care, and maintain accurate and complete documentation of all incidents.

A paramedic also is responsible for meeting the ethical standards expected of a professional emergency medical care provider. (See Chapter 7 for a detailed discussion of ethics.) Ethical standards are not laws. They are principles that identify desirable conduct by members of a particular group. Your ethical responsibilities include the following:

★ Promptly respond to both the physical and emotional needs of every patient.

liability *legal responsibility.*

Your best protection from liability is to perform systematic assessments, provide appropriate medical care, and maintain accurate and complete documentation.

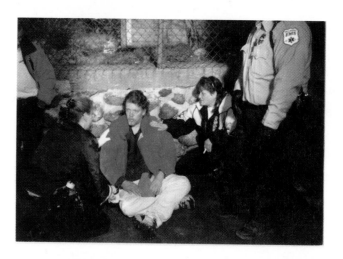

■ Figure 6-1 Each EMS response has the potential of involving EMS personnel in the legal system. (© Mark C. Ide)

★ Treat all patients and their families with courtesy and respect.

★ Maintain mastery of your skills and medical knowledge.

★ Participate in continuing education programs, seminars, and refresher training.

★ Critically review your performance, and constantly seek improvement.

★ Report honestly and with respect for patient confidentiality.

★ Work cooperatively with and respect other emergency professionals.

In addition to the paramedic's legal and ethical duties, he will encounter moral issues on a day-to-day basis. Morality, unlike legal obligations, is the principle of right and wrong as governed by individual conscience. Remember, always strive to meet the highest legal, ethical, and moral standards when providing patient care.

THE LEGAL SYSTEM

Sources of Law

In the United States, there are four primary sources of law: constitutional law, common law, legislative (or statutory) law, and administrative (or regulatory) law.

constitutional law *law based on the U.S. Constitution.*

Constitutional law is based on the Constitution of the United States. The U.S. Constitution sets forth our basic governmental structures, which include the executive (the president), legislative (Congress), and judicial (the Supreme Court) branches. Constitutional law also protects people against governmental abuse. For example, the Fourth Amendment to the Constitution protects people from unreasonable searches and seizures by the government.

common law *law that is derived from society's acceptance of customs and norms over time. Also called case law or judge-made law.*

Common law, which also is referred to as "case law" or "judge-made law," originated with the English legal system and was adopted by Americans in the 1700s. It was derived from society's acceptance of customs and norms over time. Common law changes and grows over the years as established principles are tested and adapted to meet new situations. It is a fundamental principle of our legal system that precedents set by the courts should be followed by other courts. This means that cases with similar facts should be decided in the same way.

For example, the U.S. Supreme Court issued a decision in the case of *Miranda v. Arizona* in 1966. The Court said that a person who is taken into police custody must be informed prior to interrogation that (1) he has the right to remain silent, (2) anything he says can be used against him in court, (3) he has the right to the presence of an attorney, and (4) if he cannot afford an attorney, one will be appointed to him if he so desires. In 2000, the Supreme Court upheld the rules set forth in *Miranda,* affirming that a confession will not be admissable at trial if it is found that the defendant was not advised of his rights before making his statement.

Legislative law (or statutory law) does not come from court decisions. It is created by law-making or legislative bodies. Statutes are enacted at the federal, state, and local levels by the legislative branches of government. Examples of legislative bodies include the U.S. Congress, state assemblies, city councils, and district boards. Legislative law is written in a very clear and concise manner and takes precedence over common-law decisions.

Administrative law (or regulatory law) is enacted by an administrative or governmental agency at either the federal or state level. Administrative agencies, such as the Occupational Safety and Health Administration (OSHA), will take a statute enacted by a legislative body and will produce rules and regulations necessary to implement it. The agency is given the authority to make regulations based on that statute; enforce rules, regulations, and statutes under its authority; and hold administrative hearings to carry out penalties for any violations of its rules.

> **legislative law** *law created by law-making bodies such as Congress and state assemblies. Also called statutory law.*

> **administrative law** *law that is enacted by governmental agencies at either the federal or state level. Also called regulatory law.*

Categories of Law

The United States has two general categories of law: civil law and criminal law. **Criminal law** deals with crime and punishment. It is an area of law in which the federal, state, or local government will prosecute an individual on behalf of society for violating laws meant to protect society. Homicide, rape, and burglary are examples of criminal wrongs. Violations of criminal laws are punished by imprisonment, a fine, or a combination of the two.

Civil law deals with noncriminal issues, such as personal injury, contract disputes, and matrimonial issues. In civil litigation, which involves conflicts between two or more parties, the *plaintiff* (person initiating the litigation) will seek to recover damages from the *defendant* (person against whom the complaint is made). **Tort** law, which is a branch of civil law, deals with civil wrongs committed by one individual against another (rather than against society). Tort law claims include negligence, medical malpractice, assault, battery, and slander.

Note that the United States has a *federal court system* and a *state court system*. The federal court system was created by the U.S. Constitution. Generally, only cases that involve a question of federal law or cases in which the parties are citizens of different states will be heard in a federal court. The state court system is the location for most of the cases in which a paramedic may become involved. In *trial courts,* a judge or jury determines the outcome of individual cases. *Appellate courts* hear appeals of decisions by trial courts or other appeals courts. The decisions of appellate courts may set precedents for later cases.

> **criminal law** *division of the legal system that deals with wrongs committed against society or its members.*

> **civil law** *the division of the legal system that deals with noncriminal issues and conflicts between two or more parties.*

> **tort** *a civil wrong committed by one individual against another.*

ANATOMY OF A CIVIL LAWSUIT

If you have ever been served with legal papers, you know that being sued or even being called to testify at a trial can be very unsettling. A basic understanding of the legal system can help. The following is a brief description of the components of a civil lawsuit:

★ *Incident.* For example, a person is driving on a road and fails to see a stop sign. When he passes through the intersection, he hits another car and that driver sustains several injuries.

★ *Investigation.* The injured driver's attorney makes a preliminary inquiry into the facts and circumstances surrounding the incident to determine if the case has merit.

★ *Filing of the complaint.* The injured driver (now called the "plaintiff") commences the lawsuit by filing a complaint with the court. The complaint contains information such as the names of the parties, the legal basis for the claim, and the damages sought by the plaintiff. A copy of the complaint is served on the defendant.

 Review

Content

Components of a Civil Lawsuit

- Incident
- Investigation
- Filing of complaint
- Answering of complaint
- Discovery
- Trial
- Decision
- Appeal
- Settlement

★ *Answering the complaint.* The defendant's attorney then prepares an answer, which addresses each allegation made in the complaint. The answer is then filed with the court, and a copy is given to the plaintiff's attorney.

★ *Discovery.* Before any lawsuit appears in front of a judge or jury, both parties to an action participate in pretrial discovery. This is the stage of the lawsuit when all relevant information about the incident is shared so that parties can prepare trial strategies. Discovery may include:

–*An examination before trial,* which is also called a "deposition," that allows a witness to answer questions under oath with a court stenographer present.

–*An interrogatory,* used by either side, is a set of written questions that requires written responses.

–*Requests for document production* entitles each side to request relevant documents, including the patient care report, records of the receiving hospital, any subsequent medical records, police records, and other records necessary to help prove or defend the lawsuit.

★ *Trial.* A trial will be commenced at the lowest level of court in the state. In many states, they are called "superior" courts. At the trial, each side will be given the opportunity to present all relevant evidence and testimony from witnesses.

★ *Decision.* After deliberations, the judge or jury determines the guilt or liability of the defendant and then decides the amount of damages to award the plaintiff, if any.

★ *Appeal.* After the jury's decision is entered by the court, either party may be entitled to an appeal. Generally, grounds for an appeal are limited to errors of law made by the court. Appeals will not be heard at the lower-level court, but by the higher-level appellate court.

★ *Settlement.* This can occur at any stage of the lawsuit. Generally, the defendant will offer the plaintiff an amount of money that is less than the amount for which he is being sued. The plaintiff may then agree to accept the reduced amount on the condition, for example, that he will no longer pursue the case.

LAWS AFFECTING EMS AND THE PARAMEDIC

Most of the laws that affect EMS and paramedics are state laws. Although these laws vary from state to state, they share common principles.

Scope of Practice

scope of practice *range of duties and skills paramedics are allowed and expected to perform.*

The range of duties and skills paramedics are allowed and expected to perform is called the **scope of practice.** Usually, the scope of practice is set by state law or regulation and by local medical direction. Often, a state will have a general "medical practice act" that governs the practice of medicine and all health care professionals. These acts prescribe how and to what extent a physician may delegate authority to a paramedic. As you learned in Chapter 3, paramedics may function only under the direct supervision of a licensed physician through a delegation of authority. Generally, paramedics should follow orders given by on-line and off-line medical direction. However, you should not blindly follow orders that you know are medically inappropriate.

Circumstances in which an order from medical direction may be legitimately refused include: when you are ordered to provide a treatment that is beyond the scope of your training and inconsistent with established protocols or procedures, and when you

⌐○ —————
You may function as a paramedic only under the direct supervision of a licensed physician through a delegation of authority.

are ordered to administer a treatment that you reasonably believe would be harmful to the patient. For example, imagine that a paramedic is en route to the hospital with a 200-pound (100-kg) patient who is having 15 multifocal premature ventricular contractions (PVCs) per minute. The treatment protocol for such a condition is to administer 1.0 to 1.5 mg/kg of lidocaine, or 100 to 150 mg to a 200-pound patient. The on-line physician orders the paramedic to administer 1 gram (1,000 mg) of lidocaine. The paramedic knows this amount of medication would seriously harm the patient. What should he do? He should first raise the concern with the physician. If the physician still insists, the paramedic should refuse to follow the order and document the incident thoroughly on the patient care report.

In addition, every EMS system should have a policy in place to guide paramedics in dealing with intervener physicians (on-scene licensed physicians who are professionally unrelated to the patient and who are attempting to assist with patient care). Generally, such a policy requires that certain conditions be met before the paramedic should allow the intervener physician to assume control of patient care. That is, the physician must be properly identified to the paramedic, licensed to practice medicine in the state, willing to accept the responsibility of continuing medical care until the patient reaches the hospital, and willing to document the intervention as required by the local EMS system.

Licensure and Certification

Other laws that directly affect the paramedic's ability to practice relate to certification and licensure requirements. *Certification* refers to the recognition granted to an individual who has met predetermined qualifications to participate in a certain activity. It is usually given by a certifying agency (not necessarily a government agency) or professional association. For example, after completing an approved paramedic program in New York State, a student who passes an approved written and practical examination will become a certified New York State paramedic.

Licensure is a process used to regulate occupations. Generally, a governmental agency, such as a state medical board, grants permission to an individual who meets established qualifications to engage in a particular profession or occupation. Certification or licensure, or perhaps both, may be required by your state or local authorities for you to practice as a paramedic.

Most states have laws that govern paramedic practice and set forth the requirements for certification, licensure, recertification, and relicensure. It is your responsibility to understand fully the EMS laws and regulations in your state.

Motor Vehicle Laws

As with other EMS-related laws, motor vehicle laws vary from state to state. Generally, there are special motor vehicle laws that govern the operation of emergency vehicles and the equipment they carry. These laws apply to areas such as vehicle maintenance and use of the siren and emergency lights. It is important that you become familiar with the laws of your state. Keep up-to-date with local regulations, too.

Mandatory Reporting Requirements

Each state enacts different laws designed to protect the public. For example, most states have laws that require a health care worker to report to local authorities any suspected spousal abuse, child abuse and neglect, or abuse of the elderly. In many states, violent crimes, such as sexual assault, gunshot wounds, and stab wounds, must be reported to law enforcement. Emergencies that threaten public health, such as animal bites and communicable diseases, also must be reported to the proper authorities. The content of such reports and to whom they must be made is set by law, regulation, or policy. Become familiar with the circumstances under which you are required to make a report. If you fail to make a required report, you may be criminally and civilly liable for your inaction.

 Review

Content

Commonly Mandated Reports

- Spouse abuse
- Child abuse and neglect
- Elder abuse
- Sexual assault
- Gunshot and stab wounds
- Animal bites
- Communicable diseases

Legal Protection for the Paramedic

In addition to the laws that protect patients, legislative bodies have enacted laws to protect paramedics. For example, some jurisdictions have enacted laws that criminally punish a person who commits assault or battery against a paramedic while he is providing medical care. Others have laws prohibiting the obstruction of paramedic activity.

immunity *exemption from legal liability.*

Immunity, or exemption from legal liability, is another form of protection. Governmental immunity is a judicial doctrine that prohibits a person from bringing a lawsuit against a government without its consent. However, most states today have waived their immunity rights, and courts are becoming increasingly likely to strike down the ones that still exist. This type of liability protection, even if allowed under law, generally serves to protect only the government agency, not the individual paramedic. Therefore, you should not rely on governmental immunity to protect you from claims of negligence.

Good Samaritan laws *laws that provide immunity to certain people who assist at the scene of a medical emergency.*

Virtually every state has **Good Samaritan laws,** which provide immunity to people who assist at the scene of a medical emergency. Though these laws vary from state to state, generally, they protect a person from liability if that person acts in good faith, is not negligent (most states will cover acts of simple negligence but not ones of gross negligence), acts within his scope of practice, and does not accept payment for services. The Good Samaritan laws of many states have been expanded to protect both paid and volunteer prehospital personnel.

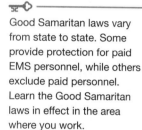

Good Samaritan laws vary from state to state. Some provide protection for paid EMS personnel, while others exclude paid personnel. Learn the Good Samaritan laws in effect in the area where you work.

As a paramedic, you should also become familiar with local laws and regulations governing the use of physical restraints for dangerous or violent patients. There also may be regulations governing entry into restricted areas such as military installations, nuclear power plants, and sites with hazardous materials. Since the laws affecting paramedic practice vary from state to state, your agency should obtain the advice of an attorney in order to minimize potential exposure to liability.

Other laws are designed to protect the paramedic in the event of exposure to bloodborne or airborne pathogens. For example, the Ryan White Comprehensive AIDS Resources Emergency Act (Ryan White CARE Act) requires hospitals and EMS agencies to create a notification system to provide information and assist the paramedic when an exposure occurs. This law allows the paramedic who has been exposed to certain diseases (such as hepatitis B, AIDS, and tuberculosis) access to medical records to determine if the patient has tested positive for, or is exhibiting signs and symptoms of, an infectious disease. The Ryan White CARE Act is a federal law, but many states have enacted similar or even more comprehensive laws to protect paramedics who may have been exposed to infectious diseases. It is important for each agency to appoint an infection control officer and for this individual to implement protocols and an appropriate infection control plan.

LEGAL ACCOUNTABILITY OF THE PARAMEDIC

As a paramedic, you are required to provide a level of care to your patients that is consistent with your education and training and equal to that of any other competent paramedic with equivalent training. You also are expected to perform your duties in a reasonable and prudent manner, as any other paramedic would in a similar situation. Any deviation from this standard might open you to allegations of negligence and liability for any resulting damages.

NEGLIGENCE AND MEDICAL LIABILITY

negligence *deviation from accepted standards of care recognized by law for the protection of others against the unreasonable risk of harm.*

Negligence is defined as a deviation from accepted standards of care recognized by law for the protection of others against the unreasonable risk of harm. It can result in legal accountability and liability. In the health care professions, negligence is synonymous with malpractice.

Components of a Negligence Claim

In a negligence claim against a paramedic, the plaintiff must establish and prove four particular elements in order to prevail: a duty to act, a breach of that duty, actual damages to the patient or other individual, and proximate cause (causation of damages).

First, the plaintiff must establish that the paramedic had a **duty to act.** That is, he must prove that the paramedic had a formal contractual or informal legal obligation to provide care. Note that the act of voluntarily assuming care of a patient may imply that there was a duty to act, which creates a continuing duty to act. For example, in some states if an off-duty paramedic witnesses a person choking, he may be under no legal duty to act. However, if that paramedic initiates care, then he has a duty to continue care. The rationale behind this rule is if bystanders see that a victim is being helped, they may walk away. If the paramedic rendering assistance walks away after initiating treatment, but not completing it, the patient may actually be left in a worse condition than if the paramedic never tried to help.

Duties that are expected of the paramedic include:

★ Duty to respond to the scene and render care to ill or injured patients

★ Duty to obey federal, state, and local laws and regulations

★ Duty to operate the emergency vehicle reasonably and prudently

★ Duty to provide care and transportation to the expected standard of care

★ Duty to provide care and transportation consistent with the paramedic's scope of practice and local medical protocols

★ Duty to continue care and transportation through to appropriate conclusions

Second, the plaintiff must prove there was a **breach of duty** by the paramedic. A paramedic always must exercise the degree of care, skill, and judgment that would be expected under like circumstances by a similarly trained, reasonable paramedic in the same community. The **standard of care** specific to the paramedic's practice is generally established by court testimony and referenced to published codes, standards, criteria, and guidelines applicable to the situation. A breach of duty may occur by **malfeasance, misfeasance,** or **nonfeasance:**

★ *Malfeasance,* or the performance of a wrongful or unlawful act by the paramedic. For example, a paramedic commits malfeasance if he assaults a patient.

★ *Misfeasance,* or the performance of a legal act in a manner that is harmful or injurious. For example, a paramedic commits misfeasance when he inadvertently intubates a patient's esophagus, fails to confirm tube placement, and leaves the tube in place.

★ *Nonfeasance,* or the failure to perform a required act or duty. For example, it would be an act of nonfeasance to fail to fully immobilize a collision patient who is complaining of neck and back pain.

In some cases, negligence may be so obvious that it does not require extensive proof. Unlike criminal cases, which require proof "beyond a reasonable doubt," civil cases require only a proof of guilt by a "preponderance of evidence." In most cases, the burden of proving negligence rests on the plaintiff. As a result, when it is difficult to do so, a plaintiff may sometimes invoke the doctrine of *res ipsa loquitur,* which is Latin for "the thing speaks for itself."

Review

The Four Elements of Negligence

- Duty to act
- Breach of that duty
- Actual damages
- Proximate cause

duty to act *a formal contractual or informal legal obligation to provide care.*

breach of duty *an action or inaction that violates the standard of care expected from a paramedic.*

Always exercise the degree of care, skill, and judgment expected under like circumstances by a similarly trained, reasonable paramedic in the same community.

standard of care *the degree of care, skill, and judgment that would be expected under like or similar circumstances by a similarly trained, reasonable paramedic in the same community.*

malfeasance *a breach of duty by performance of a wrongful or unlawful act.*

misfeasance *a breach of duty by performance of a legal act in a manner that is harmful or injurious.*

nonfeasance *a breach of duty by failure to perform a required act or duty.*

res ipsa loquitur *a legal doctrine invoked by plaintiffs to support a claim of negligence; it is a Latin term that means "the thing speaks for itself."*

To support a claim of *res ipsa loquitur*, the complainant must prove that the damages would not have occurred in the absence of somebody's negligence, the instruments causing the damages were under the defendant's control at all times, and the patient did nothing to contribute to his own injury. After the doctrine of *res ipsa loquitur* is invoked in court, the burden of proof shifts from the plaintiff to the defendant.

For example, a classic situation in which *res ipsa loquitur* might be used occurs when a patient has an appendectomy and wakes to find that a surgical instrument has been left inside his abdomen. To prove negligence in this case, the plaintiff's attorney would show that the damage would not have occurred without the physician's negligence, that the surgical instrument was under the physician's control at all relevant times, and that the patient did not contribute to the injury. Many cases in which *res ipsa loquitur* would be successful are settled out-of-court.

Another situation in which little proof is required occurs when the paramedic violates a statute and injury to a plaintiff results. Some laws state that if a statute is violated and an injury results, a person will be guilty of *negligence per se*, or automatic negligence. For example, if a paramedic, who is driving in nonemergency mode, fails to stop at a red light and hits a pedestrian, the paramedic's negligence is obvious. He violated vehicle and traffic statutes that prohibit a vehicle from running a red light, and he is therefore guilty of *negligence per se*.

actual damages *refers to compensable physical, psychological, or financial harm.*

After a duty to act and a breach of that duty have been proven, **actual damages** is the third required element of proof in a negligence claim. That is, the plaintiff must prove that he was actually harmed in a way that can be compensated by the award of damages. This is an essential component. A lawsuit cannot be won if the paramedic's action caused no ill effects. The plaintiff must prove that he suffered compensable physical, psychological, or financial damage such as medical expenses, lost wages, lost future earnings, conscious pain and suffering, or wrongful death.

In addition, the plaintiff may seek punitive (punishing) damages. These are awarded only when a defendant commits an act of gross negligence or willful and wanton misconduct. An act of ordinary negligence, such as accidentally allowing an IV to infiltrate, will not support an award of punitive damages. If punitive damages are awarded to the plaintiff, most insurance policies will not cover them. Therefore, the paramedic may become personally liable for any punitive damages awarded to the plaintiff.

proximate cause *action or inaction of the paramedic that immediately caused or worsened the damage suffered by the patient.*

Finally, to prove negligence, the plaintiff must show that the paramedic's action or inaction was the **proximate cause** of the damages; that is, the action or inaction of the paramedic immediately caused or worsened the damage suffered by the plaintiff. For example, a cardiac patient who breaks his arm during an ambulance collision while en route to the hospital will likely be able to prove that his injuries resulted from the incident; that is, the collision was the proximate cause of his injuries. However, a patient with a sprained wrist who happens to suffer a stroke while in the ambulance would have difficulty proving the ambulance ride was the proximate cause of the stroke.

Proximate cause may also be thought of in terms of "foreseeability." To show the existence of proximate cause, the plaintiff needs to prove that the damage to the patient was reasonably foreseeable by the paramedic. This is usually established by expert testimony. For example, imagine that a paramedic negligently crashes into a telephone pole with the ambulance. As a result, two people are injured—the patient who was in the back of the ambulance and, two blocks away, a baby who was dropped by his mother when the loud crash startled her. It should be easy for the patient to prove proximate cause, because it was reasonably foreseeable that an ambulance crash could hurt passengers. However, if the woman who dropped her baby sued the paramedic, she probably would not be able to establish proximate cause. Although the crash was the reason her baby was injured, it was not a foreseeable injury resulting from the ambulance crash.

High Risks for Lawsuits Most lawsuits filed against EMS personnel allege negligence or a failure to act. Many involve allegations of misplaced endotracheal tubes, problems related to patient restraint, or medication errors and omissions. Be aware of high-risk areas in EMS practice, make sure that you closely adhere to your system's treatment protocols, and document your care in detail.

Defenses to Charges of Negligence

If you are accused of negligence, you may be able to avoid liability if you can establish a defense to the plaintiff's claim. The following is a list of potential defenses to negligence:

★ *Good Samaritan laws.* If the paramedic can establish that his actions were protected by a Good Samaritan law, liability may be avoided. Note that such laws generally do not protect providers from acts of gross negligence, reckless disregard, or willful or wanton conduct, and they do not prohibit the filing of lawsuits.

★ *Governmental immunity.* These laws do not offer much protection for the individual paramedic accused of negligence. Though governmental immunity laws vary from state to state, the current legal trend is toward limiting this type of protection.

★ *Statute of limitations.* This is a law that sets the maximum time period during which certain actions can be brought in court. After the time limit is reached, no legal action can be brought regardless of whether or not a negligent act occurred. Statutes of limitations vary from state to state, so carefully review the laws in your state. Note that they may vary for different negligent acts and for cases involving children.

★ *Contributory or comparative negligence.* Some state laws will reduce or eliminate a plaintiff's award of damages if the plaintiff is found to have caused or worsened his own injury. For example, imagine that a patient involved in a car crash complained of neck pain but refused to let the paramedics properly immobilize his spine. The paramedics explained the risks of refusing treatment, but the patient signed a "release-from-liability" form anyway. Later, the patient learns that he has permanent spinal-cord damage and sues the paramedics for negligence. Many courts will find that the paramedics were not negligent because, by refusing necessary treatment, the patient contributed to the exacerbation of his own injury.

To protect yourself against claims of negligence, you should receive appropriate education, training, and continuing education; receive appropriate medical direction, both on-line and off-line; always prepare accurate, thorough documentation; have a professional attitude and demeanor at all times; always act in good faith; and use your own common sense. In addition, it is essential for all paramedics to be covered by liability insurance. Although many employers and agencies carry coverage, it is a good idea to obtain your own because your agency's coverage may be inadequate.

It is essential for all paramedics to be covered by liability insurance.

SPECIAL LIABILITY CONCERNS

Medical Direction

If a paramedic makes a mistake in the field and is sued by the injured patient, it is possible that the patient will also sue the paramedic's medical director and the on-line physician. The on-line physician may be liable to a patient for giving the paramedic medically incorrect orders or advice, for the refusal to authorize the administration of a medically necessary medication, or for directing an ambulance to take a patient to an inappropriate medical facility.

A paramedic's medical director may be liable to the patient for the negligent supervision of the paramedic. In order for the patient to be successful in this type of claim, he would have to prove that the physician breached a duty to supervise the paramedic and that breach was the proximate cause of the patient's injuries. Examples include: the medical director's failure to establish medication protocols or standing orders consistent with the current standards of medical practice for the paramedic to use in the field; the medical director observed and then failed to correct a paramedic's poor intubation technique; or the medical director received complaints of inappropriate care by a paramedic and then failed to effectively investigate and resolve the problem.

Borrowed Servant Doctrine

As a paramedic, you may find yourself in the position of supervising other emergency care providers, such as EMT-Basics or EMT-Intermediates. When doing so, it will be your responsibility to make sure they perform their duties in a professional and medically appropriate manner. Depending on the degree of supervision and the amount of control you have, you may be liable for any negligent act they commit. This is called the "borrowed servant" doctrine. For it to apply, the paramedic accused of negligence must have taken the employees of another employer under his control and exercised supervisory powers over them.

Civil Rights

In addition to suing you for negligence, a patient may be able to sue you under certain circumstances for violating his civil rights if you fail to render care for a discriminatory reason. As a paramedic, you may not withhold medical care for reasons such as race, creed, color, gender, national origin, or in some cases, ability to pay. Also, all patients should be provided with appropriate care regardless of their status, condition, or disease (including AIDS/HIV, tuberculosis, and other communicable diseases).

Off-Duty Paramedics

Liability also may arise in a situation in which an off-duty paramedic renders assistance at the scene of an illness or injury. Generally, any person who provides basic emergency first aid to another person would be protected from liability under a Good Samaritan law. However, when the off-duty paramedic provides advanced life support, a problem may arise. In most states, paramedics cannot practice advanced skills unless they are practicing within an EMS system. To perform paramedic skills and procedures that require delegation from a physician while off-duty may constitute the crime of practicing medicine without a license. Learn the law in your jurisdiction.

PARAMEDIC-PATIENT RELATIONSHIPS

The relationship you establish with your patient is a very important one. Not only must you provide the best medical care, but you also have legal and ethical duties to protect the patient's privacy and treat him with honesty, respect, and compassion.

CONFIDENTIALITY

All records related to the emergency care rendered to a patient must be kept strictly confidential. Keeping patient **confidentiality** means that any medical or personal information about a patient—including medical history, assessment findings, and treatment—will not be released to a third party without the express permission of the patient or legal guardian. However, there are specific circumstances under which a patient's confidential information may be released:

confidentiality *the principle of law that prohibits the release of medical or other personal information about a patient without the patient's consent.*

★ *Patient consents to the release of his records.* A patient may request a copy of his medical records for any reason. If the patient is a child, consent for release of medical records must be obtained from the child's parent or other legal guardian. The request should be accepted only if it is in writing, specifically authorizes the agency to release the records, and contains the patient's signature (or other authorized signature). If the request so directs, it is permissible to forward the records to the patient's physician, insurance company, attorney, or any other party the patient specifies. Be sure your agency retains a copy of the consent document.

★ *Other medical care providers have a need to know.* For example, it is not a breach of patient confidentiality to discuss the patient's condition with on-line medical direction or to give a patient report to an emergency department nurse upon arrival at the hospital. This is permitted because it allows medical care appropriate for the patient to be continued. It is not acceptable, however, to discuss confidential patient information with medical providers who have no responsibility for the patient's care.

★ *EMS is required by law to release a patient's medical records.* Records may be requested by a court order that is signed by a judge, or they may be requested by *subpoena* (a command to appear at a certain time and place to give testimony). When an agency receives a court order or subpoena, it is good practice to consult with an attorney to make sure the order is valid and for assistance with compliance. Failure to comply with a court order or subpoena may result in severe penalties.

★ *There are third-party billing requirements.* For EMS agencies that bill patients for services, it is generally necessary to release certain confidential information to receive reimbursement from private insurance companies, Medicaid, or Medicare. If possible, the agency should obtain patient authorization for this purpose.

The law provides penalties for the breach of confidentiality. The improper release of information may result in a lawsuit against the paramedic for defamation (libel or slander), breach of confidentiality, or invasion of privacy. If found guilty, the paramedic may be responsible for paying money damages to the patient.

Legal Notes

HIPAA The Health Insurance Portability and Accountability Act (HIPAA) enhances the confidentiality of medical records and mandates that EMS personnel be educated as to the requirements of the law. HIPAA also provides methods to assure that EMS personnel who have been exposed to a communicable disease are notified in a timely fashion.

Health Insurance Portability and Accountability Act (HIPAA)

The Health Insurance Portability and Accountability Act of 1996 (HIPAA) changed the methods EMS providers use to file for insurance and Medicare payments. It also adds important new layers of privacy protection for EMS patients. The privacy protections provide, among other things, that all EMS employees be trained in HIPAA compliance. Furthermore, EMS providers must develop administrative, electronic, and physical barriers to unauthorized disclosure of patients' protected health information. Disclosures of information—except for purposes of treatment, obtaining payment for services, health care operations, and disclosures mandated or permitted by law—must be preauthorized in writing. HIPAA requires providers to post notices in prominent places advising patients of their privacy rights and provides both civil and serious criminal penalties for violations of privacy.

Patients are given the right to inspect and copy their health records, restrict use and disclosure of their individually identifiable health information, amend their health records, require a provider to communicate with them confidentially, and account for disclosures of their protected health information except for treatment, payment, health care operations, and legally required reporting purposes. The requirements of HIPAA are detailed and every EMS provider must become familiar with them.

Defamation

defamation *an intentional false communication that injures another person's reputation or good name.*

Defamation occurs when a person makes an intentional false communication that injures another person's reputation or good name. A patient may sue a paramedic for defamation if the paramedic communicates an untrue statement about a patient's character or reputation without legal privilege or consent. Defamation can occur in written form or through verbal statements.

libel *the act of injuring a person's character, name, or reputation by false statements made in writing or through the mass media with malicious intent or reckless disregard for the falsity of those statements.*

Libel is the act of injuring a person's character, name, or reputation by false statements made in writing or through the mass media with malicious intent or reckless disregard for the falsity of those statements. Allegations of libel can be avoided by completing an accurate, professional, and confidential patient care report. Do not use slang and value-loaded words or phrases in your report (for example, do not refer to a patient as "stupid" or use any derogatory race-based terms). Since many states consider the patient care report part of the public record, never write anything on it that could be considered libelous.

slander *act of injuring a person's character, name, or reputation by false or malicious statements spoken with malicious intent or reckless disregard for the falsity of those statements.*

Slander is the act of injuring a person's character, name, or reputation by false or malicious statements spoken with malicious intent or reckless disregard for the falsity of those statements. An allegation of slander can be avoided by limiting oral reporting of a patient's condition to appropriate personnel only. Note that many EMS systems record ambulance-hospital radio transmissions. In addition, scanners, which give the public access to EMS transmissions, are common in the United States. Therefore, information transmitted over the radio should be limited to essential matters of patient care. In most cases, the patient's name and insurance status should not be transmitted over the radio.

Invasion of Privacy

A paramedic may be accused of invasion of privacy for the release of confidential information, without legal justification, regarding a patient's private life, which might reasonably expose the patient to ridicule, notoriety, or embarrassment. That includes, for example, the release of information regarding HIV status or other sensitive medical information. The fact that released information is true is not a defense to an action for invasion of privacy.

CONSENT

By law, you must get a patient's consent before you can provide medical care or transport. **Consent** is the granting of permission to treat. More accurately, it is the granting of permission to touch. It is based on the concept that every adult human being of sound mind has the right to determine what should be done with his own body. Touching a patient without appropriate consent may subject you to charges of assault and battery.

A patient must be **competent** in order to give or withhold consent. A competent adult is one who is lucid and able to make an informed decision about medical care. He understands your questions and recommendations, and he understands the implications of his decisions made about medical care. Although there is no absolute test for determining competency, keep the following factors in mind when making a determination: the patient's mental status, the patient's ability to respond to questions, statements regarding the patient's competency from family or friends, evidence of impairment from drugs or alcohol, or indications of shock.

Informed Consent

Conscious, competent patients have the right to decide what medical care to accept. However, for consent to be legally valid, it must be **informed consent,** or consent given based on full disclosure of information. That is, a patient must understand the nature, risks, and benefits of any procedures to be performed. Therefore, before providing medical care, you must explain the following to the patient in a manner he can understand:

★ Nature of the illness or injury

★ Nature of the recommended treatments

★ Risks, dangers, and benefits of those treatments

★ Alternative treatment possibilities, if any, and the related risks, dangers, and benefits of accepting each one

★ Dangers of refusing treatment and/or transport

Informed consent must be obtained from every competent adult before treatment may be initiated. Conscious, competent patients may revoke consent at any time during care and transport. In most states, a patient must be 18 years of age or older in order to give or withhold consent. Generally, a child's parent or legal guardian must give informed consent before treatment of the child can begin.

Expressed, Implied, and Involuntary Consent

There are three more types of consent: expressed, implied, and involuntary. **Expressed consent** is the most common. It occurs when a person directly grants permission to treat—verbally, nonverbally, or in writing. Often, the act of a patient requesting an ambulance is considered an expression of a desire to be treated. However, just because the patient consents to a ride to the hospital does not mean he has consented to all types of treatment (such as the initiation of an IV and/or the administration of medications). You must obtain consent for each treatment you plan to provide. Consent from the patient does not always need to be granted verbally. It may be expressed by allowing care to be rendered.

Unconscious patients cannot grant consent. When treating them or any patient who requires emergency intervention but is mentally, physically, or emotionally unable to grant consent, treatment depends on **implied consent** (sometimes called "emergency doctrine"). That is, it is assumed that the patient would want life-saving treatment if he were able to give informed consent. Implied consent is effective only until the patient no longer requires emergency care or until the patient regains competence.

By law, you must get a patient's consent before you can provide medical care or transportation.

consent *the patient's granting of permission for treatment.*

competent *able to make an informed decision about medical care.*

informed consent *consent for treatment that is given based on full disclosure of information.*

expressed consent *verbal, nonverbal, or written communication by a patient that he wishes to receive medical care.*

implied consent *consent for treatment that is presumed for a patient who is mentally, physically, or emotionally unable to grant consent. Also called emergency doctrine.*

Occasionally, a court will order patients to undergo treatment, even though they may not want it. This is called **involuntary consent.** It is most commonly encountered with patients who must be held for mental-health evaluation or as directed by law enforcement personnel who have the patient under arrest. It also is used on occasion to force patients to undergo treatment for a disease that threatens the community at large (tuberculosis, for example). Law-enforcement personnel often will accompany patients who are undergoing court-ordered treatment.

Consent issues also can arise when a paramedic is called by law-enforcement officials to treat a sick or injured prisoner or arrestee. The officers may tell you that they have the legal authority to give consent to treatment for the patient simply because the patient is in police custody. However, a competent adult in police custody does not necessarily lose the right to make medical decisions for himself. In fact, many prisoners have successfully sued health care providers for rendering treatment without consent. Generally, forced treatment is limited to emergency treatment necessary to save life or limb or treatment ordered by the court. Be sure that you are familiar with your local protocols and laws on this issue.

Special Consent Situations

In the case of a **minor** (depending on state law, this is usually a person under the age of 18), consent should be obtained from a parent, legal guardian, or court-appointed custodian. The same is true of a mentally incompetent adult. If a responsible person cannot be located, and if the child or mentally incompetent adult is suffering from an apparent life-threatening injury or illness, treatment may be rendered under the doctrine of implied consent.

Generally, an **emancipated minor** is considered an adult. This is a person under 18 years of age who is married, pregnant, a parent, a member of the armed forces, or financially independent and living away from home. As an adult, an emancipated minor may legally give informed consent. Anyone else under the age of 18 may not grant informed consent.

Withdrawal of Consent

A competent adult may withdraw consent for any treatment at any time. However, refusal must be informed. That is, the patient must understand the risks of not continuing treatment or transport to the hospital in terms he can fully understand. A common example of a patient withdrawing consent occurs after a hypoglycemic patient regains full consciousness with the administration of dextrose. The patient should be encouraged—*but may not be forced*—to go to the emergency department. If he is competent, the patient may refuse transport. In such cases, advanced life support measures, such as IV fluids, which were initiated when the patient was unconscious should be discontinued. The patient also should complete a release-from-liability form (Figure 6-2 ▪).

Sometimes patients choose to accept one recommended treatment, but refuse others. For example, a patient involved in a motor vehicle crash may refuse to be fully im-

Cultural Considerations

Religious and Cultural Beliefs Religious and cultural beliefs impact a patient's health care decisions. Some, such as Christian Scientists, prefer to use prayer instead of traditional health care and may refuse treatment on religious grounds. Similarly, Jehovah's Witnesses believe that blood transfusions are prohibited by biblical teachings.

REFUSAL OF TREATMENT AND TRANSPORTATION

I, THE UNDERSIGNED HAVE BEEN ADVISED THAT MEDICAL ASSISTANCE ON MY BEHALF IS
NECESSARY AND THAT REFUSAL OF SAID ASSISTANCE AND TRANSPORTATION MAY RESULT IN
DEATH, OR IMPERIL MY HEALTH. NEVERTHELESS, I REFUSE TO ACCEPT TREATMENT OR
TRANSPORT AND ASSUME ALL RISKS AND CONSEQUENCES OF MY DECISION AND RELEASE
GOLD CROSS AMBULANCE COMPANY AND ITS EMPLOYEES FROM ANY LIABILITY ARISING FROM
MY REFUSAL.

_____
SIGNATURE OF PATIENT

_____
WITNESSED BY

_____
DATE SIGNED

Figure 6-2   Example of a "release-from-liability" form.

mobilized but ask to be transported to the hospital. It is very important for you to do everything in your power to be sure he understands why spinal precautions are necessary and what may happen if they are not taken. If a competent adult continues to refuse care, be sure to thoroughly document his reason for refusal and your attempts to convince him to change his mind. Have the patient and a witness sign a release-from-liability form.

Refusal of Service

Not every EMS run results in the transportation of a patient to a hospital. Emergency care should always be offered to a patient, no matter how minor the injury or illness may be. However, often, the patient will refuse. If this occurs, you must:

★ Be sure that the patient is legally permitted to refuse care; that is, the patient must be a competent adult.

★ Make multiple and sincere attempts to convince the patient to accept care.

★ Enlist the help of others, such as the patient's family or friends, to convince the patient to accept care.

★ Make certain that the patient is fully informed about the implications of his decision and the potential risks of refusing care.

★ Consult with on-line medical direction.

★ Have the patient and a disinterested witness, such as a police officer, sign a release-from-liability form.

★ Advise the patient that he may call you again for help, if necessary.

★ Attempt to get the patient's family or friends to stay with the patient.

★ Document the entire situation thoroughly on your patient care report.

Remember, the refusal of care must be informed. That is, the patient must be told of and understand all possible risks of refusal. Decisions not to transport should involve medical direction. It is a good idea to put the patient directly on the phone with the on-line physician. If all efforts fail, be sure to thoroughly document the reasons for refusal and your efforts to change the patient's mind. If an on-line physician was involved, it is

Refusal of care by a patient
must be informed and
properly documented.

Patients with Mental Disorders Several types of mental disorders are frequently encountered with problem patients. In addition to intoxication with alcohol or drugs, many problem patients suffer from personality disorders. These disorders cloud judgment and significantly impact interactions with others.

a good idea to obtain his signature on your patient care report. (See Figure 6-3 ■ for an example of an EMS patient refusal checklist.)

Problem Patients

As a paramedic, you will occasionally encounter a "problem patient," one who is violent, a victim of a drug overdose, an intoxicated adult or minor, or an ill or injured minor with no adult available to provide consent for medical treatment. Such a patient can present you with a medical–legal dilemma. For example, consider the patient who has allegedly taken an overdose of medication. Concerned family members may panic and activate the EMS system. However, upon your arrival at the scene, you find the patient alert, oriented, denying that he has taken any medication, and refusing to give consent for treatment or transport.

In a case such as this, attempt to develop trust and some rapport with the patient. If he continues to refuse, and remains alert and oriented, a refusal form should be completed and witnessed by a police officer. If the patient will not sign the form, have a police officer or family member sign it, indicating that the patient verbally refused care. If, however, the situation becomes dangerous, or you have reason to suspect the patient has tried to injure himself, police officers or family members should consider legal measures to force the patient to receive treatment.

The intoxicated person who refuses treatment and transport also poses a problem for the paramedic. Every effort should be made to encourage the patient to accept care and transport to the hospital. If the patient refuses, explain to him in a calm and detailed manner the implications of refusal. However, if you determine that the patient cannot understand the nature of his illness or the consequences of his refusal, then he may not refuse treatment because he is not competent to do so. Involve law enforcement at this point. If the patient is competent to make such a decision, then have him sign a refusal form. Your conversation with the patient and his refusal should be witnessed by a disinterested third party such as a police officer.

Regardless of the type of problem patient, always document the encounter in detail. Your records should include a description of the patient, the results of any physical examination (or reasons for the lack of one), important statements made by the patient and other persons at the scene, and the names and addresses of any witnesses. If you are going to include an important statement from the patient or witnesses in your patient care report, put the exact statement in quotation marks.

Ideally, a police officer should respond to the scene of all problem patients and should either sign the patient care report as a witness or, if the paramedic's safety is at risk, accompany the patient and paramedic to the emergency department.

Involve the police and document in detail any encounter with a "problem patient."

LEGAL COMPLICATIONS RELATED TO CONSENT

There are many legal complications related to consent to treatment. If the paramedic does not obtain the proper consent to treat or fails to continue appropriate treatment, he may be liable for damages based on a tort cause of action, such as abandonment, assault, battery, or false imprisonment.

EMS PATIENT REFUSAL CHECKLIST

PATIENT's NAME: _____ AGE: _____

LOCATION OF CALL: _____ DATE: _____

AGENCY INCIDENT #: _____ AGENCY CODE: _____

NAME OF PERSON FILLING OUT FORM: _____

I. **ASSESSMENT OF PATIENT** (Check appropriate response for each item)

    1.   Oriented to: Person? ☐ Yes ☐ No
                           Place? ☐ Yes ☐ No
                           Time? ☐ Yes ☐ No
                           Situation? ☐ Yes ☐ No

    2.   Altered level of consciousness? ☐ Yes ☐ No

    3.   Head injury? ☐ Yes ☐ No

    4.   Alcohol or drug ingestion by exam or history? ☐ Yes ☐ No

II. **PATIENT INFORMED** (Check appropriate response for each item)

☐ Yes ☐ No   Medical treatment/evaluation needed

☐ Yes ☐ No   Ambulance transport needed

☐ Yes ☐ No   Further harm could result without medical treatment/evaluation

☐ Yes ☐ No   Transport by means other than ambulance could be hazardous in light of patient's illness/injury

☐ Yes ☐ No   Patient provided with Refusal Information Sheet

☐ Yes ☐ No   Patient accepted Refusal Information Sheet

III. **DISPOSITION**

☐ Refused all EMS assistance

☐ Refused field treatment, but accepted transport

☐ Refused transport, but accepted field treatment

☐ Refused transport to recommended facility

☐ Patient transported by private vehicle to_____

☐ Released in care or custody of self

☐ Released in care or custody of relative or friend

    Name: _____ Relationship: _____

☐ Released in custody of law enforcement agency

    Agency: _____ Officer: _____

☐ Released in custody of other agency

    Agency: _____ Officer: _____

IV. **COMMENTS:** _____

_____

_____

_____

■ Figure 6-3   Some EMS systems have checklists for procedures to follow when a patient refuses care.

Abandonment

abandonment *termination of the paramedic-patient relationship without assurance that an equal or greater level of care will continue.*

Abandonment is the termination of the paramedic-patient relationship without providing for the appropriate continuation of care while it is still needed and desired by the patient. You cannot initiate patient care and then discontinue it without sufficient reason. You cannot turn the care of a patient over to personnel who have less training than you without creating potential liability for an abandonment action. For example, a paramedic who has initiated advanced life support should not turn the patient over to an EMT-Basic or an EMT-Intermediate for transport.

Abandonment can occur at any point during patient contact, including in the field or in the hospital emergency department. Physically leaving a patient unattended, even for a short time, may also be grounds for a charge of abandonment. If, for example, you leave a patient at a hospital without properly turning over his care to a physician or nurse, you may be liable for abandonment. It is always a good idea to have the nurse or physician to whom you have passed responsibility for patient care sign your patient care report.

Assault and Battery

assault *an act that unlawfully places a person in apprehension of immediate bodily harm without his consent.*

Failure to obtain appropriate consent before treatment could leave the paramedic open to allegations of assault and battery. **Assault** is defined as unlawfully placing a person in apprehension of immediate bodily harm without his consent. For example, your patient states that he is scared of needles and refuses to let you start an IV. If you then show him an IV catheter and bring it toward his arm as if to start an IV, you may be liable for assault.

battery *the unlawful touching of another individual without his consent.*

Battery is the unlawful touching of another individual without his consent. It would be battery to actually start an IV on a patient who does not consent to such treatment. A paramedic can be sued for assault and battery in both criminal and civil contexts.

False Imprisonment

false imprisonment *intentional and unjustifiable detention of a person without his consent or other legal authority.*

False imprisonment may be charged by a patient who is transported without consent or who is restrained without proper justification or authority. It is defined as intentional and unjustifiable detention of a person without his consent or other legal authority, and may result in civil or criminal liability. Like assault and battery, a charge of false imprisonment can be avoided by obtaining appropriate consent.

This is a particular problem with psychiatric patients. In most cases, you can avoid allegations of false imprisonment by having a law enforcement officer apprehend the patient and accompany you to the hospital. If no officer is available, you should attempt to consult with medical direction and carefully judge the risks of false imprisonment against the benefits of detaining and treating the patient. You should determine whether medical treatment is immediately necessary and whether the patient poses a threat to himself or to the public when you are making your decision to treat or transport.

REASONABLE FORCE

reasonable force *the minimal amount of force necessary to ensure that an unruly or violent person does not cause injury to himself or others.*

If it is safe to do so, you may use a reasonable amount of force to control an unruly or violent patient. The definition of **reasonable force** depends on the amount of force necessary to ensure that the patient does not cause injury to himself, you, or others. Excessive force can result in liability for the paramedic. Force used as punishment will be considered assault and battery for which the patient may be able to recover damages and the paramedic may face criminal charges. When you believe it is necessary to use force, involve law enforcement if possible.

The use of restraints may be indicated for a combative patient. Restraints must conform to your local protocols. Restraining devices typically used by EMS providers include straps, jackets, and restraining blankets. In this circumstance, an EMS team's goal is to use the least amount of force necessary to safely control the patient while causing him the least amount of discomfort. If the use of restraints is indicated, involve law enforcement officials.

PATIENT TRANSPORTATION

The transportation of patients to a health care facility is an integral part of the patient-care continuum. During transportation to a health care facility, be sure to maintain the same level of care as was initiated at the scene. This means that if you, as a paramedic, initiate advanced emergency care procedures, you must either ride with the patient to the hospital or ensure that another paramedic will accompany the patient. If you fail to do so, and the patient is harmed as a result, you may be liable for abandonment.

One of the greatest areas of potential liability for paramedics is emergency vehicle operations. It is essential that you become familiar with your state and local laws. The laws that provide exceptions from driving rules and regulations may allow you, for example, to drive at a rate of speed in excess of a posted speed limit, but if you are negligent at any time during the operation of your vehicle, you will not be protected from liability.

Another issue that will arise is patient choice of destination. If you work in a small area with only one hospital, you are not likely to encounter difficulties. However, many paramedics work in areas that have many hospitals and medical centers to choose from. Over the past few years, increasing numbers of lawsuits involving facility selection have been brought by patients. Some have sued paramedics themselves, claiming negligence based on the failure to transport to the nearest or most appropriate hospital.

An additional issue you may need to address involves the patient's insurance company protocols. In some situations, it may be appropriate to respect a patient's choice of facility based on his insurance company's facility-choice protocols. Local restrictions by insurance companies and health care maintenance organizations may determine under what conditions and to what facilities patient transport may be authorized and paid for. While most areas are not yet being confronted with restrictions on service provision, it may be only a matter of time. However, never put patient care in jeopardy by transporting to a less-appropriate facility because of insurance concerns.

In general, facility selection should be based on patient request, patient need, and facility capability. Local written protocols, the paramedic, on-line medical direction, and the patient should all play a role in facility selection. The patient's preference, however, should be honored unless the situation or the patient's condition dictates otherwise.

RESUSCITATION ISSUES

Advances in medical technology have saved and prolonged thousands of lives. However, in some instances, the use of sophisticated medical technology may only prolong pain, suffering, and death. When a person is seriously injured or gravely ill, family members must make difficult decisions regarding the intensity of medical care to be provided, including the use or withdrawal of life-support systems.

Generally, you are under obligation to begin resuscitative efforts when summoned to the scene of a patient who is unresponsive, pulseless, and apneic (not breathing). There are times, however, when you will determine that resuscitation is not indicated. This occurs with patients who have a valid Do Not Resuscitate (DNR) order, with patients who are obviously dead (decapitated, for example), with patients with obvious tissue decomposition or extreme dependent lividity (gravitational pooling of blood in dependent areas of the body), or with a patient who is at a scene that is too hazardous to enter.

Always follow your state laws, local protocols, and medical direction. The role of medical direction should be clearly delineated and included in your agency's protocols.

Patient restraint has become a particularly thorny legal issue for EMS personnel. Because physical restraint has been associated with significant problems, all EMS systems must have detailed protocols and standing orders that specifically deal with restraint.

During transport of a patient to a health care facility, be sure to maintain the same level of care as was initiated at the scene.

If you are authorized to determine that resuscitative efforts are not indicated, be sure to thoroughly document your decision and the criteria upon which it was based.

ADVANCE DIRECTIVES

To improve communication between patients, their family members, and physicians regarding such matters, the federal government enacted the Patient Self-Determination Act of 1990. This act requires hospitals and physicians to provide patients and their families with sufficient information to make informed decisions about medical treatment and the use of life-support measures, including cardiopulmonary resuscitation (CPR), artificial ventilation, nutrition, hydration, and blood transfusions.

Patients and their families are therefore more likely than ever to have prepared a written statement of the patient's own preference for future medical care, or an **advance directive.** An advance directive is a document created to ensure that certain treatment choices are honored when a patient is unconscious or otherwise unable to express his choice of treatments. They come in a variety of forms. The most common encountered in the field are: living wills, durable powers of attorney for health care, Do Not Resuscitate orders, and organ donor cards.

The types of advance directives recognized in each state are governed by state law and local protocols. Medical direction must establish and implement policies for dealing with advance directives in the field. Those policies should clearly define the obligations of a paramedic who is caring for a patient with an advance directive. They should also provide for reasonable measures of comfort to the patient and emotional support to the patient's family and loved ones. Some states do not allow paramedics to honor living wills in the field, but do allow them to honor valid Do Not Resuscitate orders. Be sure you are familiar with your state law and local policies.

Review

Advance Directives

- Living wills
- Durable powers of attorney for health care
- DNR orders
- Organ donor cards (such as found on a driver's license)

Living Will

A **living will** is a legal document that allows a person to specify the kinds of medical treatment he wishes to receive should the need arise (Figure 6-4 ■). For example, many states allow patients to include in living wills their wishes concerning dying in a hospital or at home, receiving CPR, and donation of their organs and other body parts. In addition, patients with prolonged illnesses sometimes invoke the right to choose a person who may make health care decisions for them in the event that their mental functions become impaired. They might formalize this decision by way of a special notation in a living will. (They may also do this through execution of a document called a "Durable Power of Attorney for Health Care" or "Health Care Proxy.") Living wills, once signed and witnessed, are effective until they are revoked by the patient.

Be sure you know your local protocols concerning living wills. If any question arises on scene, contact medical direction for instructions.

Do Not Resuscitate Orders

A **Do Not Resuscitate (DNR) order** is a common type of advance directive (Figure 6-5 ■). Usually signed by the patient and his physician, the DNR order is a legal document that indicates to medical personnel which, if any, life-sustaining measures should be taken when the patient's heart and respiratory functions have ceased. DNR orders generally direct EMS personnel to withhold CPR in the event of a cardiac arrest. When you honor a DNR order, do not simply pack up your equipment and leave the scene. You still may have the patient's family and loved ones to attend to. Provide emotional support as appropriate.

LIVING WILL

I, _____ _____ , make the following Living Will declaration to my family, physicians, hospitals, and other health-care providers and any Court or Judge:

After thoughtful consideration and while I am of sound mind, I make this statement as an expression of my settled and firm wishes if the time comes when I can no longer take part in decisions about my own future health.

My Wishes. If at any time I have a terminal condition, and in the opinion of my attending or treating physician there is no reasonable probability that I will recover and the condition can be expected to cause my death within a relatively short time if medical procedures which serve only to prolong the process of dying are not used, or if I am in a persistent vegetative state in which I have no voluntary action or cognitive behavior and cannot communicate or interact purposefully and which is a permanent and irreversible condition of unconsciousness, **I request that I be allowed to die naturally and not be kept alive by artificial means.** I ask that all life-prolonging procedures, including medical assistance to eat and drink when it is highly unlikely that I will regain the capacity to eat and drink without medical assistance, be withheld or withdrawn in such a situation.

Resuscitation. It is my further wish that no cardiopulmonary resuscitation shall thereafter be administered to me if I sustain a cardiac or respiratory arrest. In those circumstances I consent to an order not to resuscitate, and direct that such an order be placed in my medical record.

I direct that these decisions shall be carried into effect even if I am unable to personally reconfirm or communicate them, without seeking judicial approval or authority.

I recognize that there may be instances besides those described above for which life-sustaining treatment should be withheld or withdrawn and this instrument shall not be construed as an exclusive enumeration of these circumstances.

Revocation and Responsibility. This instrument and its instructions may be revoked by me at any time and in any manner. However, no physician, hospital, or other health-care provider who withholds or withdraws life-sustaining treatment in reliance upon this Living Will or upon my personally communicated instructions shall have any liability or responsibility to me, my estate, or any other persons for having withheld or withdrawn treatment.

I intend this declaration be accepted in the circumstances described as an exercise of my legal right to refuse medical treatment even if I am unable to personally reconfirm or communicate that. It is made in the presence of the witnesses who have signed below in my presence.

Signed on (date): _____

Signature: _____

Witness: _____

Witness: _____

Figure 6-4 Example of a "living will."

133

PREHOSPITAL DO NOT RESUSCITATE ORDERS

ATTENDING PHYSICIAN

In completing this prehospital DNR form, please check part A if no intervention by prehospital personnel is indicated. Please check Part A and options from Part B if specific interventions by prehospital personnel are indicated. To give a valid prehospital DNR order, this form must be completed by the patient's attending physician and must be provided to prehospital personnel.

A) _____ **Do Not Resuscitate (DNR):**
No Cardiopulmonary Resuscitation or Advanced Cardiac Life Support be performed by prehospital personnel

B) _____ **Modified Support:**
Prehospital personnel administer the following checked options:
_____ Oxygen administration
_____ Full airway support: intubation, airways, bag/valve/mask
_____ Venipuncture: IV crystalloids and/or blood draw
_____ External cardiac pacing
_____ Cardiopulmonary resuscitation
_____ Cardiac defibrillator
_____ Pneumatic anti-shock garment
_____ Ventilator
_____ ACLS meds
_____ Other interventions/medications (physician specify)
_____

Prehospital personnel are informed that (print patient name)_____
should receive no resuscitation (DNR) or should receive Modified Support as indicated. This directive is medically appropriate and is further documented by a physician's order and a progress note on the patient's permanent medical record. Informed consent from the capacitated patient or the incapacitated patient's legitimate surrogate is documented on the patient's permanent medical record. The DNR order is in full force and effect as of the date indicated below.

_____   _____

Attending Physician's Signature   _____

_____   _____

Print Attending Physician's Name   Print Patient's Name and Location
(Home Address or Health Care Facility)

_____

Attending Physician's Telephone

_____   _____

Date   Expiration Date (6 Mos from Signature)

Figure 6-5   Example of an EMS "Do Not Resuscitate" order.

DNR orders pose a particular problem in the field. Paramedics are often called to nursing homes or residences where they find a patient in cardiac arrest and in need of resuscitation. As a rule, you are legally obligated to attempt resuscitation. If a physician has written a specific order to avoid it, the paramedics should not have been summoned. Even so, people tend to panic and will call for help. Valid DNR orders should be honored as your protocols allow. Note, however, that if there is any doubt as to the patient's wishes, resuscitation should be initiated.

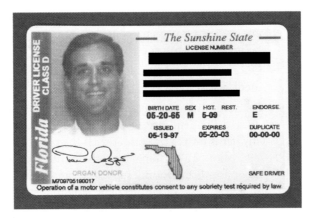

■ Figure 6-6 An indication that a person is willing to be an organ donor may appear on the driver's license.

Occasionally, you may be requested to treat a patient as a "slow code" or "chemical code only." This is not legally permitted. Cardiac resuscitation is an all-or-nothing proposition. Treating a cardiac arrest with only medications would mean abandoning airway management and defibrillation. To do so, even at the request of the family, amounts to negligence and must be avoided.

Potential Organ Donation

Over the past few years, advances in medicines have led to an increased number of organ transplants and a higher survival rate of transplant patients. As organs and tissues are in very high demand and short supply, many EMS systems are now becoming a vital link in the organ procurement and transplant process. Some have developed protocols that specifically address organ viability after a patient's death. These include providing circulatory support through IV fluids and CPR and ventilatory support via endotracheal tube. Whether or not your EMS has protocols in place for potential organ donation, it is important for you to consult with on-line medical direction when you have identified a patient as a potential donor (Figure 6-6 ■).

Some states require that relatives of a recently deceased person be asked about the possibility of organ donation. Become familiar with your state's laws on organ donation.

DEATH IN THE FIELD

Whether you arrive at the scene of a patient who has died prior to your arrival or you make an authorized decision to terminate resuscitative efforts, a death in the field must be appropriately dealt with and thoroughly documented. Paramedics should carefully follow state and local protocols. It is also important for the paramedic to contact on-line medical direction for guidance.

CRIME AND ACCIDENT SCENES

Since it may be your duty as a paramedic to treat a patient found at a crime scene, you should be aware of crime-scene preservation issues. However, you must not sacrifice patient care to preserve evidence or to become involved in detective work. You can best assist investigating officers by properly treating the patient and by doing your best to avoid destroying any potential evidence. As a paramedic, your responsibilities at a crime scene include the following:

★ If you believe a crime may have been committed on scene, immediately contact law enforcement if they are not already involved.

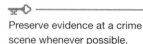

Preserve evidence at a crime scene whenever possible.

★ Protect yourself and the safety of other EMS personnel. This should always be your primary consideration. You will not be held liable for failing to act if a scene is not safe to enter.

★ Once a crime scene has been deemed safe, initiate patient contact and medical care.

★ Do not move or touch anything at a crime scene unless it is necessary to do so for patient care. Observe and document the original placement of any items moved by your crew. If the patient's clothing has holes made by a gunshot or a stabbing, leave them intact, if possible. If the patient has an obvious mortal wound, such as decapitation, try not to touch the body at all. Do your best to protect any potential evidence.

★ If you need to remove items from the scene, such as an impaled weapon or bottle of medication, be sure to document your actions and notify investigating officers.

You should treat the scene of an accident in the same way. Your goals are to ensure your own safety and the safety of your crew and to treat your patients as medically indicated. Use the resources available to you, and be prepared to summon additional personnel and rescue equipment as necessary.

DOCUMENTATION

The importance of developing and maintaining superior documentation skills and habits cannot be overemphasized. As a paramedic, you must recognize that the treatment of your patient does not end until you have properly documented the entire incident from initial response to the transfer of patient care to the hospital emergency department staff.

A complete, well-written patient care report is your best protection in a malpractice action. In fact, a well-written report may actually discourage a plaintiff from filing a malpractice case in the first place. In general, a plaintiff's attorney will request copies of all medical records, including the paramedic's report, before filing a lawsuit. If the paramedic's report is sloppy, incomplete, or otherwise not well written, this may encourage the plaintiff to sue, even if the paramedic's conduct was not negligent.

A well-documented patient care report has the following characteristics:

★ *It is completed promptly after patient contact.* It should be made in the course of business, not long after the event. Any delay could cause you to forget important observations or treatments. If possible, a copy of the completed report should be left with the emergency department staff before you leave the hospital. This copy will become part of the patient's permanent medical records. Proper documentation is so important that some EMS systems now require paramedics to dictate their reports, which are later transcribed and placed in the patient's permanent records (Figure 6-7 ■).

Note: Never delay patient care to attend to a patient care report.

★ *It is thorough.* The report should paint a clear and complete picture of the patient's condition and the care that was provided. Its main purpose is not simply to record patient data, but also to support the diagnosis and treatment that you provided to the patient. All actions, procedures, and

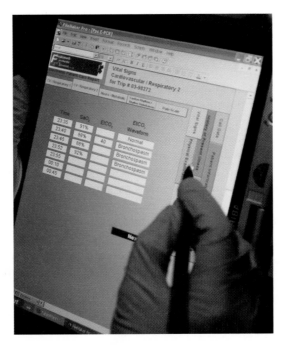

■ Figure 6-7 Some EMS systems require paramedics to dictate their patient care reports, which are later transcribed and placed in the patient's medical records. *(© Jeff Forster)*

administered medications should be documented as well. Remember: "If you didn't write it down, you didn't do it."

★ *It is objective.* Avoid the use of emotional and value-loaded words. Not only are they irrelevant to patient care, but they also may be the cause of a libel suit against you.

★ *It is accurate.* Be as precise as possible, avoiding the use of abbreviations and jargon that are not commonly understood. Also try to limit your report to information that you have personally seen or heard. If you need to document something that you do not have personal knowledge of, be sure to indicate the source of your information. Document your observations, not your assumptions, and do not draw a medical conclusion that you are not competent to make. For example, you cannot conclusively diagnose a patient as having pneumonia. You can, however, report your suspicion of pneumonia and document findings that are consistent with this condition.

★ *It maintains patient confidentiality.* Your agency should have well-defined policies regarding the release of patient information. Whenever possible, patient consent should be obtained prior to release of information.

The medical record should never be altered. An intentional alteration amounts to an admission of guilt by the paramedic. If a patient care report is found to be incomplete or inaccurate, a written amendment should be attached to the report. The date and time the amendment was written, not the date of the original report, should be noted on the addendum. Also, be sure to send a copy of the addendum to the receiving hospital so that it will become a part of the patient's medical records.

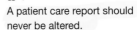

A patient care report should never be altered.

Medical records need to be maintained for a period of time that is prescribed by state law. For example, in New York State patient care reports must be maintained by an EMS agency for a period of 6 years, or 3 years after the patient reaches the age of 18, whichever is longer. Be sure to become familiar with the record retention requirements in your state.

Summary

The very nature of a paramedic's job requires interaction with law enforcement authorities and frequent involvement in situations that can give rise to litigation. For example, not only will police be called to the same emergencies to which paramedics are called, such as motor-vehicle collisions or scenes where violence caused injuries, but paramedics also may become material witnesses to crimes or domestic disputes. It is therefore in your best interest to learn and follow all state laws and local protocols related to your practice as a paramedic.

Also be sure to receive good training and keep current by attending continuing medical education programs and conferences, reading industry journals, and obtaining recertification or relicensure as required by state law.

Remember, a paramedic is not immune from allegations of negligence or malpractice. However, the potential for liability may be limited or avoided by adhering to the following guidelines:

- ★ Always obtain informed consent before initiating treatment and/or transport.
- ★ Practice only those skills and procedures that a reasonable and prudent paramedic would, given the same or similar circumstances.
- ★ Practice only those procedures that you are trained to perform and are directly authorized to perform by a medical-control physician or by approved local standing orders.
- ★ Prepare accurate, legible, and complete medical records that thoroughly document the entire EMS incident, from initial response to the transfer of patient care to hospital emergency department staff.
- ★ Discuss patient information with only those who need to know. Limit writings and oral reports to information essential to patient care.
- ★ Purchase and maintain malpractice insurance, and see that your employer does the same.
- ★ Be nice to your patients and their families.

Always act in good faith and use your common sense. High-quality patient care and high-quality documentation are always your best protection from liability.

High-quality patient care and high-quality documentation are always your best protection from liability.

You Make the Call

You and the rest of the crew of EMS Unit 116 receive a call to assist an unconscious 5-year-old girl. Upon arriving at the scene, you are met by the child's babysitter, who states that for the past hour the child had been acting "strangely," after which she fell asleep and would not wake up. The babysitter also tells you that the child had been playing in her bedroom alone all afternoon. You ask the babysitter to call the child's parents immediately. She tells you that they are unreachable but are expected home in approximately 20 minutes.

While your partner searches the child's room, you assess the patient and note the following physical findings: respiratory depression, hypotension, bradycardia, and constricted pupils. Quickly searching, your partner finds an empty bottle of Darvocet under the child's bed. You now suspect a narcotic overdose and determine that the child needs immediate medical intervention and transport to an appropriate medical facility. You prepare to start an IV, when the babysitter tells you that she will not consent to treatment and tells you to wait for the parents to return home. A neighbor arrives on scene and insists that the child's parents would want only the family physician to treat her, and begs you to drive her there.

1. You believe that the child needs emergency care, but the child's parents are unavailable. What should you do?
2. If you decide to treat the child without consent, can you be sued for doing so?
3. What would you do if the parents returned home and refused to grant permission for treatment?

See Suggested Responses at the back of this book.

Review Questions

1. _____ _____ originated with the English legal system and was adopted by Americans in the 1700s.
   a. common law
   b. civil law
   c. criminal law
   d. constitutional law

2. _____ _____ is enacted by an administrative or governmental agency at either the federal or state level.
   a. civil law
   b. criminal law
   c. legislative law
   d. administrative law

3. The _____ _____ is the location of most of the cases in which a paramedic may become involved.
   a. appellate court system
   b. state court system
   c. federal court system
   d. supreme court system

4. On-scene licensed physicians who are professionally unrelated to the patient and who are attempting to assist with patient care are called:
   a. intervener physicians.
   b. direct control physicians.
   c. on-line medical control.
   d. indirect control physicians.

5. Legislative statutes that generally protect the person who provides care at no charge at the scene of a medical emergency are called:
   a. medical practice laws.
   b. scope of practice laws.
   c. Good Samaritan laws.
   d. standard of care laws.

6. In a negligence claim against a paramedic, the plaintiff must establish and prove four particular elements in order to prevail. Which of the following is not one of those elements?
   a. proximate cause
   b. duty to act
   c. level of compensation
   d. breach of the duty to act

7. The law provides penalties for the breach of confidentiality. The improper release of information may result in a lawsuit against the paramedic for:
   a. defamation.
   b. invasion of privacy.
   c. breach of confidentiality.
   d. all of the above.

8. This court-ordered type of consent is most commonly encountered with patients who must be held for mental-health evaluation or as directed by law enforcement personnel who have the patient under arrest.
   a. implied
   b. expressed
   c. involuntary
   d. guardianship

9. _____ is the termination of the paramedic-patient relationship without providing for the appropriate continuation of care while it is still needed and desired by the patient.
   a. libel
   b. slander
   c. neglect
   d. abandonment

10. A well-documented patient care report is:
    a. accurate.
    b. objective.
    c. thorough.
    d. all of the above.

See Answers to Review Questions at the back of this book.

Further Reading

The Ambulance Service Guide to HIPAA Compliance. Mechanicsburg, PA: Page, Wolfberg, & Wirth, 2003.

Cohn, B. M., and A. J. Azzara. *Legal Aspects of Emergency Medical Services.* Philadelphia: W. B. Saunders, 1998.

Lee, N. G. *Legal Concepts and Issues in Emergency Care.* Philadelphia: W. B. Saunders, 2001.

Louisell, D., and H. Williams. *Medical Malpractice.* New York: Matthew Bender, 1995.

Page, J. O. "Anatomy of a Lawsuit." *JEMS* 14 (1989).

Schneid, Thomas D. *Fire and Emergency Law Case Book.* Albany, NY: Delmar Publishing, 1997.

On the Web

Visit Brady's Paramedic Website at **www.bradybooks.com/paramedic**.

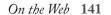

Ethics in Advanced Prehospital Care

Objectives

After reading this chapter, you should be able to:

1. Define ethics and morals. (p. 144)
2. Distinguish between ethical and moral decisions in emergency medical service. (pp. 144–151)
3. Identify the premise that should underlie the paramedic's ethical decisions in out-of-hospital care. (p. 146)
4. Analyze the relationship between the law and ethics in EMS. (p. 144)
5. Compare and contrast the criteria used in allocating scarce EMS resources. (pp. 155–156)
6. Identify issues surrounding advance directives in making a prehospital resuscitation decision. (pp. 151–153)
7. Describe the criteria necessary to honor an advance directive in your state. (pp. 151–153)
8. Given several narrative circumstances, make decisions in keeping with the ethical principles associated with EMS. (pp. 140–156)

Key Terms

Case Study

Mrs. Weinberg has fractured her hip. Her right lower extremity is obviously shortened and externally rotated. Fortunately, she has no apparent life-threatening injuries. As you and your partner tend to her, you notice that she seems more anxious than other patients you have seen with a similar problem. When your partner goes to the ambulance to retrieve additional pillows, she whispers to you, "I would really prefer if you took care of me."

"Why?" you ask.

She rolls up her sleeve and shows you a tattoo of a number on her left forearm. "This is why," she says. "When I was a little girl back in Germany, I was in a Nazi concentration camp. Your partner reminds me of the men who worked there. They killed my family, and they almost killed me. Could you take care of me on the way to the hospital?"

You do not have much time to think about this question, but you promise to help. Before you leave the scene, you approach your partner discreetly. "Heinz," you say to him, "this patient is a concentration camp survivor. Apparently your blond hair, blue eyes, and German accent remind her of the men who killed her family. Would you mind driving to the hospital on this call? I realize you enrolled in an exchange program to gain experience in patient care here in the United States, but there will be other calls." Heinz has no objection, so he drives to the hospital, and you take care of Mrs. Weinberg in the back of the ambulance.

After the call, the two of you discuss what happened. "Boy," you say, "I've never had a patient make a request like that. I think it was really great of you to accommodate her. Did it make you uncomfortable?" "No," he says, "but it surprised me." You agree that the best way to make Mrs. Weinberg comfortable was to switch places. You also agree that the two of you handled a difficult situation gracefully.

Later, when you think about the call a little more, you realize that this situation was truly a first for you. Is it right, you wonder, to accommodate a request like this? Heinz was not going to harm her. Were you assuaging her fears or validating her prejudices? What if the patient had been an elderly man who asked you to switch places with your black partner? Would the patient's ignorance have been enough of a reason to accommodate him? What if the patient had been a neo-Nazi skinhead who insisted on having a white person care for him?

Was the situation just a matter of being courteous, as you first thought? After all, no one was hurt, and it was only a minor inconvenience for you and your partner to switch positions. Or was it actually a matter of ethics? You realize you are not quite sure how to determine the best thing to do under circumstances like these. It is time, you realize, to brush up on your ethics.

INTRODUCTION

When asked what the most difficult part of the job is, most paramedics do not say "ethics." Nonetheless, in one recent survey almost 15 percent of advanced life support calls in an urban EMS system generated some ethical conflict.[1] In another survey, EMS providers responded that they frequently have ethical problems related to patients refusing care, conflicts regarding hospital destination, and difficulties with advance directives.[2] Other aspects of prehospital care present potential ethical problems. These include patient confidentiality, consent, the obligation to provide care, and research.

Although ethical problems often have a legal aspect, most ethical problems are solved in the field and not in a courtroom. However, there are times when ethical problems spill over into the legal arena and become the subject of legislation or regulations. The federal government, for instance, recently instituted rules to protect patients who are unable to consent to emergency care.

Ethical issues often begin with specific circumstances and lead to broad general rules or principles for behavior. This chapter examines how the most common principles and approaches are applied to common prehospital situations.

OVERVIEW OF ETHICS

morals *social, religious, or personal standards of right and wrong.*

ethics *the rules or standards that govern the conduct of members of a particular group or profession.*

Ethics and morals are closely related concepts. **Morals** are generally considered to be social, religious, or personal standards of right and wrong. **Ethics** more often refers to the rules or standards that govern the conduct of members of a particular group or profession, and how our institutions should function. Both ethics and morals address a question Socrates asked: "How should one live?"

RELATIONSHIP OF ETHICS TO LAW AND RELIGION

Ethics and the law have a great deal in common, but they are distinctly separate disciplines (Figure 7-1 ■). Although ethical discussions have an unfortunate tendency to degenerate into arguments about what is legal and who might be liable, ethics is not the same as law. In general, laws have a much narrower focus than ethics. Laws frequently describe what is wrong in the eyes of society. Ethics goes beyond examining what is wrong. It also looks at what is right, or good, behavior. As a result, the law frequently has little or nothing to say about ethical problems. In fact, laws themselves can be unethical. For example, for many years laws existed and were enforced that perpetuated racial segregation in the United States. These were ethically wrong and, ultimately, made legally wrong.

Even though ethics and the law are different, ethical discussions can sometimes benefit from techniques developed by the law over the centuries. In particular, the law emphasizes impartiality, consistent procedures, and methods to identify and balance conflicting interests.

Just as ethics differs from the law, it also differs from religion. In a pluralistic society such as ours, ethics must be understood by and applied to people who hold a broad range of religious beliefs, or no religious beliefs at all. Thus, ethics cannot derive from

[1] Adams, J. G., R. Arnold, L. Siminoff, and A. B. Wolfson. "Ethical Conflicts in the Prehospital Setting." *Annals of Emergency Medicine* 21 (1992).

[2] Heilicser, B., C. Stocking, and M. Siegler. "Ethical Dilemmas in Emergency Medical Services: The Perspective of the Emergency Medical Technician." *Annals of Emergency Medicine* 27 (1996).

Cultural Considerations

Cultural Responses to Illness and Injury The population of North America has certainly become a cultural blend. You can see it in the different ways people respond to serious illness or injury. Some may look at an illness as a disease process with predictable results. Others may look at it as destiny. Others will simply attribute an illness to God's will. In some cultures, certain illnesses and injuries are believed to be the work of the devil or a result of witchcraft, curses, or spells. To those who believe, such interpretations are as real and as plausible as any other. For them, the only successful treatment possible may involve countering the effects of the curse or spell in question. Thus, they may not have much confidence that your skilled prehospital care will make much of a difference.

Paramedics must recognize that people of different cultural backgrounds respond to illnesses and injuries in different ways. Never criticize or chastise patients for beliefs that differ from yours. These beliefs are so culturally ingrained that a single contact with an EMS provider is unlikely to change them. It is important to acknowledge such beliefs and never to ridicule those who hold them.

Relationship of Ethical and Legal Issues with Medicine

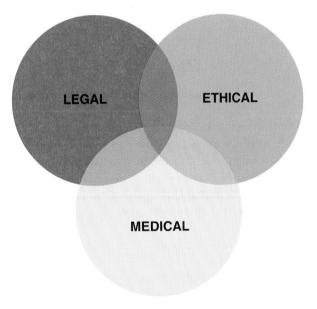

■ Figure 7-1 The relationship of ethical and legal issues and medicine.

a single religion. It is true, however, that religion can enhance and enrich one's ethical principles and values.

MAKING ETHICAL DECISIONS

There are many different approaches one can use to determine how a medical professional should behave under different circumstances. One approach is to say that each person must decide how to behave and whatever decision that person makes is okay. This approach is known as *ethical relativism*. People sometimes say they believe in ethical relativism. However, when questioned, they typically admit they do not find it satisfactory. For example, no reasonable person would say that it was acceptable for the Nazis to behave as they did.

A similar approach is to say, "Just do what is right." This sounds fine but in reality does not answer the question of how a health care professional should act. This occurs because different people have different beliefs about what is "right." Ethics and morality overlap, but professional ethics go beyond what one individual thinks is right or wrong. Even the Golden Rule—"Do unto others as you would have them do unto you"—is not a sufficient guideline. What happens when the person making the decision has desires and values that are radically different from the patient's? It becomes clear that reason and logic must be used and emotion must be excluded as much as possible from the decision-making process.

Another approach is to say that people should just fulfill their duties. This is known as the *deontological method*. A very simple example of this approach is someone who says, "Just follow the Ten Commandments." Unfortunately, although the Ten Commandments provide useful instruction, they do not provide enough guidance for medical professionals who must make difficult ethical decisions in health care situations.

A very different approach is *consequentialism*. Followers of this school of thought believe that actions can be judged as good or bad only after we know the consequences of those actions. Utilitarians, who believe that the purpose of an action should be to bring the greatest happiness to the greatest number of people, are consequentialists. One difficulty with the utilitarians' approach is determining what constitutes happiness. Another challenge arises when the happiness of one person is in conflict with the happiness of another person. Utilitarianism offers a "bankbook" approach to resolving these conflicts, asking the decision maker to weigh relative "amounts" of happiness.

CODES OF ETHICS

Over the years, a number of organizations have drafted codes of ethics for the members of their organizations. The American Medical Association has a code of ethics for physicians. The American College of Emergency Physicians has a code of ethics specifically for emergency physicians. The American Nurses Association and Emergency Nurses Association both have codes for practitioners in their fields. The National Association of EMTs adopted a code of ethics for EMTs in 1978 (see Chapter 4). Most codes of ethics address broad humanitarian concerns and professional etiquette. Few provide solid guidance on the kind of ethical problems commonly faced by practitioners.

IMPACT OF ETHICS ON INDIVIDUAL PRACTICE

Only by consistently displaying ethical behavior will paramedics gain and maintain the respect of their colleagues and their patients. It is vital that individual paramedics exemplify the principles and values of their profession. Paramedics must understand and agree to abide by the responsibilities, both implicit and explicit, of their profession. Occasionally, this can be a problem. A paramedic is expected to work, for example, in an uncontrolled environment that is sometimes dangerous. A person who is unwilling to enter a scene until every risk has been totally eliminated is not acting in accordance with the expectations of the profession. Conversely, a paramedic is expected to refrain from entering a hazardous area until the risks have been made manageable. Common sense should help in resolving conflicts such as these.

THE FUNDAMENTAL QUESTIONS

The single most important question a paramedic has to answer when faced with an ethical challenge is "What is in the patient's best interest?" Most of the time the answer to this question is obvious: The patient wants reassurance, relief from pain, and prompt, safe transport to a hospital emergency department. But sometimes the answer to this question is not so obvious. For example, what is in the best interest of a terminally ill patient who goes into cardiac arrest? Is it to resuscitate him? Or is it to not start resuscitation in order to prevent further suffering?

Under ideal circumstances, a written statement describing the patient's desires will be available. In many states, such a statement (which meets other specified state and local requirements) is in fact required before a paramedic may elect not to start resuscitation efforts. In less extreme circumstances, the patient may state verbally what he wishes you to do and not do. As long as the patient is competent and the desires are consistent with good practice, the paramedic is obligated to respect the patient's desires.

Traditionally, family members have been an important source of information for physicians in determining the wishes of a patient. This approach, however, is not necessarily appropriate in the field. In the hospital or especially in the years before a hospital admission, physicians are able to spend time with the patient and the patient's family and develop a relationship with them. In the field, paramedics typically do not know the patient or the family. There is usually not enough time for a paramedic to develop the same kind of relationship that physicians do in their practices. Additionally, the family is under a great deal of stress when the paramedic encounters them.

For these reasons and others, a paramedic must be very cautious in accepting a family's description of what a patient desires. The paramedic must also take into consideration the state and local laws regarding patient resuscitation desires and documentation of those desires.

It may sometimes be difficult for a paramedic to agree with a patient's wishes, but it is important that he respect them. Only by demonstrating "good faith" in following a patient's wishes does a paramedic show respect for the patient. A paramedic must also realize that the family may not agree with the patient's desires. This may lead family members to substitute their own desires for the patient's. This is another reason why the paramedic should not necessarily accept a family's description of a patient's desires at face value.

FUNDAMENTAL PRINCIPLES

A common approach to resolving problems in bioethics today is to employ four fundamental principles or values. These principles are **beneficence, nonmaleficence, autonomy,** and **justice.**

Beneficence is related to a more familiar term, *benevolence.* Both come from Latin and concern doing good. However, *benevolence* means the *desire* to do good (usually the main reason people become paramedics), whereas *beneficence* means actually *doing* good (the paramedic's obligation to the patient).

Maleficence means doing harm, the opposite of *beneficence. Nonmaleficence* means *not* doing harm. Few medical interventions are without risk of harm. Under the principle of nonmaleficence, however, the paramedic is obligated to minimize that risk as much as possible. This includes, for example, making the scene safe and protecting the patient from impaired or unqualified health care providers. The Latin phrase, *primum non nocere,* which means "first, do no harm," sums up nonmaleficence very well.

Autonomy refers to a competent adult patient's right to determine what happens to his own body, including treatment for medical illnesses and injuries. The paramedic has an obligation to respect this right of self-determination. Under ordinary conditions, a patient must give consent before the paramedic can begin treatment. There are, of course, exceptions to this, including the patient who is not competent

beneficence *the principle of doing good for the patient.*

nonmaleficence *the obligation not to harm the patient.*

autonomy *a competent adult patient's right to determine what happens to his own body.*

justice *the obligation to treat all patients fairly.*

First, do no harm (*primum non nocere*).

and for whom the doctrine of implied consent applies. But the competent patient must receive accurate information in order to make an informed decision. This implies that the paramedic must be truthful in describing to the patient his condition and the risks and benefits of treatment for it. It also implies respect for the patient's privacy.

Justice refers to the paramedic's obligation to treat all patients fairly. For example, the paramedic should provide necessary emergency care to all patients without regard to sex, race, ability to pay, or cultural background, among other conditions.

RESOLVING ETHICAL CONFLICTS

Even if everyone agreed upon the same principles and procedures for resolving ethical difficulties, there would still be disagreements in specific situations. These disagreements can be resolved at different levels. Even the government sometimes takes action when issues become very important to the public. For example, there are now laws to protect the rights of hospitalized patients and members of managed-care organizations. Many states have implemented laws or regulations that allow for the use of advance directives. The federal government has instituted rules to protect the rights of patients in emergency research when they are unable to consent.

The health care community has also responded to the challenge. Long before the federal government instituted rules regarding consent in emergency research, hospitals and universities set up institutional review boards (IRBs). These groups serve to protect the rights of subjects participating in research projects. Hospitals throughout the world have had ethics committees for many years to assist in clarifying patients' desires and in weighing competing interests in ethically challenging situations.

The paramedic, however, cannot depend on these institutions to assist in the field. He needs to have a system for resolving these conflicts, one that will allow him to weigh the various factors, including all relevant facts, principles, and values, that lead to responsible, defensible actions. One such system or method of resolving ethical issues before or after they arise is illustrated in the following scenario:

> You are the official representative of your service to the regional EMS coordinating agency. At the most recent meeting, the head nurse for the emergency department of the largest hospital in the county mentioned how recent cutbacks in support staff had led to more difficulty retrieving patients' medical records in a timely manner. This has led to a number of difficulties in treating patients. As a result, the ED was considering asking incoming ambulances to give patients' names and dates of birth on the radio. This would give the ED staff additional time to search for the patient's medical records.
>
> After the meeting, you consider the issue's ethical aspects. First, you identify the problem, which in this case is: Is it justifiable to breach patient confidentiality in order to expedite the retrieval of medical records? Second, you list the possible actions that might be taken in this situation. Possibilities include:
>
> • Provide all patients' names and dates of birth on the radio.
> • Continue the current policy of identifying patients only by age and sex.
> • Provide selected patients' names and dates of birth on the radio.

To reason out an ethical problem, first state the action in a universal form. Then list the implications or consequences of the action. Finally, compare them to relevant values (Figure 7-2 ■). The application of this method to the scenario described would be as follows:

✓ Review

Solving an Ethical Problem

1. State the action in a universal form.
2. List the implications or consequences of the action.
3. Compare them to relevant values.

Content

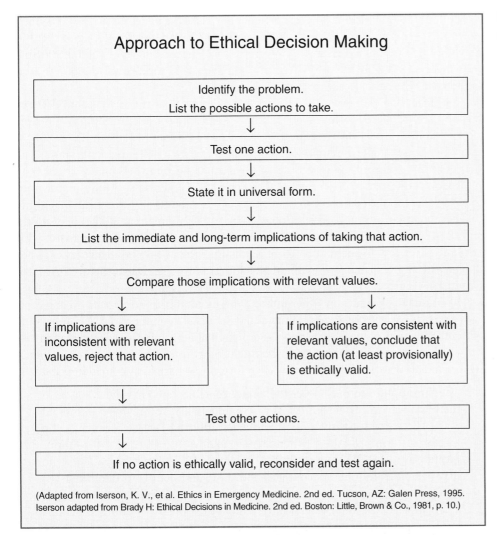

Figure 7-2 An approach to ethical decision making.

Approach to Ethical Decision Making

Identify the problem.
List the possible actions to take.

↓

Test one action.

↓

State it in universal form.

↓

List the immediate and long-term implications of taking that action.

↓

Compare those implications with relevant values.

↓　　　　　　　　　　↓

If implications are inconsistent with relevant values, reject that action.

If implications are consistent with relevant values, conclude that the action (at least provisionally) is ethically valid.

↓

Test other actions.

↓

If no action is ethically valid, reconsider and test again.

(Adapted from Iserson, K. V., et al. Ethics in Emergency Medicine. 2nd ed. Tucson, AZ: Galen Press, 1995. Iserson adapted from Brady H: Ethical Decisions in Medicine. 2nd ed. Boston: Little, Brown & Co., 1981, p. 10.)

To state an action in a universal form, describe what should be done, who should do it, and under what conditions. For example, EMS (who) will volunteer names and dates of birth for all patients (what) on the radio (condition).

The immediate implications are that the ED will be able to get records sooner for patients who have records at that hospital. There will be no change for most patients because hospital records are often irrelevant to emergency care. The ED admitting staff may be able to admit patients more quickly. However, patients' names and dates of birth will be broadcast to thousands of people listening with scanners. The long-term consequences are that people with scanners will learn more about patients who go to the hospital via EMS. Because private information may be broadcast, patients may become reluctant to call EMS. Conceivably, there may be more burglaries at homes of patients who use EMS.

Finally, compare those consequences to values that are relevant. A list of values that pertain to this case might include: beneficence, nonmaleficence, autonomy, and confidentiality. That is, if EMS provided names and dates of birth for all patients on the radio, what would be the benefit to the patient (beneficence)? A few patients might be cared for sooner because their records arrived sooner. Most patients will see no benefit because they have no records at that hospital or time is not a significant issue (such as for a laceration that requires sutures).

Autonomy suffers under this arrangement because the patient is not given the opportunity to consent (or decline). The patient's name and date of birth go out over the air without his permission. And, in this case, nonmaleficence and confidentiality are intertwined. There is potential for harm to the patient and to future patients who lose faith in the EMS system's ability to maintain privacy.

So, since the possible consequences of providing all patients' names and dates of birth on the radio are not compatible with the values we consider important and relevant, you must go back and test another action using this same method.

When you evaluate the choice of continuing the current policy of identifying all patients over the radio only by age and sex, you may find the following consequences: People listening to scanners can learn facts about patients EMS is transporting, but no more than they have in the past; a few patients may get care that is delayed or less than optimal because their hospital records do not arrive quickly enough; and the ED staff are still stressed because they cannot get records in a timely manner. A comparison with relevant values reveals that patient confidentiality and patient confidence in EMS are unchanged, but the patients who might benefit from earlier arrival of their records may be suffering.

Continue to evaluate any other options you listed. In this case, the third and final one is: Provide selected patients' names and dates of birth on the radio. A comparison with relevant values shows that there is some potential benefit for selected patients, a breach of confidentiality for patients who might benefit, and no breach of confidentiality for patients who would not benefit. Therefore, the scenario may conclude as follows:

> The third option sounds closer to being acceptable, but you might wonder if there is a way to further limit loss of confidentiality. You revise your rule to read, "EMS broadcasts the initials and dates of birth of selected patients who meet predetermined criteria when there is no other private means of communication available." This strictly limits the loss of confidentiality to patients who may benefit from it and encourages both EMS and the ED to find other less public means of identifying patients. For example, paramedics could broadcast a patient's age, sex, and hospital card number or, if the patient does not have a hospital identification card available and time allows, someone at the scene could telephone the ED to relay the patient's name and date of birth privately.

The method just described is useful when you come upon a new ethical problem and time is not an issue. In situations where time is limited, an abbreviated method can sometimes be used (Figure 7-3 ■). First, ask yourself whether the current problem is similar to other problems for which you have already formulated a rule. Then, if the answer is yes, follow that rule. If the answer is no, determine if you can do something to buy time. Finally, if you can find a reasonable way to postpone dealing with the issue for a while, do so. If you cannot, analyze the best rule you have against three tests suggested by Iserson:[3] the *impartiality test*, the *universalizability test*, and the *interpersonal justifiability test*:

- ★ *Impartiality test*—asks whether you would be willing to undergo this procedure or action if you were in the patient's place. This is really a version of the Golden Rule (Do unto others as you would have them do unto you), which helps to reduce the possibility of bias.

- ★ *Universalizability test*—asks whether you would want this action performed in all relevantly similar circumstances, which helps the paramedic to avoid shortsightedness.

Content

✓ Review

Quick Ways to Test Ethics

- Impartiality test
- Universalizability test
- Interpersonal justifiability test

---

[3] Iserson, K. V., et al. *Ethics in Emergency Medicine.* 2nd ed. Tucson, AZ, Galen Press, 1995.

Quick Approach to New Ethical Problems

Consider the ethical problem.

*Do you already have a rule for dealing with this problem?

*Or, can you reasonably extend a rule to apply to the situation?

If yes to either of the above, follow the rule.

If no to the above,

*Can you buy time to consider a solution without causing significant risk to the patient?

*If you cannot, then apply the impartiality test, the universalizability test, or the interpersonal justifiability test.

(Based on Iserson, K. V., et al. Ethics in Emergency Medicine. 2nd ed. Tucson, AZ: Galen Press, 1995.)

■ Figure 7-3   A quick approach to new ethical problems.

★ *Interpersonal justifiability test*—asks whether you can defend or justify your actions to others. It helps to ensure that an action is appropriate by asking the paramedic to consider whether other people would think the action reasonable.

When there is little time to consider a new ethical problem, these three questions can help a paramedic navigate murky waters, allowing him to find an acceptable solution in a short time.

ETHICAL ISSUES IN CONTEMPORARY PARAMEDIC PRACTICE

The first part of the chapter built a foundation for ethical decision making by describing and demonstrating methods for dealing with these types of issues. The following discussion is meant to help you apply those principles to several commonly encountered situations. It also describes some of the ethical considerations to take into account in less common situations you may face.

RESUSCITATION ATTEMPTS

Consider the following scenario:

> You are leaving the emergency department (ED) in your ambulance when an approximately 50-year-old woman jumps out of a window on the third floor of the hospital and lands on the road in front of you. Your partner stops the vehicle, and you get your equipment to begin assessment and management of the patient. As you reach her, a breathless aide runs out the door and says, "Don't do anything! She's got a DNR order!" How does this affect the care you administer?
>
> You have virtually no time to think about what to do for this woman, who is bleeding on the street and appears unresponsive. Your instincts say, treat her now and let the hospital sort things out later if she survives.

In this case, your instincts are probably steering you in the right direction for a number of reasons. First, every state that has laws or rules regarding Do Not Resuscitate (DNR) orders requires that you see the order and verify its legitimacy in some manner. In this case, the order is not available for you to see so you are under no legal obligation to withhold care.

Second, if the patient is alive (as she appears to be), even a valid DNR order would not prevent you from assessing the patient and administering basic care, including comfort care.

Third, the principle of nonmaleficence says do no harm. Refraining from helping her might cause irreversible harm, including perhaps death. The principles of beneficence and nonmaleficence both urge you to help the patient. The potential conflict arises when you consider autonomy. The competent patient of legal age has a right to determine what happens to her body. You have some reason to believe she has determined that she does not wish resuscitation efforts if her heart stops but, in this case, the accuracy of this information cannot be verified.

The conclusion of the scenario is as follows:

Considering the lack of verifiable information and the severe time limitations you are facing, you and your partner go ahead and assess the patient. You find that she responds to verbal stimuli by moaning, her airway is open, ventilations are adequate, and she has several lacerations and apparent fractures. Since you are literally in front of the hospital, you limit your interventions to quick immobilization on a spine board with bleeding control and oxygen by mask. You rapidly move her to the ED and turn her over to the team there.

Later you discover that she had originally been admitted for evaluation of new onset seizures. When the doctors told her she might have a brain tumor, she signed a DNR form. Fortunately, no tumor was found and her prognosis is actually quite good. The trauma team finds no life-threatening injuries from her fall and expects her to be able to begin psychiatric treatment before she leaves the hospital. This additional information makes you very glad you decided to go ahead with treatment.

More and more states are passing laws or regulations allowing prehospital personnel to withhold certain treatment when the patient has a DNR order. A valid order consists of a written statement describing interventions a particular patient does not wish to have that is recognized by the authorities of that state. Before following a DNR order, the paramedic must be aware of several things.

First, the order must meet state and local requirements regarding wording and witnesses (a standardized form is usually available). Also, there may be a time limit on how long a DNR order is valid in certain jurisdictions. A patient with a valid prehospital DNR order may be required to wear or have nearby a particular means of identification, such as a bracelet with a special symbol. There should be a clear description of which interventions are to be withheld and under which circumstances. And finally, every patient is still entitled to reasonable measures intended to make the patient more comfortable (comfort care). Similarly, the family and loved ones are entitled to emotional support from EMS providers. (See Chapter 6 for legal aspects of DNR orders.)

Paramedics spend a great deal of time and energy learning how to assess and treat patients with life-threatening problems. It becomes difficult, then, for a paramedic to watch someone die without doing something to try to stop it. You must nonetheless respect the patient's wishes when a competent patient has clearly communicated what he really wants. DNR orders make this easier because they typically must be signed or approved by a physician, increasing the likelihood that the decision was thoroughly thought through.

When there is no such order, however, it becomes more difficult for the paramedic to determine what the patient's wishes truly are. Family members may be able to describe the patient's desires, but they can have conflicts of interest that make their statements less credible. For example, the patient may have accepted his impending death before his family has. They may want you to attempt resuscitation when that was clearly against the patient's expressed wishes. A less common situation is one in which the patient wishes all resuscitation efforts, but the family does not because they do not wish to prolong their own suffering or they have other less noble motivations.

The general principle for paramedics to follow in cases such as these is: "When in doubt, resuscitate." This usually satisfies the principles of beneficence and nonmaleficence, admittedly perhaps at the expense of autonomy, but one of the biggest advantages to this approach is that, unlike the alternative, it is not irreversible. If you refrain from attempting resuscitation, it is certain that the patient will die. If you attempt resuscitation, there is no guarantee the patient will survive, but the patient can be removed from life-sustaining equipment later if that is deemed appropriate. Another advantage is that there will be more time later to sort out competing interests.

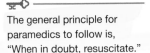

The general principle for paramedics to follow is, "When in doubt, resuscitate."

What about not attempting resuscitation when the situation appears futile? This option may appear attractive at first glance. After a little investigation, though, the issue becomes much more complex. How would a reasonable person or society define "futile"? This is an issue that has received a good deal of attention and the conclusion is that, except at the extreme ends of the spectrum, there is no consensus on what constitutes a futile attempt at resuscitation.

In addition, there is the issue of who would actually make the decision that a resuscitation attempt is futile in a particular case. Is it the experienced paramedic who has seen very few lives saved under similar circumstances or the new paramedic who is still excited about the prospect of saving lives every day? How can it be fair to have such wide disparities in such an important decision? Clearly, the concept of futility does not provide a useful guide for whether or not to attempt resuscitation.

Another related topic is what to do when an advance directive is presented to you after you have begun resuscitation. Once you have verified the validity of the order and the identity of the patient, you are obligated ethically (and perhaps legally, depending on your state) to cease resuscitation efforts. This can be a very difficult situation for you emotionally, but you have an obligation to respect the patient's autonomy and stop doing something to him that he did not want. Follow your local protocols regarding procedures for cessation of resuscitation efforts.

CONFIDENTIALITY

Consider this scenario:

> You are called at one o'clock in the morning to a local hotel for a man reported to be unresponsive (but breathing) at the front desk. When you arrive, one of the guests at the hotel meets you at the front door. He tells you that he tried to call the front desk from his room to request a wake-up call but got no answer. When he went to the front desk, he found the clerk slumped over in his chair, apparently unconscious, with what smelled like alcohol on his breath.
>
> When you approach the patient, you see an approximately 25-year-old male who appears to be unresponsive. His skin appears normal, and he is moving air well. He does not respond when you call him by the name on his name plate, which is Howard. He has a strong, regular radial pulse that is within normal limits. You do not smell anything except for a faint minty odor. When you shake his shoulder and call his name again, he moans. Further shaking and shouting eventually bring him to the point where his eyes are open, he is looking around, and he asks, "Who are you?"

You explain to Howard that you were called by a concerned guest who could not wake him up. Howard says he is fine now and does not want to go to a hospital. He is alert and oriented to person, place, and time. He denies any complaints, takes no medications, and has no past medical history. His vital signs are within normal limits. He denies any alcohol intake or use of any other drugs. The physical exam is unremarkable.

By your protocols and standard operating procedures, you have no reason to attempt to force the patient to go to a hospital. You complete the appropriate documentation for a refusal of transport and are leaving the lobby when the guest who called 911 stops you. "Aren't you going to take him to the hospital?" he asks. No, you reply, he does not want to go. "But what if there's a fire in the hotel and he's passed out and unable to help guests evacuate?"

This makes you stop and think, and you begin to weigh the rights of the hotel guests against the rights of your patient.

Your obligation to the patient is to maintain as confidential the information you obtained as a result of your participation in this medical situation. Clearly, the most beneficial thing you can do for his privacy is not to notify anyone about his condition. Additionally, there are questions regarding what you could accurately report. The patient denies alcohol and drug intake, and you could find no objective signs to dispute his claim. He might just be a heavy sleeper. Reporting that he is or may be under the influence of alcohol or drugs might lead to the loss of his job and to legal trouble for you.

However, what if there is an emergency in which the desk clerk's assistance is needed and he is unable to provide it? That is an unlikely, though certainly a conceivable, possibility. However, there is no clear and present danger that would require you to report. In fact, you may, depending on the state you're in, have a legal obligation to maintain confidentiality under circumstances such as these.

There are a number of reasons to respect confidentiality in general. In an emergency, a patient typically has little choice about who is going to come to his aid. He is assuming that he can be honest with these strangers who have come to help him because they will protect his privacy. If that trust was routinely violated without sufficient cause, patients might very well be embarrassed or humiliated. This would undermine the public's trust in EMS and any particular patient's trust in the paramedics and others coming into his home. If word got around that private information was being made public, patients might not be forthcoming in giving their medical histories, potentially leading to disastrous consequences. For example, a man who had recently taken sildenafil (Viagra) for erectile dysfunction might deny taking it before you give him nitroglycerin. This drug interaction is potentially serious, possibly even fatal.

There are nonetheless times when it is appropriate and necessary to breach confidentiality. Every state has laws requiring the reporting of certain health facts such as births, deaths, particular infectious diseases, child neglect and abuse, and elder neglect and abuse. These last requirements have the most applicability to EMS. They are considered justifiable reasons to breach confidentiality because, in the eyes of society, the benefit to someone who is defenseless (protection from harm and perhaps even death) and to the public (a safer environment for children) outweighs the right to privacy of a particular person. A valid court order is also considered a reasonable justification for breaching confidentiality. So is a clear threat by a patient to a specific person, as well as informing other health care professionals who will care for the patient.

Clearly, patient confidentiality is an important principle, but not an inviolable one. When determining whether it is appropriate to breach confidentiality, take into account the probability of harm, the magnitude of the expected harm, and alternative methods of avoiding harm that do not require encroaching on confidentiality.

In the previous scenario, factors do not justify breaching confidentiality. The person who called 911 for emergency assistance, however, is under no such obligation. The scenario comes to an end as follows:

> When you inform the guest that you are unable to discuss the case with anyone because of confidentiality, he replies, "Well, you may not be able to do anything about it, but I can. I'm calling the manager!"

CONSENT

Consider this scenario:

> Bob, a 58-year-old male, has been having crushing substernal pain radiating to his left arm for several hours. He also is pale, sweaty, and nauseated. He denies shortness of breath. His condition remains unchanged after you give him oxygen and nitroglycerin. When you ask Bob which hospital he wants to go to, he tells you, "I'm not going to any hospital." Surprised, you find it difficult to understand why someone in this much pain would not want to go to a hospital. You try to enlist the help of relatives over the telephone (Bob lives alone), but they are unable to persuade the patient. He has no regular physician, so that option is not available to you. Finally, you decide to try on-line medical direction. While you are waiting for the physician to come to the phone, you wonder: If the patient continues to refuse, can you force him to go? How can you act in the best interest of a patient who refuses to accept what you feel certain is best for him?

A competent patient of legal age has the fundamental right to decide what health care he will receive and will not receive. This is at the core of patient autonomy. To exercise this right, a patient must have the information necessary to make an informed decision, the mental faculties to weigh the risks and benefits of various treatment options, and the freedom from restraints that might hamper his ability to exercise his options (such as threats).

It is sometimes appropriate to use the doctrine of implied consent to force the patient to go to the hospital. For the paramedic to use this approach, the patient must be unable to give consent. Typically, the doctrine is invoked when the patient is unable to communicate, but it also can be employed when the patient is incapacitated because of drugs, illness, or injury. In this scenario, however, the patient shows no signs of being incapacitated. He is alert; oriented to person, place, and time; aware of his surroundings; and making judgments and answering questions in a manner completely compatible with competence. The fact that the patient refuses something you recommend does not, in itself, necessarily indicate that he is incompetent.

Before you leave the patient, you must not only do the things you need to do to protect yourself legally, but you must also assure yourself that the patient truly understands the issues at hand and is able to make an informed decision. As difficult as it may be for the paramedic, if the patient is able to do these things, he may have to accept the patient's desires and leave him.

ALLOCATION OF RESOURCES

Paramedics do not usually think of themselves as guardians of finite resources, but occasionally they are. The most obvious example of this is when there are more patients present than the paramedic is able to manage, such as in a multiple-casualty incident (MCI). While learning how to provide emergency medical care for multiple patients at the same scene, you might ask: What are the ethics of triage?

There are several possible approaches to consider in parceling out scarce resources. Patients could all receive the same amount of attention and resources (true parity). They could receive resources based on need. Or they could receive what someone has determined they've earned.

The civilian method of triage, where the most seriously injured patients receive the most care, is based on need. This is intended to produce the most good for the most people. However, other methods of triage are in use. Military triage, for example, has traditionally concentrated on helping the least seriously injured because this approach produces the greatest number of soldiers who can return to duty. When the President or Vice President visits a town or city, there is typically an ambulance dedicated for the dignitary's use, if needed. The ambulance is not to be used for anyone else. Because these officials are so important and because so many others need them, the typical order of care is changed.

A controversy exists in emergency medicine as to whether or not celebrities should be treated ahead of others. The argument for doing so typically emphasizes the disorder brought to the ED by the presence of a celebrity and the need to get the person out of the ED as quickly as possible to restore normal operation. The argument against takes the position that giving preferential treatment to a celebrity is an affront to justice and fairness.

All of these methods have their proponents for different situations. The key to resolving the issue of allocation of scarce resources is to examine the competing theories in light of the circumstances at hand.

OBLIGATION TO PROVIDE CARE

By virtue of membership in a profession, a paramedic takes on a responsibility to help others. The public, through the government, grants certain privileges to professionals in return for the expectation of professional behavior. As a practitioner of prehospital emergency medicine, the paramedic has even greater responsibilities. Those who provide emergency care have a special obligation to help all those in need. Many other health care professionals are free to pick and choose their patients, accepting only those who have health insurance or who can themselves pay for the services delivered by the health care professional. This is not the case in emergency medicine.

Paramedics, like other emergency professionals, are obligated to provide medical care for those in need without regard to ability to pay. They also have an ethical obligation to prevent and report instances of patient "dumping," where those without insurance are transferred against their will to public or charity hospitals.

A particular issue arises regarding the patient who is a member of a managed-care organization such as a health maintenance organization (HMO). The HMO may insist that the patient be treated at a particular facility with which the HMO has a contract. This must not be allowed to interfere with the patient's emergency care. The paramedic, like every other member of the EMS system, has an obligation to act in the patient's best interest, even when that goes against the HMO's economic interests.

Legal Notes

Intervening Outside Your EMS System The paramedic functions under the auspices of the EMS medical director as detailed in system protocols and standing orders. Providing ALS skills or interventions outside of your EMS system can lead to possible legal problems and litigation.

A very different aspect of providing care has to do with offering assistance when off duty. Although only two states require paramedics, among others, to stop and render help when they come upon someone in need of emergency care, there is still a strong ethical obligation to do so. This does not extend to situations where the paramedic would put himself in danger (such as getting into a car teetering on the edge of a cliff), if assisting would interfere with important duties owed to others (such as leaving young children unattended in a car), or when someone else is already providing assistance. In return, society offers limited liability in the form of Good Samaritan statutes in every state in the United States.

TEACHING

Many paramedics act as preceptors in their EMS systems. Two issues raised by this role are whether or not patients should be informed that a student is working on them and how many attempts a student should be allowed to have in performing critical interventions before the preceptor steps in.

When patients call for EMS, they generally expect to receive care from individuals who have finished their education and who hold credentials qualifying them to work. If a system decides not to inform patients of the presence of students, the system runs the risk of being accused of concealing important information from patients.

To avoid this problem, EMS systems with students working in them should make sure students are clearly identified as such by the uniform they wear. The preceptor should also, when appropriate, inform patients of the presence of a student and request the patient's consent before the student performs a procedure. This sounds more cumbersome than it actually is. Patients who are unable to consent obviously do not fall into this category; implied consent is invoked in this case. (Iserson discusses a societal obligation to allow this in a related context.[4]) And patients who are able to consent are frequently very understanding of the student's need for experience. As long as the preceptor stresses that he is overseeing the student, the vast majority of patients usually give their consent.

Another issue related to students is how many attempts they should be allowed in order to perform procedures such as intravenous placement and endotracheal intubation before the preceptor steps in. Factors to consider include: the student's skill level (as determined by classroom practice on mannequins and previous field experience), the anticipated difficulty of the procedure (some patients are obviously going to be more difficult to intubate or start an IV on), and the relative importance of the procedure (not all IVs are equally important). It is important to have a limit, at least initially, for the number of times a student will be allowed to attempt a procedure. Such a number will need to be decided by each system in consultation with the medical director.

PROFESSIONAL RELATIONS

As a health care professional, the paramedic answers to the patient. As a physician extender, the paramedic answers to a physician medical director. As an employee (or volunteer), the paramedic answers to the EMS system. These competing interests can sometimes make life difficult. Each can lead to ethical challenges.

In general, there are three potential sources of conflict between paramedics and physicians. One possibility is a case in which a physician orders something the paramedic

---

[4] Iserson, K. V. "Law versus Life: The Ethical Imperative to Practice and Teach Using the Newly Dead Emergency Department Patient." *Annals of Emergency Medicine*, 25.

believes is contraindicated. For example, suppose a physician ordered a paramedic to transport a critical blunt-trauma patient without attempting any intravenous access, either at the scene or en route during the anticipated 45-minute transport. This order runs counter to standard medical practice. The patient will have spent more than an hour since the trauma without receiving any intravenous fluid or intravenous access.

A different situation arises when the physician orders something the paramedic believes is medically acceptable but not in the patient's best interests. For example, imagine you are transporting a patient with stable vital signs who is complaining of abdominal pain. In accordance with your protocols, you and your partner have each tried twice to start an IV line without success. The patient's veins are some of the worst you have ever seen, and you have no expectation that you will be successful on further attempts. The patient experienced considerable pain with each attempt and is now crying, asking you not to try any more. The physician, however, insists you continue attempts to gain access.

A third potential source of conflict is the situation in which the physician orders something the paramedic believes is medically acceptable, but morally wrong. For example, say you are ordered to stop CPR on a young male found in cardiac arrest after blunt trauma. His initial rhythm of asystole has remained unchanged, and you know it is almost always associated with death. Nonetheless, although there is a very slim chance of recovery for the patient if you continue your resuscitation efforts, you would not be able to live with yourself if you did not at least try.

In each of the three cases, it is certainly appropriate for the paramedic to start by confirming the order and asking the physician to repeat it. If the order is confirmed, the medic would be prudent to ask the physician for an explanation, given the controversial nature of the orders in the first two situations (in the third, the physician's thoughts and goals are fairly clear). The next steps will depend on the physician's explanation, the patient's condition, the need for the intervention in the judgment of the paramedic, the feasibility of performing the intervention (like gaining IV access), and the amount of time available to discuss the issue.

Ultimately, the paramedic must determine for himself how the patient's interests are best served. This typically does not lead to conflict, but on occasion the paramedic may run into situations like the ones previously described. In these cases, the medic must consider the competing interests of beneficence, nonmaleficence, autonomy, and justice; the roles of the physician and the paramedic; the relative confidence (or lack thereof) the paramedic has in his own medical and ethical judgment; how far the paramedic is willing to go as an advocate for his patient; and the degree of risk acceptable to the paramedic in contravening physician orders.

It is important for the paramedic to understand that no matter what decision he makes, he will have to defend it. The explanation that he was just following the doctor's orders (or, conversely, just doing what he felt was right) will not be sufficient in and of itself. A paramedic is expected to be more than a robot. He is expected to simultaneously be a physician extender, working under a physician's license, and a clinician with the ability and independence to recognize and question inappropriate orders. The paramedic should also understand that he is not expected to act in ways he feels are immoral. However, if the individual's morals are significantly out of step with the expectations of the profession, he needs to reconsider his profession.

Disagreements with physician orders happen rarely. Usually they are the result of poor communication (such as saying one thing while meaning another or static interfering with the radio transmission) or lack of sufficient information. Conflicts with physicians that reach the level in the previous examples are fortunately rare. When they happen, the paramedic must be willing to be an advocate for the patient and act in the patient's best interests.

RESEARCH

EMS research is only in its infancy, but it will clearly become more important and more common as the field establishes the foundation necessary to introduce, modify, and justify field interventions. As this occurs, paramedics will become instrumental in implementing research protocols and gathering data. It is essential that a paramedic participating in a research project understand the importance of gaining expressed patient consent or following federal, state, and local regulations regarding implied consent.

The goal of patient care is to improve the patient's condition. The goal of research, however, is to help future patients by gaining knowledge about a specific intervention. The two goals are not the same, so patients must be protected from untoward outcomes as much as possible.

One very important way of protecting the patient is by gaining the patient's expressed consent. There are several difficulties with this. One is the concern that a patient experiencing an emergency may not be able to truly consent because of the emotional pressures he is feeling. This pressure may occur in spite of the paramedic's best efforts to explain matters calmly and impartially.

Another concern is with the patient who is unable to consent. An excellent example of this occurs in cardiac arrest research. By the very nature of the problem being studied, the investigators will be unable to gather consent from the patient. In this case, the federal government has strict rules, for example, about community notification before the study begins and gaining consent from the patient or an appropriate family member as soon as possible after a patient is entered into the study. A paramedic participating in such a study needs to be familiar with these rules and their implications.

Although many interventions have been tested and found to be life saving, there are unfortunately documented instances of patients denied treatment for life-threatening conditions in the name of research in the United States (e.g., the Tuskegee syphillis research project). The paramedic has an obligation to prevent such things from happening in EMS research.

Summary

Ethical challenges in EMS are more common than is generally believed. Issues such as patient refusal of care, confidentiality, consent, and advance directives provide some of the most common difficulties. Less common problems include obligation to provide care, teaching, and research.

Ethics shares some common ground with religion and the law, but stands apart from them both. Modern bioethics recognizes four fundamental principles or values to consider in ethical decision making: beneficence, nonmaleficence, autonomy, and justice. The paramedic needs to have a system that can compare the consequences of his choices with those values (and other relevant values) and lead to the selection of an ethical choice.

Perhaps the single most important question a paramedic has to answer when faced with an ethical challenge is: "What is in the patient's best interest?"

You Make the Call

You are transporting a 32-year-old male, Phil Cornock, who has a long history of kidney stones and has all the classic signs of having another one now. He is in severe pain and is unable to find a comfortable position. You know that although this condition can be excruciating, it is not generally life threatening. He is allergic to the only narcotic analgesic you can administer for pain. He asks you, "Can't you use the lights and sirens to get to the hospital faster?" Your service's policy regarding the use of lights and sirens restricts their use to cases in which the paramedic believes there is a significant threat to life or limb. This patient's condition does not qualify. You wonder, though, whether you should use the lights and sirens to speed up transport since the patient is in severe pain.

1. What potential benefits are there in yielding to the patient's request (beneficence)?
2. What potential harm is there in yielding to the patient's request (nonmaleficence)?
3. How does justice come into play in this situation?
4. How should paramedics in general respond when a patient requests an intervention that is not medically indicated?

See Suggested Responses at the back of this book.

Review Questions

1. _____ are generally considered to be social, religious, or personal standards of right and wrong.
   a. ethics
   b. morals
   c. standards
   d. principles

2. _____ means not doing harm.
   a. autonomy
   b. maleficence
   c. nonmaleficence
   d. beneficence

3. These groups serve to protect the rights of subjects participating in research projects.
   a. IRBs
   b. HMOs
   c. EMS
   d. CQI

4. This quick way to test ethics asks whether you would be willing to undergo a particular procedure or action if you were in the patient's place.
   a. impartiality test
   b. navigation test
   c. universalizability test
   d. interpersonal justifiability test

5. Every state has laws requiring the reporting of certain health facts such as:
   a. births.
   b. deaths.
   c. child neglect and abuse.
   d. all of the above.

See Answers to Review Questions at the back of this book.

Further Reading

American College of Emergency Physicians. "Code of Ethics for Emergency Physicians." *Annals of Emergency Medicine* 30 (1997).

Beauchamp, T., and J. F. Childress, eds. *Principles of Biomedical Ethics.* 5th ed. New York: Oxford University Press, 2001.

Iserson, K.V., et al. *Ethics in Emergency Medicine.* 2nd ed. Tucson, AZ: Galen Press, 1995.

Mappes, T., and D. Degrazia. *Biomedical Ethics.* 5th ed. Columbus: McGraw-Hill, 2000.

Veatch, R., and H. Flack. *Case Studies in Allied Health Ethics.* Upper Saddle River, N.J.: Prentice Hall, 1997.

On the Web

Visit Brady's Paramedic Website at **www.bradybooks.com/paramedic.**

General Principles of Pathophysiology

Objectives

After reading this chapter, you should be able to:

Part 1: The Cell and the Cellular Environment (begins on p. 166)
1. List types of tissue. (p. 169)
2. Discuss cellular adaptation, injury, and death. (pp. 174–180)
3. Describe the cellular environment and factors that precipitate disease in the human body. (pp. 180–200)

Part 2: Disease—Causes and Pathophysiology (begins on p. 200)
1. Analyze disease risk. (pp. 200–205)
2. Describe environmental risk factors and combined effects and interaction among risk factors. (pp. 200–201)
3. Discuss familial diseases and associated risk factors. (pp. 201–205)
4. Discuss hypoperfusion. (pp. 205–219)
5. Define cardiogenic, hypovolemic, neurogenic, anaphylactic, and septic shock. (pp. 214–219)
6. Describe multiple organ dysfunction syndrome. (pp. 219–221)

Part 3: The Body's Defenses against Disease and Injury (begins on p. 221)
1. Define the characteristics of the immune response. (pp. 225–239)
2. Discuss induction of the immune system. (pp. 226–230)
3. Discuss fetal, neonatal, and geriatric immune function. (pp. 238–239)
4. Describe the inflammation response and its systemic manifestations. (pp. 223–225, 240–253)

5. Discuss the role of mast cells, the plasma protein system, and cellular components as part of the inflammation response. (pp. 241–251)

6. Describe the resolution and repair from inflammation. (pp. 251–252)

7. Discuss the effects of aging on the mechanisms of self-defense. (pp. 252–253)

8. Discuss hypersensitivity. (pp. 253–258)

9. Describe deficiencies in immunity and inflammation. (pp. 258–260)

10. Describe homeostasis as a dynamic steady state. (p. 262)

11. Describe neuroendocrine regulation. (pp. 263–266)

12. Discuss the interrelationships between stress, coping, and illness. (pp. 266–269)

Key Terms

ABO blood groups, p. 230
acidosis, p. 195
acquired immunity, p. 225
active transport, p. 188
adenosine triphosphate (ATP), p. 168
aerobic metabolism, p. 210
afterload, p. 207
AIDS, p. 259
albumin, p. 193
alkalosis, p. 196
allergy, p. 253
anabolism, p. 179
anaerobic metabolism, p. 210
anaphylactic shock, p. 217
anaphylaxis, p. 217
anatomy, p. 171
anion, p. 185
antibiotics, p. 221
antibody, p. 225
antigen, p. 225
antigen-antibody complex, p. 233
antigen-presenting cells (APCs), p. 237
antigen processing, p. 237
apoptosis, p. 180
atrophy, p. 175
autoimmunity, p. 253
B lymphocytes, p. 226
bacteria, p. 221
basophils, p. 248
buffer, p. 186
cardiac contractile force, p. 207
cardiac output, p. 207
cardiogenic shock, p. 214
cascade, p. 244
catabolism, p. 179
catecholamines, p. 207

cation, p. 185
cell, p. 166
cell-mediated immunity, p. 226
cell membrane, p. 167
cellular swelling, p. 179
chemotactic factors, p. 243
chemotaxis, p. 243
clonal diversity, p. 231
clonal selection, p. 231
coagulation system, p. 244
colloids, p. 193
compensated shock, p. 213
complement system, p. 244
connective tissue, p. 169
contraction, p. 252
cortisol, p. 264
crystalloids, p. 193
cytokines, p. 237
cytoplasm, p. 168
cytotoxic, p. 236
debridement, p. 251
decompensated shock, p. 213
degranulation, p. 242
dehydration, p. 183
delayed hypersensitivity, p. 236
delayed hypersensitivity reaction, p. 254
diapedesis, p. 247
diffusion, p. 186
dilation, p. 175
dissociate, p. 185
diuretic, p. 199
dynamic steady state, p. 262
dysplasia, p. 176
edema, p. 189

electrolyte, p. 185
endotoxins, p. 222
eosinophils, p. 248
epithelial tissue, p. 169
epithelialization, p. 251
erythrocytes, p. 191
exotoxins, p. 222
extracellular fluid (ECF), p. 181
exudate, p. 247
facilitated diffusion, p. 188
fatty change, p. 179
fibroblasts, p. 250
filtration, p. 189
general adaptation syndrome (GAS), p. 261
granulation, p. 251
granulocytes, p. 248
granuloma, p. 250
haptens, p. 228
hematocrit, p. 191
hemoglobin, p. 191
hemoglobin-based oxygen-carrying solutions (HBOCs), p. 193
histamine, p. 243
HIV, p. 259
HLA antigens, p. 228
homeostasis, p. 171
humoral immunity, p. 226
hydrostatic pressure, p. 189
hyperplasia, p. 175
hypersensitivity, p. 253
hypertonic, p. 186
hypertrophy, p. 175
hypoperfusion, p. 206
hypotonic, p. 186
hypovolemic shock, p. 215
hypoxia, p. 176

Case Study

Medic-1 is an advanced life support (ALS) unit that serves a suburban community. Today, it is staffed by paramedics Terry Martinez and Mark Westbrook. In addition, paramedic student Steve Matthews is riding as a part of his field internship. The paramedics have just backed into the station with three sacks of groceries when a frantic teen runs up to them. He says that his neighbor is having some sort of problem and wants the paramedics to come and take a look.

The crew gets back into the unit and drives the short distance to the scene. Upon arrival they find a 34-year-old female seated in a porch swing in moderate distress. She is anxious and slightly confused. Between breaths, she complains of a tightness in her chest and difficulty swallowing. She denies any significant event that might have led to her symptoms. Her medical history is unremarkable as is her family history.

On physical exam, the paramedics find her to be cold, pale, and diaphoretic. Her voice is hoarse and she is having obvious difficulty breathing. Her pulse is rapid and weak. The paramedics continue their assessment. Her airway is patent. Breath sounds are present but diminished at the bases. Scattered wheezes are heard throughout both lung fields. The peripheral pulses are weak, but equal. In addition, the paramedics note a characteristic "wheal and flare" rash, consistent with hives, on her chest and abdomen.

Based upon their assessment, the paramedics feel the patient's signs and symptoms are consistent with an anaphylactic reaction. As they begin treatment, Mark explains to Steve the underlying pathophysiology. The patient's mental status change is most likely due to inadequate ventilation. Mark states that, in many instances, an obvious cause for an anaphylactic reaction cannot be identified.

Mark quickly describes how the body reacts to a foreign substance with an exaggerated immune response. The presence of the offending substance causes specialized cells to release histamine and other potent substances. These in turn cause the signs and symptoms seen. For example, histamine causes constriction of the bronchioles, resulting in wheezing and decreased air movement. It also causes the capillaries to become "leaky," causing the wheal and flare rash of urticaria (hives). Based upon their understanding of the pathophysiological processes involved in the current emergency, the paramedics begin a treatment plan.

First they move the patient to the stretcher and begin assisting ventilations with a bag-valve-mask unit and 100 percent oxygen. An IV of normal saline is quickly placed in the patient's left forearm. The patient's blood pressure is 80/60, her pulse rate is 120 beats per minute, and her respiratory rate is 44 breaths per minute. Furthermore, her mental status is deteriorating.

Because of the rapid progression of the anaphylactic reaction, the paramedics administer 0.5 mg of epinephrine 1:10,000 intravenously per standing orders. They follow this with a 250 mL bolus of normal saline. Epinephrine will reverse many of the adverse effects of histamine. The fluid bolus will help replace intravascular fluid lost to interstitial spaces. Later, the patient receives 50 milligrams of diphenhydramine (Benadryl) intravenously. This is a potent antihistamine and serves to blunt the adverse effects of histamine and other substances released in the course of the anaphylactic reaction.

Because patients suffering severe anaphylactic reactions often deteriorate quite rapidly, the paramedics ready the intubation equipment and obtain vials of midazolam (Versed) and succinylcholine (Anectine) in case rapid sequence intubation is required. Fortunately, the patient responds favorably to the epinephrine. She is prepared for transport. En route, Terry administers 125 milligrams of methylprednisolone (Solu-Medrol) intravenously. Although the effects of this drug will not be seen in the prehospital phase of treatment, it will ultimately improve the patient's overall condition through various mechanisms.

Upon arrival at the hospital, the patient is much improved. Her mental status is improved and the hives have disappeared. She remains tachycardic from both the anaphylactic reaction and the epinephrine administered by the paramedics. While in the emergency department, she redevelops some wheezing as the effects of the epinephrine wear off. The emergency physician orders the administration of 0.5 mg of albuterol (Ventolin) in 2.5 milliliters of normal saline via a small volume nebulizer. The patient's wheezes disappear following the treatment. Because of the severe nature of the reaction, she is admitted to the emergency department's Clinical Decision Unit for 23 hours. She ultimately does well and goes home the next day with a prescription for an antihistamine and a steroid dose pack.

INTRODUCTION

As a paramedic, you will assess your patient (noting the patient's complaints, signs, and symptoms) and plan a course of treatment. If you understand basic human physiology (how the body functions normally) and pathophysiology (how the body functions in the presence of disease or injury), you will be far more able to understand the probable causes of common assessment findings and, consequently, far more able to choose effective treatments.

General principles of physiology and pathophysiology are presented in this chapter, which is divided into three parts:

Part 1: The Cell and the Cellular Environment
Part 2: Disease—Causes and Pathophysiology
Part 3: The Body's Defenses against Disease and Injury

Part 1: The Cell and the Cellular Environment

THE NORMAL CELL

cell *the basic structural unit of all plants and animals. A membrane enclosing a thick fluid and a nucleus. Cells are specialized to carry out all of the body's basic functions.*

The fundamental unit of the human body is the **cell** (Figure 8-1 ■). It contains all necessary components to turn essential nutrients into energy, remove waste products, reproduce, and carry on other essential life functions.

There are two kingdoms of cells: *prokaryotes* and *eukaryotes*. Prokaryotes are the cells of lower plants and animals such as blue-green algae and bacteria. Their structure is very simple, with an indistinct nucleus that is not encased in a membrane, and containing no other internal structures. Eukaryotes are the cells of higher plants and animals such as

■ Figure 8-1   The cell.

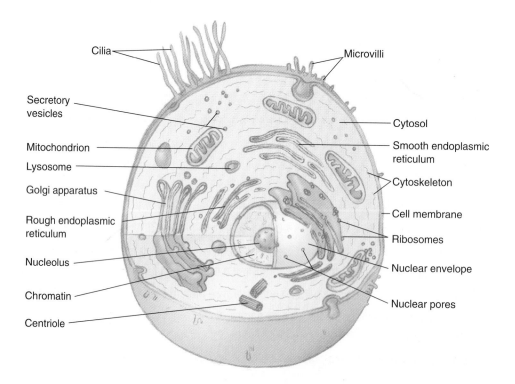

most algae, fungi, protozoa—and humans. Eukaryotes are, of course, more complex than prokaryotes. The cell structure discussed on the following pages relates to the eukaryotes.

CELL STRUCTURE

A cell is something like a small, self-sustaining city. Within the cell, specialized structures perform specific functions. In a normal cell, all the structures and functions work together to maintain a normal, balanced environment. Each cell has three main elements: the cell membrane, the cytoplasm, and the organelles.

The Cell Membrane

The **cell membrane** (sometimes called the *plasma membrane*) is the outer covering that encircles and protects the cell.

The membrane is selectively permeable, or **semipermeable,** which means that it allows certain substances to pass from one side to another but does not allow others to pass. Vital functions of the cell membrane, made possible by its selective permeability, include electrolyte and fluid balance and the transfer of enzymes, hormones, and nutrients into and out of the cell. These functions will be discussed in greater detail later.

Without the cell membrane, the interior contents of a cell would become exposed to the extracellular environment and quickly die. That is why the cellular membrane of bacteria is the site targeted by many antibiotic drugs—because destroying the cell membrane kills the cell.

 Review

Main Elements of the Cell

Cell membrane
Cytoplasm
Organelles

cell membrane   *also* plasma membrane; *the outer covering of a cell.*

semipermeable   *able to allow some, but not all, substances to pass through. Cell membranes are semipermeable.*

The Root CYT

To understand the discussion of cells, take note of the root *cyt*—which means "cell." Words with this root you will encounter in this chapter include:

cytoplasm—thick fluid that fills a cell.

cytosol—clear liquid portion of the cytoplasm in a cell.

cytoskeleton—structure of protein filaments that supports the internal structure of a cell.

erythrocyte—red blood cell.

leukocyte—white blood cell.

thrombocyte—blood cell responsible for clotting; also called a *platelet.*

lymphocyte—a type of leukocyte, or white blood cell, that attacks foreign substances as part of the body's immune response.

phagocyte—a cell that has the ability to ingest other cells and substances such as bacteria and cell debris.

phagocytosis—ingestion and digestion of bacteria and other substances by phagocytes.

monocyte—white blood cell with a single nucleus; the largest normal blood cell.

granulocyte—white cell with multiple nuclei that has the appearance of a bag of granules.

cytokine—protein produced by a white blood cell that instructs neighboring cells to respond in a genetically preprogrammed fashion.

cytotoxin—substance that is poisonous to cells.

cytotoxic—poisonous (toxic) to cells.

The Cytoplasm

cytoplasm *the thick fluid, or protoplasm, that fills a cell.*

Cytoplasm is the thick, viscous fluid that fills and gives shape to the cell, also called *protoplasm*. The clear liquid portion of the cytoplasm is called *cytosol*. Substances dissolved in the cytosol are mainly electrolytes, proteins, glucose (sugar), and lipids (fatty substances). Structures of various sizes and functions are dispersed throughout the cytosol.

The Organelles

organelles *structures that perform specific functions within a cell.*

Structures that perform specific functions within the cell are called **organelles.** Six of the most important organelles are the *nucleus*, the *endoplasmic reticulum*, the *Golgi apparatus, mitochondria, lysosomes,* and *peroxisomes*. A brief discussion of a few of their functions provides an idea of the complex activity that takes place within a cell.

nucleus *the organelle within a cell that contains the DNA, or genetic material; in the cells of higher organisms, the nucleus is surrounded by a membrane.*

* ★ *Nucleus.* The **nucleus** contains the genetic material, deoxyribonucleic acid (DNA), and the enzymes necessary for replication of DNA. DNA determines our inherited traits and also plays a critical ongoing role within our bodies. DNA must be constantly copied and transferred to the cells.

* ★ *Endoplasmic reticulum.* The endoplasmic reticulum is a network of small channels that has both rough and smooth portions. Rough endoplasmic reticulum functions in the synthesis (building) of proteins. Smooth endoplasmic reticulum functions in the synthesis of lipids, some of which are used in the formation of cell membranes, and carbohydrates.

* ★ *Golgi apparatus.* The Golgi apparatus is located near the nucleus of most cells. It performs a variety of functions including synthesis and packaging of secretions such as mucus and enzymes.

* ★ *Mitochondria.* The mitochondria are the energy factories, sometimes called the "powerhouses," of the cells. They convert essential nutrients into energy sources, often in the form of **adenosine triphosphate (ATP).**

adenosine triphosphate (ATP) *a high-energy compound present in all cells, especially muscle cells; when split by enzyme action it yields energy. Energy is stored in ATP.*

* ★ *Lysosomes.* Lysosomes contain digestive enzymes. Their functions include protection against disease and production of nutrients, breaking down bacteria and organic debris that has been taken into the cells, and releasing usable substances such as sugars and amino acids.

* ★ *Peroxisomes.* Peroxisomes are similar to lysosomes. Especially abundant in the liver, they absorb and neutralize toxins such as alcohol.

A wide variety of other structures and functions exist within the cell. Within the nucleus, for example, there are one or more smaller organelles called *nucleoli* (plural of *nucleolus*). Another component of the nucleus is *chromatin* (tangles of chromosome filaments containing DNA). Additional organelles exist in the cytoplasm (cytosol) outside the nucleus, including the *cytoskeleton* (a structure of protein filaments that supports the internal structure of the cell), *ribosomes* (granular structures that manufacture proteins—some float free, others attach to the surface of the endoplasmic reticulum, which creates the "rough" endoplasmic reticulum), *vesicles* (which play a role in transferring and storing secretions from the rough endoplasmic reticulum and Golgi complex), and *centrioles* (which play a role in cell division). On the surface of some cells are *microvilli* (folds on the cell surface), and, on some cells, whiplike *cilia* and *flagella* (which move fluids across cell surfaces and move cells through the surrounding extracellular fluid).

CELL FUNCTION

All the cells of the human body have the same general structure and contain the same genetic material but, through a process called *differentiation*, or *maturation*, cells become specialized. Eventually, cells perform specific functions that are different from the functions performed by other cells. There are seven major functions of cells:

- ★ *Movement* is performed by muscle cells. Skeletal muscles move arms and legs. The smooth muscle around blood vessels causes them to dilate or constrict as necessary. Other smooth muscle moves food and wastes through the digestive tract. Cardiac muscle causes the chambers of the heart to contract. (See Muscle Tissue in the next section.)

- ★ *Conductivity* is the function of nerve cells that creates and transmits an electrical impulse in response to a stimulus.

- ★ *Metabolic absorption* is a function of cells of the intestines and kidneys, which take in nutrients that pass through the body.

- ★ *Secretion* is performed by glands that produce substances such as hormones, mucus, sweat, and saliva. exocrine glands, salivary glands

- ★ *Excretion* is a function all cells perform as they break down nutrients and expel wastes. external

- ★ *Respiration* is the function by which cells take in oxygen, which is used to transform nutrients into energy.

- ★ *Reproduction* is the process by which cells enlarge, divide, and reproduce themselves, replacing dead cells and enabling new tissue growth and healing of wounds. Some cells, such as nerve cells, cannot reproduce—for instance, a severed spinal cord cannot repair itself.

TISSUES

Tissue refers to a group of cells that perform a similar function. The following are the four basic types of tissue:

- ★ **Epithelial tissue** lines internal and external body surfaces and protects the body. In addition, certain types of epithelial tissue perform specialized functions such as secretion, absorption, diffusion, and filtration. Examples of epithelial tissue are skin, mucous membranes, and the lining of the intestinal tract.

- ★ **Muscle tissue** has the capability of contraction when stimulated. The three types of muscle tissue (Figure 8-2 ■) are:
  - –*Cardiac muscle* is tissue that is found only within the heart. It has the unique capability of spontaneous contraction without external stimulation.
  - –*Smooth muscle* is the muscle found within the intestines and encircling blood vessels. Smooth muscle is generally under the control of the involuntary, or autonomic, component of the nervous system.
  - –*Skeletal muscle* is the most abundant muscle type. It allows movement and is mostly under voluntary control.

- ★ **Connective tissue** is the most abundant tissue in the body. It provides support, connection, and insulation. Examples of connective tissue include bones, cartilage, and fat. Blood is also sometimes classified as connective tissue.

- ★ **Nerve tissue** is tissue specialized to transmit electrical impulses throughout the body. Examples of nerve tissue include the brain, the spinal cord, and peripheral nerves.

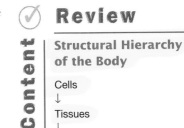

Review

Structural Hierarchy of the Body

Cells
↓
Tissues
↓
Organs
↓
Organ systems
↓
Organism

tissue *a group of cells that perform a similar function.*

epithelial tissue *the protective tissue that lines internal and external body tissues. Examples: skin, mucous membranes, the lining of the intestinal tract.*

muscle tissue *tissue that is capable of contraction when stimulated. There are three types of muscle tissue: cardiac (myocardium, or heart muscle), smooth (within intestines, surrounding blood vessels), and skeletal, or striated (allows skeletal movement). Skeletal muscle is mostly under voluntary, or conscious, control; smooth muscle is under involuntary, or unconscious, control; cardiac muscle is capable of spontaneous, or self-excited, contraction.*

connective tissue *the most abundant body tissue; it provides support, connection, and insulation. Examples: bone, cartilage, fat, blood.*

nerve tissue *tissue that transmits electrical impulses throughout the body.*

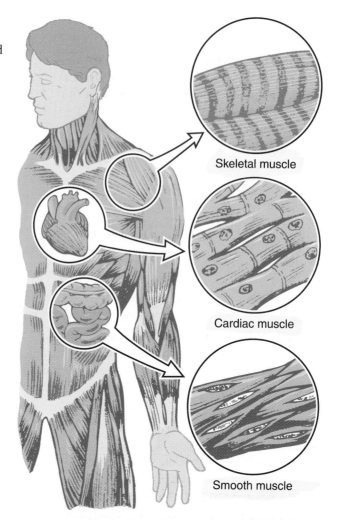

■ Figure 8-2   The three types of muscle. Skeletal muscle, also called voluntary muscle, is found throughout the body. Cardiac muscle is limited to the heart. Smooth muscle, occasionally called involuntary muscle, is found within the intestines and surrounding the blood vessels.

Skeletal muscle

Cardiac muscle

Smooth muscle

organ   *a group of tissues functioning together. Examples: heart, liver, brain, ovary, eye.*

organ system   *a group of organs that work together. Examples: the cardiovascular system, formed of the heart, blood vessels, and blood; the gastrointestinal system, comprising the mouth, salivary glands, esophagus, stomach, intestines, liver, pancreas, gallbladder, rectum, and anus.*

 Review

Organ Systems

Cardiovascular
Respiratory
Gastrointestinal
Genitourinary
Reproductive
Nervous
Endocrine
Lymphatic
Muscular
Skeletal

ORGANS, ORGAN SYSTEMS, AND THE ORGANISM

A group of tissues functioning together is an **organ.** For example, the pancreas consists of epithelial tissue, connective tissue, and nervous tissue. Together, these tissues perform the essential functions of the pancreas. These functions include production of certain digestive enzymes and regulation of glucose metabolism.

A group of organs that work together is referred to as an **organ system.** The following are important organ systems:

★ *Cardiovascular System.* The cardiovascular system consists of the heart, blood vessels, and blood. It transports nutrients and other essential elements to all parts of the body.

★ *Respiratory System.* The respiratory system consists of the lungs and associated structures. It provides oxygen to the body, while removing carbon dioxide and other waste products.

★ *Gastrointestinal System.* The gastrointestinal system consists of the mouth, salivary glands, esophagus, stomach, intestines, liver, pancreas, gallbladder, rectum, and anus. It takes in complex nutrients and breaks them down into a form that can be readily used by the body. It also aids in the elimination of excess wastes.

★ *Genitourinary System.* The genitourinary system consists of the kidneys, ureters, bladder, and urethra. It is important in the elimination of various waste products. It also plays a major role in the regulation of water, electrolytes, blood pressure, and other essential body functions.

★ *Reproductive System.* The reproductive system provides for reproduction of the organism. In the female, it consists of the ovaries, fallopian tubes, uterus, and vagina. In the male, it consists of the testes, prostate, seminal vesicles, vas deferens, and penis.

★ *Nervous System.* The nervous system consists of the brain, spinal cord, and all of the peripheral nerves. It controls virtually all bodily functions and is the seat of intellect, awareness, and personality.

★ *Endocrine System.* The endocrine system is a control system closely associated with the nervous system. It consists of the pituitary gland, pineal gland, pancreas, testes (male), ovaries (female), adrenal glands, thyroid gland, and parathyroid glands. There is evidence that other organs—such as the heart, kidney, and intestines—have endocrine functions. As noted earlier, the endocrine system exerts its effects through the release of chemical messengers called hormones.

★ *Lymphatic System.* The lymphatic system is often considered a part of the cardiovascular system. It consists of the spleen, lymph nodes, lymphatic channels, thoracic duct, and the lymph fluid itself. It is important in fighting disease, in filtration, and in removing waste products of cellular metabolism.

★ *Muscular System.* The muscular system is responsible for movement, posture, and heat production. It consists, primarily, of the skeletal muscles.

★ *Skeletal System.* The skeletal system consists of the bones, cartilage, and associated connective tissue. It provides for support, protection, and movement. The bone marrow is the site for production of various blood cells, including the red blood cells and certain types of white blood cells.

The sum of all cells, tissues, organs, and organ systems is the **organism.** The failure of any component, from the cellular level to the organ-system level, can result in the development of a serious medical emergency.

SYSTEM INTEGRATION

The human body is not just a static structure of bones, cavities, and tubes. It is a dynamic organization in which cells, tissues, organs, and organ systems perform functions essential to the preservation of the organism. **Homeostasis** is the term for the body's natural tendency to keep the internal environment and metabolism steady and normal. At the cellular level, the body will strive to maintain a very constant environment, because cells do not tolerate extreme environmental fluctuations.

A significant amount of energy is needed to maintain the order that is evident in the structures (**anatomy**) and functions (**physiology**) of the organism. Potential energy is stored in the biochemical bonds of cells and tissues in plants and animals, and the kinetic energy necessary to maintain homeostasis is obtained by the breaking of those bonds. Food provides energy substrates such as sugar, fats, and proteins which, when broken down, produce the energy for the maintenance of homeostasis. **Metabolism is the term used to refer to the building up** (*anabolism*) **and breaking down** (*catabolism*) of biochemical substances to produce energy.

The body's cells interact and intercommunicate, rather like a multicellular "social" organism. Communication between the cells consists of electrochemical messages. When something interferes with the normal sending or receiving of these messages, a disease process can begin or advance.

organism *the sum of all the cells, tissues, organs, and organ systems of a living being. Examples: the human organism, a bacterial organism.*

homeostasis *the natural tendency of the body to maintain a steady and normal internal environment.*

The failure of any component of an organism—from the cellular level to the organ system level—can result in a serious medical emergency.

anatomy *the structure of an organism; body structure.*

physiology *the functions of an organism; the physical and chemical processes of a living thing.*

metabolism *the total changes that take place during physiological processes.*

When something interferes with the electrochemical messages cells send to each other, a disease process can begin or advance.

Many intercellular messages are conveyed by substances secreted by various body glands. *Endocrine glands,* sometimes called ductless glands (including the pituitary, thyroid, parathyroid, and adrenal glands, the Islets of Langerhans in the pancreas, the testes, and the ovaries), secrete hormones directly into the circulatory system, where they travel to the target organ or tissue. *Exocrine glands* secrete substances such as sweat, saliva, mucus, and digestive enzymes onto the epithelial surfaces of the body (the skin or linings of body cavities and organs) via ducts.

Several types of signaling take place among cells. *Endocrine signaling* (via hormones distributed throughout the body) is one mode of intercellular communication. *Paracrine signaling* (nonendocrine, nonhormonal) involves secretion of chemical mediators by certain cells that act only on nearby cells. In *autocrine signaling,* cells secrete substances that may act upon themselves. In *synaptic signaling,* cells secrete specialized chemicals called neurotransmitters, such as norepinephrine, acetylcholine, serotonin, and dopamine, that transmit signals across synapses, the junctions between neurons.

These chemical signals—in the form of hormones and neurotransmitters—are received by various kinds of receptors. Receptors can be nerve endings, sensory organs, or proteins that interact with, and then respond to, the chemical signals and other stimuli. Many of the medications administered by paramedics act upon these receptors. *Chemoreceptors* respond to chemical stimuli. Chemoreceptors within the brain respond to increasing levels of CO_2 in the cerebrospinal fluid, stimulating respiratory centers in the brainstem to increase the rate and depth of respirations. *Baroreceptors* respond to pressure changes. Baroreceptors in the arch of the aorta and in the carotid sinuses along the carotid artery sense changes in blood pressure, which then cause the cardiac centers in the medulla to alter the heart rate. *Alpha* and *beta adrenergic receptors* on the surfaces of cells in the bronchi, heart, and blood vessels respond to neurotransmitters and medications, resulting in a variety of cardiovascular and respiratory responses.

As the previous examples demonstrate, when normal intercellular communication is interrupted and normal metabolism is disturbed, the body will respond in various ways to compensate and attempt to restore the normal metabolism, (i.e., homeostasis).

Each organ system plays a role in maintaining homeostasis. An example is the body's response to the accumulation of cellular carbon dioxide that occurs during exercise. The respiratory system immediately attempts to return the internal environment to its normal state by increasing the respiratory rate and depth to eliminate excess carbon dioxide—which is why runners pant.

The organization of the human body is very complex, with constant interactions occurring within and among the systems to maintain homeostasis. When disease interrupts these interactions, it can cause both local effects (at the specific site of the illness or injury) and systemic effects (throughout the body). When this happens, body cells and systems will respond to restore normal conditions.

To understand how human systems interact, physiologists sometimes view them from an engineering perspective. Various body systems respond to *inputs,* or stressors, that may be sensed by other systems. The system receiving the input responds in some fashion, creating an *output.* The portion of the system creating the output, be it a cell or an organ, is known as the *effector.* For example, consider a large laceration to an extremity with severe blood loss. The drop in blood pressure resulting from the blood loss is sensed by the baroreceptors, which in turn cause messages to be sent from the cardiac center in the medulla to the heart, resulting in an increase in the rate and strength of contractions in an attempt to restore normal blood pressure. By definition, the input would be the drop in pressure sensed by the baroreceptors; the effector would be the heart, which increased its rate in response to signals from the medulla; and the output would be the resultant increase in blood pressure.

This kind of feedback is essential for maintaining stability within a system and homeostasis for the organism. When the output of a system corrects the situation that

When normal metabolism is disturbed the body attempts to restore normal metabolism (i.e., homeostasis).

✓ Review

Effects of Disease

Local (at the site of the illness or injury)
Systemic (throughout the body)

Content

created the input, it is said to loop, or feed back on the input, and a **negative feedback loop** exists—"negative" because the feedback negates the input caused by the original stressor. To elaborate on the example of the baroreceptors, the output or increase in blood pressure resulting from the increased heart rate feeds back on, or cancels out, the original input (low blood pressure), and the heart (effector) no longer has to maintain an elevated rate. This particular feedback loop is known as the baroreceptor reflex mechanism.

Unfortunately, the grim reality of this model is that blood loss often overwhelms the heart's ability to respond with an increased rate. At that point, the system has lost the ability to compensate, and, as a paramedic, you must intervene by administering fluids and taking other necessary therapeutic measures. When the outputs of effector organs are ineffective in correcting the input condition, *decompensation* is said to have occurred.

In the case of decompensation, the feedback system doesn't or can't restore homeostasis. The opposite problem can occur when the feedback system goes too far and overcompensates for the original problem. To prevent this, it is important for the body to have some way to stop the output—to restore the heart rate to normal, because the inability to control the pulse rate would cause instability in the cardiovascular system and danger to the organism. In fact, the body does have numerous means of controlling or halting output. (Some of these output-halting mechanisms will be discussed later in the chapter.)

Biological systems generally employ negative feedback loops to maintain stability. Positive feedback systems do exist in human physiology. (Positive feedback enhances, rather than negates, the effects of input.) An example would be some short-lived positive feedback loops involved in follicular (egg) development in females. However, these loops work in conjunction with negative feedback loops to maintain stability.

Feedback activity must be orchestrated and synchronized to maintain homeostasis. Two systems work together to maintain homeostasis and to integrate the responses of different systems: the nervous system and the endocrine system. They are functionally and anatomically coupled to allow for this integration. For example, the pituitary gland of the endocrine system is joined with the hypothalamus of the nervous system by a stalklike structure called the infundibulum. This allows for rapid communication between these two body control systems.

There are important temporal (time-related) differences in the responses of these two systems. Nervous system response is generally rapid in onset but short-lived. An example is the baroreceptor reflex mechanism, mentioned earlier, which is primarily mediated by the nervous system. Conversely, endocrine responses generally take longer—that is, they have a slower onset of action but a longer duration. For example, the pituitary gland secretes antidiuretic hormone (ADH) in response to low blood pressure. ADH acts on the renal (kidney) tubules, causing water to be reabsorbed into the blood instead of being eliminated from the body. This causes an increase in intravascular fluid volume that compensates for the decrease in intravascular volume caused by the blood loss.

All these responses are stimulated by pathological alterations or events. Such reactions, including the inflammatory and immune responses which will be discussed later in this chapter, often occur in both trauma and disease.

As a paramedic, it is vital that you understand the various responses of the body to trauma and disease in the context of interacting systems so that you can recognize clinical indicators of pathology. For example, the classic duet of tachycardia with hypotension is a prelude to the "dance with death"—shock (as explained in the next section). The greater your understanding of pathophysiology, the more confidence you will have in your assessments and in making patient care decisions.

Pathophysiology

Pathology, from the root *patho* meaning "disease," is the study of disease and its causes. **Pathophysiology** is the study of how diseases alter or result from an alteration in the

negative feedback loop *body mechanisms that work to reverse, or compensate for, a pathophysiological process (or to reverse any physiological process, whether pathological or nonpathological).*

 Review

Control Systems

Content

Nervous system
Endocrine system

As a paramedic, it is vital that you understand the responses of the body to trauma and disease so that you can recognize clinical indicators of pathology. For example, the classic duet of tachycardia with hypotension is a prelude to the "dance with death." The greater your understanding of pathophysiology, the more confidence you will have in your assessments and patient care decisions.

pathology *the study of disease and its causes.*

pathophysiology *the physiology of disordered function.*

Understanding Pathophysiology The term *pathophysiology* is defined as "the physiology of disordered function." But, before you can understand disordered function, you must first understand normal function. It is for this reason that paramedic education, and medical education in general, always begins with instruction in normal anatomy and physiology. One must first understand the normal before studying the abnormal.

At several points during your career you will encounter patient conditions or diseases that were not addressed in your initial paramedic education. When this occurs, go to a reputable medical source and read about the condition in question. Various signs and symptoms will be attributed to the condition. But always look beyond this to find what the underlying pathophysiological process is—if it is known. If you are able to understand this, then you will truly understand the disease or condition in question. In some instances you may not have the detailed knowledge of normal anatomy and physiology necessary to understand the pathophysiology. In this case, you must first review the normal anatomy and physiology and then review the pathophysiology. Only then will you fully understand the clinical findings (signs, symptoms, lab results, x-ray findings). Finally, with this knowledge, the treatment will almost seem intuitive.

Keep in mind that our understanding of pathophysiology, as a consequence of basic science and clinical outcomes research, is constantly expanding. This has resulted in changes and improvements in how we care for patients.

In shock, many physiological changes occur before the classic signs, hypotension and rapid pulse, become evident. Therefore, you must treat for shock promptly based on the mechanism of injury and early, subtle signs and symptoms, without waiting for the classic signs to appear.

normal physiological processes of the human body. The concept "disease" may include both medical illness and injury.

As a paramedic, you should realize that our understanding of pathophysiology, as a consequence of basic science and clinical outcomes research, is constantly expanding. This has resulted in many changes and improvements in how we care for patients.

One example of this is the assessment and management of shock. From the origin of EMS until the mid-1980s, emergency department and EMS personnel depended on hypotension with tachycardia (low blood pressure with an accelerated pulse rate) as the primary indicators of shock in trauma and medical patients. Basic scientific research has revealed the pathophysiology of shock to be a cellular event, with many compensatory mechanisms occurring before a patient actually presents with hypotension and tachycardia. A patient with this combination of vital signs has already been in shock for an undetermined amount of time without any intervention, and will probably not have a good outcome. Clinical research validated what had been deduced from basic scientific research, and the standard of care shifted from using the presence of hypotension and tachycardia to using the mechanism of injury and, earlier, more subtle clinical signs and symptoms as the catalysts for responding to shock before it has advanced beyond the stage where it can be effectively reversed.

In this chapter, we will discuss the elements of physiology and pathophysiology: more about the cell (its function and environment), the role of genetics, the interplay and integration of systems to maintain homeostasis, and the impact of system disorders that result in stress, disease, and death. You will confirm, as you read, that an understanding of the cell is critical to an understanding of all these topics.

HOW CELLS RESPOND TO CHANGE AND INJURY

Keep in mind the concept of homeostasis: the body's tendency to maintain a constantly balanced environment and to correct or compensate for any change that upsets the balance. In this section, we will look at a variety of mechanisms by which cells respond to change and potential or actual injury.

CELLULAR ADAPTATION

Cells, tissues, organs, and even entire organ systems can adapt to both normal and injurious (pathological) conditions. For example, the growth of the uterus during pregnancy is a response to a normal change in condition. Dilation of the left ventricle after a myocardial infarction is an example of response to a pathological condition.

Adaptation to external stressors results in alterations in structure and function at the cellular level. These alterations are classified as atrophy, hypertrophy, hyperplasia, metaplasia, and dysplasia.

Many of these cellular adaptations are successful, at least in the short run, but may also be part of the process of a disease. Therefore, it is sometimes hard to distinguish an adaptive change that is a successful response to a functional demand from one that is pathological in nature.

 Review

Content

Cellular Adaptations

Atrophy
Hypertrophy
Hyperplasia
Metaplasia
Dysplasia

Atrophy

The size of an individual cell is generally determined by its workload. The cell's size will be sufficient to meet the demands placed on it by the body without wasting energy or vital nutrients. If demands decrease, cell size will also decrease to meet the demands efficiently, using minimal energy and nutrients. The cell will use less oxygen and ATP, due to its decrease in size, and the number of organelles within the cytoplasm will decrease. The process of decreasing size and increasing efficiency is known as **atrophy.**

In addition to a decrease in workload, a variety of other causes of atrophy have been identified. Atrophy may occur as a result of disuse, lack of stimulation, lack of nervous impulses, decreased nutrient supply, ischemia (lack of oxygen), or a decreased vascular (blood) supply.

Atrophy generally affects the cells found in skeletal muscle, the heart, the brain, and sex organs.

atrophy   a decrease in cell size resulting from a decreased workload.

Hypertrophy

When there is an increase in workload, a cell will often respond, in the opposite direction from atrophy, as **hypertrophy.** Hypertrophy is an increase in the size of the cell and its functional mass, including an increase in the number of organelles. The increased functional mass allows the cell to meet the increased demand. Hypertrophy of the myocardium (heart muscle) gradually occurs in response to aerobic exercise. When the heart enlarges as a consequence of a pathological event, such as after an AMI (acute myocardial infarction, or heart attack), the term applied is **dilation.** In a dilated state, the heart muscle cells have increased in size, often with a decrease in the force of contraction.

It is thought that cells that undergo hypertrophy are those that must enlarge in mass because they are unable to increase their numbers through division as in hyperplasia, described in the following section. Hypertrophy most commonly affects cells of the heart and kidneys (enlarged heart, enlarged kidney).

hypertrophy   an increase in cell size resulting from an increased workload.

dilation   enlargement. In reference to the heart, an abnormal enlargement resulting from pathology.

Hyperplasia

Another type of response to an increased workload is **hyperplasia.** Hyperplasia is an increase in the number of cells through cell division. Cell division and duplication also includes duplication of the genetic material (DNA) and the nucleus in a process called **mitosis.** Cells capable of undergoing hyperplasia include epithelial, glandular, and epidermal cells. Others, such as skeletal, cardiac, and nerve tissues, cannot divide by mitosis and therefore cannot undergo hyperplasia.

Hyperplasia is very commonly seen along with hypertrophy, because the demands placed on cells in a specific area often affect cells and tissues throughout the body, some of which respond through hypertrophy and others of which respond through hyperplasia.

hyperplasia   an increase in the number of cells resulting from an increased workload.

mitosis   cell division with division of the nucleus; each daughter cell contains the same number of chromosomes as the mother cell. Mitosis is the process by which the body grows.

Metaplasia

metaplasia *replacement of one type of cell by another type of cell that is not normal for that tissue.*

Sometimes, damaged or destroyed cells of one type are replaced by cells of another type in a process called **metaplasia.** Metaplasia often involves replacement of one type of epithelial cell with another type of epithelial cell.

This process can be seen in chronic inflammation or irritation of the respiratory tract from inhalation of irritants, commonly cigarette smoke. The irritants in the smoke will damage and destroy the ciliated columnar epithelial cells of the trachea and larger airways. The response by the body will be to replace these cells with stratified squamous epithelial cells. The squamous epithelium is less likely to be damaged by the carcinogens in the smoke. However, the squamous epithelial cells do not secrete mucus or have cilia, thus causing loss of a vital protective mechanism. In addition, the stratified squamous epithelial cells have a higher tendency to become malignant (cancerous).

Metaplasia is reversible if the causative factor is removed in time. If the person stops smoking before a malignancy (cancer) develops, the body will replace the stratified squamous cells with normal ciliated columnar cells.

Dysplasia

dysplasia *a change in cell size, shape, or appearance caused by an external stressor.*

The last adaptive mechanism of cellular response is **dysplasia.** Dysplasia is an abnormal change in cell size, shape, and appearance due to some type of external stressor. (Dysplasia is related to hyperplasia and is often called abnormal or atypical hyperplasia.)

With dysplasia, the external stressor is usually chronic inflammation due to chronic irritation of the tissue. The changes seen result from the irritation and inflammation of the cells. As a result, there is cellular proliferation to protect underlying cells. If the irritant is removed early on, then the cellular changes are often reversible.

Dysplastic cells have a high tendency to cause malignant (cancerous) changes if they are present for an extended period of time. For example, dysplasia of the female cervix potentially leads to cervical cancer.

✓ Review

Forms of Cellular Injury

Hypoxia
Chemicals
Infectious agents
Inflammatory reactions
Physical agents
Nutritional factors
Genetic factors

CELLULAR INJURY

In addition to the cellular adaptations just described, there is an enormous variety of cellular responses to injury or insult. In this section, we will discuss the seven most common mechanisms of cellular injury—hypoxia, chemicals, infectious agents, immunologic/inflammatory reactions, physical agents, nutritional factors, and genetic factors—and provide examples of the ways cells respond to these types of injury in the effort to restore homeostasis.

Hypoxic Injury

hypoxia *oxygen deficiency.*

The most common cause of cellular injury is **hypoxia,** or oxygen deficiency. Hypoxia can have various causes, usually a deficit in the respiratory or cardiovascular system. Such causes include an inadequate amount of oxygen being taken into the lungs (as from a lack of oxygen in the environment, an occluded airway, or inadequate respiration), a condition that prevents oxygen in the lungs from passing into the bloodstream (as with emphysema), inadequate pumping of blood throughout the body (as in congestive heart failure), or by a blockage in the arterial system that prevents oxygenated blood from reaching the cells (as in myocardial infarction or stroke). A blockage or reduction of the delivery of oxygenated blood to the cells is known as **ischemia.**

ischemia *a blockage in the delivery of oxygenated blood to the cells.*

Ischemia can also result if there is a deficiency of red blood cells to carry the oxygenated hemoglobin, a deficiency in hemoglobin in the blood, or a lack of available binding sites as occurs in patients with carbon monoxide poisoning. As the cell becomes progressively more ischemic, the intracellular metabolism becomes *anaerobic* (without oxygen). With anaerobic metabolism, there is a marked decrease in cellular ATP production and an increase in the production of harmful acids, primarily lactic acid. The cell and some of its organelles then begin to swell due to increased levels of sodium that result from the breakdown of the sodium-potassium ATPase pump. In those cells that use fats as their primary sources of energy, fat may accumulate within the cells, worsening the swelling.

If oxygen is supplied to the cell in time, the injury is reversible. But if oxygen is not supplied, the cell begins to break down and the cell membrane ruptures, releasing lysosomes and digestive enzymes into the extracellular environment. As a result, the cellular injury has progressed from reversible to irreversible. The result is the cellular and tissue death called *infarction*.

Patients suffering a heart attack should be thought of as having myocardial ischemia. Myocardial infarction is irreversible, and we hope to intervene before this occurs.

Chemical Injury

Cellular injury due to chemical products is very common. Deadly chemicals can be found under our sink, in our walls, in our work environment, and everywhere around us. Harmful chemical agents include heavy metals such as lead, carbon monoxide, ethanol (alcohol), drugs (misused medicinal drugs as well as street drugs), and insecticides, among others. Some, such as cyanide, cause cell damage and death within minutes. Others, such as common air pollutants, cause injury through prolonged exposure.

Children make up a large percentage of the population affected by chemicals. From accidental ingestion of poisons, such as cleaning products, to ingestion of lead-based-paint chips, to ingestion of ethanol products, children lead the way. However, persons of all ages can suffer injury from chemical agents.

Chemicals can damage the body in many ways. Injuries to the cells cause disruption of the cellular membrane resulting in enzymatic reactions, alteration of coagulation, and eventually death of the cell.

Infectious Injury

Infectious, or disease-causing, agents are a common cause of cellular injury. A healthy person harbors many microorganisms (living things so tiny they are invisible to the naked eye) in various body sites. These include bacteria, viruses, fungi, and parasites. The vast majority are harmless, and some are even useful to their human hosts. Only a few cause infection or disease. Those that do are known as **pathogens.**

The body has a variety of entry-blocking barriers and mechanisms that ward off most pathogens. The chief barrier is the skin. Mucous secretions trap pathogens and are another important barrier. Normal bacteria, enzymes, gastric acids, and other body substances destroy many pathogens. Coughing, sneezing, vomiting, and elimination of urine and feces also rid the body of pathogens.

When a pathogen does succeed in invading the body, three things can happen: First, it may multiply and spread, overwhelming the body's defenses. Second, the body and the pathogen may battle to a draw, producing a chronic infection that is kept in check but is not destroyed by the body. Third, the body's defenses, with or without the assistance of medical treatment, may defeat and destroy the pathogen.

The greater the number of body cells invaded or destroyed by a pathogen, the greater the risk of serious or permanent damage to the body. An example would be a localized infection of the hand as compared with widespread peritonitis of the abdominal cavity.

The degree of damage or injury that can be created by a pathogen depends on its numbers, its virulence (or pathogenicity), and the body's ability to contain or destroy it. Virulence is dependent on three factors: first, the pathogen's ability to invade and destroy cells; second, its ability to produce toxins; and third, its ability to produce hypersensitivity (allergic) reactions.

pathogen *a microorganism capable of producing infection or disease.*

 Review

Content

Pathogens vs. the Body: Three Possible Outcomes

Pathogen wins.
Pathogen and body battle to a draw.
Body defeats pathogen.

Immunologic/Inflammatory Injury

Protective responses of the body can cause cell injury and even death. The body's responses to cell injury are inflammation and immune responses in which the body attacks invading foreign substances. Sometimes an exaggerated immune response called *hypersensitivity* (allergy), or even a life-threatening *anaphylactic* response, may develop. Any immune response, whether mild or severe, not only attacks foreign cells, but it also tends to injure healthy body cells in the same area, in particular damaging or interfering with the function of the cell membrane. Once the foreign cells are destroyed, the injured body cells will generally begin to repair themselves.

Immunological responses will be discussed in greater detail later in this chapter and in the chapter on allergies and anaphylaxis, Volume 3, Chapter 5.

Injurious Physical Agents

Cellular damage can be caused by physical agents. Extreme variances in temperature, whether hot or cold, can cause injury to the epidermis and underlying tissue, as from a burn or frostbite. Electrical burns, including lightning injuries, cause severe cellular damage. Hyperthermia and hypothermia (exposure to unusually warm or cool environmental temperatures) can also cause cell damage by altering body temperature, breathing patterns, and so on.

Other physical agents that can cause cellular damage include atmospheric pressure changes (for example, in a blast injury or deep-sea-diving injury), exposure to ionizing radiation (x-rays, nuclear radiation), illumination (eyestrain from fluorescent lighting, skin cancers from ultraviolet radiation), noise (hearing impairment), and mechanical stresses (blunt or penetrating trauma, irritation to the skin, repetitive-motion injuries, and overexertion back injuries).

Injurious Nutritional Imbalances

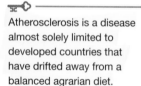
Atherosclerosis is a disease almost solely limited to developed countries that have drifted away from a balanced agrarian diet.

Improper nutrition contributes to one of the most widely publicized forms of cellular injury: atherosclerosis caused by the deposition of lipids, cholesterol, and calcium inside arteries. Many nutritionists identify excessive intake of saturated fats and cholesterol as major contributing causes. Others place the blame on excessive carbohydrate (glucose) intake, which triggers increased insulin secretion, which in turn stimulates production of cholesterol by the liver. Whatever the underlying causes, the result is a narrowing diameter of the arteries, which decreases the amount of oxygenated blood that reaches target cells, increasing the risk of ischemia to vital organs such as the heart and brain.

Problems other than atherosclerosis can also be caused or exacerbated by nutritional imbalances. In diabetic patients, an imbalance between insulin levels and carbohydrate intake causes complex, often severe metabolism problems.

While excessive intake of nutrients may cause problems such as those previously mentioned, insufficient intake of nutrients can cause other problems. The cells require proteins, carbohydrates, lipids, vitamins, and minerals for their metabolism and survival. Deficient intake of any of these nutrients can cause cellular damage and illness.

More commonly in less-developed countries, less commonly in the United States, malnutrition and starvation lead to cellular injury and diseases such as beriberi, scurvy, and rickets, which are all caused by vitamin deficiencies in the diet.

Injurious Genetic Factors

Genes, the basic units of heredity, are composed of DNA. A large number of genes attach to form double-stranded helical molecules of DNA. Molecules of DNA are carried on long threadlike strands called *chromosomes.* The DNA resides in the nucleus of the cells. Some cellular dysfunctions are caused by genetic predisposition, either defective genes or altered chromosomes that the person is born with. Genetic cell injuries can involve alterations to the nucleus or the cell membrane, the shape of the cell, the receptors on the cell membrane, or the transport mechanisms that carry substances across the cell membrane.

A person's genetic makeup is determined at conception, and the interaction of genes and environmental factors determine that person's development. Some diseases are mainly environmental; for example, invasion of the body by bacteria. Other diseases are mainly genetic; for example, sickle cell disease, which is due to a genetic defect. Many diseases result from the combined effects of environmental and genetic factors, including certain metabolic disorders such as diabetes.

Manifestations of Cellular Injury

There are two aspects of the metabolism that take place within cells: anabolism and catabolism. **Anabolism** is the constructive or "building up" phase of metabolism—the processes in which the cell takes in nonliving substances from the blood and the extracellular environment and converts them into the living cytoplasm of the cell. **Catabolism** is the destructive, or "breaking down," phase of metabolism—the processes in which the cell converts complex substances into simpler substances, usually with an accompanying release of energy.

When cells are injured, metabolism goes awry. A chief consequence is that substances, not all of which are in the cells normally, *infiltrate* or *accumulate* in the cells to an abnormal degree. This can occur from one of three causes: (1) endogenous substances (substances normally found in the cells) are anabolized (produced) in excess; (2) endogenous substances are not properly catabolized (broken down); or (3) harmful exogenous substances (substances from outside the cell, such as heavy metals, mineral dusts, or microorganisms) are taken into and remain in the cells.

When the cells attempt to catabolize the accumulated substances, excessive amounts of metabolites (products of catabolism) are excreted into the extracellular environment. Large numbers of phagocytes (specialized white blood cells) migrate to the area to ingest the excreted metabolites, and this causes swelling of the tissues, as may be seen in enlargement of the liver or spleen.

A variety of substances can accumulate in the cells, including water, lipids, carbohydrates, glycogen, proteins, pigments, calcium, and urate, causing a variety of effects from diabetic disorders to moles and skin color changes to arthritic conditions. Regardless of the type or agent of injury, among the most commonly seen effects of cell injury and accumulation are cellular swelling and fatty change.

Cellular swelling, resulting from a permeable or damaged cellular membrane, is the most frequent result of cellular injury. The cellular swelling is caused by an inability to maintain stable intra- and extracellular fluid and electrolyte levels (which will be explained in more detail later).

Another response that frequently accompanies cellular swelling is the **fatty change,** in which lipids (small fat vesicles) invade the area of injury. Fatty change with swelling is an ominous sign of impending cellular destruction. The fatty deposits commonly occur in vascular organs such as the kidney and heart, but most commonly in the liver. These deposits begin to cause disruption of the cellular membrane and metabolism and interfere with the vital functions of the affected organs. If the injury does not involve the circulatory system, cellular damage may be contained in the immediate area. If the circulatory system is involved, chemical mediators and lysosomes from the local injury response can enter into the circulatory system, potentially causing systemic injury.

Systemic signs and symptoms of cellular injury include general feelings of fatigue and malaise, an altered appetite (increased or decreased hunger), fever associated with the inflammatory response, an increased heart rate associated with fever, and pain. Laboratory blood chemistry tests may reveal a high leukocyte (white blood cell) count, resulting from the immune response, as well as the presence of certain cellular enzymes indicating specific sites of cellular injury, such as the skeletal muscle, bone, heart, brain, liver, kidney, or pancreas.

anabolism *the constructive phase of metabolism in which cells convert nonliving substances into living cytoplasm.*

catabolism *the destructive phase of metabolism in which cells break down complex substances into simpler substances with release of energy.*

cellular swelling *swelling of a cell caused by injury to or change in permeability of the cell membrane with resulting inability to maintain stable intra- and extracellular fluid and electrolyte levels.*

fatty change *a result of cellular injury and swelling in which lipids (fat vesicles) invade the area of injury; occurs most commonly in the liver.*

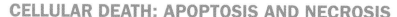

apoptosis *response in which an injured cell releases enzymes that engulf and destroy itself; one way the body rids itself of damaged and dead cells.*

Cellular death leads to one of two processes: apoptosis or necrosis. If the cellular injury or insult is confined to a local region, **apoptosis** may occur. Apoptosis is the body's way of ridding itself of destroyed or nonfunctional cells. It occurs as a result of both normal and pathological tissue changes. The word is Greek, meaning "falling apart." Simply stated, the injured cell releases digestive enzymes that will engulf and destroy itself. By eliminating damaged and dead cells, apoptosis allows tissues to repair and possibly regenerate.

necrosis *cell death; a pathological cell change. Four types of necrotic cell change are* coagulative, liquefactive, caseous, *and* fatty. Gangrenous necrosis *refers to tissue death over a wide area.*

The other process that may follow cellular death is **necrosis.** Unlike apoptosis, necrosis is always a pathological process. Four types of necrotic cell change may occur: coagulative, liquefactive, caseous, and fatty. In *coagulative necrosis,* the transparent viscous albumin of the cell becomes firm and opaque, like a cooked egg white. It generally results from hypoxia and commonly occurs in the kidneys, heart, and adrenal glands. In *liquefactive necrosis,* the cells become liquid and contained in walled cysts. This is common in the ischemic death of neurons and brain cells. In *caseous necrosis,* common in tubercular lung infection, incompletely digested cells take on a cottage-cheese-like consistency. In *fatty necrosis,* commonly occurring in the breast and abdominal structures, fatty acids combine with calcium, sodium, and magnesium ions to create soaps (a process called *saponification*). The dead tissue is opaque and white.

Review

Content

Results of Cell Death

Apoptosis (usually normal)
Necrosis (always
  pathological)
  –Coagulative
  –Liquefactive
  –Caseous
  –Fatty
Gangrenous necrosis (over
  a wide area)
  –Dry gangrene
  –Wet gangrene
  –Gas gangrene

Gangrenous necrosis refers to tissue death over a wide area. *Dry gangrene* results from coagulative necrosis and affects the skin, most commonly of the lower extremities, turning it dry, shrunken, and black. *Wet gangrene* results from liquefactive necrosis and usually affects internal organs. *Gas gangrene* is the result of a bacterial infection of injured tissue, generating gas bubbles in the cells. By attacking red blood cells, gas gangrene can cause death from shock.

There are several key differences between apoptosis and necrosis. In apoptosis, cells shrink. In necrosis, cells swell and rupture. Apoptosis appears to be a form of normal bodily housekeeping. Destroyed cells are cleared away and digested by phagocytes, permitting repair and regeneration. Necrosis is always pathological. Dead cells take on a different physical form (becoming hardened or liquefied) and destroy or interfere with normal physiological processes. Apoptosis has specificity. It occurs in scattered, single cells. Necrosis lacks specificity. It will destroy not only the injured cells but also neighboring cells.

THE CELLULAR ENVIRONMENT: FLUIDS AND ELECTROLYTES

Some fluid and electrolyte derangements can result in death.

Many pathological conditions, both medical and traumatic, adversely affect the fluid and electrolyte balance of the body. Certain disease processes, such as diabetic ketoacidosis and heat emergencies, are associated with certain electrolyte abnormalities. Severe derangements in fluid and electrolyte status can result in death. For this reason, as a paramedic, you need to have a good understanding of the fluids and electrolytes present in the human body.

WATER

total body water (TBW) *the total amount of water in the body at a given time.*

Water is the most abundant substance in the human body. In fact, water accounts for approximately 60 percent of the total body weight (the average for all ages). The total amount of water in the body at any given time is referred to as the **total body water (TBW).** In an adult weighing 70 kilograms (154 pounds), the amount of total body water would be approximately 42 liters (11 gallons) (Figure 8-3 ■).

15% of body weight. Extracellular fluid (4.5% intravascular; 10.5% interstitial)

60% of body weight: Total body water

45% of body weight: Intracellular fluid

Water is distributed into various compartments of the body (Table 8–1). These compartments are separated by cell membranes. The largest compartment is the *intracellular compartment*. This compartment contains the **intracellular fluid (ICF),** which is all of the fluid found inside body cells. Approximately 75 percent of all body water is found within this compartment. The *extracellular compartment* contains the remaining 25 percent of all body water. It contains the **extracellular fluid (ECF),** all of the fluid found outside the body cells.

There are two divisions within the extracellular compartment. The first contains the **intravascular fluid**—the fluid found outside of cells and within the circulatory system. It is essentially the same as the blood plasma. The remaining compartment contains the **interstitial fluid**—all the fluid found outside of the cell membranes, yet not within the circulatory system. For example, minute amounts of fluid are found in the

THE MAJORITY

intracellular fluid (ICF) *the fluid inside the body cells.*

extracellular fluid (ECF) *the fluid outside the body cells. Extracellular fluid is comprised of intravascular fluid and interstitial fluid.*

intravascular fluid *the fluid within the circulatory system; blood plasma.*

interstitial fluid *the fluid in body tissues that is outside the cells and outside the vascular system.*

Table 8–1	Body Fluid Compartments	
Compartment	Percentage of Total Body Water	Volume in 70-kg Adult
Intracellular fluid	75.0%	31.50 L
Extracellular fluid	25.0%	10.50 L
Interstitial fluid	17.5%	7.35 L
Intravascular fluid	7.5%	3.15 L

synovial fluid that lubricates the joints, the aqueous humor of the eye, secretions including saliva, gastric juices, bile, and so on.

Total body water and its distribution vary with age and physiological condition. At birth, an infant's TBW is about 75 to 80 percent of its body weight, compared to the 65 percent TBW of the average adult. Infants have a higher TBW for two reasons. First, infants have less fat than adults. (Fat does not absorb water, so the less fat in the body, the more water.) Second, water is essential for the high rates of metabolism that are necessary to promote growth in the infant. The TBW slowly decreases to approximately 70 to 75 percent by age 1. Diarrhea is especially worrisome in the infant, because it can mean the loss of a significant percentage of TBW. In addition, body systems that compensate for fluid loss are still immature, so that infants can rapidly become dangerously dehydrated and subject to electrolyte imbalances. By late childhood the TBW decreases to 65 to 70 percent.

By early adulthood, the TBW of males and females begins to differ. In adult males, TBW constitutes approximately 65 to 70 percent of the body weight, while in adult females the average TBW is 60 to 65 percent. The gender difference is the result of hormonal differences that result in the male's greater muscle mass and the female's greater percentage of body fat.

As the human body ages, the loss of muscle mass, increased percentage of fat, and the body's decreasing ability to regulate fluid levels lowers the TBW to around 45 to 55 percent. Due to a decreasing ability to regulate electrolytes and fluid levels, the elderly, like the very young, are at high risk for dehydration and disorders related to electrolyte imbalances.

Hydration

solvent *a substance that dissolves other substances, forming a solution.*

Water is the universal **solvent.** That is, most substances dissolve in water. When they do, various chemical changes take place. For this reason, the water content of the body is crucial to virtually all of the body's biochemical processes. Normally, the total volume of water in the body, as well as the distribution of fluid in the three body compartments, remains relatively constant. This occurs despite wide fluctuations in the amount of water that enters and is excreted from the body on a daily basis. The water coming into the body is referred to as intake. The water excreted from the body is referred to as output. To maintain relative homeostasis, the intake must equal the output, as shown in the following text.

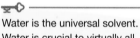

Water is the universal solvent. Water is crucial to virtually all of the body's biochemical processes.

Intake

digestive system:

liquids	1,000 mL
food (solids)	1,200 mL
metabolic sources:	300 mL
TOTAL:	2,500 mL

Output

lungs (water vapor):	400 mL
kidneys (urine):	1,500 mL
skin (perspiration):	400 mL
intestines (feces):	200 mL
TOTAL:	2,500 mL

Several mechanisms work to maintain a relative balance between input and output. For example, as explained earlier, when the fluid volume drops, the pituitary gland secretes antidiuretic hormone (ADH), which causes the kidney tubules to reabsorb more water into the blood and to excrete less urine. This process helps to restore the fluid volume to normal values.

Thirst also regulates fluid intake. The sensation of thirst normally occurs when body fluids decrease, stimulating the person to take in more fluids orally. Conversely, when too many fluids enter the body, the kidneys are activated and more urine is excreted, thus eliminating excess fluid. The body also maintains fluid balance by shifting water from one body space to another.

Dehydration   **Dehydration** is an abnormal decrease in the total body water and can result from several factors:

★ *Gastrointestinal losses* result from prolonged vomiting, diarrhea, or malabsorption disorders.

★ *Increased insensible loss* is loss of water through normal mechanisms that is difficult to detect or measure (e.g., perspiration, water vapor from the lungs, saliva). These can be increased in fever states, during hyperventilation, or with high environmental temperatures.

★ *Increased sweating* (also called perspiration or diaphoresis) can result in significant fluid loss. This can occur with many medical conditions or high environmental temperatures.

★ *Internal losses* are commonly called "third-space" losses because fluid is lost from intravascular or intracellular spaces into the interstitial space. With dehydration, fluid is typically lost from the intravascular compartment into the interstitial compartment, which effectively takes it out of the circulating volume. This can occur with peritonitis, pancreatitis, or bowel obstruction. It can also occur in poor nutritional states where there is not enough protein in the vascular system to retain water.

★ *Plasma losses* occur from burns, surgical drains and fistulas, and open wounds.

Dehydration rarely involves only the loss of water. More commonly, there is also a loss of electrolytes. At the hospital, fluid replacement will be based on both fluid and electrolyte deficits, once the patient's electrolyte abnormalities are determined through laboratory testing.

Clinically, the dehydrated patient will exhibit dry mucous membranes and poor skin **turgor.** There often is excessive thirst. As it becomes more severe, dehydration will be accompanied by an increased pulse rate, decreased blood pressure, and orthostatic hypotension (increased pulse and decreased blood pressure on rising from a supine position). In infants, the anterior fontanelle may be sunken and the diaper may be dry or reveal the presence of highly concentrated (dark yellow, strong-smelling) urine. The absence of tears in a crying infant, a capillary refill time greater than 2 seconds, dry mucosa, and a decrease in urinary output are signs that indicate severe dehydration. The treatment for dehydration is replacement of fluid.

Overhydration   **Overhydration** can occur as well. The major sign of overhydration is edema. Patients with heart disease may manifest overhydration much earlier than patients without heart disease. In severe cases of overhydration, overt heart failure may be present. Treatment is directed at removing the excessive fluid.

dehydration   *excessive loss of body fluid.*

 Review

Some Causes of Dehydration

Vomiting
Diarrhea
Perspiration
Peritonitis
Malnutrition
Burns
Open wounds

Dehydration usually involves loss of both water and electrolytes.

turgor   *normal tension in a cell; the resistance of the skin to deformation. (In a normally hydrated person, the skin, when pinched, will quickly return to its normal formation. In a dehydrated person, the return to normal formation will be slower.)*

overhydration   *the presence or retention of an abnormally high amount of body fluid.*

How to Read Chemical Notation

To describe chemical substances and reactions, scientists use chemical notation, a kind of "shorthand." Every chemical element has a one- or two-letter abbreviation. Just four elements—hydrogen, oxygen, carbon, and nitrogen—make up over 99 percent of the body's atoms. These are called the "major elements." Nine "trace elements" account for the remaining less-than-1 percent.

Major Element	Symbol	Percent	Trace Element	Symbol
Hydrogen	H	62.0%	Calcium	Ca
Oxygen	O	26.0%	Chlorine	Cl
Carbon	C	10.0%	Iodine	I
Nitrogen	N	1.5%	Iron	Fe
			Magnesium	Mg
			Phosphorus	Ph
			Potassium	K
			Sodium	Na
			Sulfur	S

An atom is the smallest particle of an element. A molecule is a combination of atoms. The notation for a molecule combines the notations of the included elements. A subscript number after an element indicates the number of atoms of that element. If there is just one atom, there is no number. For example:

$NaCl$ (Sodium chloride, or table salt. A sodium chloride molecule has
   1 sodium atom and 1 chlorine atom.)
H_2O (Water. A water molecule has 2 hydrogen atoms and 1 oxygen atom.)
H_2CO_3 (Carbonic acid. A carbonic acid molecule has 2 hydrogen, 1 carbon,
   and 3 oxygen atoms.)

Ions

Each atom is made up of even smaller particles: electrons (that have a negative electrical charge), protons (that have a positive electrical charge), and neutrons (that are uncharged). Protons and neutrons are in the inner core, or nucleus, of the atom while electrons occupy outer orbits around the nucleus. Sometimes an atom of an element can lose one or more of its outer electrons or can capture one or more extra electrons from another element.

An ion is an atom that has lost one or more negatively charged electrons and now has a positive charge, or an atom that has gained one or more electrons and now has a negative charge. A superscript plus ($^+$) indicates a positively charged cation. A superscript minus ($^-$) indicates a negatively charged anion. For example:

Na^+ (A sodium ion has lost an electron and has a positive charge.)
Ca^{++} (A calcium ion has lost two electrons and has a double positive charge.)
Cl^- (A chloride ion has gained an electron and has a negative charge.)

Electrolytes are substances that form ions when they break down, or dissociate, in water. Remember that the body and its blood are mostly water. The ions formed by dissociation of electrolytes in the body's fluids is a major factor in body metabolism.

Chemical Reactions

Notations for chemical reactions use a plus sign (+) to indicate substances that are combined and an arrow (→) to show the direction of the reaction. The reactants are usually on the left, with the product of the reaction on the right.

$$2H + O \rightarrow H_2O$$
(2 hydrogen atoms + 1 oxygen atom → 1 water molecule)

In some circumstances, a reaction may be reversible. That is, separate elements may synthesize (combine), or the synthesized substance may dissociate (break down) into separate components. A two-directional arrow (↔) shows that a reaction is reversible and can be read in either direction.

$$CO_2 + H_2O \leftrightarrow H_2CO_3$$
Read as: (carbon dioxide + water → carbonic acid) or
(carbonic acid → water + carbon dioxide).

Notice that no atoms are gained or lost in a chemical reaction. In the previous example, the two oxygen atoms in CO_2 and the single oxygen atom in H_2O combine to equal the three oxygen atoms in H_2CO_3. The hydrogen and carbon atoms are also equal on both sides of the reaction.

Up and down arrows (↑↓) are used to indicate an increase or decrease in the substance that follows the arrows. For example:

↑ H^+ (an increase in hydrogen ions)
↓ CO_2 (a decrease in carbon dioxide)

The various chemical substances present throughout the body can be classified either as electrolytes or nonelectrolytes. **Electrolytes** are substances that **dissociate** into electrically charged particles when placed into water. The charged particles are referred to as **ions.** Ions with a positive charge are called **cations,** while ions with a negative charge are called **anions.**

An example of this would be the dissociation of the drug sodium bicarbonate when placed into water. Sodium bicarbonate is a neutral salt. When placed into water, it dissociates into two charged particles, as shown below.

$$NaHCO_3 \rightarrow Na^+ + HCO_3^-$$
sodium bicarbonate → sodium cation + bicarbonate anion
neutral salt → cation + anion

Sodium bicarbonate is an example of an electrolyte that is taken into the body as a medication. However, there are many naturally occurring electrolytes present in the body.

The most frequently occurring cations include:

★ *Sodium (Na$^+$).* Sodium is the most prevalent cation in the extracellular fluid. It plays a major role in regulating the distribution of water because water is attracted to and moves with sodium. In fact, it is often said that "water follows sodium." Sodium is also important in the transmission of nervous impulses. An abnormal increase in the relative amount of sodium in the body is called *hypernatremia,* while an abnormal decrease is referred to as *hyponatremia.*

★ *Potassium (K$^+$).* Potassium is the most prevalent cation in the intracellular fluid. It is also important in the transmission of electrical impulses. An abnormally high potassium level is called *hyperkalemia,* while an abnormally low potassium level is referred to as *hypokalemia.*

electrolyte *a substance that, in water, separates into electrically charged particles.*

dissociate *separate; break down. For example, sodium bicarbonate, when placed in water, dissociates into a sodium cation and a bicarbonate anion.*

ion *a charged particle; an atom or group of atoms whose electrical charge has changed from neutral to positive or negative by losing or gaining one or more electrons. (In an atom's normal, nonionized state, its positively charged protons and negatively charged electrons balance each other so that the atom's charge is neutral.)*

cation *an ion with a positive charge—so called because it will be attracted to a cathode, or negative pole.*

anion *an ion with a negative charge—so called because it will be attracted to an anode, or positive pole.*

★ *Calcium (Ca^{++})*. Calcium has many physiological functions. It plays a major role in muscle contraction as well as nervous impulse transmission. An abnormally increased calcium level is called *hypercalcemia,* while an abnormally decreased calcium level is called *hypocalcemia.*

★ *Magnesium (Mg^{++})*. Magnesium is necessary for several biochemical processes that occur in the body and is closely associated with phosphate in many processes. An abnormally increased magnesium level is called *hypermagnesemia;* an abnormally decreased magnesium level is called *hypomagnesemia.*

The most frequently occurring anions include:

★ *Chloride (Cl$^-$)*. Chloride is an important anion. Its negative charge balances the positive charge associated with the cations. It also plays a major role in fluid balance and renal function. Chloride has a close association with sodium.

★ *Bicarbonate (HCO$_3^-$)*. Bicarbonate is the principal **buffer** of the body. This means that it neutralizes the highly acidic hydrogen ion (H$^+$) and other organic acids. (Buffering will be discussed in more detail later in this chapter.)

★ *Phosphate (HCO$_4^-$)*. Phosphate is important in body energy stores. It is closely associated with magnesium in renal function. It also acts as a buffer, primarily in the intracellular space, in much the same manner as bicarbonate.

Many other compounds carry negative charges. Among these are some of the proteins, certain organic acids, and other compounds. Electrolytes are usually measured in *milliequivalents* per liter (mEq/L).

Nonelectrolytes are molecules that do not dissociate into electrically charged particles. These include glucose, urea, proteins, and similar substances.

OSMOSIS AND DIFFUSION

As discussed earlier, the various fluid compartments are separated by cell membranes. These membranes are semipermeable, allowing the passage of certain materials while restricting the passage of others. Compounds with small molecules, such as water (H$_2$O), pass readily through the membrane; larger compounds, such as proteins, are restricted. This selective movement of fluids results from the presence of pores (openings) in the membrane. Electrolytes do not pass as readily as water through the membrane. This is due not so much to their size as to their electrical charge.

When solutions on opposite sides of a semipermeable membrane are equal in concentration, the relationship is said to be **isotonic.** When the concentration of a given solute (dissolved substance) is greater on one side of the membrane than on the other, it is said to be **hypertonic.** When the concentration is less on one side of the cell membrane, as compared to the other, it is referred to as **hypotonic.** This difference in concentration is known as the **osmotic gradient.**

The natural tendency of the body is to keep the balance of electrolytes and water equal on both sides of the cell membrane. This is an example of homeostasis. If one side of a cell membrane has an increased quantity of a given electrolyte (is hypertonic), there will be a shift of the electrolyte from that side and a shift of water from the other side to restore balance in concentration—the balanced state.

The tendency of molecules to move from an area of higher concentration to an area of lower concentration is referred to as **diffusion** and does not require energy (Figure 8-4 ■). The diffusion of a solute (usually an electrolyte) across a cell membrane from

buffer *a substance that tends to preserve or restore a normal acid-base balance by increasing or decreasing the concentration of hydrogen ions.*

isotonic *equal in concentration of solute molecules; solutions may be isotonic to each other.*

hypertonic *having a greater concentration of solute molecules; one solution may be hypertonic to another.*

hypotonic *having a lesser concentration of solute molecules; one solution may be hypotonic to another.*

osmotic gradient *the difference in concentration between solutions on opposite sides of a semipermeable membrane.*

diffusion *the movement of molecules through a membrane from an area of greater concentration to an area of lesser concentration.*

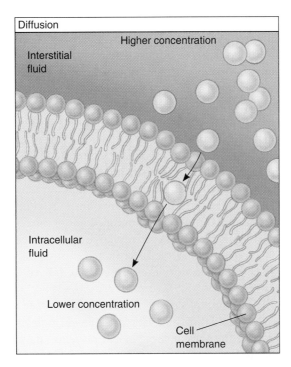

■ Figure 8-4   Diffusion is the movement of a substance from an area of greater concentration to an area of lesser concentration.

the area of higher concentration to the area of lower concentration continues until the natural balance is again attained. This movement from an area of higher concentration to an area of lower concentration is termed a movement *with the osmotic gradient.*

Water also moves across the cell membrane so as to dilute the area of increased electrolyte concentration. The movement of water is more rapid than the movement of electrolytes. This form of diffusion (the passage of any solvent, usually water, through a membrane) is referred to as **osmosis** (Figure 8-5 ■). It occurs in the direction opposite to the direction of solute movement. For example, if a semipermeable membrane separates solutions of water and sodium, and if the concentration of sodium is two times higher on one side of the membrane than on the other, then two things will occur. Sodium will diffuse from the area of higher concentration (the hypertonic side) to the area of lesser concentration (the hypotonic side). Concurrently, water will diffuse in the opposite direction. That is, water will leave the hypotonic side and diffuse across the

osmosis   *the passage of a solvent such as water through a membrane.*

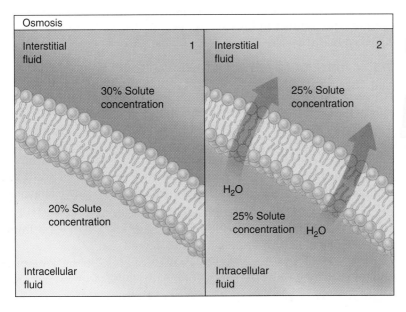

■ Figure 8-5   Osmosis is the movement of water from an area of higher WATER concentration to an area of lesser WATER concentration. Because water is a solvent, it moves from an area of lower SOLUTE concentration to an area of higher SOLUTE concentration.

membrane to the hypertonic side. These actions will continue until the concentration of water and sodium on both sides has equalized.

In addition to diffusion, two other mechanisms—active transport and facilitated diffusion—can transport substances across cell membranes. **Active transport** is the movement of a substance across the cell membrane *against the osmotic gradient* (that is, toward the side that already has more of the substance).

For example, the body requires cells of the myocardium to be negatively charged on the inside of the cells as compared to the outside. However sodium, with its positive charge, tends to diffuse passively into the cell. This would destroy the negative charge inside the cell. In order to maintain the desired negative charge, sodium ions are actively pumped out of the cell, while potassium ions are pumped into the cell, by a mechanism known as the sodium-potassium pump. (Sodium and potassium ions are both positive, but more sodium ions are pumped out of the cell than potassium ions are pumped in, creating the desired negative charge inside the cell.)

Active transport is faster than diffusion, but it requires the expenditure of energy, which diffusion does not. Proteins are moved across the cell membrane in a similar fashion.

Certain molecules can move across the cell membrane by another process known as **facilitated diffusion.** Glucose is an example of such a molecule. Facilitated diffusion requires the assistance of "helper proteins," parts of a membrane transport system, on the surface of the cell membrane. These proteins, once activated, bind to the glucose molecule. Following binding, the protein changes its configuration and transports the glucose molecule to the inside of the cell, where it is released. Depending on the substance being transported, facilitated diffusion may or may not require energy.

Water Movement between Intracellular and Extracellular Compartments

The mechanisms by which water and solutes move across cell membranes, as previously described, assure that the **osmolality** of body water, both within and outside the cells, is normally in equilibrium. (The term *osmolality* refers to the concentration of solute per kilogram of water; a related term, **osmolarity,** refers to the concentration of solute per liter of water. The terms are often used interchangeably.) Sodium, the most abundant ion in the extracellular fluid, is responsible for the osmotic balance of the extracellular space. Potassium plays the same role in the intracellular space.

Generally, the osmolality of intracellular fluid does not change very rapidly. However, when there is a change in the osmolality of extracellular fluid, water will move from the intracellular to the extracellular compartment, or vice versa, until osmotic equilibrium is regained.

Water Movement between Intravascular and Interstitial Compartments

Within the extracellular compartment, movement of water between the plasma in the intravascular space and the interstitial space is primarily a function of forces at play in the capillary beds.

In general, the movement of water and solutes across a cell membrane is governed by **osmotic pressure.** Osmotic pressure is the pressure exerted by the concentration of solutes on one side of a semipermeable membrane, such as a cell membrane or the thin wall of a capillary. Osmotic pressure can be thought of as a "pull" rather than a "push," because a hypertonic concentration of solutes tends to pull water from the other side of the membrane.

Generally, this is a two-way street as solutes move out of a space while water moves into the space to balance the concentration of solutes on both sides of the membrane.

active transport *movement of a substance through a cell membrane against the osmotic gradient; that is, from an area of lesser concentration to an area of greater concentration, opposite to the normal direction of diffusion.*

facilitated diffusion *diffusion of a substance such as glucose through a cell membrane that requires the assistance of a "helper," or carrier protein.*

osmolality *the concentration of solute per kilogram of water. See also osmolarity.*

osmolarity *the concentration of solute per liter of water (often used synonymously with osmolality).*

osmotic pressure *the pressure exerted by the concentration of solutes on one side of a membrane that, if hypertonic, tends to "pull" water (cause osmosis) from the other side of the membrane.*

However, there is a somewhat different osmotic mechanism that operates between the plasma inside a capillary and the interstitial space outside the capillary. Blood plasma generates **oncotic force,** which is sometimes called *colloid osmotic pressure.* Plasma proteins are colloids, large particles that do not readily move across the capillary membrane. They tend to remain within the capillary. At the same time, there is very little water in the interstitial space. The small amount of water that does get into the interstitial space is usually taken up by the lymph system. Therefore, since there is little water outside the capillary, and because plasma proteins do not readily move outside the capillary, the forces governing movement of water between the capillary and the interstitial space are almost all on one side, governed by the plasma on the inside of the capillary.

Another force inside the capillaries is **hydrostatic pressure,** which is the blood pressure, or force against the vessel walls, created by contractions of the heart. Hydrostatic pressure does tend to force some water out of the plasma and across the capillary wall into the interstitial space, a process that is called **filtration.** Hydrostatic pressure (a force that favors filtration, pushing water out of the capillary) and oncotic force (a force opposing filtration, pulling water into the capillary) together are responsible for **net filtration,** which is described in *Starling's hypothesis:*

Net filtration = (Forces favoring filtration) − (Forces opposing filtration)

Net filtration in a capillary is normally zero. It works this way: As plasma enters the capillary at the arterial end, hydrostatic pressure forces water to cross the capillary membrane into the interstitial space. This loss of water increases the relative concentration of plasma proteins. By the time the plasma reaches the venous end of the capillary, the oncotic force exerted by the increased concentration of plasma proteins is great enough to pull the water from the interstitial space back into the capillary. The outcome is that water is retained in the intravascular space and does not remain in the interstitial space.

Edema

Edema is the accumulation of water in the interstitial space. It occurs when there is a disruption in the forces and mechanisms that normally keep net filtration at zero (retaining water in the vascular system as plasma flows through the capillaries, according to Starling's hypothesis, previously described) or a disruption in the forces that would normally remove water from the interstitial space.

The mechanisms that most commonly result in accumulation of water in the interstitial space are a decrease in plasma oncotic force, an increase in hydrostatic pressure, increased permeability of the capillary membrane, and lymphatic obstruction.

  ★ *A decrease in plasma oncotic force* may result from a loss or decrease in production of plasma proteins (albumins, globulins, and clotting factors). Plasma proteins are synthesized in the liver, so a liver disorder may be responsible for decreased production. Plasma loss from open wounds, hemorrhage, and burns may also cause a loss of plasma proteins. The result is that oncotic force is reduced to the point that some of the water lost through hydrostatic pressure is not regained.

  ★ *An increase in hydrostatic pressure* can result from venous obstruction, salt and water retention, thrombophlebitis, liver obstruction, tight clothing at the extremities, or prolonged standing. The increase in hydrostatic pressure forces more water into the interstitial space than the oncotic force can recover.

  ★ *Increased capillary permeability* generally results from the mechanisms of inflammation and immune response. These can result from allergic

oncotic force *a form of osmotic pressure exerted by the large protein particles, or colloids, present in blood plasma. In the capillaries, the plasma colloids tend to pull water from the interstitial space across the capillary membrane into the capillary. Oncotic force is also called* colloid osmotic pressure.

hydrostatic pressure *blood pressure or force against vessel walls created by the heartbeat. Hydrostatic pressure tends to force water out of the capillaries into the interstitial space.*

filtration *movement of water out of the plasma across the capillary membrane into the interstitial space.*

net filtration *the total loss of water from blood plasma across the capillary membrane into the interstitial space. Normally, hydrostatic pressure forcing water out of the capillary is balanced by oncotic force pulling water into the capillary for a net filtration of zero.*

edema *excess fluid in the interstitial space.*

reactions, burns, trauma, or cancer. The greater permeability allows plasma proteins to escape from the capillaries, permitting water to remain in the interstitial space through the osmotic pressure of increased interstitial proteins and the reduction of oncotic force within the capillaries.

★ *Lymphatic channel obstruction* can result from infection. Lymphatic channels are also sometimes removed through surgery. The loss of lymphatic channels interferes with the normal absorption of interstitial fluid by the lymphatic system. For example, removal of axillary lymph nodes in the treatment of breast cancer can result in edema of the arm.

Edema can be localized or generalized. Local swelling may appear at the site of an injury (e.g., a sprained ankle) or within a certain organ system such as the brain (cerebral edema), lungs (pulmonary edema), heart (pericardial effusion), or abdomen (ascites). A generalized edema may present as dependent edema, in which gravity pulls water to the lowest areas; for example, in the feet and ankles when standing or in the sacral area when supine. You can identify dependent edema by pressing a finger over a bony prominence. A pit may remain after you remove your finger, and this is called *pitting edema.*

Edema is not only a sign of an underlying disease or problem; edema itself causes problems. It interferes with the movement of nutrients and wastes between tissues and capillaries. It may diminish capillary blood flow, depriving tissues of oxygen. In turn, this may slow the healing of wounds, promote infection, and facilitate formation of pressure sores. Edema affecting organs such as the brain, lung, heart, or larynx may be life threatening.

Body water that is retained in the interstitial spaces is body water that is not available for metabolic processes in the cells. Therefore, even though the total body water is normal, edema can cause a relative condition of dehydration.

The body has regulatory mechanisms that help to maintain homeostasis by controlling total body water and water distribution. Antidiuretic hormone (ADH), also known as *vasopressin,* is the chief regulator of water retention and distribution. Throughout the body, a network of sensors detects fluctuations in fluid and changes in the osmolar concentration of plasma. Osmoreceptors are located in the anterior hypothalamus. If there is an increase of 1 to 2 percent in osmolality—that is, if there is relatively less fluid in the plasma—the osmoreceptors will stimulate the release of ADH in an attempt to retain more fluid. Another type of receptor, baroreceptors, will detect both high and low pressure levels. Baroreceptors located in the carotid sinus, aortic arch, and kidney detect increases and decreases in pressure. Signals from the baroreceptors are relayed to the hypothalamus which, again, will stimulate release of ADH as needed.

Definitive treatment of edema requires treatment of the underlying cause. Supportive care may include applying compression stockings, restricting salt intake, improving nutritional status, avoiding prolonged standing, and taking diuretics. Little can be done in the prehospital setting except elevation of edematous limbs.

INTRAVENOUS THERAPY

Intravenous (IV) therapy is the introduction of fluids and other substances into the venous side of the circulatory system. It is used to replace blood lost through hemorrhage, for electrolyte or fluid replacement, and for introduction of medications directly into the vascular system.

Blood and Blood Components

To understand IV therapy, it is necessary to understand the function of blood and its components. The blood is the fluid of the cardiovascular system. An adequate amount

Edema is not only a sign of underlying disease. Edema itself causes problems. Edema of the brain, lung, heart, or larynx may be life threatening.

Little can be done to treat edema in the prehospital setting except elevation of edematous limbs.

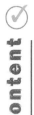

✓ **Review**

Blood Components

Liquid portion (plasma)
Formed elements (blood
   cells)

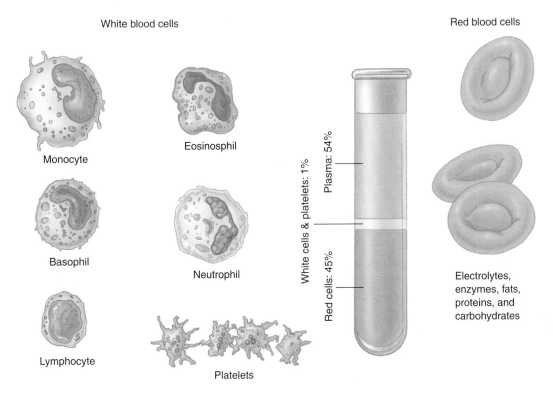

White blood cells

Monocyte

Eosinosphil

Basophil

Neutrophil

Lymphocyte

Platelets

Red blood cells

Plasma: 54%

White cells & platelets: 1%

Red cells: 45%

Electrolytes, enzymes, fats, proteins, and carbohydrates

■ Figure 8-6   Blood components.

of blood is required for the transport of nutrients, oxygen, hormones, and heat. Blood consists of the liquid portion, or plasma, and the formed elements, or blood cells (Figure 8-6 ■).

Plasma   Plasma is made up of approximately 92 percent water, 6 to 7 percent proteins, and a small portion consisting of electrolytes, lipids, enzymes, clotting factors, glucose, and other dissolved substances.

Formed Elements   The formed elements include the red blood cells, or **erythrocytes;** the white blood cells, or **leukocytes;** and the platelets, or **thrombocytes.** More than 99 percent of the blood cells are erythrocytes. Erythrocytes contain hemoglobin and are responsible for transporting oxygen to the body's peripheral cells. **Hemoglobin** is an iron-based compound that binds with oxygen in the pulmonary (lung) capillaries and transports the oxygen to the peripheral tissues where it can be unloaded and taken into the cells. Factors such as pH (to be discussed later in this chapter) and oxygen concentration affect the amount of oxygen that can be transported by hemoglobin.

The leukocytes are responsible for immunity and fighting infection. The thrombocytes play a major role in blood clotting. The viscosity (thickness) of the blood is determined by the ratio of plasma to formed elements. The greater the proportion of formed elements within the plasma, the greater the viscosity.

The plasma can be separated from the formed elements by centrifugation. That is, blood can be placed in a test tube inside a centrifuge and spun at high speed. The heavier cells, the erythrocytes, will be forced to the bottom of the tube, leaving the plasma portion at the top. Usually, the erythrocytes will account for approximately 45 percent of the blood volume. The percentage of blood occupied by erythrocytes is referred to as the **hematocrit** (Figure 8-7 ■).

plasma   *the liquid part of the blood.*

erythrocytes   *red blood cells, which contain hemoglobin, which transports oxygen to the cells.*

leukocytes   *white blood cells, which play a key role in the immune system and inflammatory (infection-fighting) responses.*

thrombocytes   *platelets, which are important in blood clotting.*

hemoglobin   *an iron-based compound that binds with oxygen and transports it to the cells.*

hematocrit   *the percentage of the blood occupied by erythrocytes.*

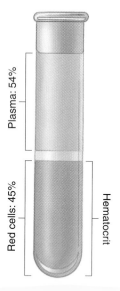

■ **Figure 8-7** The percentage of the blood occupied by the red blood cells is termed the hematocrit.

Be alert for signs and symptoms of transfusion reaction. If they occur, immediately stop the transfusion.

Fluid Replacement

The most desirable fluid for blood loss replacement is whole blood. There are several reasons for this. First, blood contains hemoglobin, which can transport oxygen. In addition, it is the most natural replacement. However, even in the hospital setting, the routine use of whole blood is not practical (Table 8–2). Blood is a precious commodity, and it must be conserved so that it can benefit the most people. Because of this, blood is often fractionated, or separated into parts. The red cells are packaged separately as packed red blood cells. The white cells are used for other purposes. Plasma is packaged as fresh frozen plasma for use when plasma or clotting factors are needed. Thus, with the exception of true hemorrhagic shock (resulting from blood loss), where whole blood is the fluid of first choice, packed red blood cells are now more frequently used than whole blood.

Before blood, or blood products, can be administered to a patient, they must be typed and cross-matched to prevent a severe allergic reaction. The exception to this is fresh frozen plasma, which does not require cross-matching. If there is not adequate time for typing and cross-matching, O-negative blood (type O, Rh negative), the universal donor, can be administered.

Transfusion Reaction

Blood and blood products are not used in the field. However, on occasion, you may be called upon to transport a patient with blood infusing. Because of this, you must be able to recognize the signs and symptoms of a transfusion reaction. Transfusion reactions occur when there is a discrepancy between the blood type of the patient and the blood type of the blood being transfused. In addition to the ABO and Rh types, there are many minor types that can cause a transfusion reaction. Common signs and symptoms of a transfusion reaction include fever, chills, hives, hypotension, palpitations, tachycardia, flushing of the skin, headaches, loss of consciousness, nausea, vomiting, or shortness of breath.

If a transfusion reaction is suspected, IMMEDIATELY stop the transfusion and save the substance being transfused. A rapid IV fluid infusion should be started to prevent renal damage. Quickly assess the patient's mental status. Administer oxygen and contact medical direction. The medical direction physician may request the administration of mannitol (Osmotrol), diphenhydramine (Benadryl), or furosemide (Lasix). These drugs are used to maintain renal function, which is often severely compromised during a transfusion reaction.

In addition to overt reaction, you must always be alert for signs of fluid overload and congestive heart failure secondary to transfusion. This is evidenced by increased dyspnea, pulmonary congestion, edema, and altered mental status. If fluid overload is suspected, stop the infusion and start a crystalloid solution at a TKO (to-keep-open) rate. Administer oxygen and contact the medical direction physician.

Table 8–2	Resuscitation Fluids			
	Resuscitation Fluid Used			
Diagnosis	**1st Choice**	**2nd Choice**	**3rd Choice**	**4th Choice**
Hemorrhagic Shock	Whole blood	Packed RBCs	Plasma or plasma substitute	Lactated Ringer's or normal saline
Shock Due to Plasma Loss (Burns)	Plasma	Plasma substitute	Lactated Ringer's or normal saline	—
Dehydration	Lactated Ringer's or normal saline	—	—	—

Intravenous Fluids

Intravenous fluids are the most common products used in prehospital care for fluid and electrolyte therapy. Intravenous fluids occur in two standard forms—colloids and crystalloids. An important new type of intravenous fluid is the hemoglobin-based oxygen-carrying solutions (HBOCs).

Hemoglobin-Based Oxygen-Carrying Solutions (HBOCs) Hemoglobin-Based Oxygen-Carrying Solutions (HBOCs) represent a major development in the field of emergency and critical care. These products differ from other intravenous fluids in that they have the capability to transport oxygen. HBOCs contain long chains of *polymerized hemoglobin*. This hemoglobin is obtained from either expired donated human blood or bovine (cow) blood. The hemoglobin is removed from the red blood cells and then repeatedly filtered to remove any infectious substances or antigenic proteins. Finally, the individual hemoglobin molecules are joined together in a large chain through a chemical process known as polymerization. HBOCs are compatible with all blood types and do not require blood typing, testing, or cross-matching.

hemoglobin-based oxygen-carrying solutions (HBOCs) *intravenous fluids that have the capability to transport oxygen and are compatible with all blood types.*

★ *PolyHeme* is an HBOCs derived from expired donated human blood. PolyHeme contains 50 grams of hemoglobin per unit, which is the same as human blood. PolyHeme must be refrigerated, and the shelf life is one year.

★ *Hemopure* is an HBOCs derived from bovine (cow) blood. It has been widely used in South Africa. Hemopure does not require refrigeration and has a shelf life of 3 years.

Colloids **Colloids** contain proteins, or other high-molecular-weight molecules, that tend to remain in the intravascular space for an extended period of time. In addition, as described earlier, colloids have oncotic force (colloid osmotic pressure), which means they tend to attract water into the intravascular space from the interstitial space and the intracellular space. Thus, a small amount of a colloid can be administered to a patient with a greater-than-expected increase in intravascular volume. The following are examples of colloids:

colloids *substances, such as proteins or starches, consisting of large molecules or molecule aggregates that disperse evenly within a liquid without forming a true solution.*

★ *Plasma protein fraction (Plasmanate)* is a protein-containing colloid. The principal protein present is **albumin,** which is suspended along with other proteins in a saline solvent.

★ *Salt-poor albumin* contains only human albumin. Each gram of albumin holds approximately 18 milliliters of water in the bloodstream.

★ *Dextran* is not a protein, but a large sugar molecule with osmotic properties similar to albumin. It comes in two molecular weights: 40,000 and 70,000 Daltons. Dextran 40 has 2 to 2.5 times the colloid osmotic pressure of albumin.

★ *Hetastarch (Hespan)*, like dextran, is a sugar molecule with osmotic properties similar to protein. It does not appear to share many of dextran's side effects.

albumin *a protein commonly present in plant and animal tissues. In the blood, albumin works to maintain blood volume and blood pressure and provides colloid osmotic pressure, which prevents plasma loss from the capillaries.*

Colloid replacement therapy, at present, does not have a role in prehospital care except under rare circumstances. The colloid products are expensive and have a short shelf life.

crystalloids *substances capable of crystallization. In solution, unlike colloids, they can diffuse through a membrane, such as a capillary wall.*

Crystalloids **Crystalloids** are the primary compounds used in prehospital intravenous fluid therapy. There are multiple fluid preparations. It is often helpful to classify them according to their **tonicity** relative to plasma:

tonicity *solute concentration or osmotic pressure relative to the blood plasma or body cells.*

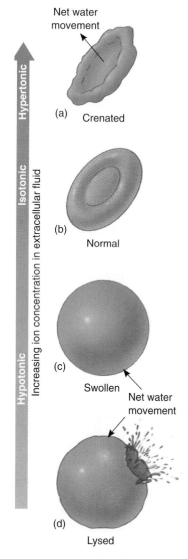

Net water movement

(a) Crenated

(b) Normal

(c) Swollen

Net water movement

(d) Lysed

Hypertonic

Isotonic

Hypotonic

Increasing ion concentration in extracellular fluid

■ Figure 8-8 The effects of hypertonic, isotonic, and hypotonic solutions on red blood cells.

The three most commonly used fluids in prehospital care are lactated Ringer's, normal saline, and D_5W.

★ *Isotonic solutions* have electrolyte composition similar to the blood plasma. When placed into a normally hydrated patient, they will not cause a significant fluid or electrolyte shift. Examples: normal saline (0.9 percent sodium chloride, also written as 0.9 percent NaCl), lactated Ringer's.

★ *Hypertonic solutions* have a higher solute concentration than the cells. These fluids will tend to cause a fluid shift out of the interstitial space and intracellular compartment into the intravascular space when administered to a normally hydrated patient. Later, there will be a diffusion of solute in the opposite direction. Examples: plasmanate, dextran.

★ *Hypotonic solutions* have a lower solute concentration than the cells. When administered to a normally hydrated patient, they will cause a movement of fluid from the intravascular space into the interstitial space and intracellular compartment. Later, solutes will move in an opposite direction. Example: 5 percent dextrose in water (D_5W).

Intravenous replacement fluids should be chosen based on the needs of the patient and the patient's underlying problem. This is typically guided by laboratory studies obtained in the hospital. However, these studies are not available in the prehospital setting. Hemorrhage occurs so fast that there is usually not time for a significant fluid shift to occur between the intravascular space and interstitial/intracellular spaces. Because of this, isotonic replacement fluids, such as lactated Ringer's and normal saline, should be used (Figure 8-8 ■).

Certain conditions, such as gastroenteritis (characterized by diarrhea, vomiting, and fever), can cause a patient to lose water more rapidly than sodium. These patients will have a deficit in total body water (TBW) due to reduced water intake, excessive water loss, or a combination of both. When water is lost in this manner, the level of sodium in the serum can increase, resulting in hypernatremia (elevated sodium levels). Patients with hypernatremia primarily need water. Because of this, hypotonic intravenous solutions, such as 0.45 percent sodium chloride (half-normal saline), are often chosen, because they provide the needed water with less sodium. However, it is important to point out that, even in cases of hypernatremia, initial fluid replacement therapy should be with an isotonic solution until adequate blood pressure and adequate tissue perfusion have been restored.

Some replacement fluids contain a single element, such as sodium chloride or dextrose, while others contain multiple elements. Solutions such as lactated Ringer's are designed so that the concentration of electrolytes is very similar to that of the plasma. As a result, these solutions are referred to as balanced salt solutions.

The most commonly used solutions in prehospital care are lactated Ringer's solution, 0.9 percent sodium chloride (normal saline), and 5 percent dextrose in water (D_5W).

★ *Lactated Ringer's* is an isotonic electrolyte solution of sodium chloride, potassium chloride, calcium chloride, and sodium lactate in water.

★ *Normal saline* is an electrolyte solution of sodium chloride in water. It is isotonic with the extracellular fluid.

★ *D_5W* is a hypotonic glucose solution used to keep a vein open and to supply calories necessary for cell metabolism. While it will have an initial effect of increasing the circulatory volume, glucose molecules rapidly diffuse across the vascular membrane. Water follows the glucose into the interstitial space, resulting in an increase in interstitial water.

Both lactated Ringer's solution and normal saline are used for fluid replacement, because their administration causes an immediate expansion of the circulatory volume. However, as was noted earlier, due to the movement of electrolytes and water, two thirds of either of these solutions is lost into the interstitial space within 1 hour.

ACID-BASE BALANCE

Acid-base balance is a dynamic relationship that reflects the relative concentration of hydrogen ions (H^+) in the body. Hydrogen ions are acidic and the concentration of these within the body must be maintained within fairly strict limits. Any deviation in the hydrogen ion concentration adversely affects all of the biochemical events that occur in the body. The hydrogen ion concentration is dynamic, changing from second to second.

THE pH SCALE

The total number of hydrogen ions present in the body at any given time is very high. Because of this, the **pH** system of measurement is used. The pH scale is inversely related to hydrogen ion concentration. That is, the greater the hydrogen ion concentration, the lower the pH. The lower the hydrogen ion concentration, the higher the pH.

The pH scale is *logarithmic*, with each number representing a value 10 times that of its neighboring number, so that pH 6 represents a hydrogen ion concentration 10 times as great as that represented by pH 7. The following formula represents pH:

$$pH = \log \frac{1}{[H^+]}$$

The pH scale ranges from 1 to 14. A pH of 1 means that only hydrogen ions are present. A pH of 14 means that there are virtually no hydrogen ions present. The pH of water is 7.0, which is a neutral pH. The pH of the body is normally 7.35 to 7.45 (Table 8–3).

Because hydrogen ions are acidic, a pH below 7.35 is referred to as **acidosis.** A substance that produces negatively charged ions that can neutralize the positively charged

pH *abbreviation for* potential of hydrogen. *A measure of relative acidity or alkalinity. Since the pH scale is inverse to the concentration of acidic hydrogen ions, the lower the pH the greater the acidity and the higher the pH the greater the alkalinity. A normal pH range is 7.35 to 7.45.*

acidosis *a high concentration of hydrogen ions; a pH below 7.35.*

Table 8–3	The pH Scale and Hydrogen Ion Concentrations		
pH		**Example**	**Hydrogen Ion Concentration***
Acidic	0	Hydrochloric acid	10^{-0} (1.0)
	1	Stomach secretions	10^{-1} (0.1)
	2	Lemon juice	10^{-2} (0.01)
	3	Cola drinks	10^{-3} (0.001)
	4	White wine	10^{-4} (0.0001)
	5	Tomato juice	10^{-5} (0.00001)
	6	Coffee, urine, saliva	10^{-6} (0.000001)
Neutral	7	Distilled water	10^{-7} (0.0000001)
Basic	8	Blood, semen	10^{-8} (0.00000001)
	9	Bile	10^{-9} (0.000000001)
	10	Bleach	10^{-10} (0.0000000001)
	11	Milk of magnesia	10^{-11} (0.00000000001)
	12	Ammonia water	10^{-12} (0.000000000001)
	13	Drain opener	10^{-13} (0.0000000000001)
	14	Lye	10^{-14} (0.00000000000001)

*Hydrogen ion concentrations are expressed in moles per liter, a quantity based on molecular weight.

hydrogen ions (or other acids) is called an *alkali* or a *base*. An excess of alkaline (base) substances or a deficit of acids will produce a pH above 7.45, which is referred to as **alkalosis.** In humans, a variation of only 0.4 of a pH unit in either direction from normal (6.9 or 7.8) can be fatal.

BODILY REGULATION OF ACID-BASE BALANCE

The body is constantly producing hydrogen ions (acids) through metabolism and other biochemical processes. To maintain the acid-base balance, these hydrogen ions must be constantly eliminated from the body. There are three major mechanisms to remove hydrogen ions from the body. The fastest mechanism is often referred to as the *buffer system* or the *bicarbonate buffer system.*

The two components of the bicarbonate buffer system are bicarbonate ion (HCO_3^-) and carbonic acid (H_2CO_3). These two compounds are in equilibrium with hydrogen ion (H^+), as follows: In some circumstances hydrogen ion will combine with bicarbonate ion to produce carbonic acid. In other circumstances, carbonic acid will dissociate into bicarbonate ion and hydrogen ion:

$$H^+ + HCO_3^- \leftrightarrow H_2CO_3$$
Hydrogen ion + bicarbonate ion $\leftrightarrow$ carbonic acid

In a healthy individual, for every molecule of carbonic acid, there are 20 molecules of bicarbonate ion. Any change in this 20:1 ratio is immediately corrected without significant change in the total body pH. This occurs in the following manner: An increase in hydrogen ion (acidosis) is corrected as the excess hydrogen ions combine with bicarbonate ions to form carbonic acid. (Thus, an increase in hydrogen ion leads to an increase in carbonic acid—driving the previous equation to the right.) Conversely, when there is a deficit in hydrogen ions (alkalosis), carbonic acid will dissociate into bicarbonate ion and hydrogen ion. [Thus, a decrease in hydrogen ion leads to a decrease in carbonic acid—driving the previous equation to the left (Figure 8-9 ■).]

$$\text{Increased Acid: } \uparrow H^+ + HCO_3^- \rightarrow \uparrow H_2CO_3$$
$$\text{Decreased Acid: } \downarrow H^+ + HCO_3^- \rightarrow \downarrow H_2CO_3$$

Carbonic acid is a weak acid that is better tolerated by the body than pure hydrogen ion. However, the body carries this reaction further. Any increase in carbonic acid must also be eliminated.

The elimination of excess carbonic acid takes place as follows: Carbonic acid is unstable and will eventually dissociate into carbon dioxide and water. This normally slow process is speeded by the blood's erythrocytes, which contain an enzyme called *carbonic anhydrase.* Carbonic anhydrase causes carbonic acid to be converted to carbon dioxide and water very rapidly—so rapidly that carbonic acid exists for only a fraction of a second before it is converted into carbon dioxide and water. Most buffering of acid in the body occurs in the erythrocytes.

The enzyme also works in a reverse fashion, which allows carbon dioxide and water to be quickly converted into carbonic acid. The reaction proceeds in accordance with *LeChetalier's Principle.* Given an excess of carbon dioxide on the right hand side of the equilibrium, a stress is placed on it such that it must shift to the left, which is sometimes referred to as a mass action effect. The net effect of this is the generation of more hydrogen ion, and acidosis. The clinical application of this is that when a patient is said to hypoventilate, that is, retain CO_2, then the accumulation (stress) of increased CO_2 forces the equilibrium to shift to the left, causing what is known as respiratory acidosis. So, with the aid of carbonic anhydrase, an equilibrium eventually is attained between hydrogen ion and carbon dioxide. The following equation illustrates this relationship.

$$H^+ + HCO_3^- \leftrightarrow H_2CO_3 \leftrightarrow H_2O + CO_2$$

hydrogen ion + bicarbonate ion $\leftrightarrow$ carbonic acid $\leftrightarrow$ water + carbon dioxide

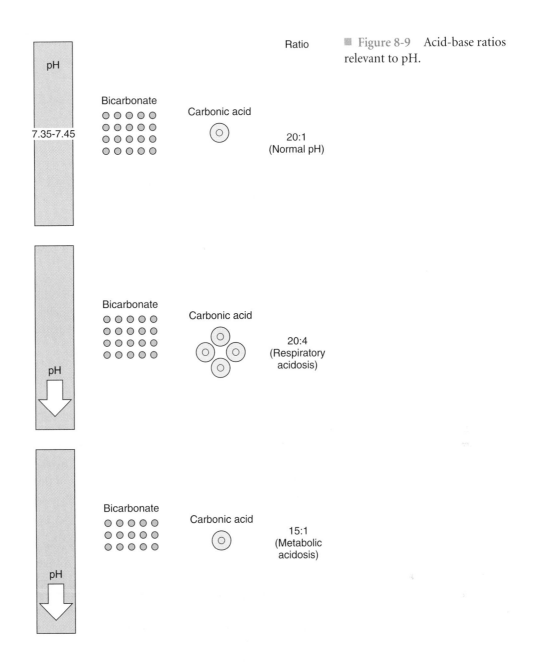

Ratio

Bicarbonate   Carbonic acid

20:1
(Normal pH)

Bicarbonate   Carbonic acid

20:4
(Respiratory acidosis)

Bicarbonate   Carbonic acid

15:1
(Metabolic acidosis)

Thus, an increase in hydrogen ion (acid) would result in an increase in carbonic acid. With the aid of carbonic anhydrase, carbonic acid would quickly dissociate into water and carbon dioxide. Conversely (since the reaction can move in either direction), an increase in CO_2 causes an increase in hydrogen ion concentration and a decrease in pH (increase in acidity), as shown below.

$$\uparrow H^+ \leftrightarrow \uparrow CO_2$$

In conjunction with the bicarbonate buffer system previously described, the body regulates acid–base balance by two other mechanisms, respiration and kidney function. Increased respirations cause increased elimination of CO_2, which results in a decrease in hydrogen ions and an increase in pH. Conversely, decreased respirations cause CO_2 to be retained. This causes an increase in hydrogen ions and a decrease in pH (Figure 8-10 ■).

The kidneys also can regulate the pH by altering the concentration of bicarbonate ion (HCO_3^-) in the blood. Increased elimination of HCO_3^- results in a lowered pH. (There is less bicarbonate ion to combine with and eliminate hydrogen ion.) Conversely retention of HCO_3^- causes an increase in pH. (There is more bicarbonate ion to combine

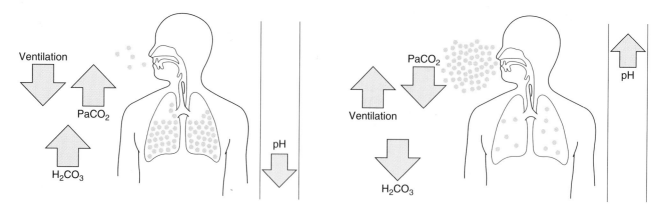

Figure 8-10   The respiratory component of acid-base balance.

with and eliminate hydrogen ion.) In addition, the kidneys affect the acid-base balance by removing or retaining various chemicals. Normally, the kidneys remove larger metabolic acids, excreting them in the urine, resulting in an increase in pH.

ACID-BASE DERANGEMENTS

As previously noted, an increase in hydrogen ion (as occurs, for example, in cardiac arrest) drives the equation described earlier to the right. Hydrogen ion is immediately combined with bicarbonate ion. This combination results in the formation of carbonic acid, which then dissociates into carbon dioxide and water with the assistance of carbonic anhydrase. Carbon dioxide is eliminated by the lungs, and water is eliminated through the kidneys. Any change in a component of this equation affects the other components. For example:

$$\uparrow H^+ + HCO_3^- \rightarrow \uparrow H_2CO_3 \rightarrow H_2O + \uparrow CO_2$$

Conversely, if the amount of carbon dioxide is increased, the equation is driven in the other direction, resulting in an increase in hydrogen ion (acid).

$$\uparrow CO_2 + H_2O \rightarrow \uparrow H_2CO_3 \rightarrow \uparrow H^+ + HCO_3^-$$

Both types of acid-base derangements, alkalosis and acidosis, can be divided into two categories based on the underlying causes. Changes in the concentration of CO_2 result from changes in respiratory function. Thus, an acidosis caused by retained CO_2 is referred to as *respiratory acidosis*. An alkalosis caused by the excess removal of CO_2 is called *respiratory alkalosis*. However, if acidosis results from the production of metabolic acids, such as lactic acid, then *metabolic acidosis* is said to exist. If an alkalosis is caused by the excess elimination of hydrogen ion, it is termed *metabolic alkalosis*.

Respiratory Acidosis

Respiratory acidosis is caused by the retention of CO_2. This can result from impaired ventilation due to problems occurring either in the lungs or in the respiratory center of the brain. The CO_2 level is increased and the pH is decreased.

$$\downarrow RESPIRATION = \uparrow CO_2 + H_2O \rightarrow \uparrow H_2CO_3 \rightarrow \uparrow H^+ + HCO_3^-$$

Treatment is directed at improving ventilation.

Respiratory Alkalosis

Respiratory alkalosis results from increased respiration and excessive elimination of CO_2. This can occur with anxiety or following ascent to a high altitude. The CO_2 level is decreased and the pH is increased.

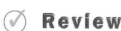

Review

Acid-Base Derangements

Respiratory acidosis
Respiratory alkalosis
Metabolic acidosis
Metabolic alkalosis

respiratory acidosis *acidity caused by abnormal retention of carbon dioxide resulting from impaired ventilation.*

respiratory alkalosis *alkalinity caused by excessive elimination of carbon dioxide resulting from increased respirations.*

$$\uparrow \text{RESPIRATION} = \downarrow CO_2 + H_2O \rightarrow \downarrow H_2CO_3 \rightarrow \downarrow H^+ + HCO_3^-$$

Treatment, if required, consists of increasing the CO_2 level by emotionally supporting the patient and coaching him to reduce his respiratory rate.

Metabolic Acidosis

Metabolic acidosis results from the production of metabolic acids such as lactic acid, which consume bicarbonate ion. In addition, it can result from dehydration (as from diarrhea, vomiting), diabetes, and medication usage. The pH is decreased, and the CO_2 level is normal.

$$\uparrow H^+ + HCO_3^- \rightarrow \uparrow H_2CO_3 \rightarrow H_2O + \uparrow CO_2$$

In addition to treating the underlying cause, treatment includes ventilation, which causes the elimination of CO_2 and, subsequently, hydrogen ion (Figure 8-11 ■). On rare occasions, an IV bolus of sodium bicarbonate ($NaHCO_3$) may be required.

Metabolic Alkalosis

Metabolic alkalosis occurs much less frequently than metabolic acidosis. It is usually caused by the administration of **diuretics,** loss of chloride ions associated with prolonged vomiting, or the overzealous administration of sodium bicarbonate. The pH is increased and the CO_2 level is normal.

$$\downarrow H^+ + HCO_3^- \rightarrow \downarrow H_2CO_3 \rightarrow H_2O + \downarrow CO_2$$

Treatment consists of correcting the underlying cause.

metabolic acidosis *acidity caused by an increase in acid, often because of increased production of acids during metabolism or from causes such as vomiting, diarrhea, diabetes, or medication.*

metabolic alkalosis *alkalinity caused by an increase in plasma bicarbonate resulting from causes including diuresis, vomiting, or ingestion of too much sodium bicarbonate.*

diuretic *an agent that increases urine secretion and elimination of body water.*

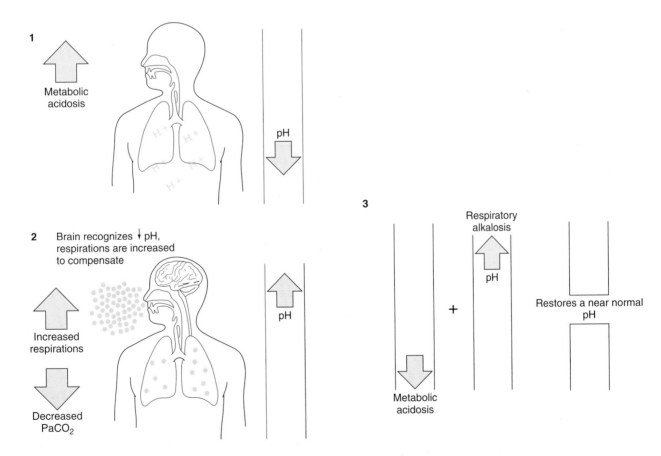

■ Figure 8-11   Compensation for metabolic acidosis begins with an increase in respirations.

Usually, both a respiratory and a metabolic component are present in an acid-base derangement. The type of acid-base derangement present can only be determined by arterial blood gas studies. These, of course, are only available in the hospital setting. Arterial blood gases report the pH, $PaCO_2$, PaO_2, bicarbonate concentration, and oxygen saturation. Pulse oximetry is now available for field use and is quite accurate in determining oxygen saturation levels. It does not, however, provide any information about the patient's underlying acid-base status.

Part 2: Disease—Causes and Pathophysiology

GENETIC AND OTHER CAUSES OF DISEASE

When we think of disease, we are likely to think first of infections caused by pathogens, including bacteria, viruses, fungi, and parasites. In recent years, great strides have been made in the medical treatment of infectious diseases, but many diseases result from genetic causes, which have been far more difficult to identify and treat. The picture is additionally complicated by the fact that many diseases result from a combination of genetic and environmental factors (including lifestyle factors) as well as factors such as age and gender.

Even a family history of a particular disease does not necessarily mean that the disease has a purely genetic origin, because families also share environmental and lifestyle factors that may cause or contribute to the family disease. While family history points to the possibility of genetic causes, these cannot be confirmed, much less treated, until scientists are able to make definitive identifications of the defective genes or chromosomes that cause or contribute to particular diseases.

At present, there is increasing progress in identifying and understanding genetic and other noninfectious causes of disease. Many promising advances toward gene therapies (the replacement of defective genes with normal genes) and other therapies for diseases have been made.

GENETICS, ENVIRONMENT, LIFESTYLE, AGE, AND GENDER

As noted earlier, our inherited traits are determined by molecules of deoxyribonucleic acid, or DNA, which form structures called genes, which reside on larger structures called chromosomes within the nuclei of all our cells. We inherit our genetic structure from our parents. Every one of a person's somatic cells (all the cells except the sex cells) contains 46 chromosomes. The sex cells, however, contain only 23 chromosomes each. The sex cells contribute these 23 chromosomes to the offspring. Thus, the offspring receives 23 chromosomes from the father and 23 chromosomes from the mother, resulting in a total of 46 chromosomes. Occasionally one or more of a person's genes or chromosomes is abnormal, and this may cause a congenital disease (one we are born with) or a propensity toward acquiring a disease later in life.

Some diseases are thought to be purely genetic. For example, cystic fibrosis, which affects mainly people of European origin, and sickle cell disease, which affects mainly people of African origin, are known to be caused by disorders of single genes. They affect different populations to a different degree because of the evolutionary history of those populations. A genetic disease may be caused by a single defective gene or by several defective genes or chromosomes. Single-gene causes are, obviously, easier for medical researchers to identify and potentially devise treatments for than are other, more complex genetic causes of disease.

Other diseases are caused by a combination of genetic and environmental factors and are called *multifactorial disorders*. For example, Type II (adult-onset) diabetes has

Every human somatic cell contains 46 chromosomes (23 pairs).

Most disease processes are multifactorial in origin.

a very high correlation with family history of the disease. However, it is also affected by environmental and lifestyle factors such as a high-fat or high-carbohydrate diet and lack of exercise, which results in obesity, and with age. (There is a higher incidence of Type II diabetes in overweight people, and the disease tends to appear in middle age or later.) Heart disease, which is highly correlated with family history and age, also has a gender/hormonal factor: Women appear to be somewhat protected from heart disease before menopause, when their bodies are still producing estrogen. Following menopause, women quickly "catch up" with men in the development of heart disease.

Clinical practitioners and epidemiologists study disease, respectively, from the point of view of their effects on individuals and from the point of view of their effects on populations as a whole.

Review

Causative Analysis of Disease

Clinical Factors:

Host

Agent

Environment

Epidemiological Factors:

Incidence

Prevalence

Mortality

★ *Effects on Individuals.* Physicians and other clinical practitioners study the effects of diseases on individuals, and find it instructive to view the development of diseases as products of the interactions among three factors: *host, agent,* and *environment.* This establishes a framework for determining how one, or a combination, of these factors may precipitate a disease state. Genetic predisposition, gender, and ethnic origin are determinants related to the host. These may interact with a specific agent, in a specific type of environment, to cause illness. The agent may be a bacterium, toxin, gunshot, or other pathophysiological process. The environment may be defined by the local climate, socioeconomic or demographic features, culture, religion, and associated factors. Determination of how the host, agent, and environment interact may yield solutions to curing a disease process. Injury and trauma are now being viewed as "diseases," in the sense of how the interaction of host, agent, and environment may contribute to an understanding of what, heretofore, have been perceived as social problems.

★ *Effects on Populations.* Epidemiologists, who study the effects of diseases on populations, generally report disease data with three basic measures: *incidence, prevalence,* and *mortality. Morbidity,* a term commonly used in discussing disease statistics, can be more precisely reported as incidence and prevalence. Incidence is the number of new cases of the disease that are reported in a given period of time, usually 1 year. Prevalence is the proportion of the total population who are affected by the disease at a given point in time. (Prevalence is higher than incidence, as those who acquire the disease each year are added to those who already have the disease.) *Mortality* is the rate of death from the disease.

Epidemiologists and clinical practitioners are now collaborating to study risk factors, such as the relationship between smoking and lung cancer. Risk factor analysis is both statistical and complex. Although the correlation of smoking to lung cancer is extremely high, not everyone who smokes develops lung cancer, and not everyone who develops lung cancer has been a smoker. Risk factor analysis would compare the number of smokers to nonsmokers among lung cancer cases, the pack/year (number of packs per day × number of years) history of the smokers with lung cancer, factors that might have aggravated or mitigated the effects of smoking, and so on.

FAMILY HISTORY AND ASSOCIATED RISK FACTORS

It is important for those who have a family history of a particular disease not to conclude that acquiring the disease is their destiny and there is nothing they can do about it. This is not always true. Most diseases with a genetic component that come on during adulthood also have associated risk factors that can be modified to prevent, delay, or reduce the impact of the disease.

Consider the variety of possible risk factors for disease: People who live in less-developed countries are often at higher risk for disease from microorganisms flourishing in their water supply and disease transmission caused by poor sanitation. Physical conditions commonly seen in larger U.S. cities as well as rural areas, such as inadequate housing, poor nutrition, and little or no medical attention, potentiate disease transmission. Chemical factors such as smoke, smog, illicit drug use, occupational chemical exposure, and additives in our food are causative agents for a variety of diseases.

Personal habit is among the most publicized—and controllable—causes of disease in our society. For example, predisposing factors for cardiovascular disease include smoking, excessive alcohol consumption, inactivity, and obesity. Unfortunately, changes in individual lifestyle often occur only after a disease has already manifested itself. As we age, the predisposing factors and causative agents take their toll. The body's ability to defend itself against disease decreases due to the effects of aging on our immunological system and other compensatory mechanisms.

Following is a discussion of some of the most common diseases in which both genetics and other risk factors play a role. You will notice, as you read, that the causation of various diseases varies widely, and that while the causes are known for some diseases, the causes of other diseases are still not clearly understood.

Immunologic Disorders

A number of immunologic disorders, such as rheumatic fever, allergies, and asthma, are more prevalent among those with a family history of the disorder but also involve other risk factors.

Rheumatic fever is an inflammatory reaction to an infection but is not an infection itself. There seems to be a hereditary factor, but inadequate nutrition and crowded living conditions are contributing factors.

Allergies often have a family history factor (and some allergies can be passed from the mother to the fetus during pregnancy). However, allergic reactions are triggered by exposure to allergens and can usually be controlled by avoiding or reducing the presence of allergens as well as with medication.

Asthma sufferers may inherit the propensity for airway-narrowing in response to various stimuli, but other triggering factors may be identified and, perhaps, controlled, including stress, overexertion, exposure to cold air, and stimuli such as pollens, dust mites, cockroach detritus, and smoke.

Cancer

A wide variety of family history and environmental factors are included among the risk factors for cancer. Some kinds of cancer, such as breast and colorectal cancer, tend to cluster in families and seem to have a combination of genetic and environmental causes. Others, such as lung cancer, are more strongly identified with environmental causes.

For *breast cancer,* the greatest risk factor is age, with the majority occurring after age 60 and the greatest risk after age 75. A history of breast cancer in a first-degree relative (mother, sister, or daughter) increases the risk by two or three times. Some progress has been made in identifying genes for certain breast cancers. Lifestyle factors such as lack of exercise and obesity may contribute slightly to the incidence of breast cancer, but this has not been proven.

As with breast cancer, *colorectal cancer* risk factors include age (with the incidence rising after age 40 and peaking between 60 and 75) and family history (incidence in a first-degree relative increases the risk by two or three times). There are gender factors, with rectal cancer being more common in men and colon cancer more common in women. Diet may also be a risk factor, although recent studies have failed to confirm a link between a high-fat, low-fiber diet and colorectal cancer. (However, a high-fat, low-fiber diet has been positively linked to heart disease and other health problems.)

The causes of *lung cancer* are overwhelmingly environmental. Smoking has been identified as the main cause of 90 percent of lung cancers in men and 70 percent of lung cancers in women. Lung cancer can also be caused by inhaling substances such as asbestos, arsenic, and nickel, usually in the workplace.

Endocrine Disorders

The most common endocrine disorder is *diabetes mellitus,* which is a leading cause of blindness, heart disease, kidney failure, and premature death. The causes of diabetes are complex and still not well understood.

There are two major types of diabetes: Type I and Type II. Type I diabetes usually occurs before age 40, sometimes in childhood. Although it is less prevalent than Type II diabetes (accounting for about 20 percent of diabetes cases), it is more severe. In the Type I diabetic, the pancreas produces no or almost no insulin, which is required for the cellular utilization of glucose, the body's chief source of energy. Type I diabetics must take insulin daily. There is some association of Type I diabetes with family history (siblings of Type I diabetics have a 6 percent risk compared to 0.3 percent in the general population), and medical researchers have pinpointed some possible genetic factors. Other causative factors may include autoimmunity disorders and viral infections that invade the pancreas and destroy the insulin-producing cells.

Type II diabetes accounts for about 80 percent of all diabetes cases. It usually occurs after age 40 and the incidence increases with age. It clusters much more strongly in families than does Type I diabetes (siblings have a 10 to 15 percent risk). In contrast to Type I diabetes, in which there is a total lack of insulin, Type II diabetes is associated with a decreased insulin receptor response or a decrease in insulin production. Diet and exercise may also be factors, since the majority of Type II diabetics are obese. Type II diabetes can often be controlled with diet and exercise or with oral medications.

Hematologic Disorders

Hereditary coagulation disorders have been studied by geneticists and physicians in great detail. There are many causes of hereditary hematological disorders such as gene alteration and histocompatibility (tissue interaction) dysfunctions.

Hemophilia is a bleeding disorder that is caused by a genetic clotting factor deficiency. It can be mild, but if severe it can cause not only serious bruising but bleeding into the joints, which can lead to crippling deformities. A slight bump on the head can cause bleeding within the skull, often resulting in brain damage and death. The heredity is sex-linked (associated with the sex chromosomes), inherited through the mother, and affects male children almost exclusively. There is no cure, but administration of concentrated clotting factors can improve the condition.

Hemochromatosis is another genetic disorder, but this time caused by a histocompatibility complex dysfunction. It is marked by an excessive absorption and accumulation of iron in the body, causing weight loss, joint pain, abdominal pain, palpitations, and testicular atrophy in males. It is treated by removing blood from the body at intervals.

Not all blood disorders are genetic. Environmental factors, for example, can cause *anemia* (reduction in circulating red blood cells). For example, some antihypertensive medications and other drugs may cause a drug-induced hemolytic (red-blood-cell-destroying) anemia.

Cardiovascular Disorders

The cardiovascular system can be greatly affected by genetic disorders. Disorders such as *prolongation of the QT interval* (a delay between depolarization and repolarization of the ventricles as revealed in an electrocardiogram) and *mitral-valve prolapse* (an upward ballooning of the valve between the left ventricle and atrium that allows blood to regurgitate back into the atrium when the ventricle contracts) tend to cluster in families.

The American Heart Association lists heredity as a major risk factor for cardiovascular disease. Those with parents who have *coronary artery disease* (deposits on the walls of the coronary arteries that reduce blood flow to the heart muscle) have an approximately fivefold risk of developing the disease. This is why it is important to ask about family history of congenital heart disease (CHD), hypertension, and stroke when assessing patients with possible cardiovascular disease. However, environmental factors, such as a diet high in saturated fats and cholesterol (or a diet high in carbohydrates) and lack of exercise, also play a large role in cardiovascular disease.

Hypertension (high blood pressure) is a major risk factor, not only for cardiac disease but also for stroke and kidney disease. Studies of family history show that approximately 20 to 40 percent of the causation of hypertension is genetic. The remaining causative factors, then, are environmental, and may include high sodium ingestion, lack of physical activity, stress, and obesity.

Not all cardiac disorders have a genetic component. For example, *cardiomyopathy* (disease affecting the heart muscle) is thought to occur secondarily to other causes such as infectious disease, toxin exposure, connective tissue disease, or nutritional deficiencies, which may be partially or totally environmental.

Renal Disorders

Renal (kidney) failure is caused by a variety of factors (primarily hypertension) which may eventually require a patient to receive dialysis treatment several times a week. As the location of dialysis treatment shifts from medical centers to homes and community satellite centers, EMS personnel are increasingly being called to deal with the complications of dialysis. These include problems with vascular access devices (shunts, fistulas), localized infection and sepsis, and electrolyte abnormalities (hyperkalemia), which can result in cardiac arrest.

Rheumatic Disorders

Gout is a condition that may have both genetic and environmental causes. It is characterized by severe arthritic pain caused by deposit of crystals in the joints, most commonly the great toe. The crystals form as the result of an abnormally high level of uric acid in the blood that may be caused when the kidneys do not excrete enough uric acid or by high production of uric acid. High production of uric acid may be caused by a hereditary metabolic abnormality. Although the underlying cause may be genetic, attacks of gout can be triggered by environmental factors such as trauma, alcohol consumption, ingestion of certain foods, stress, or other illnesses. Patients with gout also have a tendency to develop *kidney stones*.

Gastrointestinal Disorders

Gastrointestinal disorders have a variety of causes, and the causes of some are not known. *Lactose intolerance,* for example, is usually identified by the inability of the patient to tolerate milk and some other dairy products. The patient lacks lactase, the enzyme that usually breaks down lactose in the digestive tract. This enzyme deficiency may be congenital (inborn) or may develop later on.

Crohn's disease is a chronic inflammation of the wall of the digestive tract that usually affects the small intestine, the large intestine, or both. The cause is not known, but medical researchers have focused on immune system dysfunction, infection, and diet as the major probabilities. A similar disorder is ulcerative colitis, in which the large intestine becomes inflamed and develops ulcers. As with Crohn's disease, the cause is not known, but an overactive immune response is suspected, and heredity seems to play a role.

Peptic ulcers develop when the normal protective structures and mechanisms, such as mucous production, break down and areas in the lining of the stomach or

As dialysis treatment shifts from medical centers to homes and community centers, EMS personnel are increasingly being called to deal with complications of dialysis.

duodenum are inflamed by stomach acid and digestive juices. Environmental factors, bacterial infection (by *Helicobacter pylori*), diet, stress, and alcohol consumption are thought to play roles in the development of peptic ulcers. Many medications, particularly nonsteroidal anti-inflammatory medications, are associated with ulcer formation.

Cholecystitis is an inflammation of the gallbladder that usually results from blockage by a gallstone. There may be a genetic predisposition for gallstone formation. Gallstones are more prevalent in women and in some groups such as Native Americans and Mexican Americans. Other risk factors include age, a high-fat diet, and obesity.

Obesity can be defined as being more than 20 percent over the ideal body weight. Obesity has both an environmental and familial risk transmission. Research has shown that children whose parents are obese have a much-increased chance of developing obesity. Environmental factors such as proper nutrition and exercise may not be modeled or taught by obese parents, but there also seems to be a genetic factor to many cases of obesity. Obesity has been linked to, or defined as a cause for, diseases such as hypertension, heart disease, and vascular diseases.

Neuromuscular Disorders

Diseases of the nervous and muscular systems also have a variety of causes. *Huntington's disease* (which results in uncontrollable jerking and writhing movements) and muscular dystrophy (which results in progressive muscle weakness) are both known to be caused by genetic defects.

Multiple sclerosis (which affects the nerves of the eye, brain, and spinal cord) seems to have some hereditary factor with clustering among close relatives. Its exact cause is unknown, but it seems to result when the virus-triggered autoimmune response begins to attack the myelin sheath that protects the nerves.

Alzheimer's disease is thought to cause about 50 percent of dementias, or progressive mental deterioration. Its cause is unknown, but it does cluster strongly in families and appears to be either caused or influenced by specific gene abnormalities.

Psychiatric Disorders

Genetic and biological causes of psychiatric disorders are being studied and increasingly understood. An example is *schizophrenia*, which affects about 1 percent of the population worldwide and is more prevalent than Alzheimer's disease, diabetes, or multiple sclerosis. The schizophrenic loses contact with reality and suffers from hallucinations, delusions, abnormal thinking, and disrupted social functioning. People who develop schizophrenia are now thought to be "biologically vulnerable" to the disease, but what makes them vulnerable is not fully understood. The cause may be a genetic predisposition or some problem that occurs before, during, or after birth or a viral infection of the brain.

Another common psychiatric disorder is *manic-depressive illness*, also called *bipolar disorder*, in which the person experiences alternating periods of depression and mania or excitement. It can be mild or severe enough to interfere with the patient's ability to work or function socially. Manic-depressive illness affects about twice as many people as schizophrenia. It is believed to be hereditary, but the exact gene deficit has not yet been discovered.

Many disease processes have a genetic cause.

HYPOPERFUSION

Hypoperfusion (shock) is a condition that is progressive (that is, it triggers a self-worsening cycle of pathophysiological events) and fatal if not corrected. It can occur for many reasons such as trauma, fluid loss, myocardial infarction, infection, allergic reaction, spinal cord injury, and other causes. Although causes differ, all forms of shock have the same underlying pathophysiology at the cellular and tissue levels.

THE PHYSIOLOGY OF PERFUSION

As discussed earlier, all body cells require a constant supply of oxygen and other essential nutrients, while waste products, such as carbon dioxide, must be constantly removed. It is the circulatory system, in conjunction with the respiratory and gastrointestinal systems, that provides the body's cells with these essential nutrients and removal of wastes. This is accomplished by the passage of blood through the capillaries, the small vessels that interface with body cells, while oxygen and carbon dioxide, nutrients and wastes, are exchanged by movement across the capillary walls and cell membranes. This constant and necessary passage of blood through the body's tissues is called **perfusion.**

Inadequate perfusion of body tissues is **hypoperfusion,** which is commonly called **shock.** Shock occurs first at a cellular level. If allowed to progress, the tissues, organs, organ systems, and ultimately the entire organism is affected.

Components of the Circulatory System

Perfusion is dependent on a functioning and intact circulatory system. The three components of the circulatory system are listed below. A derangement in any one of these can adversely affect perfusion (Figure 8-12 ■).

★ The pump (heart)
★ The fluid (blood)
★ The container (blood vessels)

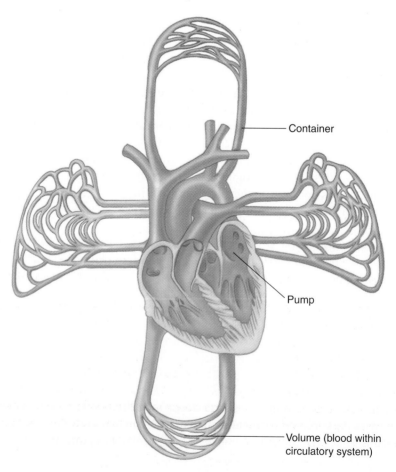

Container

Pump

Volume (blood within circulatory system)

All body cells require a constant supply of oxygen and other nutrients.

perfusion *the supplying of oxygen and nutrients to the body tissues as a result of the constant passage of blood through the capillaries.*

hypoperfusion *inadequate perfusion of the body tissues, resulting in an inadequate supply of oxygen and nutrients to the body tissues. Also called* shock.

shock *see hypoperfusion.*

■ Figure 8-12 Components of the circulatory system.

The Pump The heart is the pump of the cardiovascular system. It receives blood from the venous system, pumps it to the lungs for oxygenation, and then pumps it to the peripheral tissues. The amount of blood ejected by the heart in one contraction is referred to as the **stroke volume.** Factors affecting stroke volume include:

★ Preload

★ Cardiac contractile force

★ Afterload

Preload is the amount of blood delivered to the heart during diastole (when the heart fills with blood between contractions). Preload depends on venous return. The venous system is a capacitance, or storage, system. That is, it can be contracted or expanded, to some extent, as needed to meet the physiological demands of the body. When additional oxygenated blood is required, the venous capacitance is reduced, thus increasing the amount of blood delivered to the heart. The greater the preload, the greater the stroke volume.

Preload also affects **cardiac contractile force.** The greater the volume of preload, the more the ventricles are stretched. The greater the stretch, up to a certain point, the greater will be the subsequent cardiac contraction. This is referred to as the *Frank-Starling mechanism* and can be illustrated through the example of a rubber band. The more the rubber band is stretched, the greater will be its velocity when released.

In addition, cardiac contractile strength is affected by circulating hormones called **catecholamines** (epinephrine and norepinephrine) controlled by the sympathetic nervous system. Catecholamines enhance cardiac contractile strength by action on the beta-adrenergic receptors on the surface of the cells.

Finally, stroke volume is affected by **afterload.** Afterload is the resistance against which the ventricle must contract. This resistance must be overcome before ventricular contraction can result in ejection of blood. Afterload is determined by the degree of peripheral vascular resistance (defined later). This, in effect, is due to the amount of vasoconstriction present. The arterial system can be expanded and contracted to meet the metabolic demands of the body. The greater the resistance offered by the arterial system, the less the stroke volume.

The amount of blood pumped by the heart in 1 minute is referred to as the **cardiac output.** It is a function of stroke volume (milliliters per beat) and heart rate (beats per minute). Cardiac output is usually expressed in liters per minute. It can be defined by this equation:

$$\text{Stroke volume} \times \text{Heart rate} = \text{Cardiac output}$$

The foregoing equation illustrates the factors that can affect cardiac output. An increase in stroke volume or an increase in heart rate can increase cardiac output. Conversely, a decrease in stroke volume or a decrease in heart rate can decrease cardiac output. The blood pressure is dependent upon both cardiac output and peripheral vascular resistance.

$$\text{Cardiac output} \times \text{Peripheral vascular resistance} = \text{Blood pressure}$$

Peripheral vascular resistance is the pressure against which the heart must pump. Since the circulatory system is a closed system, increasing either cardiac output or peripheral vascular resistance will increase blood pressure. Likewise, a decrease in cardiac output or a decrease in peripheral vascular resistance will decrease blood pressure.

The body strives to keep the blood pressure relatively constant by employing *compensatory mechanisms* and negative feedback loops. As noted earlier, baroreceptors in the carotid sinuses and in the arch of the aorta closely monitor blood pressure. If blood pressure increases, the baroreceptors send signals to the brain that cause the blood pressure to return to its normal values. This is accomplished by decreasing the heart rate, decreasing the preload, or decreasing peripheral vascular resistance.

stroke volume *the amount of blood ejected by the heart in one contraction.*

preload *the amount of blood delivered to the heart during diastole (when the heart fills with blood between contractions); in cardiac physiology, defined as the tension of cardiac muscle fiber at the end of diastole.*

The venous system is a capacitance, or storage, system.

cardiac contractile force *the strength of a contraction of the heart.*

catecholamines *epinephrine and norepinephrine, hormones that strongly affect the nervous and cardiovascular systems, metabolic rate, temperature, and smooth muscle.*

afterload *the resistance a contraction of the heart must overcome in order to eject blood; in cardiac physiology, defined as the tension of cardiac muscle during systole (contraction).*

cardiac output *the amount of blood pumped by the heart in 1 minute (computed as stroke volume × heart rate).*

peripheral vascular resistance *the resistance of the vessels to the flow of blood: increased when the vessels constrict, decreased when the vessels relax.*

The baroreceptors are also stimulated if the blood pressure falls. The heart rate is increased, as is the strength of the cardiac contractions. There is also arteriolar constriction, venous constriction (which results in decreased container size), and overall increased peripheral vascular resistance. Also, the adrenal medulla (the inner portion of the adrenal gland) is stimulated. This results in the secretion of epinephrine and norepinephrine, which further enhance the response.

The Fluid   Blood is the fluid of the cardiovascular system. It is a viscous fluid; that is, it is thicker and more adhesive than water. As a result, blood flows more slowly than water. Blood, which consists of the plasma and the formed elements (red cells, white cells, and platelets), transports oxygen, carbon dioxide, nutrients, hormones, metabolic waste products, and heat.

An adequate amount of blood is required for perfusion. Since the cardiovascular system (the heart and blood vessels) is a closed system, the volume of blood present must be adequate to fill the container, as described in the following section.

The Container   Blood vessels (arteries, arterioles, capillaries, venules, and veins) serve as the container of the cardiovascular system. The blood vessels can be thought of as a continuous, closed, and pressurized pipeline by which blood moves throughout the body. While the heart functions as the pump of the circulatory system, the blood vessels—under the control of the autonomic nervous system—can regulate blood flow to different areas of the body by adjusting their size as well as by selectively rerouting blood through the microcirculation.

While the arteries and veins, like the heart, are subject to direct stimulation from sympathetic portions of the autonomic nervous system, the *microcirculation* (comprised of the small vessels: the arterioles, capillaries, and venules) is primarily responsive to local tissue needs. The capability of some vessels in the capillary network to adjust their diameter permits the microcirculation to selectively supply undernourished tissue, while temporarily bypassing tissues with no immediate need. Capillaries have a sphincter at the origin of the capillary (between arteriole and capillary), called the *precapillary sphincter*, and another at the end of the capillary (between capillary and venule), called *the postcapillary sphincter*. The precapillary sphincter responds to local tissue conditions, such as acidosis and hypoxia, and opens as more arterial blood is needed. The postcapillary sphincter opens when blood is to be emptied into the venous system.

Blood flow through the vessels is regulated by two factors: peripheral vascular resistance and pressure within the system. Peripheral vascular resistance, as noted earlier, is the resistance to blood flow. Vessels with larger inside diameters offer less resistance, while vessels with smaller inside diameters offer greater resistance. Peripheral vascular resistance is governed by three factors—the length of the vessel, the diameter of the vessel, and blood viscosity.

There is very little resistance to blood flow through the aorta and arteries, but a significant change in peripheral resistance occurs at the arterioles and precapillary sphincters. This is because the inside diameter of the arteriole is much smaller, as compared to that of the aorta and arteries. Additionally, the arteriole has the ability to make a pronounced change in its diameter, as much as fivefold. It tends to do this in response to local tissue needs and autonomic nervous signals.

Contraction of the venous side of the vascular system results in decreased capacitance and increased cardiac preload. The arterial system, however, provides systemic vascular resistance. An increase in arterial tone increases resistance, which increases blood pressure.

Oxygen Transport

Oxygen is brought into the body via the respiratory system. During inspiration, approximately 500 to 800 mL of atmospheric air is taken in through the upper and lower airways, coming to rest in the alveoli of the lungs.

The precapillary sphincter responds to local tissue demands such as acidosis and hypoxia.

Surrounding the alveoli are capillaries that are perfused by the pulmonary circulation. The blood that comes into the pulmonary capillaries is oxygen-depleted blood that was returned from the body to the right atrium of the heart, then pumped by the right ventricle of the heart into the pulmonary arteries and thence into the pulmonary capillaries.

The air in the alveoli contains a concentration of about 13.6 percent oxygen. This is less than the 21 percent concentration of oxygen in atmospheric air because of various factors, including the fact that some air always remains in the alveoli from earlier respirations and oxygen is constantly being absorbed from this air. Nevertheless, alveolar air is far richer in oxygen than blood that enters the pulmonary capillaries.

Another way of stating this is that the *partial pressure of oxygen* present in air in the alveoli of the lungs is greater than the partial pressure of oxygen in the blood within the pulmonary circulation. (In a mix of gases, the portion of the total pressure exerted by each component of the mix is known as the *partial pressure* of that component.) For this reason, oxygen from the alveoli diffuses across the alveolar-capillary membrane and into the bloodstream—from the area of greater partial pressure to the area of lower partial pressure.

The red blood cells "pick up" this oxygen while passing through the pulmonary capillary bed. Oxygen binds to the hemoglobin molecules of the red blood cells, which serve as the primary carriers of oxygen within the bloodstream. Normally, between 95 and 100 percent of the hemoglobin is saturated with oxygen. The oxygen-enriched blood then circulates back to the heart through the venous side of the pulmonary circulation. Passing through the left atrium and into the left ventricle, the oxygen-enriched blood is pumped throughout the body via the systemic circulation.

Upon reaching capillaries throughout the body, the oxygen-rich blood interfaces with the tissues. The tissues contain cells that are oxygen-deficient as a result of normal metabolic activity. Since the partial pressure of oxygen is greater in the bloodstream than in the cells, oxygen will diffuse from the red blood cells across the capillary wall-cell membrane barrier, into the cells and tissues.

Overall, the movement and utilization of oxygen in the body is dependent upon the following conditions:

★ Adequate concentration of inspired oxygen

★ Appropriate movement of oxygen across the alveolar/capillary membrane into the arterial bloodstream

★ Adequate number of red blood cells to carry the oxygen

★ Proper tissue perfusion

★ Efficient off-loading of oxygen at the tissue level

The dependence on this set of conditions for oxygen movement and utilization is known as the *Fick Principle*.

Waste Removal

The waste products of cellular metabolism are expelled from the cells and carried away by the blood. Carbon dioxide leaves the bloodstream during the oxygen-carbon dioxide exchange, which occurs through the alveolar/capillary membranes. Carbon dioxide is ultimately eliminated by exhalation from the lungs. Some cellular waste products are expelled into the interstitial fluid and picked up by the lymphatic system. These ultimately flow through the lymph channels into the thoracic duct. The thoracic duct empties the waste products into the venous side of the circulatory system. Other wastes are cleansed from the blood by the kidneys and excreted as urine. Finally, some cellular waste products are emptied into the gastrointestinal system and expelled in the feces.

There is some local control of both tissue perfusion and waste removal. When the amounts of metabolic waste products (such as lactic acid) increase, the tissues subsequently become acidotic. This local acidosis causes nearby precapillary sphincters to relax,

 Review

Content

Fick Principle

The movement and utilization of oxygen by the body is dependent upon:
–Adequate concentration of inspired oxygen
–Appropriate movement of oxygen across the alveolar/capillary membrane into the arterial bloodstream
–Adequate number of red blood cells to carry the oxygen
–Proper tissue perfusion
–Efficient off-loading of oxygen at the tissue level

thus opening the capillaries and increasing perfusion of the affected tissues. This provides increased capacity for waste elimination and response to local metabolic demands.

THE PATHOPHYSIOLOGY OF HYPOPERFUSION

Causes of Hypoperfusion

Hypoperfusion (shock) is almost always a result of inadequate cardiac output. A number of factors can decrease effective cardiac output. These include:

* ★ Inadequate pump
    * –Inadequate preload
    * –Inadequate cardiac contractile strength
    * –Inadequate heart rate
    * –Excessive afterload
* ★ Inadequate fluid
    * –Hypovolemia (abnormally low circulating blood volume)
* ★ Inadequate container
    * –Dilated container without change in fluid volume (inadequate systemic vascular resistance)
    * –Leak in container

Occasionally, hypoperfusion can develop even when cardiac output is adequate. This can happen when cell metabolism is so excessive that the body cannot increase perfusion enough to meet the cells' metabolic requirements. It can also happen when abnormal circulatory patterns develop, so that circulating blood is bypassing critical tissues.

As mentioned earlier, the conditions that lead to hypoperfusion can result from a number of underlying causes, such as infection, trauma and hemorrhage, loss of plasma through burns, severe cardiac dysrhythmia, central nervous system dysfunction, and many others. But the outcome is always the same: inadequate delivery of oxygen and essential nutrients to, and removal of wastes from, all the tissues of the body, especially the critical tissues (brain, heart, kidneys).

Shock at the Cellular Level

Shock is a complex phenomenon. The causes vary. The signs and symptoms vary. At the simplest level, however, shock is inadequate tissue perfusion. Additionally, all types of shock have this in common: The ultimate outcome is impairment of cellular metabolism. Two characteristics of impaired cellular metabolism in any type of shock are impaired oxygen use and impaired glucose use.

Impaired Use of Oxygen   One characteristic of any type of shock is that the cells are either not receiving enough oxygen or are unable to use it effectively. This may be caused by hypoperfusion resulting from reduced cardiac function, inadequate blood volume, or vasodilation (pump, fluid, or container problems). It may result from insufficient red cells to carry the oxygen, from fever that increases cellular oxygen demand, or chemical disruption of cellular metabolism.

When the cells don't receive enough oxygen or cannot use it effectively, they change from **aerobic metabolism** to **anaerobic metabolism,** a far less efficient means of producing energy—as explained in the following text.

The primary energy source for the cells is glucose, taken into the cell with the aid of insulin. Glucose does not provide energy until it is broken down inside the cell. The

Review

Physiological Classifications of Shock

Inadequate pump (cardiogenic)

Inadequate fluid (hypovolemic)

Inadequate container (distributive/neurogenic)

At the simplest level, shock is inadequate tissue perfusion.

Review

Characteristics of Impaired Cellular Metabolism in Shock

Impaired use of oxygen

Impaired use of glucose

aerobic metabolism   *the second stage of metabolism, requiring the presence of oxygen, in which the breakdown of glucose (in a process called the Krebs or citric acid cycle) yields a high amount of energy. Aerobic means "with oxygen."*

anaerobic metabolism   *the first stage of metabolism, which does not require oxygen, in which the breakdown of glucose (in a process called glycolysis) produces pyruvic acid and yields very little energy. Anaerobic means "without oxygen."*

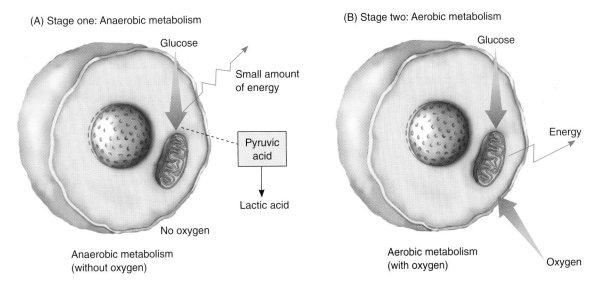

(A) Stage one: Anaerobic metabolism

Glucose

Small amount of energy

Pyruvic acid

Lactic acid

No oxygen

Anaerobic metabolism (without oxygen)

(B) Stage two: Aerobic metabolism

Glucose

Energy

Oxygen

Aerobic metabolism (with oxygen)

■ Figure 8-13   Glucose breakdown. (a) Stage one, glycolysis, is anaerobic (does not require oxygen). It yields pyruvic acid, with toxic byproducts such as lactic acid, and very little energy. (b) Stage two is aerobic (requires oxygen). In a process called the Krebs or citric acid cycle, pyruvic acid is degraded into carbon dioxide and water, which produces a much higher yield of energy.

first stage of glucose breakdown, called glycolysis, is anaerobic (does not require oxygen). Glycolysis produces pyruvic acid but yields very little energy. Thus, by itself, glycolysis is an inefficient utilization of glucose. Therefore, in a normal state of metabolism, a second stage of glucose breakdown is required. During this second stage, which is aerobic (requires oxygen), pyruvic acid is further degraded into carbon dioxide, water, and energy in a process termed the Krebs or citric acid cycle. The energy yield of this second-stage aerobic process is much higher than from the first-stage anaerobic process (Figure 8-13 ■).

During shock, or any condition in which the cells do not receive adequate oxygen or cannot use it effectively, glucose breakdown can only complete the first-stage, anaerobic process of glycolysis and cannot enter into the second-stage, aerobic, citric acid cycle. This causes an accumulation of the end product of glycolysis, pyruvic acid. In these cases, pyruvic acid is quickly degraded to lactic acid. If oxygen is promptly restored to the cells, lactic acid will be reconverted to pyruvic acid. However, if time elapses and the cellular hypoxia is not corrected, lactic acid and other metabolic acids will accumulate. One outcome is that the acidic condition of the blood reduces the ability of hemoglobin in red blood cells to bind with and carry oxygen, which compounds the problem of cellular oxygen deprivation.

The energy that is produced during glucose breakdown is in the form of the chemical adenosine triphosphate (ATP), which is essential to all the metabolic processes in the cells. As just noted, the amount of energy, or ATP, produced during first-stage, anaerobic glycolysis is very small. Without oxygen, when the process of glucose breakdown stops after glycolysis (during which very little energy has been produced), cellular stores of ATP are used up much faster than they can be replaced, so that all of the processes of cellular metabolism are gravely impaired.

Because of changes to the internal cell and because blood flow has been slowed by the decreased pumping action and vasodilation, sludging of the blood occurs. This further impedes blood flow. Thus, the normal diffusion of nutrients and wastes in and out of the cells is disrupted and the balance of the cellular electrolytes is altered. Lysosomes, the organelles that assist in digestion of nutrients, are normally enclosed by a membrane that prevents the digestive enzymes from damaging other cell components. Now the lysosomes rupture, releasing the lysosomal enzymes into the cell. The sodium-potassium pumping mechanism fails, changing the electrical charge of the cells' internal environment. There is an increase in sodium and water (since water follows sodium) inside the cells, causing cellular edema. The cell membrane then ruptures, allowing lysosomal enzymes and other cellular contents to leak into the interstitial spaces. Cellular death soon follows.

Impaired Use of Glucose   The same factors that reduce delivery of oxygen to the cells also reduce delivery of glucose to the cells. In addition, uptake of glucose by the cells may be disrupted by fever, cell damage, or the presence of bacteria, toxins, histamine, or other substances produced or activated by the body's immune and inflammatory responses to disease or injury. Compensatory mechanisms activated by shock may also be responsible for substances that inhibit glucose uptake, including catecholamines and the hormones cortisol and growth hormone.

Glucose that is prevented from entering the cells remains in the blood, resulting in a condition of high serum glucose, or hyperglycemia. Since glucose is the substance from which cells produce energy, the consequences of reduced glucose delivery and uptake are critical.

In the absence of an adequate supply of glucose, certain body cells can create fuel for energy production by converting other substances to glucose. One source is glycogen, the form of glucose that cells store and hold in reserve. Cells convert glycogen to glucose in a process called *glycogenolysis*. However, there is very little stored glycogen in cells other than the liver, kidneys, and muscles. When glycogen reserves are depleted, which typically occurs in 4 to 8 hours, the cells will then derive energy from the breakdown of fats (*lipolysis*) and from the conversion of noncarbohydrate substrates, such as amino acids from proteins, to glucose (*gluconeogenesis*). The energy costs of glycogenolysis and lipolysis are high and contribute to the failure of cells. But the depletion of proteins in gluconeogenesis will ultimately cause organ failure.

In addition, the anaerobic breakdown of proteins produces ammonia, which is toxic to the cells, and urea, which leads to uric acid, which is also toxic to cells. Finally, when cellular metabolism is impaired, the waste products of metabolism build up in the cells, further impairing cell function and damaging cell membranes.

Impaired use of oxygen and glucose soon leads to cellular death. Cellular death will ultimately lead to tissue death; tissue death will lead to organ failure; and organ failure will lead to death of the individual.

Compensation and Decompensation

Usually, the body is able to compensate for any of the changes previously described. However, when the various compensatory mechanisms fail, shock develops and may progress.

Compensation   In shock, the fall in cardiac output, detected as a decrease in arterial blood pressure by the baroreceptors, activates several body systems that attempt to reestablish a normal blood pressure—a process known as *compensation*. The sympathetic nervous system stimulates the adrenal gland of the endocrine system to secrete the catecholamines epinephrine and norepinephrine. These chemicals profoundly affect the cardiovascular system, causing an increased heart rate, increased cardiac contractile strength, and arteriolar constriction—all of which serve to elevate the blood pressure.

Another compensatory mechanism, the *renin-angiotensin system*, aids the body in maintaining an adequate blood pressure. When the renin-angiotensin system is activated by a fall in blood pressure, the enzyme *renin* is released from the kidneys into the systemic circulation. Renin acts on a specialized plasma protein called *angiotensin* to produce a substance called *angiotensin I*. Angiotensin I is converted to *angiotensin II* by

Cellular death will ultimately lead to tissue death, tissue death to organ failure, and organ failure to death of the individual.

Ⓧ **Review**

The Stages of Shock

Compensated
Decompensated
   (progressive)
Irreversible

an enzyme found in the lungs called *angiotensin converting enzyme (ACE)*. Angiotensin II is a potent vasoconstrictor. As angiotensin II causes the diameter of the vascular container to decrease, the blood pressure increases. Angiotensin II also stimulates the production of aldosterone, a hormone secreted by the adrenal cortex (outer layer of the adrenal gland) which, in turn, stimulates the kidneys to reabsorb sodium, and, subsequently, water (as noted earlier, "water follows sodium") into peritubular capillaries. The intravascular volume is maintained and elimination of water by the kidneys is reduced.

Another endocrine response by the pituitary gland results in the secretion of antidiuretic hormone (ADH), which also causes the kidneys to reabsorb water, creating an additive effect to that of aldosterone.

The spleen, capable of storing over 300 mL of blood, can expel up to 200 mL of blood into the venous circulation, consequently increasing blood volume, preload, cardiac output, and blood pressure in response to a sudden drop in blood pressure.

Some passive compensatory responses also occur, with beneficial fluid shifts taking place as a result of simple diffusion. With volume loss, the hydrostatic pressure in capillary beds is reduced, and water from the interstitial spaces diffuses into the capillaries.

All of the forementioned mechanisms work to compensate for the shock state, and may be able to restore normal circulatory volume—if excessive bleeding is managed and the shock state has not progressed too far. In this case, the patient is said to be in **compensated shock.**

Once normal circulatory function and blood pressure are reestablished, the blood pressure will "feed back" on all of the compensatory mechanisms so that all systems can return to normal. In this way, negative feedback loops work to maintain stability by "signaling" the systems to cease the compensatory responses. In this way, stability and homeostasis are maintained.

Decompensation   If the conditions causing shock are too serious, or progress too rapidly, compensatory mechanisms may not be able to restore normal function. In those cases, *decompensation* is said to occur, and the patient is in a state of **decompensated shock,** also called **progressive shock.** During decompensated or progressive shock, medical intervention may still be able to correct the condition.

Since all of the "responding" systems have a point at which they can no longer sustain their action (i.e., a limited duration of action), the shock state may progress to a condition where correction, either by the body's own compensatory mechanisms or through medical intervention, is no longer possible. This condition is known as **irreversible shock.**

A critical factor in the downward spiral of decompensation is cardiac depression. The compensatory mechanisms that increase heart rate and contractile strength create a greatly increased demand for oxygen by the myocardium. When arterial blood pressure has fallen sufficiently, however, coronary blood flow is reduced below the level necessary to adequately perfuse the myocardium. The heart is weakened and cardiac output falls even further.

Depression of the vasomotor center of the brain is another consequence of reduced blood pressure. In early shock, as previously discussed, the sympathetic nervous system is stimulated to cause release of catecholamines that support the function of the circulatory system. But when blood pressure falls to a certain point, in the late stages of shock, reduced blood supply to the vasomotor center results in a slowing, then stoppage, of sympathetic activity.

Metabolic wastes, products of anaerobic metabolism, are released into the slower-flowing blood. The blood in the capillary beds becomes acidic, causing formation of minute blood clots ("sludged" blood), which further slows the flow of blood. And a more generalized, systemic acidosis develops, causing further deterioration of cells and tissues, including the capillary walls.

compensated shock *early stage of shock during which the body's compensatory mechanisms are able to maintain normal perfusion.*

decompensated shock *advanced stages of shock when the body's compensatory mechanisms are no longer able to maintain normal perfusion; also called* **progressive shock.**

irreversible shock *shock that has progressed so far that no medical intervention can reverse the condition and death is inevitable.*

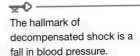

The hallmark of decompensated shock is a fall in blood pressure.

Capillary cells, like other cells, suffer from lack of oxygen and other nutrients, as well as from the ravages of acidosis. This begins to cause permeability of the capillaries and leakage of fluid into the interstitial spaces. This is another self-perpetuating process, as the decreased circulating volume and anaerobic metabolism cause further cell hypoxia and increased permeability.

Cellular deterioration progresses to tissue deterioration, which progresses to organ failure. (See Multiple Organ Dysfunction Syndrome, later in the chapter.) Medical intervention may save the patient if initiated early enough, but when enough damage has been done to cells, tissues, and organs, no known treatment can help the patient to recover. Medical therapies may support function for awhile, but death becomes inevitable.

TYPES OF SHOCK

Shock is usually classified according to the cause. Some newer terminology classifies shock as *cardiogenic* (caused by impaired pumping power of the heart), *hypovolemic* (caused by decreased blood or water volume), *obstructive* (caused by an obstruction that interferes with return of blood to the heart, such as a pulmonary embolism, cardiac tamponade, or tension pneumothorax), and *distributive* (caused by abnormal distribution and return of blood resulting from vasodilation, vasopermeability, or both, as in neurogenic, anaphylactic, or septic shock).

Another, more familiar terminology classifies shock as *cardiogenic, hypovolemic, neurogenic, anaphylactic,* and *septic.* The following discussion of types of shock uses these classifications.

Although all types of shock ultimately have the same effects on the body's cells, tissues, and organs, it is important to try to identify the underlying cause, because correcting the cause is the most important element in reversing the condition and saving the patient's life. Many of the treatments that you, as a paramedic, will provide for the shock patient will be the same, no matter what the cause or type of shock is, but some differ in important ways. For example, providing IV fluid boluses, which may be appropriate to support circulating volume in the hypovolemic patient, would not be indicated for the patient in cardiogenic shock with pulmonary edema.

Cardiogenic Shock

An inability of the heart to pump enough blood to supply all body parts is referred to as **cardiogenic shock.** Cardiogenic shock is usually the result of severe left ventricular failure secondary to acute myocardial infarction or congestive heart failure. The reduced blood pressure that accompanies this form of shock aggravates the situation by decreasing coronary artery perfusion. With decreased coronary perfusion, the heart muscle becomes even more damaged, thus establishing a vicious cycle that ultimately results in complete pump failure.

During cardiogenic shock, as noted earlier, the activation of compensatory mechanisms can actually worsen the situation. When the peripheral resistance increases in an attempt to maintain blood pressure, the myocardial workload increases. This, in turn, increases the myocardial oxygen demand, further aggravating myocardial ischemia and infarction. Cardiac output is further depressed and ejection fraction (the percentage of blood in the ventricle that is ejected with each beat) is decreased.

While the most common cause of cardiogenic shock is severe left ventricular failure, a number of other factors can have the same result. These include chronic progressive heart disease such as cardiomyopathy, rupture of the papillary heart muscles or interventricular septum, and end-stage valvular disease (mitral stenosis or aortic regurgitation).

Most patients who experience cardiogenic shock will have normal blood volume. However, some patients will be hypovolemic from an excessive use of prescribed diuretics or the severe diaphoresis that accompanies some acute cardiac events. Patients

Review

Types of Shock

Cardiogenic
Hypovolemic
Neurogenic
Anaphylactic
Septic
(*Alternative classifications of shock: Cardiogenic, Hypovolemic, Obstructive, Distributive*)

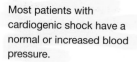

Try to identify the underlying cause of shock, because correcting the cause is the most important element in reversing the condition and saving the patient's life.

cardiogenic shock *shock caused by insufficient cardiac output; the inability of the heart to pump enough blood to perfuse all parts of the body.*

Most patients with cardiogenic shock have a normal or increased blood pressure.

may also experience relative hypovolemia (neurogenic shock) from the vasodilatory (vessel dilation) effects of drugs such as nitroglycerin.

Evaluation and Treatment   A major difference between cardiogenic and other types of shock is the presence of pulmonary edema (excess fluid in the lungs), which will probably result in a complaint of difficulty breathing. There may be diminished lung sounds as fluid enters the interstitial spaces of the lungs. As fluid levels rise, wheezes, crackles, or rales may be heard. A productive cough may develop, characterized by white- or pink-tinged foamy sputum. Cyanosis (a dusky blue-gray skin color) is typical, resulting from the decreased diffusion of oxygen across the alveolar/capillary interface, decreasing oxygen delivery to cells that are already hypoxic because of decreased blood pressure and perfusion. Other signs of shock include altered mentation (resulting from reduced perfusion of the brain) and oliguria (diminished urination resulting from compensatory mechanisms that stimulate reabsorption of water by the kidneys to enhance circulating volume).

Treatment of cardiogenic shock includes the supportive measures that should be provided for shock of any origin: Assure an open airway, administer oxygen and assist ventilations if necessary (to support oxygenation of myocardial and other body cells), and keep the patient warm (because impaired cellular metabolism is no longer producing enough energy to keep body temperature normal).

In cardiogenic shock, when pulmonary edema is present, elevate the patient's head and shoulders so that gravity can help isolate fluid and create a clear area where oxygen exchange from the alveoli can take place.

A peripheral intravenous line should be established with normal saline at a TKO rate to provide access for medications, but fluid administration should be kept to a minimum to avoid aggravating the edema. (Some patients with chronic heart failure may be on diuretics and suffering dehydration however, requiring some fluid support.) Since the heart rate may vary from bradycardic (abnormally slow) to tachycardic (abnormally fast), monitoring the heart rate is important. Atropine administration or application of an external pacer may be recommended to manage bradycardia, while extreme tachycardia may be treated by sedation and cardioversion (a type of electric shock) if the patient is awake. Dopamine may be administered to elevate the blood pressure but it will also increase heart rate. Dobutamine may be administered to increase contractile force with little effect on the heart rate. Follow local protocols.

Hypovolemic Shock

Shock due to a loss of intravascular fluid volume is referred to as **hypovolemic shock.** Possible causes of hypovolemic shock include:

★ Internal or external hemorrhage (This type of hypovolemic shock is also known as hemorrhagic shock.)

★ Traumatic injury

★ Long-bone or open fractures

★ Severe dehydration from vomiting or diarrhea

★ Plasma loss from burns

★ Excessive sweating

★ Diabetic ketoacidosis with resultant **osmotic diuresis**

Hypovolemic shock can also be due to internal third-space loss (loss from intracellular or, more commonly, from intravascular spaces into the interstitial spaces). Such a condition can occur with bowel obstruction, peritonitis, pancreatitis, or liver failure resulting in ascites (accumulation of fluid within the abdominal cavity).

Provide supportive measures for shock of any origin: Assure an open airway, administer oxygen, assist ventilations, and keep the patient warm.

hypovolemic shock   *shock caused by a loss of intravascular fluid volume.*

osmotic diuresis   *greatly increased urination and dehydration due to high levels of glucose that cannot be reabsorbed into the blood from the kidney tubules, causing a loss of water into the urine.*

Evaluation and Treatment The signs of hypovolemic shock are considered the "classic" signs of shock. The mental status becomes altered, progressing from anxiety to lethargy or combativeness to unresponsiveness. The skin becomes pale, cool, and clammy (sweaty). The blood pressure may be normal during compensated shock, but then begins to fall. The pulse may be normal in the beginning, then become rapid, finally slowing and disappearing. As the kidneys continue to reabsorb water, urination decreases. Cardiac dysrhythmias may develop in late shock, deteriorating to asystole (absence of heartbeat).

While it is accepted practice to administer crystalloid or colloid solutions to replace fluids lost through vomiting, diarrhea, burns, excessive sweating, or osmotic diuresis, the replacement of fluids in trauma patients is quite controversial. It has been demonstrated that the body provides a natural compensation for low-flow states when the systolic pressure is maintained between 70 and 85 mmHg. In a few studies, elevating the systolic blood pressure to greater than 85 mmHg has been associated with worsened outcomes. The worsened outcomes are attributed to the fact that aggressive fluid resuscitation, before the source of bleeding is repaired, causes progressive dilution of the blood, which decreases the oxygen-carrying capacity of the blood. Thus, many surgeons and EMS medical directors are now recommending administering only enough fluid to maintain a systolic blood pressure between 70 and 85 mmHg—a process called "permissive hypotension."

Prehospital care for hypovolemic shock should be guided by local protocols. As a rule, patients suffering from shock from trauma should receive airway management, supplemental oxygenation, assisted ventilations (if necessary), hemorrhage control, and rapid transport. IV access should be obtained immediately or en route. Either lactated Ringer's or normal saline should be administered in small boluses to maintain the systolic blood pressure between 70 and 85 mmHg (enough to restore a radial pulse). Patients with systolic pressures less than 40 mmHg should still receive aggressive fluid resuscitation.

Neurogenic Shock

Neurogenic shock results from injury to either the brain or the spinal cord, resulting in an interruption of nerve impulses to the arteries. The arteries lose tone and dilate, causing a relative hypovolemia. There has been no loss of fluid, but the container has been enlarged. With this inappropriate vasodilation, a disproportionate amount of blood collects in the capillary bed. This reduces venous return, cardiac output, and arterial blood pressure. Sympathetic nerve impulses to the adrenal glands are lost, which prevents the release of catecholamines and their compensatory effects. With injury high in the cervical spine, there may be interruption of impulses to the peripheral nervous system, causing paralysis and loss of sensation. The respiratory and cardiac centers of the brain may also be affected.

The usual cause of neurogenic shock is central nervous system injury. Neurogenic shock is most commonly due to an injury that has resulted in severe spinal cord injury or total transection of the cord (which may be called *spinal shock*) or injury or deprivation of oxygen or glucose to the medulla of the brain.

Evaluation and Treatment The vasodilation in neurogenic shock causes warm, red skin, and sweat gland malfunction causes dry skin—in contrast to the cool, pale, sweaty skin associated with hypovolemic shock. Because of the lack of compensatory stimulation from catecholamine release, the patient will have a low blood pressure and a slow pulse even in the early stages—again, in contrast to hypovolemic shock.

Treatment for neurogenic shock or spinal shock is similar to treatment for other types of shock and includes support of the airway, oxygenation, ventilation, maintenance of body temperature, and intravenous access. Spinal shock is characterized by hypotension, reflex bradycardia, and warm, dry skin. Because these symptoms signal a likelihood of spinal injury, cervical spine stabilization must be established on first pa-

neurogenic shock *shock resulting from brain or spinal cord injury that causes an interruption of nerve impulses to the arteries with loss of arterial tone, dilation, and relative hypovolemia.*

tient contact, and the patient must be immobilized to a backboard as quickly as possible. A thorough search for other causes of shock (e.g., internal hemorrhage) must be made before concluding that a patient's hypotension is due to spinal shock alone. Treatment of spinal shock should include intravenous fluids (especially if there has been blood or fluid loss) and medications that increase the blood pressure by increasing peripheral vascular resistance. These include norepinephrine (Levophed) and dopamine (Intropin).

Anaphylactic Shock

When a foreign substance enters the body, the immune system responds to rid the body of the invader. (See the discussion of immunity later in this chapter.) This usually happens with no noticeable effects, and the person is not even aware that an immune response is taking place. Some foreign substances (antigens) provoke an exaggerated immune response (allergic response) that will cause noticeable symptoms such as a rash (as from contact with poison ivy) or swollen, irritated airway passages (as with hay fever). In rare cases, an allergic response is very severe and life threatening. This kind of severe allergic response is called **anaphylaxis,** or **anaphylactic shock.**

An anaphylactic reaction usually occurs very rapidly. Signs and symptoms most often appear within a minute or less, but occasionally may appear an hour or more after exposure. Generally, the faster the reaction develops, the more severe it is likely to be. Death can occur before the patient can get to a hospital, so prompt intervention is critical. This is a situation when the paramedic at the scene can make the difference between life and death.

Anaphylactic reactions can be triggered by a variety of substances, including foods (especially nuts, eggs, shellfish), venoms, aspirin or nonsteroidal anti-inflammatory drugs (NSAIDS), hormones (animal-derived insulin), preservatives, and others. The most rapid and severe reactions are usually caused by substances injected directly into the bloodstream, which is one reason that penicillin injections and hymenoptera stings (e.g., from bees, wasps, hornets) are the most common causes of fatal anaphylactic reactions.

anaphylaxis *a life-threatening allergic reaction; also called* **anaphylactic shock.**

Evaluation and Treatment   Because the immune responses involved in anaphylaxis can affect different body systems, the signs and symptoms can vary widely. For example:

★ Skin
  – Flushing
  – Itching
  – Hives
  – Swelling
  – Cyanosis
★ Respiratory system
  – Breathing difficulty
  – Sneezing, coughing
  – Wheezing, stridor
  – Laryngeal edema
  – Laryngospasm
★ Cardiovascular system
  – Vasodilation
  – Increased heart rate
  – Decreased blood pressure

★ Gastrointestinal system

    –Nausea, vomiting

    –Abdominal cramping

    –Diarrhea

★ Nervous system

    –Altered mental status

    –Dizziness

    –Headache

    –Seizures

    –Tearing

The patient may present with an altered mental status that can progress to unresponsiveness, so gather a brief history as soon as possible, including previous allergic reactions and any information about what the patient may have ingested or been exposed to that could have caused the present reaction. Be sure the patient is no longer in contact with the allergen; if a stinger is in the skin, scrape it away with a fingernail or scalpel blade.

Since laryngeal edema is often a problem, protecting the patient's airway will be your first concern. Administer oxygen by nonrebreather mask or, as necessary, by endotracheal intubation. The anaphylactic response causes depletion of circulatory volume by promoting capillary permeability and leaking of fluid into interstitial spaces, so establish an IV of crystalloid solution (normal saline or lactated Ringer's) for volume support.

The primary treatment for anaphylaxis is pharmacological. In addition to oxygen, epinephrine is usually administered (if the patient has a history of anaphylaxis, he may be carrying a prescribed spring-loaded epinephrine injector), as are antihistamines (diphenhydramine), corticosteroids (methylprednisolone, hydrocortisone, dexamethasone), and vasopressors (dopamine, norepinephrine, epinephrine). Occasionally an inhaled beta agonist (albuterol) may be required. Follow local protocols.

Septic Shock

Septic shock begins with *septicemia* (also called *sepsis*), an infection that enters the bloodstream and is carried throughout the body. The person may have septicemia for some time before septic shock develops, but eventually toxins released by the invading organism overcome the compensatory mechanisms. Unless it is corrected, septic shock will cause the dysfunction of more than one organ system, resulting in multiple organ dysfunction syndrome (discussed in the next section).

Evaluation and Treatment   The signs and symptoms of septic shock are progressive. In the beginning, cardiac output is increased, but toxins causing vasodilation may prevent an increase in blood pressure. The person may seem to be sick, but not alarmingly so. By the last stages, toxins have increased permeability of the blood vessels to the point where great amounts of fluid are lost from the vasculature and blood pressure falls drastically.

Signs and symptoms can vary widely as the patient progresses from early to late stages of septic shock. Some patients may have a high fever, but others, especially the elderly or the very young, may have no fever or may even be hypothermic. The skin can be flushed, if fever is present, or very pale and cyanotic in the late stages.

The most susceptible organ system is the lungs and respiratory system, so the patient may present with breathing difficulty and altered lung sounds. The brain may be infected, resulting in altered mental status. Suspicion of septic shock is usually based on a history of recent infection or illness.

Treatment includes administration of high-flow oxygen by nonrebreather mask or endotracheal intubation, as necessary. An IV of crystalloid solution (normal saline or lactated Ringer's) should be established, and dopamine may be administered to support the blood pressure. The heart rhythm must be monitored and medications administered to correct any dysrhythmias. Follow local protocols. In the hospital, antibiotic therapy will be initiated.

MULTIPLE ORGAN DYSFUNCTION SYNDROME

In the 1970s, a syndrome of multiple organ failure began to be noticed in hospital intensive care units. Medical advances were allowing patients to survive serious illness and trauma—only to die later of complications of the original disease or injury. The syndrome was described in 1975 as *multisystem organ failure*. In 1991, the American College of Chest Physicians and the Society of Critical Care Medicine named it **multiple organ dysfunction syndrome (MODS).**

MODS is the progressive impairment of two or more organ systems resulting from an uncontrolled inflammatory response to a severe illness or injury. Sepsis and septic shock are the most common causes of MODS, with MODS being the end stage. (The progression from infection to sepsis to septic shock to MODS is known as systemic inflammatory response syndrome, or SIRS).

Actually, MODS can result from any severe disease or injury that triggers a massive systemic inflammatory response—including trauma, burns, surgery, circulatory shock, acute pancreatitis, acute renal failure, and others. Risk factors include age (>65), malnutrition, and preexisting chronic disease such as cancer or diabetes. With a mortality rate of 60 to 90 percent, MODS is the major cause of death following sepsis, trauma, and burn injuries.

Pathophysiology of MODS

MODS occurs in two stages. In primary MODS, organ damage results directly from a specific cause such as ischemia or inadequate perfusion resulting from an episode of shock, trauma, or major surgery. There are stress and inflammatory responses (discussed in detail later in this chapter) to this initial injury, but they may be mild and not readily detectable. However, during this response, neutrophils and macrophages (cells that attack and destroy bacteria, protozoa, foreign cells, and cell debris) as well as mast cells (cells that produce histamine and other components of allergic response) are thought to be "primed" by cytokines (proteins released during an inflammatory or immune response).

The next time there is an insult, such as an additional injury or ischemia or infection—even though the insult may be mild—the primed cells are activated, producing an exaggerated inflammatory response, known as secondary MODS.

Now the inflammatory response enters a self-perpetuating cycle. As inflammatory mediators are released by the injured organ, they enter the circulation, activating inflammatory responses in organ systems throughout the body. These mediators, especially cytokines such as tumor necrosis factor (TNF) and interleukin 1 (IL-1), damage the endothelium (cells that line the blood vessels, the heart, and various body cavities). Gram-negative bacteria, if present, release endotoxins that also damage endothelial cells. The injured endothelial cells release factors that aggravate the inflammation and cause vasodilation. The injured epithelium becomes permeable, allowing leakage of fluid into interstitial spaces, and loses much of its anticoagulation function, which allows formation of tiny blood clots (thrombi) in the microvasculature.

The secondary insult also triggers an exaggerated neuroendocrine response. Catecholamine release causes many of the manifestations of MODS, including tachycardia, increased metabolic rates, and increased oxygen consumption. Release of a variety of hormones contributes to the hypermetabolism and release of endorphins contributes to vasodilation. Additionally, plasma protein systems are activated: specifically, the complement system, the coagulation system, and the kallikrein-kinin system. Plasma proteins are key mediators of the inflammatory response. When activated, each of these

multiple organ dysfunction syndrome (MODS) *progressive impairment of two or more organ systems resulting from an uncontrolled inflammatory response to a severe illness or injury.*

 Review

Content

Progression to MODS

Infection
↓
Sepsis
↓
Septic shock
↓
MODS
↓
Death (if not corrected early)

systems triggers a cascade of responses with the overall result of increased vasodilation, vasopermeability, cardiovascular instability, endothelial damage, and clotting abnormalities.

As a result of the release of the inflammatory mediators and toxins and the plasma protein cascades, a massive immune/inflammatory and coagulation response develops. Vascular changes (vasodilation, increased capillary permeability, selective vasoconstriction, and microvascular thrombi) continue and worsen. Two metabolites that are released have opposing vascular effects: Prostacyclin, also called prostaglandin I_2 (PGI_2), is a vasodilator, while thromboxane A_2 (TXA_2) is a vasoconstrictor. They are released in differing amounts within different organ tissues, contributing to a maldistribution of blood flow to organs and organ systems.

As noted earlier, the release of catecholamines stimulates hypermetabolism within the body cells, which in turn creates a greatly increased oxygen demand. Because of lung damage, hypoxemia, and hypoperfusion, a severe oxygen supply/demand imbalance develops. As the cells switch from aerobic to anaerobic metabolism, fuel supplies within the cells (ATP and glucose) are used up faster than they can be replenished. Without adequate ATP, the cells lose their ability to operate the sodium-potassium pump, which is essential to cardiac function. The myocardium is profoundly weakened. Cellular lysosomes begin to break down, releasing lysosomal enzymes which damage the cell membrane and the surrounding cells. Large amounts of lactic acid are released, contributing to acidosis, which further damages the cells. The overall response is similar to that seen in septic and anaphylactic shock, except on a larger scale.

Clinical Presentation of MODS

The cumulative effects of MODS at the cellular and tissue levels begin to cause the breakdown of organ systems: The organs that fail first are not necessarily the organs where the initial insult occurred, and there is a lag time between the initial insult and the onset of organ failure. Dysfunction may develop in the pulmonary, gastrointestinal, hepatic, renal, cardiovascular, hematologic, and immune systems. There is decreased cardiac function and myocardial depression, caused by the factors discussed earlier, possibly abetted by release of myocardial depressant factor (MDF) and a decrease in beta-adrenergic receptors in the heart. The smooth muscle of the vascular system fails with consequent release of capillary sphincters and increased vasodilation.

MODS does not occur in one intense crisis. It will usually develop over a period of 2, 3, or more weeks. There is no specific therapy for MODS, and the only chance of rescuing the patient from its self-perpetuating spiral toward death is early recognition and initiation of supportive measures. For this reason, it is important to understand how MODS usually presents in the first 24 hours after initial resuscitation.

Although MODS will usually be detected in the hospital rather than the prehospital setting, there may be occasions when a patient who has not been hospitalized or has returned home from the hospital is the subject of a call to EMS, or when a patient being transported by EMS from one facility to another is suffering from MODS.

The most common presentation of MODS over time is as follows:

24 Hours after Resuscitation

★ Low-grade fever

★ Tachycardia (rapid heart rate)

★ Dyspnea (breathing difficulty)

★ Altered mental status

★ General hypermetabolic, hyperdynamic state

Within 24 to 72 Hours

★ Pulmonary (lung) failure begins

MODS will usually develop over a period of 2, 3, or more weeks.

Survival from MODS is dependent on early recognition and supportive care.

Within 7 to 10 Days

★ Hepatic (liver) failure begins

★ Intestinal failure begins

★ Renal (kidney) failure begins

Within 14 to 21 Days

★ Renal and hepatic failure intensify

★ Gastrointestinal collapse

★ Immune system collapse

After 21 Days

★ Hematologic (blood system) failure begins

★ Myocardial (heart muscle) failure begins

★ Altered mental status resulting from encephalopathy (brain infection)

★ Death

Part 3: The Body's Defenses against Disease and Injury

SELF-DEFENSE MECHANISMS

So far in this chapter, we have discussed normal body conditions (the normal cell and its environment: fluids and electrolytes, the acid-base balance) and how the body may be attacked or injured (cellular injury, infection, genetic and other causes of disease, hypoperfusion, and multiple organ dysfunction syndrome). In the remainder of the chapter, we will discuss how the body defends itself from infection and injury.

It is important to keep in mind that the body has powerful ways of defending and healing itself (restoring homeostasis) and that medical intervention is needed only when, on occasion, these natural defense mechanisms are unequal to the task and become overwhelmed.

✓ **Review**

Infectious Agents

Bacteria
Viruses
Fungi
Parasites
Prions

INFECTIOUS AGENTS

Bacteria

Bacteria are single-cell organisms that consist of internal cytoplasm surrounded by a rigid cell wall. Bacteria are prokaryotic cells which, unlike the eukaryotic cells of the human body, lack an organized nucleus and other intracellular organelles. Bacteria can reproduce independently, but they need a host to supply food and other support. Inside the body, they achieve this by binding to host cells.

Bacteria can be cultured and identified readily in most hospital laboratories. Many bacteria are categorized according to their appearance under the microscope after staining with several dyes referred to as *Gram stains*. Some bacteria stain blue, while others stain red. Bacteria that stain blue are referred to as *Gram-positive* bacteria. They are somewhat similar to each other in their structure. Bacteria that stain red are referred to as *Gram-negative* bacteria. They are also somewhat similar to each other in their structure.

Bacteria can cause many of the common infections in medicine, including middle ear infections in children, many cases of tonsillitis, and meningitis. (These kinds of infections can also be caused by viruses, which are discussed in the next section.) Most bacterial infections respond to treatment with drugs called **antibiotics.** Once

bacteria (singular **bacterium**) *single-cell organisms with a cell membrane and cytoplasm but no organized nucleus. They bind to the cells of a host organism to obtain food and support.*

antibiotics *substances that destroy or inhibit microorganisms, tiny living bodies invisible to the naked eye. (Antibiotic means "destructive to life.")*

administered, antibiotics kill or inhibit the growth of invading bacteria. As mentioned earlier, the bacterial cell membrane is the site of action for many antibiotics. Once the cell membrane is broken down, phagocytes (cells that ingest and destroy pathogens and other foreign and abnormal substances) can begin to destroy the bacterium. A variety of antibiotic drugs have been developed with mechanisms of action tailored to different types of bacteria. However, the broad variety of infectious bacteria, and their ability to develop resistance to drugs, makes developing antibiotics to battle them a difficult job.

Some bacteria protect themselves by forming a capsule outside the cell wall that protects the organism from digestion by phagocytes. Some bacteria, such as *Mycoplasmic* bacteria, have no protective capsule but rely on other mechanisms to survive and attack the body. *Mycobacterium tuberculosis,* which has no protective capsule, can actually survive and be transported by phagocytes. Other bacteria simply multiply faster than the body's defense systems can respond. Still others overpower the body's defenses by producing enzymes and toxins that attack and injure cells and produce hypersensitivity reactions.

Simple infection is not the only consequence of a bacterial invasion. Many bacteria release poisonous chemicals, or *toxins.* There are two types of toxins produced by bacteria: exotoxins and endotoxins. **Exotoxins** are proteins secreted and released by the bacterial cell during its growth. They travel throughout the body via the blood or lymph, ultimately causing problems. For example, botulism toxin, released by the bacterium *Clostridium botulinum,* blocks the release of cholinergic neurotransmitters at neuromuscular junctions and elsewhere in the autonomic nervous system, causing systemic paralysis. Another example is tetanus, which is caused by the bacterium *Clostridium tetani.* The actual infection by the bacteria themselves is mild and may be limited, for example, to the site of a puncture wound in the foot. Yet, on entering the body, the bacteria release their toxin, *tetanospasmin.* This toxin then travels through the blood to the skeletal muscles, causing the spastic rigidity classically seen in tetanus.

Endotoxins are complex molecules that are contained in the cell walls of certain Gram-negative bacteria. Endotoxins can be released during the destruction of the bacterial cell by phagocytes or even when the bacterial cell is attacked by an antibiotic, so that antibiotics cannot control the endotoxic effects of bacteria. When released, endotoxins trigger the inflammatory process and produce fever. In the bloodstream, they can cause widespread clotting within the blood vessels, capillary damage, and hypotension, as well as respiratory distress and fever—a condition known as endotoxin shock. Endotoxins can survive even when the cell that produced them is dead.

Depending on their amount and site of release, the effects of toxins can be local or systemic. When a bacterial organism enters the circulatory system, its released toxins can spread throughout the body. The systemic spread of toxins through the bloodstream is known as **septicemia,** or *sepsis,* and is a grave medical illness.

The body counters the bacterial invasion and release of enzymes and toxins through activation of the immune system. The immune system will mobilize foreign-cell-destroying macrophages (a type of white blood cell) to the site of infection in an attempt to rid the body of the foreign pathogen. As the macrophages attempt to destroy the bacteria, they release substances known as pyrogens. Pyrogens are responsible for causing the increase in temperature known as fever. Pyrogens act on the thermoregulation center in the hypothalamus to cause the increased body temperature, which is thought to aid in the destruction of pathogens.

Viruses

Most infections are caused by **viruses.** Viruses are much smaller than bacteria and can only be seen with an electron microscope. In addition, they cannot grow without the assistance of another organism. In fact, viruses are referred to as *intracellular parasites,* since they must invade the cells of the organism they infect.

exotoxins *toxic (poisonous) substances secreted by bacterial cells during their growth.*

endotoxins *molecules in the walls of certain Gram-negative bacteria that are released when the bacterium dies or is destroyed, causing toxic (poisonous) effects on the host body.*

septicemia *the systemic spread of toxins through the bloodstream. Also called* sepsis.

virus *an organism much smaller than a bacterium, visible only under an electron microscope. Viruses invade and live inside the cells of the organisms they infect.*

A virus has no organized cellular structure except a protein coat (capsid) surrounding the internal genetic material, deoxyribonucleic acid (DNA) or ribonucleic acid (RNA). With no organized cellular structure or cellular organelles, viruses are incapable of metabolism. Once inside a cell, they take over, using the various cellular enzymes to replicate and produce more viruses, which decreases synthesis of macromolecules vital to the host cell.

Some viruses develop a coating in addition to the capsid, called an envelope. The envelope and the protein capsid allow the virus to resist destruction by the phagocytes of the immune system. However, since viruses cannot reproduce outside a host cell, if the virus does not find a host cell, it will die.

The symptoms of a virus may not be readily apparent because it is hidden within the host cell. After replication is complete, the virus will sometimes destroy the host cell. In other cases, a virus will remain dormant within a cell for months or years. An example is the *varicella zoster virus,* which causes childhood chicken pox and may then remain dormant, only to cause shingles in the adult decades later. Some viruses form a long-term symbiotic (living in close association) relationship with the host cell, resulting in a persistent but unapparent infection.

Viruses do not produce toxins, but they can still cause very serious illnesses. Some viruses are capable of altering the host cell to induce a malignancy (cancer). Others, such as the *human immunodeficiency virus (HIV),* which causes AIDS, can proliferate, attacking cells of the immune system and destroying its ability to ward off infections of all types.

Unlike bacteria, viruses are very difficult to treat. Once a virus infects a cell, it can only be killed by destroying the infected cell. Drugs have not yet been developed that can selectively destroy cells infected by viruses while leaving uninfected cells unharmed. This partially explains the dilemma facing researchers trying to find a cure for AIDS. An additional problem is that some viruses mutate (change) frequently, which is why a new flu vaccine must be developed for every flu season. Fortunately, most viral illnesses are mild and fairly self-limiting. (Because viral agents must spread from cell to cell, the immune system is eventually able to "catch" them outside a host cell and destroy them.) Even so, at present, viruses usually cannot be treated with more than symptomatic care.

Other Agents of Infection

Other biological agents that cause human infection include *fungi* (the plural of *fungus*) and parasites.

Fungi, which includes yeasts and molds, are more like plants than animals. Fungi rarely cause human disease other than minor skin infections such as athlete's foot and some common vaginal infections. Fungus infections are called *mycoses.* Patients with an impaired immune system, such as HIV patients or patients with organ transplants, suffer fungal infection more commonly than healthy people. In such patients, the fungi can invade the lungs, blood, and several organs. Treatment of complicated, deep fungal infections has proven difficult, even in the hospital setting.

Parasites range in size from protozoa (single-cell animals not much larger than bacteria) to large intestinal worms. Parasites tend to be more common in developing nations than in the United States. Treatment depends upon the organism and the location.

Prions are the most recently recognized classification of infectious agents. Initially thought to be slow-acting viruses, prions differ from viruses in that they are smaller, are made entirely of proteins, and do not have protective capsids.

For more about infectious diseases, see Volume 3, Chapter 11.

THREE LINES OF DEFENSE

There are three chief lines of self-defense against infection and injury. One involves anatomical barriers. The other two—the inflammatory response and the immune response—rely on actions of the leukocytes (white blood cells). Each line of defense

Review

Three Lines of Defense

Anatomic barriers
Inflammatory response
Immune response

Content

Table 8-4	Three Lines of Defense against Infection and Injury			
	External	**Internal**	**Nonspecific**	**Specific**
Anatomical Barriers	External		Nonspecific	
Inflammatory Response		Internal	Nonspecific	
Immune Response		Internal		Specific

can be characterized as external or internal, nonspecific or specific (Table 8–4)—characterizations you may want to keep in mind as you read the following sections and compare the ways these defenses protect the body.

Before an infectious agent can attack the body, it has to get past the body's natural anatomical barrier, the epithelium (the skin and the mucous membranes that line the respiratory, gastrointestinal, and genitourinary tracts). The epithelium is more than just a physical barrier; it also provides a chemical defense against infection. The sebaceous glands of the skin secrete fatty and lactic acids, which attack bacteria and fungi. Sweat, tears, and saliva secreted by other glands contain bacteria-attacking enzymes. Various mechanical responses also work to get rid of invading substances. For example, the invader may be coughed or sneezed out of the respiratory tract, flushed out of the urinary tract, or eliminated from the gastrointestinal tract by vomiting or diarrhea.

The anatomical defenses are *external* and *nonspecific.* They are considered external because they prevent substances from penetrating the skin or the coverings of internal passageways. They are nonspecific because they defend against all invaders, such as foreign bodies, chemicals, or microorganisms, without targeting any specific type of invader.

If an invading foreign body, chemical, or microorganism penetrates the anatomical barriers and begins to attack internal cells and tissues, two other lines of defense are triggered: the inflammatory response and the immune response. These twin responses of the immune system have contrasting characteristics of speed, specificity, duration (memory), and of the plasma systems and cell types that are involved in the response (Table 8–5).

The *inflammatory response,* or *inflammation,* begins within seconds of injury or invasion by a pathogen. As noted earlier, it is nonspecific, attacking any invader by surrounding it with cells and fluids to isolate, destroy, and eliminate it. Inflammation is mediated by multiple plasma protein systems, especially the complement system, the coagulation system, and the kinin system (which will be explained later) and involves a variety of cell types as it attacks the invader.

The *immune response* develops more slowly (one type of response requires a second exposure after priming by the first exposure to the invader). The immune response is specific, in that it will develop a specialized response for each different invader. It is mediated by just one plasma protein system (immunoglobulin) and attacks the invader mainly with a single cell type (lymphocytes, which are one type of leukocyte, or white blood cell).

Table 8-5	Characteristics of the Inflammatory and Immune Responses	
	Inflammatory Response	**Immune Response**
Speed	Fast	Slow
Specificity	Nonspecific	Specific
Duration (Memory)	Transient (no memory)	Long-term (memory)
Involving Which Plasma Systems	Multiple plasma protein systems (complement, coagulation, kinin systems)	One plasma protein system (immunoglobulin)
Involving Which Cell Type	Multiple cell types (granulocytes, monocytes, macrophages)	One blood cell type (lymphocytes)

Inflammation and the immune response interact in many ways. We will discuss the immune response first, because understanding the immune response is necessary for understanding some parts of the inflammatory response.

THE IMMUNE RESPONSE

HOW THE IMMUNE RESPONSE WORKS: AN OVERVIEW

Most viruses, bacteria, fungi, and parasites—as well as noninfectious substances such as pollens, foods, venoms, drugs, and others that may enter the body—have proteins on their surface called **antigens.** The immune system detects these antigens as being foreign, or "non-self," and responds to produce substances called **antibodies** that combine with antigens to control or destroy them. This is known as the **immune response.** As part of this process, *memory cells* "remember" the antigen and will trigger an even faster and more effective response to destroy the same antigen if it enters the body again. Such long-term protection against specific foreign substances is known as **immunity.**

CHARACTERISTICS OF THE IMMUNE RESPONSE AND IMMUNITY

The immune response and immunity can be classified in various ways: natural versus acquired immunity, primary versus secondary immune responses, and humoral versus cell-mediated immunity.

Natural versus Acquired Immunity

Natural immunity is not generated by the immune response. It is inborn, part of the genetic makeup of the individual or of the species in general. For example, the measles virus cannot reproduce in canine cells, so dogs are naturally immune to measles. Conversely, canine distemper cannot thrive within human cells, so humans are naturally immune to that disease. (Some diseases such as leukemia, however, can affect more than one species.)

Acquired immunity develops as an outcome of the immune response. Acquired immunity can be either active or passive. *Active acquired immunity* is generated by the host's (infected person's) immune system after exposure to an antigen. *Passive acquired immunity* is transferred to a person from an outside source. For example, a mother may transfer antibodies through the placenta to the fetus. Or antibodies may be administered to a patient as an immune serum to aid the body's response to a dangerous invader such as rabies, tetanus, or snake venom. Active acquired immunity is long-lasting. Passive acquired immunity is temporary.

Primary versus Secondary Immune Responses

There are two phases to the immune response to an antigen, the primary immune response and the secondary immune response.

On exposure to an antigen, B lymphocyte cells (explained in the next section) produce antibodies to attack the antigen. These antibodies are called **immunoglobulins,** which are proteins present in the plasma portion of the blood. There are five classes of immunoglobulins—IgM, IgG, IgA, IgE, and IgD.

On first exposure to an antigen, after a lag-time of 5 to 7 days, the presence of IgM antibodies can be detected in the blood, with a lesser presence of IgG antibodies. This constitutes the **primary immune response,** also called the *initial immune response.* If there is no further exposure to the antigen, the antibodies are catabolized (broken down)—but the immune system has been "primed." If there is a second exposure to the antigen, the body responds much faster, and a far greater quantity of IgG antibodies is

Review

Immune Classifications

Natural vs. Acquired
Primary vs. Secondary
Humoral vs. Cell Mediated

produced. The level of IgG antibodies, with their memory for the specific antigen, will remain elevated for many years. This constitutes the **secondary immune response,** also called the *anamnestic* (or memory-assisting) *immune response.*

The primary and secondary immune responses together create active acquired immunity to the specific antigen.

Humoral versus Cell-Mediated Immunity

A special type of leukocyte (white blood cell) is the **lymphocyte.** Lymphocytes (which constitute about 20 to 35 percent of all leukocytes) are responsible for several critical functions of the immune response, including recognizing foreign antigens, producing antibodies (the immunoglobulins such as IgM and IgG, previously mentioned), and developing memory.

As lymphocytes mature, they become one of several types, including B lymphocytes and T lymphocytes. **B lymphocytes** do not attack antigens directly. Instead, they produce the antibodies (immunoglobulins) that attack antigens. B lymphocytes also develop memory, and confer long-term immunity to specific antigens. This type of immunity is called **humoral immunity.** (*Humor* refers to the blood and other fluids of the body; *humoral immunity* refers to the long-lasting antibodies and memory cells present in the blood and lymph.)

T lymphocytes do not produce antibodies. Instead, they recognize the presence of a foreign antigen and attack it directly. This type of immunity is called **cell-mediated immunity** (Figures 8-14 ■ and 8-15 ■).

Lymphocytes and the Lymph System Lymphocytes—including B lymphocytes, T lymphocytes, and secretory lymphocytes (to be discussed later)—are circulated through the body as part of the lymph system. Lymph (the fluid of the lymphatic system) consists primarily of interstitial fluid carrying proteins, bacteria, and other substances. (As discussed earlier in the chapter, most interstitial fluid reenters the bloodstream via the capillaries, but the small amount that does not reenter the capillaries is carried away by the lymph system.)

Lymph is carried through the lymphatic vessels that are parallel to but separate from the blood vessels and is filtered through *lymph nodes* in various parts of the body, Eventually, the lymph empties into one of two lymphatic ducts in the thorax. The smaller of the two is the *right lymphatic duct,* which drains lymph from the right arm and the right side of the head and right side of the thorax. The larger is the *thoracic duct,* which is located in the left thorax and receives lymph from the rest of the body. These ducts drain the lymph into the right and left subclavian veins, respectively, and the lymph then travels through the bloodstream. The cycle is completed as the lymph is returned from the blood to the tissues to the lymph system. In this way, lymph, and the lymphocytes it carries, are circulated through the blood and lymph system again and again.

The B lymphocytes and T lymphocytes carried by the blood and the lymph system are the key elements in humoral and cell-mediated immunity, which will be discussed in more detail in the next sections.

INDUCTION OF THE IMMUNE RESPONSE

The immune response must be triggered, or induced. The following sections discuss the role of antigens and immunogens, histocompatibility, and blood groups in induction of the immune response.

Antigens and Immunogens

Antigens that can trigger the immune response are called **immunogens.** Not every antigen is an immunogen. In other words, not every antigen is capable of triggering the im-

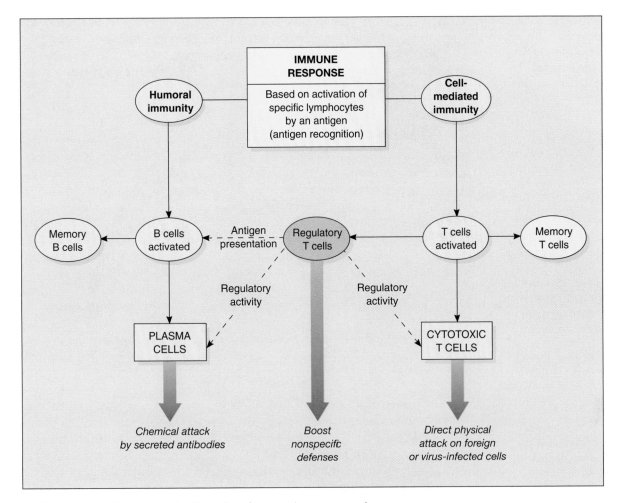

Figure 8-14 Humoral and cell-mediated immunity—an overview.

mune response. As an example, antigens are present on various helpful bacteria that reside within our bodies, but the immune response is not triggered by these antigens.

What makes a molecule an antigen is a chemical structure that is capable of reacting with existing components of the immune system, such as antibodies and T lymphocytes. However, having this chemical structure, the ability to *react* once the immune system has been triggered, is not enough to *trigger* the immune system in the first place. In order to be immunogenic—able to trigger an immune response—an antigen must have certain additional characteristics.

Characteristics of Antigenic Immunogenicity

★ Sufficient foreignness

★ Sufficient size

★ Sufficient complexity

★ Presence in sufficient amounts

As mentioned earlier, the body can distinguish between self and non-self, or foreign, antigens. Normally, the immune system is not triggered by self-antigens. In fact, the immune system does not just "tolerate" self-antigens, it actively protects them through suppression of the immune system by T lymphocytes and a special antibody called antiidiopathic antibody.

Large molecules, such as proteins, polysaccharides, and nucleic acids, are the most likely to trigger the immune response. Smaller molecules, such as amino acids,

All immunogens are antigens, but not all antigens are immunogens. In other words, only some antigens are capable of triggering an immune response.

■ Figure 8-15 (a) Humoral immune response.

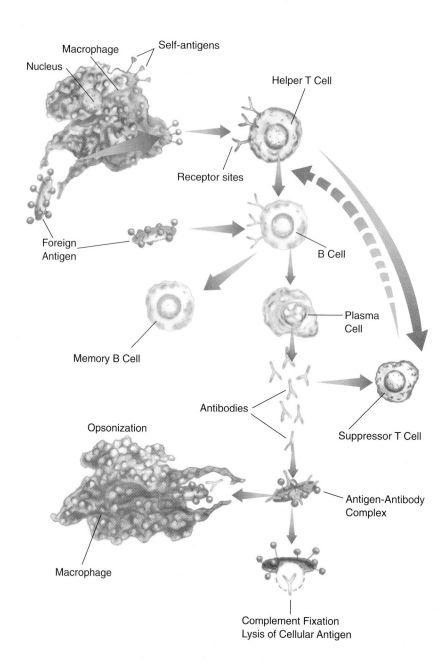

Macrophage
Self-antigens
Nucleus
Helper T Cell
Receptor sites
Foreign Antigen
B Cell
Memory B Cell
Plasma Cell
Antibodies
Opsonization
Suppressor T Cell
Antigen-Antibody Complex
Macrophage
Complement Fixation Lysis of Cellular Antigen

haptens *molecules that do not trigger an immune response on their own but can become immunogenic when combined with larger molecules.*

monosaccharides, and fatty acids, are less likely to induce the immune response. Some small molecules, however, can function as **haptens,** meaning that they can become immunogenic when combined with larger molecules.

More complex molecules, and molecules that are present in sufficient numbers, are more likely to trigger an immune response. Additionally, different routes of entry can stimulate different types of cell-mediated or humoral immune response (which dictates the route by which serum antigens may be administered: e.g., intravenous, subcutaneously, orally, intraperitoneally, intranasally). Other substances present in the body can help to stimulate the immune response. Also, as noted earlier, the person's genetic makeup can affect the ability to respond to antigens.

Histocompatibility Locus Antigens

HLA antigens *antigens the body recognizes as self or non-self; present on all body cells except the red blood cells.*

The body recognizes whether a substance is self or non-self as a result of certain antigens that are present on almost all cells of the body, except the red blood cells. These antigens are called **HLA antigens** (for *histocompatibility locus antigens*—or *human leukocyte antigens,* because leukocytes were where these antigens were originally found).

Macrophage   Nucleus   Self-antigens

Receptor sites   Helper T Cell

Foreign Antigen

Memory T Cell   Cytotoxic T Cell   Suppressor T Cell

Chemically destroys foreign cells   Produces cytokines to attract macrophages

■ Figure 8-15 (Continued) (b) Cell-mediated immune response.

HLA antigens are the antigens that the body recognizes as self or foreign. The chief genetic source of HLA antigens has been identified as genes located at several sites (loci) on chromosome 6 that are known as the **major histocompatibility complex (MHC).**

HLA antigens determine the suitability, or compatibility, of tissues and organs that will be grafted or transplanted from a donor. The more closely related the donor and recipient are, the more likely the recipient's body is to accept the graft or transplant. Why? Every person receives half of his genetic inheritance from each parent.

Like all genes, the genes that produce HLA antigens occur as pairs (alleles) on corresponding loci on pairs of chromosomes. A group of alleles on one chromosome is called a haplotype. Every person has two HLA haplotypes, one on each of the pair of chromosomes. Of each pair of chromosomes (and the HLA haplotypes they carry), the person inherits one from his father and one from his mother.

Since each parent has two haplotypes, but only one gets passed along to each child (to pair up with one from the other parent), various combinations of inherited haplotypes are possible among the children of those parents. In general, each child will share one haplotype with half their siblings, both haplotypes with a quarter of their siblings, and no haplotypes with a quarter of their siblings.

Siblings and other close relatives are generally considered first as donors of tissues and organs because they have the highest likelihood of histocompatibility, hence the least likelihood of the immune system's rejecting the graft or transplant. (Identical twins, who come from the same egg fertilized by the same sperm, have identical genetic makeups and identical haplotypes. Therefore, they are the most reliable match for grafts and transplants.)

Other factors besides HLA makeup can affect the success of a graft or transplant, so they sometimes fail, even when from a histocompatible donor. However, histocompatibility is the most important factor in graft and transplant success.

Blood Group Antigens

HLA antigens do not exist on the surface of erythrocytes (red blood cells), but other antigens, known as the blood group antigens, do. There are more than 80 of these red cell antigens that have been grouped into a number of different blood group systems. The

major histocompatibility complex (MHC) *a group of genes on chromosome 6 that provide the genetic code for HLA antigens.*

two groups that trigger the strongest immune response are the Rh system and the ABO system.

The Rh System   The **Rh blood group** is named for the rhesus monkey in which it was first identified. One of several antigens in this group is known as Rh antigen D, or the **Rh factor.** Rh factor is present in about 85 percent of North Americans (Rh positive), but absent in about 15 percent (Rh negative).

Incompatibility between Rh positive and Rh negative blood can cause harmful immune responses. For example, if a patient with Rh negative blood receives a transplant of Rh positive blood, a primary immune response is triggered. If there is a second transfusion of Rh positive blood, a severe transfusion reaction may result.

Hemolytic disease of the newborn may result from Rh incompatibility between mother and fetus. Problems will usually not occur in a first pregnancy where the mother is Rh negative and the fetus is Rh positive, because few fetal erythrocytes cross the placental barrier to the mother. However, a significant number of fetal erythrocytes do enter the mother's bloodstream at birth when the placenta separates from the uterus. These may (depending on several factors) activate a primary immune response and development of Rh antibodies. If the fetus in her next pregnancy is also Rh positive, the mother's Rh antibodies can cross the placenta and destroy the red blood cells of the fetus. This is actually a rare occurrence. Rh incompatibility occurs in only about 10 percent of pregnancies, and because not all such incompatibilities actually produce Rh antibodies in the mother, only about 5 percent of women ever have babies with hemolytic disease, even after numerous pregnancies.

The ABO System   The **ABO blood groups** are formed because there are two types of antigens that may be present on the surface of red blood cells. These antigens are named A and B. Persons with blood type A carry only A antigens on their red blood cells. Those with blood type B carry only B antigens. Those with blood type AB carry both, and those with blood type O carry neither (Table 8–6).

An immune response will be activated in a person with type A blood who receives a transfusion of type B blood, which is recognized as non-self. The same will happen when a person with type B blood receives type A blood. People with type O blood are known as *universal donors,* because type O blood has no antigens that will trigger an immune response in any other group. Those with type AB blood are known as *universal recipients,* because they have both types of antigens and will not produce antibodies in response to any other blood groups (Table 8–7).

ABO incompatibility between mother and fetus is more common than Rh incompatibility, occurring in about 20 to 25 percent of pregnancies. However, only 10 percent of ABO incompatibilities will result in hemolytic disease of the infant.

HUMORAL IMMUNE RESPONSE

Earlier, we identified the humoral immune response as the long-lasting response provided by production in the bloodstream of antibodies (immunoglobulins) and mem-

Rh blood group *a group of antigens discovered on the red blood cells of rhesus monkeys that is also present to some extent in humans.*

Rh factor *an antigen in the Rh blood group that is also known as antigen D. About 85 percent of North Americans have the Rh factor (are Rh positive) while about 15 percent do not have the Rh factor (are Rh negative). Rh positive and Rh negative blood are incompatible; that is, a person who is Rh negative can experience a severe immune response if Rh positive blood is introduced, as through a transfusion or during childbirth.*

ABO blood groups *four blood groups formed by the presence or absence of two antigens known as A and B. A person may have either (type A or type B), both (type AB), or neither (type O). An immune response will be activated whenever a person receives blood containing A or B antigen if this antigen is not already present in his own blood.*

Table 8–6	Blood Groups—ABO System	
Blood Type	**Antigen Present on Erythrocyte**	**Antibody Present in Serum**
O	None	Anti-A, Anti-B
AB	A and B	None
B	B	Anti-A
A	A	Anti-B

Table 8–7	Compatibility among ABO Blood Groups			
	Reaction with Serum of Recipient			
Cells of Donor	AB	B	A	O
AB	–	+	+	+
B	–	–	+	+
A	–	+	–	+
O	–	–	–	–

– = No reaction

+ = Reaction

ory cells by B lymphocytes (review Figure 8-15a). This is sometimes called the *internal* or *systemic immune system*. Another kind of humoral immunity is provided by secretions at the body surfaces, such as sweat and saliva, and is sometimes called the *external, mucosal,* or *secretory immune system*. These types of humoral immune responses will be discussed in the following sections.

B Lymphocytes

The blood cells that are involved in immune response, as noted earlier, are lymphocytes, which are one type of white blood cell. Lymphocytes are generated from **stem cells** in the bone marrow, from which all blood cells are generated. Lymphocytes then take one of two paths as they mature. In one path, lymphocytes that travel through the thymus gland mature into T lymphocytes, which are involved in cell-mediated immunity and will be discussed in detail later. On the other path, lymphocytes that travel through a set of lymphoid tissues, including the spleen and lymph nodes, mature into B lymphocytes, which are involved in humoral immunity.

Each mature B cell recognizes, through an antigen receptor on its surface, a single type of antigen and then produces antibodies to that antigen. But since there are many, many kinds of antigens—and since exactly which foreign antigens may ever invade the body cannot be anticipated—how does a B cell develop a receptor that is specialized to a specific antigen?

It is thought that this specialization of B cells takes place through the processes of clonal diversity and clonal selection. **Clonal diversity** is generated as the precursors of mature B cells develop in the bone marrow. During this process, a B cell precursor develops receptors for every possible kind of antigen it may ever encounter. Later, after the immature B cells have migrated into the peripheral lymphoid organs, primarily the spleen and the lymph nodes, antigen that is present in the system reacts with the appropriate receptors on the surfaces of B cell clones, which is the process of **clonal selection**.

Clonal selection activates the immature B cell, prompting it to proliferate and differentiate, the end result being the mature B cell that produces plasma cells that secrete immunoglobulin antibodies into the blood and secondary lymphoid organs. The mature B cell also produces **memory cells** that will trigger a swifter and stronger immune response if they encounter the same antigen again (the secondary immune response). The process of clonal selection is probably responsible (during the primary immune response) for the lag time of 5 to 7 days between introduction of an antigen and the first detectable appearance of antibodies in the blood.

Immunoglobulins

Immunoglobulins and Antibodies   Antibodies are proteins secreted by plasma cells that are produced by B cells in response to an antigen. All antibodies are immunoglobulins, but researchers have not yet determined whether all immunoglobulins function as antibodies.

stem cells   *undifferentiated cells in the bone marrow from which all blood cells, including thrombocytes, erythrocytes, and various types of leukocytes, develop; stem cells are also called hemocytoblasts.*

clonal diversity   *the development, by B lymphocyte precursors in the bone marrow, of receptors for every possible type of antigen.*

clonal selection   *the process by which a specific antigen reacts with the appropriate receptors on the surface of immature B lymphocytes, thereby activating them and prompting them to proliferate, differentiate, and produce antibodies to the activating antigen.*

memory cells   *cells produced by mature B lymphocytes that "remember" the activating antigen and will trigger a stronger and swifter immune response if reexposure to the antigen occurs.*

Antibodies are secreted by plasma cells in response to antigenic stimulation.

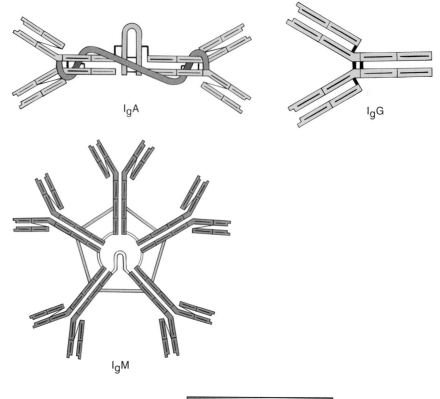

■ Figure 8-16 Some immunoglobulin (antibody) structures.

IgA

IgG

IgM

■ Figure 8-17 Antigen-antibody binding. The shape of the antigen fits the shape of the antigen-binding site on the immunoglobulin (antibody) molecule like a key in a lock.

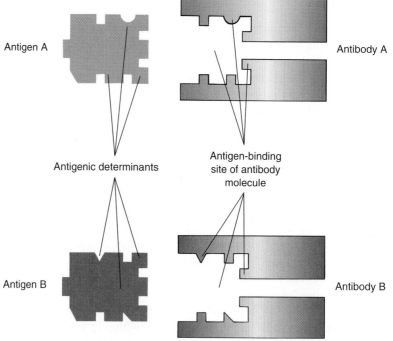

Antigen A

Antibody A

Antigenic determinants

Antigen-binding site of antibody molecule

Antigen B

Antibody B

The Structure of Immunoglobulins   The structure of immunoglobulin molecules consists of Y-shaped chains, arranged somewhat differently in the different immunoglobulin classes (Figure 8-16 ■). At the two "upper" tips of the Y are the *antigen-binding sites.* The interaction of amino acids with parts of the chain determines the shape of the immunoglobulin molecule's antigen-binding site. The shape of the antigen-binding site determines which antigen the immunoglobulin molecule will bind to—because there is an area on the antigen (the antigenic determinant) that will fit the shape of the antigen-binding site like a key in a lock (Figure 8-17 ■). In some cases, substitution of a single amino acid changes the conformation of the antigen-binding site and, therefore, the antigen it will combine with.

The Functions of Antibodies   An antibody circulates in the blood or is suspended in body secretions until it meets and binds to its specific antigen. The antibody can then have either a direct or an indirect effect on the target antigen that results in inactivation or destruction of the antigen. Both direct and indirect effects result from the binding of antibodies and antigens, forming **antigen-antibody complexes,** also called *immune complexes.*

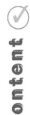

antigen-antibody complex
the substance formed when an antibody combines with an antigen to deactivate or destroy it; also called immune complex.

Direct Effects of Antibodies on Antigens

★ *Agglutination*—A soluble antibody combines with a solid antigen, causing it to clump together.

★ *Precipitation*—The antigen-antibody complex precipitates out of the blood and is carried away by body fluids.

★ *Neutralization*—The antibody, in combining with the antigen, inactivates the antigen by preventing it from binding to receptors on the surface of body cells.

Indirect Effects of Antibodies on Antigens

★ *Enhancement of phagocytosis*—*Phagocytosis* is one of the chief processes of inflammation (described later in the chapter) in which certain types of white blood cells (neutrophils and macrophages) ingest and digest foreign substances. The actions of antibodies can encourage phagocytosis.

★ *Activation of plasma proteins*—Antibodies can activate plasma proteins of the complement system (described later) that, in turn, attack and destroy antigens.

Through the direct and indirect effects previously described, antibodies serve four main functions: neutralizing bacterial toxins, neutralizing viruses, opsonizing bacteria, and activating portions of the inflammatory response.

★ *Neutralization of Bacterial Toxins.* As noted earlier, many bacteria produce harmful toxins that increase their pathogenic effect. However, bacterial toxins sow the seeds of their own destruction by triggering the humoral immune response. In this case the antigen-antibody complex is a *toxin-antitoxin complex*. Antibodies neutralize the bacterial toxins by occupying their antigenic determinant sites, which prevents them from binding to and harming tissue cells. Detection of specific antitoxins aids in the diagnosis of disease. Vaccines against diseases such as diphtheria and tetanus work by injecting a form of the bacterial toxin, which is altered to greatly reduce its toxic effects but to retain its immugenicity.

★ *Neutralization of Viruses.* Antibodies can prevent some viruses from attaching to and entering body cells. The antibodies attach to the viruses, causing agglutination or fostering phagocytosis. The effectiveness of antibodies against viruses depends on whether the virus circulates in the bloodstream (as with polio and flu) or spreads by direct cell-to-cell contact (as with measles and herpes). Antibodies against the latter may help prevent the initial infection but cannot prevent the spread or recurrence of an established infection. Vaccines are effective against some viral infections such as influenza, rubella, and polio.

★ *Opsonization of Bacteria.* Many bacteria have an outer capsule that is resistant to phagocytosis. Opsonization coats the bacteria with opsonin, a substance that makes them vulnerable to phagocytosis. Antibodies themselves are opsonins, and they also cause opsinization by a plasma protein that is a component of the complement system.

★ *Activation of Inflammatory Processes.* When the antigen-binding sites at the "upper" tips of the Y-shaped immunoglobulin molecule bind to an antigen, the "lower" tip activates elements of the inflammatory response, transmitting the information that a foreign invader has entered the body. The inflammatory response (which will be described later) enhances the attack by the immune system against the invader.

Classes of Immunoglobulins As noted earlier there are five classes of immunoglobulins. They are:

IgM—the antibody that is produced first during the primary immune response. It is the largest immunoglobulin.

IgG—the antibody that has "memory" and recognizes repeated invasions of an antigen. IgG comprises 80 to 85 percent of immunoglobulins in the blood. It is the major class of immunoglobulin in the immune response and has four subclasses. IgG is responsible for antibody functions such as agglutination, precipitation, and complement activation.

IgA—the antibody present in mucous membranes. One subclass of IgA is the predominant immunoglobulin in body secretions. The other subclass of IgA is present mostly in the blood.

IgE—the least-concentrated immunoglobulin in the circulation. It is the principal antibody that contributes to allergic and anaphylactic reactions and to the prevention of parasitic infections.

IgD—an antibody that is present in very low concentrations; little is known about its role. It is present principally on the surfaces of developing B cells.

Antibodies as Antigens A molecule that functions as an antibody in the human body can function as an antigen if it enters the body of another person or a member of another species. To function in the role of antigens, antibody molecules usually contain antigenic determinants with which the antigen-binding sites on other antibodies can combine.

The antigenic determinants on human antibody molecules are classified into three groups:

★ *Isotypic antigens* are species-specific. That is, they are the same within a given species but differ from those within other species. For example, isotypic antigens in human serum would function as antigens if injected into a rabbit.

★ *Allotypic antigens* can differ between members of the same species. The serum from a person with one form of allotype might function as an antigen in another person.

★ *Idiotypic antigenic determinants* can differ within the same individual. For example, IgG subclass 3 molecules produced against mumps and those produced against tetanus in the same person will differ from each other.

Monoclonal Antibodies Most antigens have multiple antigenic determinants, which stimulate a response from multiple clones of B lymphocytes. This is known as a *polyclonal response.* Each B cell clone secretes antibody that is slightly different from that of the other clones. Recently, researchers have been working with monoclonal antibodies. A **monoclonal antibody,** produced in the laboratory, is very pure and specific to a single antigen. Monoclonal antibodies are being put to a variety of cutting-edge and experimental uses, including identification of infectious organisms, blood and tissue typing, and treatment of autoimmune diseases and some cancers.

The Secretory Immune System

The **secretory immune system** (also known as the *external* or *mucosal immune system*) consists of lymphoid tissues beneath the mucosal endothelium. These tissues secrete substances such as sweat, tears, saliva, mucus, and breast milk. Some antibodies are present in these secretions (mostly IgA, with some IgM and IgG) and can help defend the body (or the nursing baby) against antigens that have not yet penetrated the skin or the mucous membranes.

secretory immune system *lymphoid tissues beneath the mucosal endothelium that secrete substances such as sweat, tears, saliva, mucus, and breast milk; also called the* external immune system *or the* mucosal immune system.

The secretory immune system's primary function is to protect the body from pathogens that are inhaled or ingested. Other mechanisms must be functioning adequately to complete that task. For example, gastric acid helps destroy pathogens, and mechanisms such as blinking, sneezing, coughing, and peristalsis (the wavelike muscle contractions that move substances through the passageways of the digestive system) help move pathogens out of the system.

The lymphocytes of the secretory immune system follow a different developmental path after leaving the bone marrow than do the lymphocytes of the systemic immune system. As they mature, systemic lymphocytes migrate through the spleen and lymph nodes, whereas lymphocytes of the secretory system travel through the lacrimal (tear-producing) and salivary glands and through mucosal-associated lymphoid tissues in the bronchi, breasts, intestines, and genitourinary tract.

Secretory lymphocytes circulate through the lymph system and bloodstream in a pattern that is different from the circulatory pattern of the systemic lymphocytes. Secretory lymphocytes are returned from the blood through the tissues to the mucosal-associated lymphoid tissues, rather than to the lymphoid tissues of the systemic immune system.

The secretory immune system is the body's first line of defense against pathogens, whereas the systemic immune system is the body's last line of defense.

CELL-MEDIATED IMMUNE RESPONSE

Some lymphocytes develop into B cells, which are responsible for *humoral immunity,* which we have discussed in the prior sections. Other lymphocytes develop into T cells, which are responsible for *cell-mediated immunity,* the subject of this section (Figure 8-15b).

A key difference between the two is that B cells do not attack pathogens directly. Instead, they produce antibodies that combine with antigens on the surfaces of pathogenic cells. The antibodies remain in the bloodstream for a long time and will attack the antigen again on any subsequent exposure. Thus, the humoral immunity created by B cells is long-lasting. T cells, however, do not produce antibodies. Rather, they attack pathogens directly, and the immunity they create, called cell-mediated immunity, is temporary.

Another key distinction is that one kind of T cell (helper T cells) is responsible for activating both T cells (in cell-mediated immune response) and B cells (in humoral immune response). (To compare humoral and cell-mediated responses, review Figure 8-14 as well as Figures 8-15a and 8-15b.)

T Lymphocytes and Their Major Effects

In contrast to B lymphocytes, which travel through the spleen and lymph nodes as they mature, T cells travel through the thymus gland (hence the name *T cell*).

T cells become specialized through processes that are similar to the processes described earlier for B cells: clonal diversity and clonal selection. After generation by stem cells in the bone marrow, lymphocytes destined to become T cells travel to the thymus. There, through the process of *clonal diversity,* maturing T cells develop the capacity to recognize all the antigens they will ever encounter. Later, after the T cells have migrated into the peripheral lymphoid organs, they undergo the process of *clonal selection.* In this process, the immature T cells encounter antigens that react with appropriate receptors on the surfaces of the T cells, causing them to proliferate and differentiate into five different types of mature T cells, each with distinct functions.

Five Types of Mature T Cells

★ *Memory cells* induce secondary immune responses.

★ *Td cells* transfer **delayed hypersensitivity** (allergic responses) and secrete proteins called lymphokines that activate other cells such as macrophages.

★ *Tc cells* are **cytotoxic** cells that directly attack and destroy cells that bear foreign antigens.

★ *Th cells* are *helper cells* that facilitate both cell-mediated and humoral immune processes.

★ *Ts cells* are *suppressor cells* that inhibit both cell-mediated and humoral immune processes.

As a result of this specialization, T cells are capable of attacking an antigen in a variety of ways. The major effects of cell-mediated immune response result from the specialized functions of the four types of T cells: memory, delayed hypersensitivity, cytotoxicity, and control.

Memory   Memory cells "remember" an antigen and trigger the immune response to any repeated exposure to that antigen.

Delayed Hypersensitivity   Td cells (delayed hypersensitivity cells) are involved in allergic reactions and the inflammatory response. They produce substances (lymphokines) that communicate with and influence the behavior of other cells.

Cytotoxicity   Tc cells (cytotoxic cells) mediate the direct killing of target cells, such as cells that have been infected by a virus, tumor cells, or cells in transplanted organs (Figure 8-18 ■).

Control   Th (helper) cells and Ts (suppressor) cells effect control of both humoral and cell-mediated immune responses. Th cells facilitate the response; Ts cells inhibit the response.

 Review

Five Types of Mature T Cells

Memory cells
Td cells—delayed
 hypersensitivity
Tc cells—cytotoxic
Th cells—helpers
Ts cells—suppressors

delayed hypersensitivity   *an allergic response that takes place after the elapse of some time following reexposure to an antigen.*

cytotoxic   *toxic, or poisonous, to cells.*

■ Figure 8-18   The physiology of cytotoxic T cells.

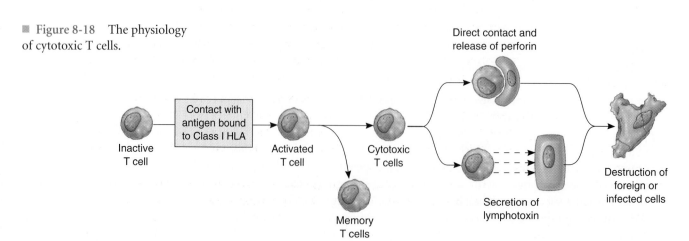

CELLULAR INTERACTIONS IN IMMUNE RESPONSE

The immune and inflammatory responses are interacting, not separate. For example:

Sequence of Events	Interaction
Macrophages released during an inflammatory response activate the helper T cells (Th cells) . . .	Inflammatory response interacting with cell-mediated immune response
. . . then the helper T cells (Th cells) activate other T cells, and they also activate B cells . . .	Cell-mediated immune response interacting with humoral immune response
. . . and delayed hypersensitivity T cells (Td cells) stimulate the production of more macrophages.	Cell-mediated immune response interacting with inflammatory response

The three key interactions that occur during an immune response (review Figures 8-15 a and b) are:

1. Antigen-presenting cells (macrophages) interact with Th (helper) cells.
2. Th (helper) cells interact with B cells.
3. Th (helper) cells interact with Tc (cytotoxic) cells.

Cytokines

Cytokines, proteins produced by white blood cells, are the "messengers" of the immune response. When released by one cell, they can bind with nearby cells, affecting their function. They can also bind with the same cell that produced them and alter the function of that cell. They help to regulate cell functions during both inflammatory and immune responses. For example, a cytokine must be released by a macrophage to facilitate activation of a helper T cell.

A cytokine that is released by a macrophage is called a **monokine** ("mono" because a macrophage is a kind of monocyte, a single-nucleus white blood cell). A cytokine that is released by a lymphocyte (a T cell or B cell) is called a **lymphokine.** Types of cytokines include proteins known as *interleukins, interferon,* and *tumor necrosis factor.*

Antigen Processing, Presentation, and Recognition

A sequence of three processes is necessary before an immune response can begin:

1. Antigen processing (by macrophages)
2. Antigen presentation (by macrophages)
3. Antigen recognition (by T cells or B cells)

More will be said later in the chapter about how macrophages are released during the inflammatory response. For now, keep in mind that a *macrophage* is a large cell (a type of white blood cell) that will ingest and destroy or partially destroy an invading organism. As it does so, the invader's antigens are released into the cytosol (fluid interior) of the macrophage cell. The ingestion of an invading organism and breakdown of its antigens is the beginning of **antigen processing.**

Once the macrophage has broken down the antigens, it then expresses these antigen fragments and "presents" them on its own surface, along with its own self-antigens. When these two markers on the surface of the macrophage—the foreign antigens and the self-antigens—are recognized by helper T cells, the helper T cells are activated (review Figure 8-15a).

Because macrophages (and other macrophagelike cells) present portions of antigen on their surfaces, they are called **antigen-presenting cells (APCs).**

cytokines *proteins, produced by white blood cells, that regulate immune responses by binding with and affecting the function of the cells that produced them or of other, nearby cells.*

monokine *a cytokine released by a macrophage.*

lymphokine *a cytokine released by a lymphocyte.*

Cytokines are often called "the hormones of the immune response."

antigen processing *the recognition, ingestion, and breakdown of a foreign antigen, culminating in production of an antibody to the antigen or in a direct cytotoxic response to the antigen.*

antigen-presenting cells (APCs) *cells, such as macrophages, that present (express onto their surfaces) portions of the antigens they have digested.*

T cell receptor (TCR) *a molecule on the surface of a helper T cell that responds to a specific antigen. There is a specific TCR for every antigen to which the human body may be exposed.*

The helper T cells recognize the presented antigen through receptors on their surfaces. There are two types of receptors. One type, called a **T cell receptor (TCR),** is antigen-specific; that is, it will respond only to one specific antigen. The other type, CD4 or CD8 receptors, will respond no matter what antigen is presented.

As discussed earlier, the body recognizes whether an antigen is self or non-self as a result of HLA antigens. For presentation of an antigen to be effective, the antigen must be in a complex with either class I or class II HLA antigens. The HLA class determines which cells will respond. Th (helper) cells respond only to class II HLA antigens. Tc (cytotoxic) cells and Ts (suppressor) cells respond only to class I HLA antigens.

In addition to the antigen-receptor interaction, another requirement for intercellular communication between the macrophage cell and the T cell is an interaction between *self-adhesion molecules* on the surface of the macrophage and the T cell. These molecules, in connecting, strengthen the interactions between the cells.

The macrophage also produces the cytokine interleukin-1 (IL-1) that helps the T cell respond to the presented antigens.

T Cell and B Cell Differentiation

T cells and B cells are not differentiated until antigens present in the system react with the appropriate receptors on the cell surfaces. As previously described, this reaction occurs as a result of antigen processing and presentation by macrophages and antigen recognition by the T or B cell. The presence of secreted cytokines is also usually necessary to facilitate the antigen-receptor reaction.

Once a reaction between antigen and T cell receptor takes place, the immature T cells proliferate and differentiate, depending on the specific receptors and antigens involved, into Th, Tc, Td, Ts, and memory cells.

After stimulation by Th cells or direct recognition of antigen, B cells will proliferate and produce antibodies differentiated as IgM, IgG, IgA, IgE, and IgD immunoglobulins (review Figure 8-15b).

Control of T Cell and B Cell Development

There are several parameters that control immune responses, activating them when needed but stopping or inhibiting them when not needed, thus preventing them from destroying the body's own tissues. As noted earlier, Ts (suppressor) cells help suppress immune responses; so do some macrophages and other monocytes.

The exact function of suppressor cells is still not fully understood. Some suppressor cells seem to affect antigen recognition, while others seem to suppress the proliferation that follows antigen recognition. Tolerance of self-antigens seems to be another function of suppressor cells.

FETAL AND NEONATAL IMMUNE FUNCTION

The human infant develops some immune response capabilities, even in utero, but the immune response system is normally not fully mature when the infant is born. For example, in the last trimester, the fetus can produce a primary immune response involving mostly IgM antibody to some infections. The ability to produce IgG and IgA antibodies is underdeveloped.

To protect the child in utero and during the first few months after birth, maternal antibodies cross the placenta into the fetal circulation. In the placenta, specialized cells called *trophoblasts* separate maternal from fetal blood. The trophoblastic cells actively transport the large immunoglobulin cells from maternal to fetal circulation. This transport is so effective that the level of antibodies in the umbilical cord is sometimes higher than in the mother's blood.

After birth, when antibodies can no longer be transported from the mother's blood, the levels of antibodies in the newborn's blood begin to drop as the immunoglobulins present at birth are catabolized, while the infant's ability to produce immunoglobulins on its own is still not fully developed. The levels are generally at their lowest at about 5 or 6 months of age (when many infants experience recurrent respiratory tract infections). Then, as the immune system matures, the levels of immunoglobulin begin to rise.

AGING AND THE IMMUNE RESPONSE

As the human body ages, immune function begins to deteriorate. B cell antibody production is affected, but the primary assault is on T cell function. The thymus, which is the organ responsible for T cell development, reaches its maximum size at sexual maturity and then decreases in size until, in middle age, it has shrunk by 65 percent. Circulating T cells do not decrease, but T cell function may diminish. Men and women over age 60 generally have decreased hypersensitivity (allergic) responses and decreased T cell response to infections.

For a summary of the immune response, see Figure 8-19 ■.

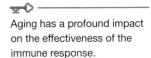

Aging has a profound impact on the effectiveness of the immune response.

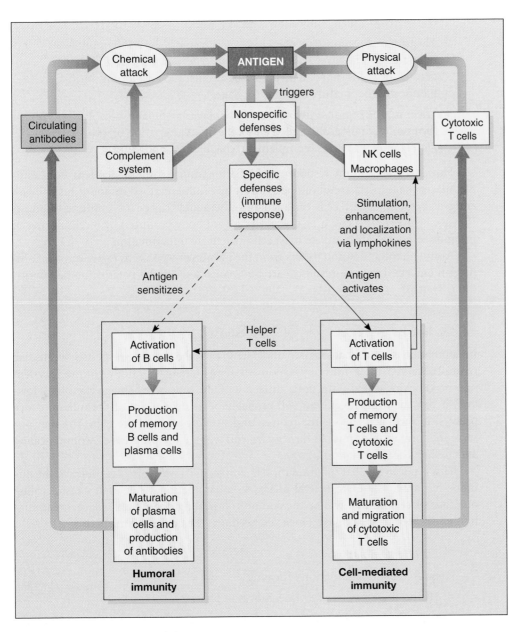

■ Figure 8-19   Summary of the immune response.

INFLAMMATION

INFLAMMATION CONTRASTED TO THE IMMUNE RESPONSE

Inflammation, also called the *inflammatory response,* is the body's response to cellular injury. It differs from the immune response in many ways. (Review Tables 8–4 and 8–5.) As you read the following sections, keep in mind that:

★ The immune response develops *slowly;* inflammation develops *swiftly.*

★ The immune response is *specific* (targets specific antigens); inflammation is *nonspecific* (it attacks all unwanted substances in the same way). In fact, inflammation is sometimes called "the nonspecific immune response."

★ The immune response is *long-lasting* (memory cells will remember an antigen and trigger a swift response on reexposure, even years later); inflammation is *temporary,* lasting only until the immediate threat is conquered—usually only a few days to 2 weeks.

★ The immune response involves *one type of white blood cell* (lymphocytes); inflammation involves *platelets and many types of white blood cells* (the granulatory cells called neutrophils, basophils, and eosinophils; the monocytes that mature into macrophages).

★ The immune response involves *one type of plasma protein* (immunoglobulins, also called antibodies); inflammation involves *several plasma protein systems* (complement, coagulation, and kinin).

However, the immune response and inflammation are interdependent. For example, macrophages that are developed during the inflammatory response must ingest antigens before helper T cells can recognize them and trigger the immune response. (Review Figures 8-15 a and b.) Conversely, IgE antibody produced by B cells during an immune response can stimulate mast cells to activate inflammation.

Although inflammation differs from the immune response in many ways, inflammation and the immune response are both considered to be part of the body's immune system.

HOW INFLAMMATION WORKS: AN OVERVIEW

Inflammation is somewhat easier to understand than the immune response, because we have all observed it. The immune response is often hidden; your body's immune system may be knocking out an infectious antigen without your ever being aware of it. However, if you cut your finger, you will probably be acutely aware of the inflammatory process. You will actually see the redness and swelling and feel the pain. You may observe the formation of pus. As days go by, you will see the progress of wound healing and, perhaps, scar formation.

This is not to say that inflammation is simple; in its way, it is as complex as the immune response. There are several phases to inflammation. After each phase, healing may take place, and that will be the end of it. If healing doesn't take place, inflammation moves into its next phase. However, healing is the goal of all the phases.

Phases of Inflammation

Phase 1: Acute inflammation →healing

(If healing doesn't take place, moves to phase 2)

Phase 2: Chronic inflammation→healing

(If healing doesn't take place, moves to phase 3)

Phase 3: Granuloma formation

Phase 4: Healing

During each phase, the components of inflammation work together to perform four functions.

The Four Functions of Inflammation (During all Phases)

★ Destroy and remove unwanted substances

★ Wall off the infected and inflamed area

★ Stimulate the immune response

★ Promote healing

ACUTE INFLAMMATORY RESPONSE

Acute inflammation is triggered by any injury, whether lethal or nonlethal, to the body's cells. As discussed earlier in this chapter, cell injury can result from causes such as hypoxia, chemicals, infectious agents (bacteria, viruses, fungi, parasites), trauma, heat extremes, radiation, nutritional imbalances, genetic factors, and even the injurious effects of the immune and inflammatory responses themselves. When cells are injured, the acute inflammatory response begins within seconds (Figure 8-20 ■).

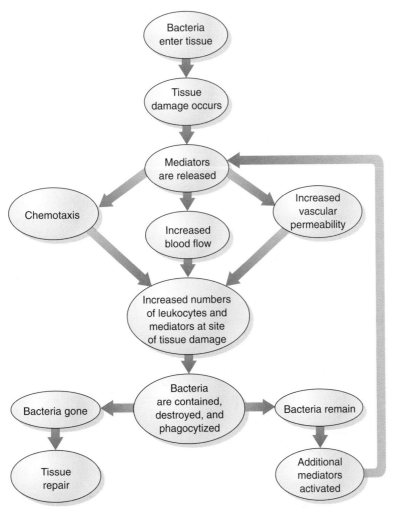

■ Figure 8-20   The inflammatory response.

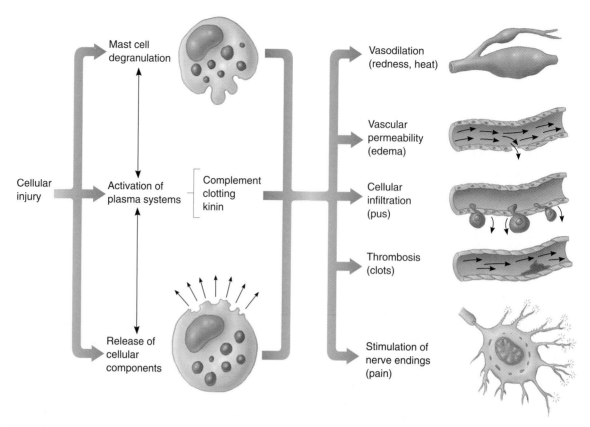

Figure 8-21   The acute inflammatory response.

The basic mechanics are always the same: (1) Blood vessels contract and dilate to move additional blood to the site. Then, (2) vascular permeability increases so that (3) white cells and plasma proteins can move through the capillary walls and into the tissues to begin the tasks of destroying the invader and healing the injury site (Figure 8-21 ▪).

MAST CELLS

Mast cells, which resemble bags of granules, are the chief activators of the inflammatory response. They are not blood cells. Instead, they reside in connective tissues just outside the blood vessels.

Mast cells activate the inflammatory response through two functions: *degranulation* and *synthesis* (Figure 8-22 ▪).

Degranulation

Degranulation is the process by which mast cells empty granules from their interior into the extracellular environment. This occurs when the mast cell is stimulated by one of the following events:

★ *Physical injury,* such as trauma, radiation, or temperature extremes

★ *Chemical agents,* such as toxins, venoms, enzymes, or a protein released by neutrophils (the latter an example of inflammatory response causing further cellular injury)

★ *Immunologic and direct processes,* such as hypersensitivity (allergic) reactions involving release of IgE antibody or activation of complement components (discussed later)

mast cells   *large cells, resembling bags of granules, that reside near blood vessels. When stimulated by injury, chemicals, or allergic responses, they activate the inflammatory response by degranulation (emptying their granules into the extracellular environment) and synthesis (construction of leukotrienes and prostaglandins).*

 Review

Mast Cell Functions

Degranulation
Synthesis

degranulation   *the emptying of granules from the interior of a mast cell into the extracellular environment.*

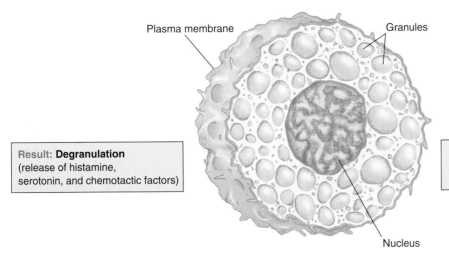

Plasma membrane

Granules

Result: Degranulation
(release of histamine, serotonin, and chemotactic factors)

Result: Synthesis
(construction of leukotrienes and prostaglandins)

Nucleus

■ Figure 8-22   Mast cell degranulation and synthesis.

During degranulation, biochemical agents in the mast cell granules are released, notably vasoactive amines and chemotactic factors.

Vasoactive Amines   **Histamine** is a vasoactive amine (organic compound) released during degranulation of mast cells. The effect of vasoactive amines is the constriction of the smooth muscle of large vessel walls and dilation of the postcapillary sphincter, resulting in increased blood flow at the injury site.

Basophils (a type of white blood cell) also release histamine, with the same effect. Additionally, **serotonin,** released by platelets, can have effects of both vasoconstriction and vasodilation that may affect blood flow to the affected site.

Chemotactic Factors   Another consequence of degranulation of mast cells is the release of various **chemotactic factors.** Chemotactic factors are chemicals that attract white cells to the site of inflammation. This attraction of white cells is called **chemotaxis.**

Synthesis

When stimulated, mast cells synthesize, or construct, two substances that play important roles in inflammation: leukotrienes and prostaglandins.

Leukotrienes   **Leukotrienes** are also known as *slow-reacting substances of anaphylaxis (SRS-A).* They have actions similar to those of histamines—vasodilation and increased permeability—as well as chemotaxis. However, they are more important in the later stages of inflammation, because they promote slower and longer-lasting effects than histamines.

Prostaglandins   Like leukotrienes, **prostaglandins** cause increased vasodilation, vascular permeability, and chemotaxis. They are also the substances that cause pain. In addition, prostaglandins act to control some inflammation by suppressing release of histamine from mast cells and suppressing release of lysosomal enzymes from some white cells.

histamine   *a substance released during the degranulation of mast cells and also released by basophils that, through constriction and dilation of blood vessels, increases blood flow to the injury site and also increases the permeability of vessel walls.*

serotonin   *a substance released by platelets that, through constriction and dilation of blood vessels, affects blood flow to an injured or affected site.*

chemotactic factors   *chemicals that attract white cells to the site of inflammation, a process called* **chemotaxis.**

leukotrienes   *also called* slow-reacting substances of anaphylaxis (SRS-A); *substances synthesized by mast cells during inflammatory response that cause vasodilation, vascular permeability, and chemotaxis.*

prostaglandins   *substances synthesized by mast cells during inflammatory response that cause vasodilation, vascular permeability, and chemotaxis and also cause pain.*

PLASMA PROTEIN SYSTEMS

plasma protein systems
*complex sequences of actions
triggered by proteins present in
the blood. For example,
immunoglobulins (antibodies) are
plasma proteins. Three plasma
protein systems involved in
inflammation are the complement
system, the coagulation system,
and the kinin system.*

cascade   *a series of actions
triggered by a first action and
culminating in a final action—
typical of the actions caused by
plasma proteins involved in the
complement, coagulation, and
kinin systems.*

complement system   *a group
of plasma proteins (the
complement proteins) that are
dormant in the blood until
activated, as by antigen-antibody
complex formation, by products
released by bacteria, or by
components of other plasma
protein systems. When activated,
the complement system is involved
in most of the events of
inflammatory response.*

 Review

Content

**Plasma Protein
Systems**

In immune response:
Immunoglobulins
In inflammatory response:
Complement system
Coagulation system
Kinin system

coagulation system   *a plasma
protein system, also called the*
clotting system, *that results in
formation of a protein called
fibrin. Fibrin forms a network
that walls off an infection and
forms a clot that stops bleeding
and serves as a foundation for
repair and healing of a wound.*

The actions of white blood cells and other components of inflammation are mediated by three important **plasma protein systems.** (Plasma proteins are proteins that are present in the blood.) One group of plasma proteins, the immunoglobulins, or antibodies, are key factors in the immune response, as discussed earlier. Three other plasma protein systems are critical to inflammation: the complement system, the coagulation system, and the kinin system.

Important to an understanding of these plasma protein systems is the concept of **cascade.** In a cascade, a first action is stimulated, that action causes the next action, which causes the next action, and so on until a final action has been completed.

The Complement System

The **complement system** consists of 11 proteins (numbered C-1 through C-9 plus factors B and D) and comprises about 10 percent of all the proteins that circulate in the blood. The complement proteins lie inactive in the blood until they are activated. The complement system can be activated by formation of antigen-antibody complexes, by products released by invading bacteria, or by components of other plasma protein systems.

Once the C-1 complement is activated, the *complement cascade* proceeds through the rest of the sequence of proteins. When activated, the complement system takes part in almost all of the events of the inflammatory response. The last few complements in the cascade have the ability to directly kill micro-organisms.

There are two chief pathways by which the complement cascade is activated and proceeds: the classic pathway and the alternative pathway (Figure 8-23 ■).

The Classic Pathway   In the classic pathway, the complement system is activated by formation of an antigen-antibody complex during the immune response. Complement factor C-1 is activated, and the cascade proceeds through complement factor C-9. Only a few antigen-antibody complexes are required to activate the complement cascade. The enzymes that are formed stimulate formation of increasing numbers of enzymes as the cascade proceeds, so that a very large response ensues, even from a small initial stimulus.

A number of effects that result from the complement cascade assist in destroying or limiting the damage of the invading organism. These include opsonization (coating) and phagocytosis (ingesting) of the organism, lysis (rupturing of bacterial cell membranes), agglutination (causing invading organisms to clump together), neutralization of viruses, and chemotaxis of white cells, increased blood flow, and increased permeability. Complement proteins also lodge in the tissues and help to prevent spread of the infection.

The Alternative Pathway   In some instances, the complement cascade can be activated without an intervening antigen-antibody complex formed by the immune response. Substances produced by some invading organisms are capable of reacting with complement factors B and D, which produce a substance that activates complement factor C-3, and the complement cascade then proceeds to its end.

Because the alternative pathway begins without waiting for the development of an antigen-antibody complex, it is much faster than the classic pathway and acts as part of the first line of inflammatory defense.

The Coagulation System

The **coagulation system,** also called the *clotting system,* forms a network at the site of inflammation. The network is composed primarily of a protein called *fibrin,* which is the end product of the coagulation cascade. The fibrinous network stops the spread of infectious agents and products of inflammation, keeps microorganisms "corralled" in the area of greatest phagocyte concentration, and forms a clot that stops bleeding and forms the foundation for repair and healing (Figure 8-24 ■).

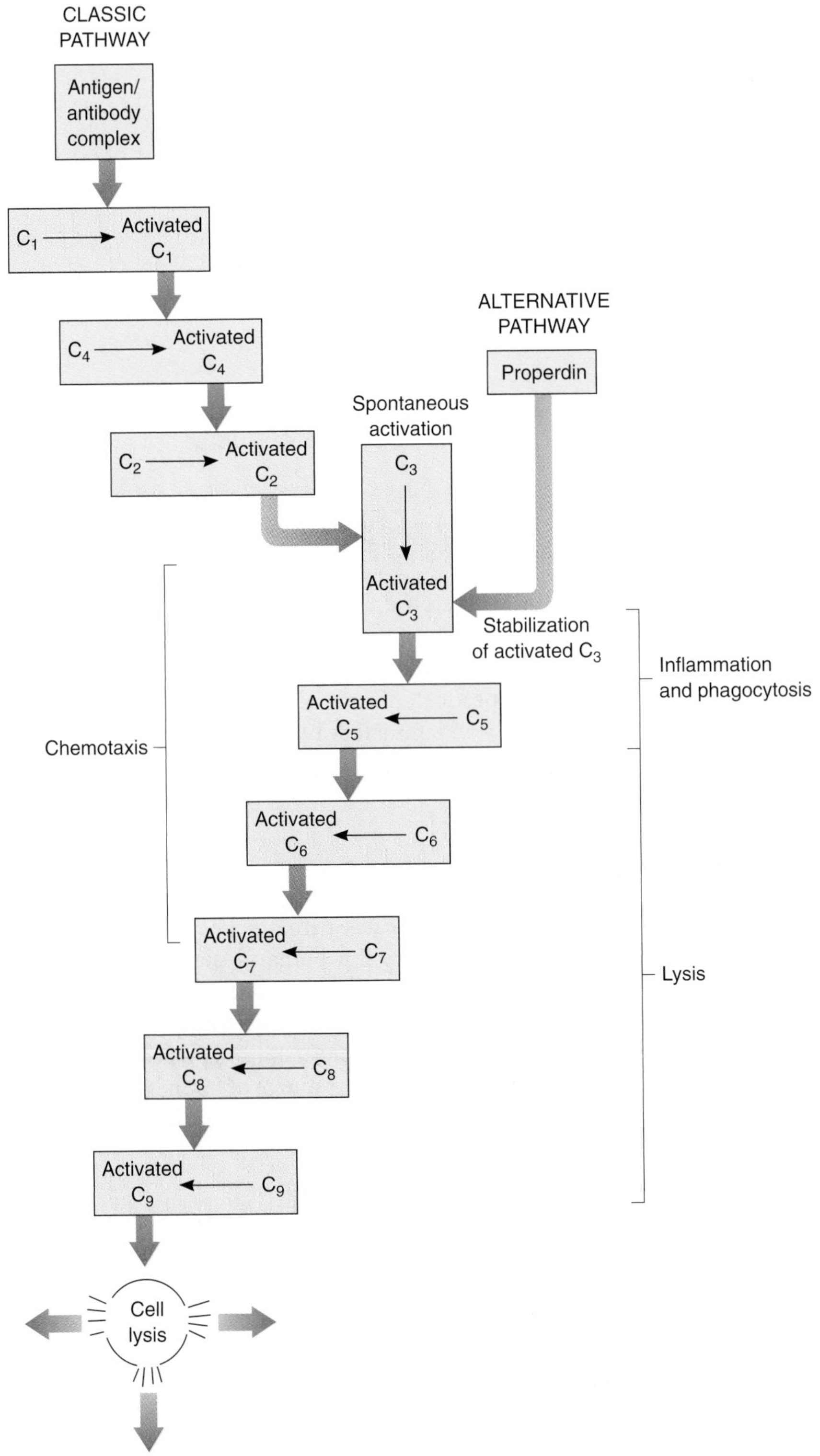

■ Figure 8-23 The complement cascade. The classic pathway is activated at C1 while the alternative pathway is activated at C3.

The *coagulation cascade* can be activated by many substances released during tissue destruction and infection. As with the complement cascade, the coagulation cascade can be activated through either of two pathways. The pathways of coagulation cascade activation are the extrinsic pathway and the intrinsic pathway. The *extrinsic pathway* of coagulation begins with injury to the vascular wall or surrounding tissues. It requires exposure of the blood to a tissue factor that originates outside the blood. The *intrinsic*

■ **Figure 8-24** The coagulation cascade.

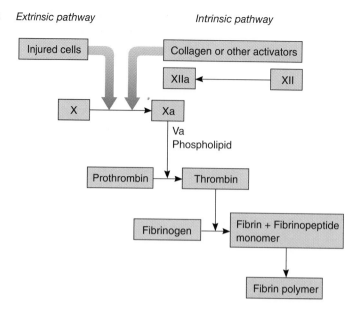

Extrinsic pathway   *Intrinsic pathway*

pathway of coagulation begins with exposure to elements in the blood itself, such as collagen from a traumatized vessel wall.

As with the complement cascade, the two pathways converge at a certain point and continue toward the same end product, fibrin. Substances produced during the complement cascade also enhance the inflammatory response, including increase of vascular permeability and chemotaxis.

The Kinin System

The **kinin system** has, as its chief product, *bradykinin,* which causes vasodilation, extravascular smooth muscle contraction, increased permeability, and possibly chemotaxis. It also works with prostaglandins to cause pain. Its effects are similar to the effects of histamine, but bradykinin works more slowly than histamine and so is probably more important during the later phases of inflammation.

The *plasma kinin cascade* is triggered by factors associated with the coagulation cascade. The sequence of the kinin cascade is conversion of prekallikrein to kallikrein, which then converts kininogen to kinin. Another source of kinin is the tissue kallikreins in saliva, sweat, tears, urine, and feces. Whatever the source, kinin is the end product, with bradykinin being the chief kinin.

Control and Interaction of Plasma Protein Systems

Control of the plasma protein systems is important for two reasons:

★ The inflammatory response is essential for protection of the body from unwanted invaders. Its functioning must be guaranteed. Therefore, there are numerous means of stimulating the inflammatory response, including those of the plasma protein systems.

★ Conversely, the inflammatory processes are powerful and potentially very damaging to the body. Therefore, they must be controlled and confined to the site of injury or infection. Obviously, there are a variety of mechanisms that regulate or inactivate inflammatory responses.

The inflammatory response is controlled at a number of levels and by a variety of mechanisms. For example, many components of inflammation are destroyed within seconds by enzymes from the blood plasma. Antagonists (substances or actions that counteract other substances or actions) exist for histamine, kinins, complement components, and other components of the inflammatory response.

---

kinin system *a plasma protein system that produces bradykinin, a substance that works with prostaglandins to cause pain. It also has actions similar to those of histamine (vasodilation and bronchospasm, increased permeability of the blood vessels, and chemotaxis) but acts more slowly than histamine, thus being more important during later stages of inflammation.*

An example of antagonistic control of inflammation is the function of histamine receptors. Histamine works by attaching itself to two types of receptors on the surface of target cells, H1 and H2 receptors. H1 receptors, when contacted by histamine, promote inflammation. H2 receptors are antagonistic to H1 receptors; when contacted by histamine, H2 receptors inhibit inflammation, mainly by suppressing leukocyte function and mast cell degranulation. In this way, the inflammatory action of histamine is triggered when needed, yet kept within bounds.

Most of the inflammatory processes interact; a substance or action that activates one element tends to activate others as well. For example, plasmin, an important factor in clot formation in the coagulation cascade, also has a role in activating the complement and kinin cascades. Conversely, controls on inflammatory processes also tend to interact. For example, a substance known as C1 esterase inhibitor inhibits plasmin activation which, in turn, tends to inhibit the coagulation, complement, and kinin cascades.

An example of what happens when interacting controls fail is the genetic deficiency of C1 esterase inhibitor. Its absence seems to permit uncontrolled activation of plasmin and triggering of the three plasma protein cascades when the patient undergoes emotional distress. This results in out-of-control effects typical of inflammation, including extreme edema of the gastrointestinal and respiratory tracts and the skin. The patient may die as a result of laryngeal swelling.

In other words, inflammatory processes have to be both reliably started and reliably stopped. Normally, this is assured by the interacting processes of activation and control.

CELLULAR COMPONENTS OF INFLAMMATION

An important term to remember in connection with inflammation is **exudate,** a collective term for all the helpful substances, including white cells and plasma, that move out of the capillaries into the tissues to attack unwanted substances and promote healing. This occurs in the sequence outlined below.

Sequence of Events in Inflammation

1. *Vascular Response.* The first response of inflammation is vascular. First, arterioles near the site constrict; then there is vasodilation of the postcapillary venules. The result is an increase in blood flow to the injury site. One result is increased pressure within the microcirculation (arterioles, capillaries, and venules), which helps to exude plasma and blood cells into the tissues.

    When plasma and blood cells move out of the microcirculation, pressure is decreased, and blood moves more sluggishly, thickening and becoming sticky. White cells migrate to the vessel walls and adhere to them—a phenomenon known as **margination** that is important in the next two events.

2. *Increased Permeability.* At the same time, chemical substances cause the endothelial cells of the vessel walls to constrict, creating openings between the cells in the vessel walls.

3. *Exudation of White Cells.* The white cells adhering to the vessel walls now squeeze out through the openings and into the tissues. Note that, ordinarily, white cells are too large to move through vessel walls. The inflammation-caused constriction of vessel-wall cells that creates openings between them and allows white cells to squeeze through is known as **diapedesis.**

Earlier, we discussed lymphocytes, which are the category of white cells involved in the immune response. The inflammatory response involves two other categories of

exudate *substances that penetrate vessel walls to move into the surrounding tissues.*

 Review

Inflammation Sequence

Content

Vascular response
Increased permeability
Exudation of white cells

margination *adherence of white cells to vessel walls in the early stages of inflammation.*

diapedesis *movement of white cells out of blood vessels through gaps in the vessel walls that are created when inflammatory processes cause the vessel walls to constrict.*

Table 8–8	Types of White Blood Cells (Leukocytes)
Lymphocytes (25–30% of all white blood cells)*	
T cells	
B cells	
Granulocytes**	
Neutrophils (55–70% of all white blood cells)	
Basophils	
Eosinophils	
Monocytes**	
Monocytes (immature) become macrophages (mature)**	

*Involved in the immune response.

**Involved in inflammation.

granulocytes *white cells with multiple nuclei that have the appearance of a bag of granules; also called* polymorphonuclear cells. *Types of granulocytes are neutrophils, eosinophils, and basophils.*

monocytes *white cells with a single nucleus; the largest normal blood cells. During inflammation, monocytes mature and grow to several times their original size, becoming macrophages.*

phagocytes *cells that have the ability to ingest other cells and substances, such as bacteria and cell debris. All granulocytes and monocytes are phagocytes.*

neutrophils *granular white blood cells (the most numerous of the white blood cells) that are readily attracted to the site of inflammation where they quickly attack and phagocytose bacteria and other undesirable substances.*

macrophages *large white blood cells (matured monocytes) that will ingest and destroy, or partially destroy, invading organisms.*

eosinophils *granular white blood cells that attack parasites and also help to control and limit the inflammatory response.*

basophils *granular white blood cells that, similarly to mast cells, release histamine and other chemicals that control constriction and dilation of blood vessels during inflammation.*

platelets *fragments of cytoplasm that circulate in the blood and work with components of the coagulation system to promote blood clotting. Platelets also release serotonin, a vasoconstrictive substance.*

white cells: granulocytes and monocytes (Table 8–8). **Granulocytes** (like mast cells, discussed earlier) have the appearance of a bag of granules, hence their name. They are also called *polymorphonuclear cells* because they have multiple nuclei. There are three types of granulocytes: *neutrophils, eosinophils,* and *basophils.* **Monocytes,** so-named because they have a single nucleus, change and mature when they become involved in inflammation. Monocytes are the largest normal blood cell. During inflammation, they grow to several times their original size, becoming *macrophages.*

All of the granulocytes and monocytes are **phagocytes,** blood cells that have the ability to ingest other cells and substances such as bacteria and cell debris. (The word comes from the Greek *phagein,* meaning "to eat," and *cyte,* for "cell"—so a phagocyte is a cell that eats.) A phagocyte behaves something like a Pac-Man® in the video game, destroying its "enemies" by swallowing them up. The most important phagocytes involved in inflammation are the neutrophils and the macrophages.

Neutrophils are the first phagocytes to reach the inflamed site. They ingest bacteria, dead cells, and cell debris, and then they die. Neutrophils can begin phagocytosis quickly because they are already mature cells. **Macrophages** come along later, because they first have to go through the process of maturing from their parent monocytes.

Eosinophils, basophils, and platelets also migrate to the site to join the inflammatory response. These cells function with assistance from plasma proteins of the complement, coagulation, and kinin systems, acting to kill microorganisms, remove the dead cells and debris, and prepare the site for healing.

Eosinophils are the primary defense against parasites. They contain large numbers of lysosomes. The eosinophils attach themselves to parasites and degranulate, depositing the caustic lysosomes, and killing the parasites by damaging their surfaces. Eosinophils also release chemicals that control the vascular effects of serotonin and histamine. Additionally, eosinophils help to control the inflammatory response, preventing it from spreading beyond the area where it is needed by degrading vasoactive amines, thereby limiting their effects.

Basophils are thought to function in the same way within the blood as mast cells do outside the blood, releasing histamines and other chemicals that control constriction and dilation of vessels.

Platelets, another cellular component of the inflammatory response, are fragments of cytoplasm that circulate in the blood. When cellular injury occurs, platelets act with components of the coagulation cascade to promote blood clotting. Platelets also release serotonin, a substance with effects similar to those of histamine.

CELLULAR PRODUCTS

As mentioned earlier, *cytokines* are proteins produced by white blood cells that act as "messengers" between cells. They are important in mediating both immune and inflammatory responses. Cytokines produced by lymphocytes are called *lymphokines*. Cytokines produced by macrophages and monocytes are called *monokines*.

Actually, cytokines are produced by a wide variety of cells, including some that are not part of the immune system. They play a wide variety of roles. Cytokines can interact in a synergistic manner (so that their combined effect is greater than the sum of their individual contributions) or they can interact in an antagonistic manner (so that they inhibit or cancel out each other's actions). Examples of the variety of sources and activities of cytokines can be found among the interleukins, lymphokines, and interferon.

Interleukins (ILs) are an important group of cytokines. They are produced by both lymphocytes and macrophages. Interleukin-1 is a lymphocyte-stimulating factor. As noted earlier, during the immune response macrophages that ingest antigens release IL-1, which assists helper T cells to respond to the antigens. It also enhances production of IL-2 by the helper T cells, which encourages antibody production. As part of the inflammatory process, IL-1 produced by macrophages induces neutrophilia, the proliferation of neutrophils.

Lymphokines are produced by T cells as a result of antigen stimulation during the immune response. In turn, these lymphokines stimulate monocytes to develop into macrophages, a critical phase of the inflammatory response. Different kinds of lymphokines have different effects. One type, called *migration-inhibitory factor (MIF)*, inhibits macrophages from migrating away from the site of inflammation. Another type, called *macrophage-activating factor (MAF)*, enhances the phagocytic activities of macrophages.

Interferon is a cytokine that is critical in the body's defense against viral infection. It is a small, low-molecular-weight protein produced and released by cells that have been invaded by viruses. It doesn't kill viruses, nor does it have any effect on a cell that is already infected by a virus. However, interferon prevents viruses from migrating to and infecting healthy cells.

SYSTEMIC RESPONSES OF ACUTE INFLAMMATION

The three chief manifestations of acute inflammation are fever, leukocytosis (proliferation of circulating white cells), and an increase in circulating plasma proteins.

Endogenous pyrogen is a fever-causing chemical that is identical to IL-1 and is released by neutrophils and macrophages. It is released after the cell engages in phagocytosis or is exposed to a bacterial endotoxin or to an antigen-antibody complex. Fever can have both beneficial and harmful effects. On one hand, an increase in temperature can create an environment that is inhospitable to some invading microorganisms. On the other hand, fever may increase susceptibility of the infected person to the effects of endotoxins associated with some Gram-negative bacterial infections.

In some infections, the number of circulating leukocytes, especially neutrophils, increases. Several components of the inflammatory response stimulate production of neutrophils, including a component of the complement system. Phagocytes produce a factor that induces production of granulocytes, including neutrophils, eosinophils, and basophils.

Plasma proteins called *acute phase reactants,* mostly produced in the liver, increase during inflammation. Their synthesis is stimulated by various interleukins. Many of these act to inhibit and control the inflammatory response.

CHRONIC INFLAMMATORY RESPONSES

Defined simply, chronic inflammation is any inflammation that lasts longer than 2 weeks. It may be caused by a foreign object or substance that persists in the wound, for example, a splinter, glass, or dirt. Or it may accompany a persistent bacterial infection. This can occur because some microorganisms have cell walls with a high lipid or wax content that resist phagocytosis. Other microorganisms can survive inside a macrophage. Still others produce toxins that persist even after the bacterium is dead, continuing to incite inflammatory responses. Inflammation can also be prolonged by the presence of chemicals and other irritants.

During chronic inflammation, large numbers of neutrophils—the phagocytes that were first on the scene during acute inflammation—degranulate and die. Now, the neutrophils are replaced by components that have taken longer to develop, and there is a large infiltration of lymphocytes from the immune response and of macrophages that have matured from monocytes. In addition to attacking foreign invaders, macrophages produce a factor that stimulates **fibroblasts,** cells that secrete collagen, a critical factor in wound healing.

As neutrophils, lymphocytes, and macrophages die, they infiltrate the tissues, sometimes forming a cavity that contains these dead cells, bits of dead tissue, and tissue fluid, a mixture called **pus.** Enzymes present in pus eventually cause it to self-digest, and it is removed through the epithelium or the lymph system.

Occasionally, when macrophages are unable to destroy the foreign invader, a **granuloma** will form to wall off the infection from the rest of the body. The granuloma is formed as large numbers of macrophages, other white cells, and fibroblasts are drawn to the site and surround it. Cells decay within the granuloma, and the released acids and lysosomes break the cellular debris down to basic components and fluid. The fluid eventually diffuses out of the granuloma, leaving a hollow, hard-walled structure buried in the tissues. Some granulomas persist for the life of the individual. Granuloma formation is common in leprosy and tuberculosis, which are caused by mycobacteria, bacteria that resist destruction by phagocytes.

Tissue repair and possible scar formation are the final stages of inflammation and will be discussed in more detail later.

fibroblasts *cells that secrete collagen, a critical factor in wound healing.*

pus *a liquid mixture of dead cells, bits of dead tissue, and tissue fluid that may accumulate in inflamed tissues.*

granuloma *a tumor or growth that forms when foreign bodies that cannot be destroyed by macrophages are surrounded and walled off.*

LOCAL INFLAMMATORY RESPONSES

All of the manifestations observed at the local inflammation site result from (1) vascular changes and (2) exudation. Redness and heat result from vascular dilation and increased blood flow to the area. Swelling and pain result from the vascular permeability that permits infiltration of exudate into the tissues.

Exudate has three functions:

★ To dilute toxins released by bacteria and the toxic products of dying cells

★ To bring plasma proteins and leukocytes to the site to attack the invaders

★ To carry away the products of inflammation (e.g., toxins, dead cells, pus)

The composition of exudate varies with the stage of inflammation and the type of injury or infection. Early exudate (serous exudate) is watery with few plasma proteins or leukocytes, as in a blister. In a severe or advanced inflammation, the exudate may be thick and clotted (fibrinous exudate) as in lobar pneumonia. In persistent bacterial infections, the exudate contains pus (purulent, or suppurative, exudate), as with cysts and abscesses. If bleeding is present, the exudate contains blood (hemorrhagic exudate).

The lesions (infected areas or wounds) that result from inflammation vary, depending on the organ affected. In myocardial infarction, cellular death results in the replacement of dead tissue by scar tissue. An infarction of brain tissue may result in liquefactive necrosis, in which the dead cells liquefy and are contained in walled cysts. In the liver, destroyed cells result in the regeneration of liver cells.

Keep in mind that inflammation can only occur in vascularized tissues (tissues to which blood can flow). When perfusion is cut off, as in a gangrenous limb or a limb distal to a tourniquet, inflammation cannot take place—and without inflammation, healing cannot take place.

RESOLUTION AND REPAIR

Healing begins during acute inflammation and may continue for as long as 2 years. The best outcome is **resolution,** the complete restoration of normal structure and function. This can happen if the damage was minor, there are no complications, and the tissues are capable of **regeneration** through the proliferation of the remaining cells. If resolution is not possible, then **repair** takes place with scarring being the end result. This happens if the wound is large, an abscess or granuloma has formed, or fibrin remains in the damaged tissues.

Both resolution and repair begin in the same way, with the **debridement** ("cleaning up") of the site of inflammation. Debridement involves the phagocytosis of dead cells and debris and the dissolution of fibrin cells (scabs). After debridement, there is a draining away of exudate, toxins, and particles from the site, and vascular dilation and permeability are reversed. At this point, either regeneration and resolution or repair and scar formation will take place.

Minor wounds with little tissue loss, like paper cuts, close and heal easily. They are said to heal by **primary intention.** More extensive wounds require more complex processes of sealing the wound, filling the wound, and contracting the wound and are said to heal by **secondary intention.**

Both resolution and repair proceed in two overlapping phases: reconstruction and maturation. Reconstruction begins 3 or 4 days after injury or infection and takes about 2 weeks. Maturation begins several days after injury or infection and can take up to 2 years.

Reconstruction

Reconstruction of a wound proceeds through four steps: initial wound response, granulation, epithelialization, and contraction.

Initial Response The first step of healing is the sealing off of the wound by a clot (scab) which contains a mesh of fibrin and trapped red and white blood cells. The fibrin mesh is formed as a result of activation of the coagulation cascade. The fibrin traps platelets, which enhance the seal. The fibrin seal creates a barrier to bacterial invasion and a framework for collagen to fill the wound.

Eventually the fibrin clot is dissolved by enzymes and cleared away through debridement by macrophages and any remaining neutrophils. The clot will then be replaced by normal tissue (in the case of resolution) or by scar tissue (in the case of repair).

Granulation Repair begins with **granulation.** Granulation tissues grow inward from the healthy connective tissues surrounding the wound. The granulation tissues are filled with capillaries. Some capillaries differentiate into venules and arterioles. Similarly, new lymph channels develop in the granulation tissues.

The granulation tissues are surrounded by macrophages. The macrophages secrete fibroblast-activating factor, which stimulates fibroblasts to enter the tissues and secrete collagen. The macrophages also secrete angiogenesis factor, which causes formation of the capillary buds, and an unidentified factor that stimulates epithelial factors to grow over the wound.

Epithelialization While granulation is taking place and the original clot, or scab, is being dissolved, **epithelialization** takes place. Epithelial cells move in under the scab, separating it from the wound surface, and providing a protective covering for the healing wound.

 Review

Outcomes of Healing

Resolution – complete restoration of normal structure
Repair – scar formation

resolution *the complete healing of a wound and return of tissues to their normal structure and function; the ending of inflammation with no scar formation.*

regeneration *regrowth through cell proliferation.*

repair *healing of a wound with scar formation.*

debridement *the cleaning up or removal of debris, dead cells, and scabs from a wound, principally through phagocytosis.*

primary intention *simple healing of a minor wound without granulation or pus formation.*

secondary intention *complex healing of a larger wound involving sealing of the wound through scab formation, granulation or filling of the wound, and constriction of the wound.*

granulation *filling of a wound by the inward growth of healthy tissues from the wound edges.*

epithelialization *growth of epithelial cells under a scab, separating it from the wound and providing a protective covering for the healing wound.*

Contraction Six to twelve days after the injury, **contraction** begins as the wound edges begin to move inward. Contraction is caused by myofibroblasts in the granulation tissues. These are similar to the collagen-secreting fibroblasts, but myofibroblasts contain parallel fiber bundles in their cytoplasm similar to those in smooth muscle cells. They exert a contractile force as they connect to neighboring cells, slowly bringing the wound edges together.

Maturation

At the end of the reconstructive phase, collagen deposition, tissue regeneration, and wound contraction are seldom completed. These processes may continue into the maturation phase, possibly for years. During **maturation,** scar tissue is remodeled; blood vessels disappear, leaving an avascular scar; and the scar tissue becomes stronger.

Only epithelial, hepatic (liver), and bone marrow cells are capable of the total regeneration by mitosis known as hyperplasia (discussed earlier in the chapter). In most wounds, healing produces new tissues that are not structured exactly like the original tissues. Typically, repaired tissues regain about 80 percent of their original strength.

Dysfunctional Wound Healing

Dysfunctional healing can result in an insufficient repair, an excessive repair, or a new infection. Causes of dysfunctional healing vary, including disease states such as diabetes, hypoxemia, nutritional deficiencies, and the use of certain drugs. Dysfunctional healing can occur during the inflammatory response or during reconstruction.

Dysfunctional Healing during Inflammation During inflammation, several factors can disrupt healing. If bleeding hasn't stopped, healing can be delayed by clotting that takes up space and inhibits granulation and by blood-cell debridement from the site. Blood is also a hospitable medium for infection, which in turn exacerbates inflammation and delays healing.

If there is excess fibrin in the wound, this, too, must be cleared away so as not to delay healing. Sometimes excess fibrin causes *adhesions,* fibrous bands that bind organs together and pose a significant problem if they occur in the abdominal, pleural, or pericardial cavities.

Other problems that can arise during inflammation include hypovolemia, which inhibits inflammation (remember that perfusion is necessary to inflammation), and anti-inflammatory steroid drugs that inhibit macrophage and fibroblast migration.

Dysfunctional Healing during Reconstruction A number of factors can disrupt the phases of reconstruction. For example, various nutritional deficiencies can inhibit collagen synthesis. Collagen synthesis can also become excessive, causing the formation of raised scars. Steroid drugs can suppress epithelialization.

Wounds can also be disrupted by pulling apart. Surgical wounds are sometimes disrupted as a result of strain or obesity. In some cases, frequently with burns, wound contraction is excessive, resulting in a deformity called *contracture.* Internal contractures may occur in cirrhosis of the liver, duodenal strictures caused by improper healing of an ulcer, or esophageal strictures from lye burns.

Positioning, exercises, surgery, and administration of drugs can sometimes help to prevent or correct the results of dysfunctional wound healing.

AGE AND THE MECHANISMS OF SELF-DEFENSE

Newborns and the elderly are particularly susceptible to problems of insufficient immune and inflammatory responses.

As noted earlier in the chapter, neonates generally go through a phase at about 5 or 6 months of age when immune system protection received from their mother is depleted and their own immune system is still immature, making them particularly susceptible to respiratory tract infections. Inflammatory responses are similarly immature in the neonate. For example, neutrophils and monocytes may not be capable of chemotaxis, the release of chemical factors that attract other white cells to the site of infection. This makes newborns prone to infections such as cutaneous abscesses and cutaneous candidiasis. As another example, the deficiency of a component of the complement cascade in infants can cause a severe, overwhelming sepsis or meningitis when infants are infected by bacteria for which they do not have transferred maternal antibody.

The elderly also have difficulties with both the immune and the inflammatory responses. As discussed earlier in the chapter, B cell and especially T cell functions of the immune system decrease markedly after age 60. The elderly are also prone to impaired wound healing. This is thought not to be due to the normal processes of aging but rather to the higher incidence of chronic diseases such as diabetes and cardiovascular disease in the elderly. Also, many elderly persons take prescribed anti-inflammatory steroids for conditions such as arthritis, and these inhibit inflammation. Decreased perfusion contributes to hypoxia in the wound bed, inhibiting inflammation and healing. Unfortunately, the elderly are also more prone to wounding as the protective fat layer diminishes and skin loses its elasticity and becomes more vulnerable to tearing. Diminished sensitivity, mobility, and balance also lead to falls and wounds.

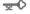

Aging has a profound impact on the effectiveness of the immune response.

VARIANCES IN IMMUNITY AND INFLAMMATION

Sometimes the immune and inflammatory systems work "too well" and sometimes not well enough. Hypersensitivity reactions are an example of the former, while immune deficiency diseases are an example of the latter.

HYPERSENSITIVITY: ALLERGY, AUTOIMMUNITY, AND ISOIMMUNITY

Immune responses are normally protective and helpful. **Hypersensitivity,** however, is an exaggerated and harmful immune response. The word *hypersensitivity* is often used as a synonym for *allergy.* However, *hypersensitivity* is also used as an umbrella term for allergy and two other categories of harmful immune response, which are defined as follows:

Three Types of Hypersensitivity

★ **Allergy**—an exaggerated immune response to an environmental antigen, such as pollen or bee venom.

★ **Autoimmunity**—a disturbance in the body's normal tolerance for self-antigens, as in hyperthyroidism or rheumatic fever.

★ **Isoimmunity**(also called *alloimmunity*)—an immune reaction between members of the same species, commonly of one person against the antigens of another person, as in the reaction of a mother to her infant's Rh negative factor or in transplant rejections.

The exact cause of such pathological immune responses is not known, but at least three factors seem to be involved: (1) the original insult (exposure to the antigen); (2) the person's genetic makeup, which determines susceptibility to the insult; and (3) an immunological process that boosts the response beyond normal bounds.

hypersensitivity *an exaggerated and harmful immune response; an umbrella term for allergy, autoimmunity, and isoimmunity.*

allergy *exaggerated immune response to an environmental antigen.*

autoimmunity *an immune response to self-antigens, which the body normally tolerates.*

isoimmunity *an immune response to antigens from another member of the same species, for example Rh reactions between a mother and infant or transplant rejections; also called alloimmunity.*

Review

Content

Four Types of Hypersensitivity Reactions

Type I—IgE reactions
Type II—Tissue-specific reactions
Type III—Immune-complex mediated reactions
Type IV—cell-mediated tissue reactions

Hypersensitivity reactions are classified as **immediate hypersensitivity reactions** or **delayed hypersensitivity reactions,** depending on how long it takes the secondary reaction to appear after reexposure to an antigen. The swiftest immediate hypersensitivity reaction is *anaphylaxis,* a severe allergic response that usually develops within minutes of reexposure. (Review anaphylactic shock earlier in this chapter. Also see Volume 3, Chapter 6 on allergies and anaphylaxis.)

Mechanisms of Hypersensitivity

Usually, when a hypersensitivity reaction takes place, inflammation is triggered that results in destruction of healthy tissues. Four mechanisms, or types, of hypersensitivity that cause this destructive reaction have been identified.

Mechanisms of Hypersensitivity Reaction

★ Type I—IgE-mediated allergen reactions
★ Type II—tissue-specific reactions
★ Type III—immune-complex-mediated reactions
★ Type IV—cell-mediated reactions

In reality, hypersensitivity reactions are not so easy to categorize. Most involve more than one type of mechanism.

Type I—IgE Reactions   As noted earlier in the chapter, IgE is the type of immunoglobulin (antibody) that contributes most to allergic and anaphylactic reactions. The first exposure to the allergen (antigen that causes allergic reaction) stimulates B lymphocytes to produce IgE antibodies. These bind to receptors on mast cells in the tissues near blood vessels. On reexposure (or after several reexposures), the allergen binds to the IgE on the mast cell, which causes degranulation of the mast cell, release of histamine, and triggering of the inflammatory process.

The potency of the inflammatory response is controlled in two ways. As discussed earlier, H1 receptors on target cells promote inflammation when contacted by histamine, while H2 receptors inhibit inflammation when contacted by histamine. Another control mechanism is the autonomic nervous system, which stimulates production of chemical mediators (epinephrine, acetylcholine) that govern release of inflammatory mediators from the mast cells and the degree to which target cells will respond to inflammatory processes.

The clinical indications of type I IgE mediated responses are the familiar signs and symptoms of allergic and anaphylactic response.

Clinical Indications of IgE Mediated Responses

★ *Skin*—flushing, itching, urticaria (hives), edema
★ *Respiratory system*—breathing difficulty, laryngeal edema, laryngospasm, bronchospasm
★ *Cardiovascular system*—vasodilation and permeability, increased heart rate, increased blood pressure
★ *Gastrointestinal system*—nausea, vomiting, cramping, diarrhea
★ *Nervous system*—dizziness, headache, convulsions, tearing

There is a genetic component to Type I, IgE mediated responses. Some individuals suffer from *atopia,* in which higher amounts of IgE are produced, and there are more receptors for IgE on the mast cells. In families where one parent has an allergy, approximately 40 percent of the offspring will also have allergies. If both parents are atopic, approximately 80 percent of their offspring will also be atopic.

Anaphylactic reactions are life threatening. Therefore, people who have reason to believe they are susceptible need to find out what specific allergens they are sensitized to so they can avoid them. A number of tests have been developed that are successful in making these identifications. Additionally, there has been some success in desensitizing some individuals by injecting small but increasing doses of the offending allergen over a long period of time. Research in desensitization techniques is ongoing.

Type II—Tissue-Specific Reactions Most cells of the body present HLA antigens, the antigens that the body recognizes as self or non-self. In addition to HLA antigens, most tissues have other antigens, but these are not the same in all tissues. They are called *tissue-specific antigens* because they exist on the cells of only some body tissues. An immune response against one of these antigens will affect only the organs or tissues that present that particular antigen; this is called a *tissue-specific reaction.*

There are four mechanisms by which Type II tissue-specific reactions attack cells. The first involves the complement system. Antibody bound to the antigen of the target cell initiates the complement cascade, which causes lysis (dissolving) of the cell's plasma membrane. The second mechanism is clearance of the target cells by macrophages. In the third mechanism, antibody bound to the antigen on the target cell also binds to cytotoxic cells, which release toxins that destroy the target cell. In the fourth mechanism, the antibody disables the target cell by occupying receptor sites on the cell, preventing them from binding to molecules that are needed for normal cell functioning.

Type III—Immune-Complex-Mediated Reactions Type III immune-complex-mediated reactions result from antigen-antibody complexes (also called *immune complexes*) that, as discussed earlier, are formed when antibody circulating in the blood or suspended in body secretions meets and binds to a specific antigen. The immune complexes generally circulate for a time before finally being deposited in vessel walls or other tissues. For this reason, which organs are affected may have very little connection with where or how the antigen or the immune complex originated.

The harmful effects of the immune complex result from the activation of the complement system. Some complement fragments are chemotactic for (attract) neutrophils. The neutrophils attempt to ingest the immune complexes but frequently fail because the complexes are bound to the tissues. During this attempt, the neutrophils release large quantities of damaging lysosomal enzymes into the tissues.

The nature and course of immune complex diseases vary tremendously. This results from the fact that immune complex formation is dynamic and constantly changing. There can be variations in the quantity and quality of circulating antigen and the antigen-antibody ratio. Also, many immune complexes bind complement components effectively, which causes complement levels in the blood to fluctuate. In some cases, the interaction between complement and the immune complexes results in dissolving the complex and mitigating its effects. As a result of these factors, immune complex diseases are characterized by tremendous variability in symptoms and periods of alternating remission and exacerbation.

Some immune complex diseases are systemic and some are localized. Systemic immune complex diseases are called *serum sickness.* They typically present with fever, enlarged lymph nodes, rash, and pain, commonly affecting the blood vessels, joints, and kidneys. *Raynaud's phenomenon* is a form of serum sickness in which temperature governs deposition of immune complexes in the peripheral circulation. Typical presentations include numbness in the fingers and toes, followed by cyanosis and gangrene or redness and pain.

Arthrus reaction is an example of a localized immune complex disease. It results from the interaction of an environmental antigen with preformed antibody lodged in the walls of blood vessels. A typical inflammatory response follows, resulting in edema, hemorrhage, clotting, and tissue damage. The antigen can enter the body through injection, ingestion, or inhalation. Examples of arthrus reactions are skin reactions following inoculations, gastrointestinal reactions to ingestion of wheat products, or hemorrhagic inflammation of the alveoli following inhalation of fungus from a source such as moldy hay.

Type IV—Cell-Mediated Tissue Reactions

Types I, II, and III hypersensitivity reactions are mediated by antibody. Type IV reactions are activated directly by T cells and do not involve antibody. There are two cell-mediated mechanisms. One involves lymphokine-producing T cells (Td cells). The other involves cytotoxic T cells (Tc cells). The lymphokine produced by Td cells activates other cells such as macrophages. The Tc cells attack antigen-bearing cells directly and destroy them with the toxins they produce.

Graft rejection and contact allergic reactions such as poison ivy are examples of Type IV reactions. There may also be Type IV components to autoimmune diseases such as rheumatoid arthritis, where the self-antigen is a protein present in joint tissues, and insulin-dependent diabetes, where the self-antigen is a protein on the cell of the pancreas that produces insulin.

Targets of Hypersensitivity

Antigens, the proteins or "markers" on the surface of cells, are the targets of the immune response and of the exaggerated immune response called hypersensitivity. As noted earlier, cells bearing these antigens can come from one of three sources: the environment, the person's own body, or another person. The source of the target antigen is what defines the type of hypersensitivity, as follows:

Type of Hypersensitivity:	*Targeted Antigen:*
Allergy	Environmental antigens
Autoimmunity	Self-antigens
Isoimmunity	Other person's antigens

In Allergy

The antigens that are the targets of allergic reaction are called *allergens.* Allergens typically occur on cells from such environmental sources as ragweed, molds, certain foods such as shellfish or peanuts, animal sources such as cat dander, cigarette smoke, and components of house dust. Often, an allergen is contained in a capsule that is too large to be phagocytosed or is surrounded by a nonallergenic coating. The actual allergen is not released until the capsule or coating is broken down by enzymes. Most allergens are low-molecular weight immunogens or haptens (which are too small to cause an immune response unless they bind with larger molecules).

In some situations, an allergen combines with components of the host tissue (tissues of the person's body) to form a new substance, called a *neoantigen,* which in its turn induces an allergic response. For example, a drug such as penicillin, which causes an allergic reaction in some people, is a hapten. It does not cause an allergic reaction until it binds to proteins on the plasma membranes of host cells. The immune system attacks the neoantigen and destroys the cell it is bound to as well. In the case of penicillin, which attaches to red blood cells, the immune response kills the red cells and causes anemia.

In Autoimmunity

The immune system normally recognizes the person's own tissues as self and tolerates the self-antigens presented by the body's own cells. If the body generated an immune response to its own tissues, it would destroy itself. Autoimmunity is a form of exactly this undesirable situation: There is a breakdown in the body's tolerance for self-antigens, and the immune system begins to attack the body's own cells.

Tolerance for self-antigens begins in the embryo when any lymphocytes that react to self-antigens are eliminated or suppressed. Several causes of a later breakdown in tolerance have been identified.

For example, some cells are *sequestered* (hidden) from the immune system by existing in areas of the body that are not drained by lymph (for example, the cornea and the testicles). If these cells become exposed to the immune system, for example during trauma, the body may recognize them as foreign and initiate an autoimmune response.

A neoantigen can trigger an immune response to the cells it is bound to. Infectious diseases can also trigger autoimmune responses in one of two ways. A foreign infectious antigen, in binding with an antibody, can form an immune complex that lodges in host tissues and causes an autoimmune response to the cells of those tissues. Additionally, a foreign antigen may resemble a self-antigen to such a degree that the antibody to the foreign antigen also attacks the self-antigen.

Suppressor T cell dysfunction is another cause of autoimmune disorders. In normal immune function, some T cells develop clones that attack self-antigens. Suppressor T cells are thought to have the function of suppressing these autoimmune responses. However, if the suppressor T cells dysfunction, the autoimmune response caused by T cell clones is able to develop.

The original insult that causes the autoimmune response is usually easy to identify, for instance an administered drug causing autoimmune anemia or a recent infection such as rubella causing autoimmune encephalitis. In other cases, the causative insult cannot be identified. In these cases, the autoimmune disease is thought to have resulted from a prior infection that is no longer traceable.

Genetic causes are actually easier to identify than pathological causes. Most autoimmune diseases are familial. All affected family members may not have the same disorder, but each may have a different autoimmune disorder or a disorder characterized by hypersensitivity responses.

In Isoimmunity   In isoimmunity, one member of a species has an immune reaction to cells from another member of the same species. In humans, two types of isoimmune disorders are most common, as discussed earlier in this chapter. One type consists of transient neonatal diseases, in which the mother becomes sensitized to fetal antigens, as in Rh negative sensitivity. The other type is encountered in the rejection of grafts or transplants from one person to another.

Autoimmune and Isoimmune Diseases

A number of diseases are recognized or suspected to have an autoimmune or isoimmune basis. Some examples are noted below.

★ *Graves' disease* is thought to be caused by an antibody that stimulates overproduction of thyroid hormone. People with Graves' disease have the symptoms of hyperthyroidism (e.g., elevated heart rate and blood pressure, increased appetite, increased activity level) plus a visibly enlarged thyroid gland (goiter), bulging eyes, and sometimes raised areas of skin over the shins. A pregnant woman with Graves' disease can pass the antibody and the disease along to the newborn.

★ *Rheumatoid arthritis* is a disease that causes inflammation of the joints and eventual destruction of the interior of the joint. Its exact cause is not known, but it is recognized as an autoimmune disorder, probably involving antibody reactions to self-antigen in the collagen of the joints.

- *Myasthenia gravis* is a disease caused by antibody response to self-antigens on acetylcholine receptors and the striations of skeletal and cardiac muscle. It is characterized by abnormal function of the neuromuscular junction, resulting in episodes of muscular weakness. Like Graves' disease, the mother's antibody can bind with receptors on the infant's muscle cells, causing neonatal muscle weakness.

- *Immune thrombocytopenic purpura (ITP)* presents with pinhead-sized red spots on the skin, unexplained bruises, and bleeding from the gums and nose and into the stool. It is characterized by a low platelet count. The exact cause is not known, but an autoimmune disorder in which antibodies destroy the person's own platelets appears to be involved. Maternal antibodies can also destroy platelets in the neonate.

- *Isoimmune neutropenia* occurs when a mother has developed antibodies that attack and severely reduce the level of neutrophils in her blood. The antibody in the maternal blood can also attack and destroy neutrophils in the blood of the neonate.

- *Systemic lupus erythematosus (SLE),* also called simply *lupus,* is an autoimmune disease in which a variety of antibodies to self-antigens are developed that then attack nucleic acids, red blood cells, coagulation proteins, lymphocytes, platelets, and many other targets within the person's own body. The disease causes episodal inflammations of joints, tendons, and other connective tissues and organs. The diversity of antibodies in maternal blood can cause a variety of problems, such as congenital heart defects, in the infant.

- *Rh and ABO isoimmunization,* or hemolytic disease of the newborn, was discussed earlier in the chapter. It is an isoimmune disease that causes severe anemia in the neonate. Immune problems occur if antigens on fetal red blood cells are different from antigens on maternal red blood cells.

DEFICIENCIES IN IMMUNITY AND INFLAMMATION

Immune deficiency disorders result from impaired function of some component of the immune system, including phagocytes, complement, and lymphocytes (T cells and B cells), with lymphocyte dysfunction being the primary cause. Immune deficiency can be congenital (inborn) or acquired (after birth). The most common manifestations of immune deficiency are recurrent infections, because the body's ability to ward off invaders has been damaged.

Congenital Immune Deficiencies

Congenital, or primary, immune deficiency develops if the development of lymphocytes in the fetus or embryo is impaired or halted. Different immune-deficiency diseases may develop, depending on whether the T cells, the B cells, or both have been affected.

In the *DiGeorge syndrome,* there is a lack or partial lack of thymus development, resulting in a severe decrease in T cell production and function. *Bruton agammaglobulinemia* is caused by impaired development of B cell precursors, resulting in B cells that cannot produce IgM or IgD antibodies. In *bare lymphocyte syndrome,* lymphocytes and macrophages are unable to produce Class I or Class II HLA antigens, which disrupts the ability of cells to recognize self or non-self substances, resulting in severe infections that are usually fatal before age 5.

Sometimes there is a defect that depresses the function of just a small portion of the immune system. For example, in *Wiskott-Aldrich syndrome,* IgM antibody production is reduced. *Selective IgA deficiency* is the most common immune deficiency. IgA is

Review

Two Types of Immune Deficiency

Congenital (inborn)
Acquired (after birth)

the antibody present in mucous membranes. People with IgA deficiency frequently suffer from sinus, lung, and gastrointestinal infections.

Some immune system deficiencies cause a decreased ability to respond to one particular antigen. For example, in *chronic mucocutaneous candidiasis,* the T lymphocytes are unable to respond against candida infections.

Acquired Immune Deficiencies

Acquired, or secondary, immune deficiencies develop after birth and do not result from genetic factors. They can be caused by or associated with pregnancy, infections, and diseases such as diabetes or cirrhosis. The elderly are more prone to acquired immune deficiencies than the young. Among the factors that can severely affect immune function are nutritional deficiencies, medical treatment, trauma, and stress. Of special interest is the fatal acquired immune disorder AIDS.

Nutritional Deficiencies   Critical deficits in calorie or protein ingestion can lead to depression of T cell production and function. Complement activity, neutrophil chemotaxis, and the ability of neutrophils to kill bacteria are also seriously affected by starvation. Zinc deficiencies and vitamin deficiencies can affect both B cell and T cell function.

Iatrogenic Deficiencies   Iatrogenic deficiencies are those that are caused by medical treatment. Some drugs depress blood cell formation in the bone marrow. Others trigger immune responses that destroy granulocytes. Immunosuppressive drugs administered in the treatment for transplants, cancer, or autoimmune diseases suppress B and T cell function and antibody production. Radiation treatment for cancer exacerbates this effect. Surgery and anesthesia also can suppress B and T cell function, with severely depressed white cell levels persisting for several weeks after surgery. Surgical removal of the spleen depresses humor response against encapsulated bacteria, depresses IgM levels, and decreases the levels of opsonins.

Deficiencies Caused by Trauma   Burn victims are especially susceptible to bacterial infection. Not only has the normal barrier presented by the skin been disrupted, but thermal burns also appear to decrease neutrophil function, complement levels, and other immune functions while increasing immunosuppressive functions, which further depress immune function.

Deficiencies Caused by Stress   It has long been suggested that persons undergoing emotional stress (major stresses such as divorce, but also minor stresses such as studying for final exams) are more prone to illness. The speculation was that stress has deleterious effects on immune function. Research into the possible mechanisms of stress-induced immune deficiency are just getting underway. (Stress and susceptibility to disease will be discussed later in the chapter.)

AIDS   AIDS is an acronym for *acquired immunodeficiency syndrome,* which has become the best known acquired immune deficiency disorder. AIDS is a syndrome of disorders that develop from infection with **HIV,** the *human immunodeficiency virus.*

HIV is a retrovirus; that is, it carries its genetic information in RNA rather than DNA molecules. As a retrovirus, HIV infects target cells by binding to receptors on their surfaces, then inserting the HIV RNA into the cell. There, the RNA is converted into DNA and becomes part of the infected cell's genetic material. HIV can remain dormant inside the host cell for years; however, once the cell is activated (and the mechanism by which this occurs is not fully understood), HIV proliferates, kills the host cell, and can then infect other cells. The result is a pervasive breakdown of the immune defenses, making the body vulnerable to a wide variety of infections and disorders.

AIDS acquired immunodeficiency syndrome, *a group of signs, symptoms, and disorders that often develop as a consequence of HIV infection.*

HIV human immunodeficiency virus, *a virus that breaks down the immune defenses, making the body vulnerable to a variety of infections and disorders.*

HIV can infect anybody, male or female, homosexual or heterosexual, mostly through the exchange of body fluids during sexual intercourse or through injection. In the United States, most cases to date have involved homosexual men and intravenous drug users. However, preventive measures (safe sex practices, including use of condoms, and clean-needle programs) have reduced the incidence of HIV/AIDS among homosexual populations and drug users. An increasing proportion of new patients are females who have acquired the infection during heterosexual intercourse. In other parts of the world, HIV/AIDS occurs equally among men and women.

The possibility of acquiring HIV/AIDS by contact with patients or accidental needle sticks fostered something of a panic among health care workers when AIDS first spread so alarmingly in the United States in the 1970s. Following recommendations by OSHA, universal precautions (body substance isolation practices) have been widely adopted—including the use of disposable gloves, protective eyewear, masks, and gowns, as appropriate, to avoid contact with any body fluids, along with improved techniques for handling needles and other sharps. These measures have proved effective in reducing the fear of HIV/AIDS infection and also in making such infections very rare among health care workers.

Until recently, more than 90 percent of those with AIDS have died within 5 years of the development of severe symptoms. This picture has improved somewhat in developed nations with the initiation of treatments involving multiple chemotherapies (treatment "cocktails") that have shown success in prolonging life, greatly improving feelings of health and well-being, and suppressing measurable blood levels of HIV.

It is not yet known if such treatments can eradicate HIV and cure AIDS. One fear is that the treatments suppress but do not totally destroy the HIV virus, which "hides" somewhere in the body, waiting to proliferate at some later date. Another fear is that HIV will develop strains that are resistant to the treatments that appear to be successful in the short term. Nevertheless, the success of these treatments has caused the first feelings of optimism since AIDS was identified. Preventive measures have also helped to greatly reduce the number of new cases reported in the United States. In some parts of the world, however, including Africa and Asia, HIV/AIDS is still spreading at an extremely alarming rate, with seriously inadequate reporting, prevention, and treatment.

Replacement Therapies for Immune Deficiencies

Advances have been made in the treatment of immune deficiencies through the use of replacement therapies, such as those listed below.

Replacement Therapies

★ *Gamma Globulin Therapy.* Gamma globulin is administered to individuals with B cell deficiencies that cause immunoglobulin (antibody) deficiencies.

★ *Transplantation and Transfusion.* HLA-matched bone marrow is transplanted into patients suffering *severe combined immune deficiencies (SCID),* which is caused by a lack of the stem cells from which T cells and B cells develop. In patients who lack a thymus or have a defective thymus, fetal thymus tissue may be transplanted. Enzyme deficiencies that cause SCID have been treated with transfusions of red blood cells that contain the needed enzyme. Other substances have been transfused into individuals to help restore T cell function and reactivity against certain antigens.

★ *Gene Therapy.* Therapies involving identification of defective genes that are responsible for immune disorders, and replacement of these defective genes with cloned normal genes, are in the early stages of development and use.

Universal precautions, including body substance isolation practices, have been effective in relieving fears of HIV/AIDS infection and in making such infections very rare among health care workers.

STRESS AND DISEASE

Stress is a word that is used a lot in modern life. You might have a stressful job, or feel stressed out by too many demands on your job, or be going through a lot of emotional stress in connection with a personal relationship. In some situations, you may be acutely aware of some of the physiological components of stress, for example sweaty palms and a pounding heart just before you have to get up and give a speech. If so, you already have a basic understanding of stress that can help you grasp the physiological and medical concepts of stress and how stress is related to disease.

CONCEPTS OF STRESS

Today, it is commonly understood that mind and body interact. It was not always so. In fact, the concept that psychological states influence physiological states—and particularly that there is a cause-effect relationship between stress and disease—date primarily from the work of Hans Selye, an Austrian-born Canadian physician and educator, in the 1940s.

General Adaptation Syndrome

Dr. Selye was not studying stress when he made his discovery. Instead, he was trying to identify a new sex hormone. He was injecting ovarian extracts into laboratory rats when he discovered the following triad of physiological effects:

Triad of Stress Effects

★ Enlargement of the cortex (outer portion) of the adrenal gland

★ Atrophy of the thymus gland and other lymphatic structures

★ Development of bleeding ulcers of the stomach and duodenum

Dr. Selye soon discovered that this triad of effects was not a response only to the ovarian extracts. The same effects occurred when he subjected the rats to other stimuli, such as cold, surgical injury, and restraint. He concluded that the triad of effects was not specific to any particular stimulus but comprised a nonspecific response to any noxious stimulus, or stressor. (**Stress** is generally defined as a state of physical and/or psychological arousal to a stimulus. Dr. Selye originally intended to use the word *stress* for the stimulus, or cause, but through a mistranslation of his work, *stress* came to mean the arousal, or effect. Dr. Selye then coined the word **stressor** for the stimulus/cause.)

Because the same responses occurred to a wide array of stimuli, Dr. Selye named it the **general adaptation syndrome (GAS).** Later, he identified three stages in the development of GAS:

Stages of GAS

★ *Stage I, Alarm.* The sympathetic nervous system is aroused and mobilized in the "fight-or-flight" response syndrome. Pupils dilate, heart rate increases, and bronchial passages dilate. In addition, blood glucose levels rise, digestion slows, blood pressure rises, and the flow of blood to the skeletal muscles increases. At the same time, the endocrine system is aroused, resulting in secretion by the pituitary and adrenal glands of hormones that enhance the body's readiness to meet the challenge.

★ *Stage II, Resistance, or Adaptation.* The person begins to cope with the situation. Sympathetic nervous system responses and circulating hormones return to normal. In most situations, this is the last stage; the stress is resolved. If the stress is very severe or prolonged, however, stress is not resolved and stage III occurs.

Mind and body interact. There is a cause-and-effect relationship between stress and disease.

stress *a state of physical or psychological arousal to stimulus.*

stressor *the stimulus or cause of stress.*

general adaptation syndrome (GAS) *a sequence of stress response stages: stage I, alarm; stage II, resistance or adaptation; stage III, exhaustion.*

 Review

Content

General Adaptation Syndrome (GAS)

Stage I—Alarm
Stage II—Resistance, or adaptation
Stage III—Exhaustion

★ *Stage III, Exhaustion.* This is the stage sometimes known as "burnout." During this stage, the triad of physiological effects described by Dr. Selye occurs. The person can no longer cope with or resolve the stress, and physical illness may ensue.

The stages of GAS begin with **physiological stress,** defined by Dr. Selye as a chemical or physical disturbance in the cells or tissue fluid produced by a change, either in the external environment or within the body itself, that requires a response to counteract the disturbance. Selye identified three components of physiological stress: (1) the stressor that initiates the disturbance, (2) the chemical or physical disturbance the stressor produces, and (3) the body's counteracting (adaptational) response.

Psychological Mediators and Specificity

Since Dr. Selye defined GAS, others who have studied adaptation to stress have refined the concept. For example, more attention has been paid to the psychological mediators of stress. Experiments have shown that there isn't a direct correlation between stressor and response. People react differently to the same stressor. One person may take in stride the same situation that greatly upsets another person, and the degree of physiological response may be governed more by the psychological, emotional, or social response to the stressor than to the stressor itself. In particular, research has demonstrated pituitary gland and adrenal cortex sensitivity to emotional/psychological/social influences.

Another way in which recent research has diverged from Dr. Selye's original hypotheses regards specificity. Dr. Selye postulated that the triad of physiological responses he identified were nonspecific, or the same for any stressor. It is now thought that, while the triad of responses he identified may occur in response to a wide variety of stressors, the total body response to different stressors must be specific; that is, targeted toward correction of the specific disturbance. For example, the body reacts to cold by shivering, and to heat through vasodilation and sweating.

Homeostasis as a Dynamic Steady State

An older definition of homeostasis states that the body maintains itself at a "constant" composition. More recently, homeostasis has been described as a **dynamic steady state.** This takes into account the concept of **turnover,** the continual synthesis and breakdown of all body substances (e.g., fats, proteins). Thus, the internal environment of the body is always changing, not constant, but the net effect of all the changes is the dynamic (always changing), yet steady (tending always toward normal balance) state.

Stressors cause a series of reactions that alter the dynamic steady state. Usually, there is a return to normal, which may be rapid or slow. If a disturbance in the dynamic steady state, for example a high blood glucose level, is prolonged and a causative stressor is no longer present, it is considered a sign of disease.

STRESS RESPONSES

Alteration of the immune system is the ultimate outcome of a stress response that resists quick and successful adaptation. The interactions of psychological, neurological/endocrine, and immunological factors that lead to this outcome are known as **psychoneuroimmunologic regulation.**

The **stress response** is initiated by a stressor. The input of the stressor into the central nervous system, as mediated by the person's psychological response, leads to production of corticotropin-releasing factor (CRF) from the hypothalamus, which in turn stimulates responses by the sympathetic nervous system and the endocrine system (neuroendocrine regulation), which then affect the immune system. This chain of events is outlined in Figure 8-25 ■ and described in the next sections.

---

physiological stress *a chemical or physical disturbance in the cells or tissue fluid produced by a change in the external environment or within the body.*

dynamic steady state *homeostasis; the tendency of the body to maintain a net constant composition although the components of the body's internal environment are always changing.*

turnover *the continual synthesis and breakdown of body substances that results in the dynamic steady state.*

psychoneuroimmunological regulation *the interactions of psychological, neurological/endocrine, and immunological factors that contribute to alteration of the immune system as an outcome of a stress response that is not quickly resolved.*

stress response *changes within the body initiated by a stressor.*

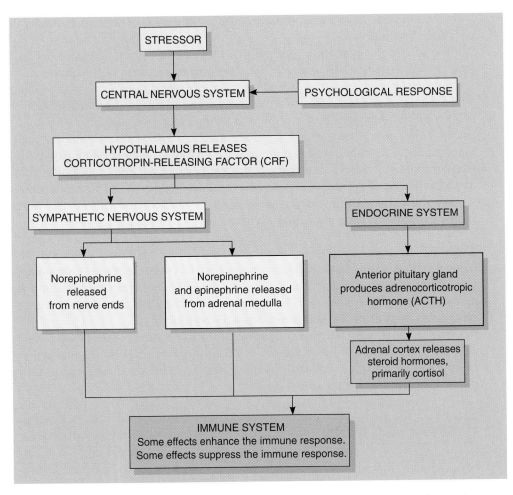

■ Figure 8-25   The stress response: effects on the sympathetic nervous, endocrine, and immune systems.

Neuroendocrine Regulation

As previously mentioned, when a person encounters a stressor and has a psychological response to the stressor, the sympathetic nervous system is stimulated by *corticotropin-releasing factor (CRF)*. In turn this stimulates release of catecholamines, cortisol, and other hormones.

Catecholamines   Sympathetic nervous system stimulation results in the release of norepinephrine (noradrenalin) and epinephrine (adrenalin), which constitute the category of hormones called *catecholamines*. The nerves of the sympathetic nervous system exit the spine at the thoracic and lumbar levels, and norepinephrine is released into the synaptic spaces (the spaces between the presynaptic ganglia and the postsynaptic nerves).

Additionally, sympathetic nervous system stimulation results in direct stimulation of the adrenal medulla, the inner portion of the adrenal gland. The adrenal medulla, in turn, releases the norepinephrine and epinephrine into the circulatory system. Approximately 80 percent of the hormones released by the adrenal medulla are epinephrine, while norepinephrine constitutes the remaining 20 percent. Once released, these hormones are carried throughout the body where their effects (preparing the body to deal with stressful situations) act on hormone receptors.

Both epinephrine and norepinephrine interact with specialized adrenergic receptors on the membranes of target organs. These receptors are located throughout the

Review

Hormones Produced in Response to Stress

Catecholamines
  (norepinephrine and
  epinephrine)
Cortisol
Beta endorphins
Growth hormone
Prolactin

Content

body. Once stimulated by the appropriate hormone, they cause a response in the organ or organs they control.

The adrenergic receptors are generally divided into four types, designated alpha 1 (α_1), alpha 2 (α_2), beta 1 (β_1), beta 2 (β_2). The α_1 receptors cause peripheral vasoconstriction, mild bronchoconstriction, and stimulation of metabolism. The α_2 receptors are found on the presynaptic surfaces of sympathetic neuroeffector junctions. Stimulation of α_2 receptors is inhibitory. These receptors serve to prevent over-release of norepinephrine in the synapse. When the level of norepinephrine in the synapse gets high enough, the α_2 receptors are stimulated and norepinephrine release is inhibited. Stimulation of β_1 receptors causes increases in heart rate, cardiac contractile force, and cardiac automaticity and conduction. Stimulation of β_2 receptors causes vasodilation and bronchodilation.

All of the effects of the catecholamines prepare the body to "fight-or-flee" in response to a stressor. Their physiological effects are summarized in Table 8–9.

cortisol *a steroid hormone released by the adrenal cortex that regulates the metabolism of fats, carbohydrates, sodium, potassium, and proteins and also has an anti-inflammatory effect.*

Cortisol Cortisol is another hormone produced in response to stress. The corticotropin-releasing factor (CRF) that stimulates the sympathetic nervous system, as previously discussed, simultaneously stimulates the anterior pituitary gland to produce *adrenocorticotropic hormone (ACTH)*, which in turn stimulates the adrenal cortex to produce a variety of steroid hormones, primarily cortisol.

One of the primary functions of cortisol is the stimulation of gluconeogenesis. It enhances the elevation of blood glucose by other hormones and also inhibits peripheral uptake and oxidation of glucose by the cells. Because of these functions, it has the overall effect of elevating blood glucose.

Table 8–9	Physiological Effects of Catecholamines
Organ	**Effects**
Brain	Increased blood flow
	Increased glucose metabolism
Cardiovascular system	Increased contractile force and rate
	Peripheral vasoconstriction
Pulmonary system	Increased ventilation
	Bronchodilation
	Increased oxygen supply
Liver	Increased glucose production
	Increased gluconeogenesis
	Increased glycogenolysis
	Decreased glycogen synthesis
Gastrointestinal and genitourinary tracts	Decreased protein synthesis
Muscle	Increased glycogenolysis
	Increased contraction
	Increased dilation of skeletal muscle vasculature
Skeleton	Decreased glucose uptake and utilization (insulin release decreased)
Adipose (fatty) tissue	Increased lipolysis
	Increased fatty acids and glycerol
Skin	Decreased blood flow
Lymphoid tissue	Increased protein breakdown (shrinkage of lymphoid tissue)

Cortisol also affects protein metabolism—increasing synthesis of proteins in the liver but increasing breakdown of proteins in the muscle, lymphoid tissue, fatty tissues, skin, and bone. The breakdown of proteins results in increased blood levels of amino acids. Cortisol also promotes lipolysis (fat breakdown) in the extremities and lipogenesis (fat synthesis and deposition) in the face and trunk.

Cortisol acts as an immunosuppressant by inhibiting protein synthesis, including synthesis of immunoglobulins (antibodies). Additionally, it reduces the numbers of lymphocytes, eosinophils, and macrophages in the blood. In large amounts, cortisol can cause lymphoid atrophy. Through a series of actions, cortisol diminishes the actions of helper T cells, which results in a decrease in B cells and antibody production. It inhibits production of interleukin-1 and interleukin-2 and, consequently, blocks cell-mediated immunity and generation of fever. It inhibits the accumulation of leukocytes at the site of inflammation and inhibits release of substances that are critical in the inflammatory response, including kinins, prostaglandins, and histamine. Cortisol also inhibits fibroblast proliferation during inflammatory response, which in turn causes poor wound healing and increased susceptibility to wound infection.

In the gastrointestinal tract, cortisol increases gastric secretions, occasionally enough to cause ulcer formation. Cortisol also suppresses the release of sex hormones, including testosterone and estradiol.

The immunosuppressive actions of cortisol seem clearly harmful, yet its production in response to stress indicates that it is beneficial in protecting against stress. Its beneficial effects in stress, however, are not well understood. It has been suggested that its promotion of gluconeogenesis helps assure an adequate source of glucose as energy for body tissues, especially nerve tissues. Pooled amino acids from protein breakdown may promote protein synthesis in some cells. Its depressive influence on inflammatory responses may play a role in decreasing peripheral blood flow and redirecting blood to critical organs or sites of injury. Suppression of immune function may also help prevent tissue damage that results from prolonged immune responses. The physiological effects of cortisol are summarized in Table 8–10.

Cortisol—produced in response to stress—has harmful immunosuppressive actions, yet seems to have a little-understood beneficial effect in protecting against stress.

Table 8-10	Physiological Effects of Cortisol
Function	**Effects**
Carbohydrate metabolism	Diminished peripheral uptake/use of glucose; promotes gluconeogenesis; elevates blood glucose levels
Protein metabolism	Increases protein synthesis in liver; depresses protein synthesis in other tissues; depresses immunoglobulin production
Inflammatory effects	Decreases blood levels of lymphocytes, macrophages, eosinophils; decreases leukocytes at inflammation site; delays healing/promotes wound infection
Lipid metabolism	Increases lipolysis in extremities, lipogenesis in face and trunk
Immune reserves	Decreases lymphoid tissue mass; decreases circulation white cells; inhibits production of interleukin-1 and interleukin-2; blocks cell-mediated immunity and generation of fever.
Digestive function	Promotes gastric secretions; at high levels causes ulceration
Urinary function	Enhances production of urine
Connective tissue function	Decreases proliferation of fibroblasts (delays healing)
Muscle function	Maintains normal contractility and work output for skeletal and cardiac muscle
Bone function	Decreases bone formation
Cardiovascular function	Maintains normal blood pressure; assists arteriole constriction; supports myocardial function
Central nervous system function	Modulates perceptual/emotional functioning and daytime arousal

Other Hormones   In addition to the catecholamines and cortisol, other hormones are associated with stress response. For example, *beta-endorphins* (endogenous opiates) are released into the blood from the pituitary gland, or possibly the central nervous system, in response to CRF stimulation. They may play a part in regulating ACTH secretion and inhibiting CRF secretion, which means that beta-endorphins may exercise a control over the stress response. The beta-endorphins also are associated with decreased pain sensitivity and increased feelings of well-being, which may help to moderate the psychological response to a stressor.

Growth hormone (GH) is released by the anterior pituitary gland. GH affects protein, lipid, and carbohydrate metabolism and immune function. Its levels have been noted to increase after stressful experiences such as electroshock, cardiac catheterization, and surgery. However, the levels of GH become depressed with prolonged stress. *Prolactin* is released by the anterior pituitary gland and is necessary for breast development and lactation. Levels of prolactin have been noted to rise after a variety of stressful stimuli. *Testosterone* is a hormone produced in the testicles and also by the adrenal cortex in both males and females. It is necessary for development of male sexual characteristics and also affects many metabolic activities. Many stressful activities lead to a decrease in testosterone, which is thought to be a result of increased cortisol levels. Some competitive sports activities, however, appear to increase testosterone levels.

Role of the Immune System in Stress

During a stress response, as noted earlier, there is a complex interaction among the nervous and endocrine systems and the immune system. As a consequence, a variety of immune-related disorders are associated with stress.

The specific mechanisms by which stress leads to immune-related disorders is the subject of ongoing research but is not yet well understood. However, research points to the substances that serve as communicators between the cells of the nervous system, the endocrine system, and the immune system—including hormones, neurotransmitters, neuropeptides, and cytokines—as the pathways of cause and effect.

The pathway is not a straight line. The directional arrows of cause and effect move forward, backward, and in circles. Many components of the immune system can be affected by the factors produced by the neuroendocrine system. Conversely, immune system products can affect components of the neuroendocrine system. Here are two examples (Figure 8-26 ■):

★ *Pathway 1: Central Nervous System to Immune System.* The central nervous system *stimulates* the hypothalamus to produce CRF Ø which *stimulates* the pituitary gland to produce ACTH Ø which *stimulates* the adrenal gland to secrete cortisol Ø which *suppresses* the development of macrophages, T cells, B cells, and natural killer (NK) cells, a lymphocyte specially adapted to recognize and kill virally infected cells and malignant cells.

★ *Pathway 2: Immune System to Central Nervous System.* During immune system response, macrophages secrete cytokines Ø which stimulate the hypothalamus to secrete CRF (which begins Pathway 1 again).

The above are only two examples of the many pathways and interactions that take place among the nervous, endocrine, and immune systems.

The suppression of immune system function that is caused by stress-related products of the sympathetic nervous and endocrine systems—especially catecholamines and cortisol—has been linked to a number of immune-mediated diseases, as listed in Table 8–11.

STRESS, COPING, AND ILLNESS INTERRELATIONSHIPS

Research has shown that the ability to cope with stress has significant effects on associated illnesses. Those who cope positively with stress have a reduced chance of becom-

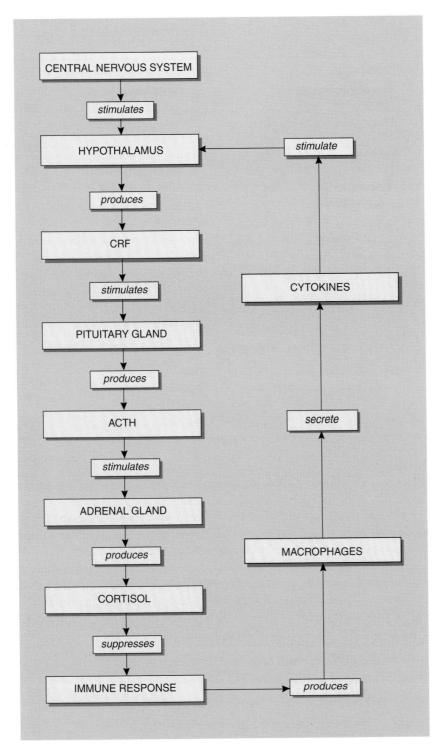

■ Figure 8-26 Interactions among the nerve, endocrine, and immune systems.

ing ill in the first place and a better chance of getting better or getting better faster if they do become ill. Conversely, those who don't cope as well with stress have a greater chance of becoming ill or of prolonging the course of illness or of not surviving an illness.

Physiological stress is caused by events that directly affect the body, such as a burn, extreme cold, or starvation. *Psychological stress* consists of the unpleasant emotions caused by life events, such as taking exams or a divorce. The effects that these stresses will have on the body depend on the individual's ability to cope with them. Some people are "thrown" by events others would perceive as relatively minor, such as a traffic

Table 8–11	Stress- and Immune-Related Diseases and Conditions
Target Organ	**Diseases and Conditions**
Cardiovascular system	Coronary artery disease
	Hypertension
	Stroke
	Dysrhythmias
Muscles	Tension headaches
	Muscle-related backaches
Connective tissues	Rheumatoid arthritis
Pulmonary system	Asthma
	Hay fever
Immune system	Immunosuppression or immune deficiency
Gastrointestinal system	Ulcer
	Irritable bowel syndrome
	Ulcerative colitis
Genitourinary system	Diuresis
	Impotence
Skin	Eczema
	Acne
Endocrine system	Diabetes mellitus
Central nervous system	Fatigue
	Depression
	Insomnia

jam or a sprained ankle. Others can take in stride events that others would find very difficult, such as loss of a job or a long-term disability.

The effects of stress, including the degree to which stress causes or affects illness, are moderated by the type, duration, and severity of the stressor in combination with the individual's perception and ability to cope with it. Stressors that are the most likely to have a negative effect on immunity and disease have been characterized as those that are not only undesirable but also are uncontrollable and that overtax the person's ability to cope.

Effective and ineffective coping has been seen to have potentially different effects in healthy persons, symptomatic persons (those who already have some manifestations of disease), and persons who are undergoing medical treatment.

Potential Effects of Stress Based on Effectiveness of Coping

★ *In a healthy person:*

  Effective coping → Transient effects, return to normal function

  Ineffective coping → Significant stress effects, illness

★ *In a symptomatic person:*

  Effective coping → Little or no effect on symptoms

  Ineffective coping → Exacerbation of symptoms, illness

★ *In a person undergoing medical treatment:*

  Effective coping → Person does not perceive the treatment itself as stressful → Treatment is more likely to have a positive effect on symptoms and the course of illness

  Ineffective coping → Person perceives the treatment itself as stressful → Treatment is more likely to have a negative effect on symptoms and the course of illness

Because of the importance of coping ability in the interplay between stress and illness, attention is increasingly being paid to providing counseling and support systems—including family members, friends, and other support networks—to assist persons who are ill or in stressful life situations. There is recognition that supporting the patient's ability to cope is a critical adjunct to medical treatment itself.

Summary

The cell is the basic unit of life. It contains all the components needed to turn nutrients into energy, remove waste products, reproduce, and carry on other essential life functions. The body's cells interact via electrochemical substances including hormones, neurotransmitters, neuropeptides, and cytokines. The cells exist in an environment of fluids and electrolytes. When something interferes with normal cell function, the normal cell environment, or normal cell intercommunication, disease can begin or advance.

Groups of cells that perform similar functions form tissues. A group of tissues functioning together is an organ. A group of organs that work together is an organ system.

Perfusion of the tissues is necessary to provide essential nutrients to the cells (especially oxygen and glucose) and to remove wastes. Inadequate perfusion, called hypoperfusion or shock, can be caused by a problem in any of the three parts of the cardiovascular system (the heart, the blood vessels, or the blood), sometimes abetted by problems with the respiratory or gastrointestinal system in which the normal intake and transfer of oxygen and glucose may be interrupted. If not corrected, positive feedback mechanisms can enhance the process of shock, creating a downward spiral toward irreversible shock, possible multiple organ dysfunction syndrome (MODS), and death.

Cells can be injured in a variety of ways, including hypoxia, chemicals, infectious agents, immunological/inflammatory injuries, and others. Diseases can be caused by genetic factors, environmental factors, or a combination of factors (multifactorial diseases).

The body responds to cellular injury in a variety of ways to restore homeostasis, the body's normal dynamic steady state. Cells can adapt through atrophy, hypertrophy, hyperplasia, metaplasia, and dysplasia. Negative feedback mechanisms work to correct, or compensate for, shock—if shock has not progressed too far.

The body's chief means of self-defense is the immune system and the immune and inflammatory responses, which work to attack and destroy infectious agents and other unwanted invaders. Occasionally, the immune response system works "too well," as in hypersensitivity reactions, or not well enough, as in immune deficiency disorders. Stress can also contribute to disease through the interactions of the nerve, endocrine, and immune systems.

Keep in mind that an understanding of the cell is essential to an understanding of all of these physiological and pathophysiological systems and processes.

You Make the Call

You have volunteered to work at a high school rodeo for your fire department. You and another paramedic take the backup EMS unit to the arena. This event brings in participants from several states. Over 300 people are expected to attend. Upon arrival at the arena, you park the unit at the designated spot and move your equipment to the "first-aid room."

Shortly after the rodeo is underway, an elderly gentleman stumbles into the first-aid room and slumps onto the treatment table. He states that he feels very weak and wants to be "checked out." You perform a quick assessment. The patient is pale but dry. His pulse rate is 110 beats per minute, blood pressure is 110/60, and his respirations are 36 per minute. You notice the characteristic odor of ketones on his breath. You ask the patient if he is diabetic. He says he is, but has not had his insulin in 2 days as he ran out of syringes. A finger stick glucose reads "HIGH." On further exam you note that the patient's mucous membranes are very dry.

1. Explain the physiological basis for the patient's apparent dehydration.
2. Describe the role of insulin in glucose transport into the cell.
3. Prepare a prehospital treatment plan given the information provided.

See Suggested Responses at the back of this book.

Review Questions

1. The clear liquid portion of the cytoplasm in a cell is called:
   a. cytosol.
   b. cytoskeleton.
   c. monocyte.
   d. granulocytes.

2. The _____ are the energy factories, sometimes called the "powerhouses," of the cells.
   a. lysosomes
   b. mitochondria
   c. Golgi apparatus
   d. Endoplasmic reticulum

3. _____ is the function of nerve cells that creates and transmits an electrical impulse in response to a stimulus.
   a. movement
   b. maturation
   c. conductivity
   d. metabolic absorption

4. _____ tissue has the capability of contraction when stimulated.
   a. nerve
   b. muscle
   c. connective
   d. epithelial

5. _____ is the term for the body's natural tendency to keep the internal environment and metabolism steady and normal.
   a. anatomy
   b. physiology
   c. metabolism
   d. homeostasis

6. _____ is the study of disease and its causes.
   a. pathology
   b. anatomy
   c. physiology
   d. pathophysiology

7. _____ is an increase in the number of cells through cell division.
   a. multiplasia
   b. metaplasia
   c. dysplasia
   d. hyperplasia

8. _____ is the constructive or "building up" phase of metabolism.
   a. anabolism
   b. apoptosis
   c. catabolism
   d. hyperplasia

9. Water accounts for approximately _____ percent of the total body weight.
   a. 40
   b. 50
   c. 60
   d. 70

10. The fluid found outside of cells and within the circulatory system is the _____ fluid.
    a. synovial
    b. interstitial
    c. intravascular
    d. extracellular

11. The most frequently occurring anions include all of the following except:
    a. chloride.
    b. calcium.
    c. phosphate.
    d. bicarbonate.

12. The mechanisms that most commonly result in accumulation of water in the interstitial space include:
    a. lymphatic obstruction.
    b. an increase in hydrostatic pressure.
    c. increased permeability of the capillary membrane.
    d. all of the above.

13. _____ are secreted by plasma cells in response to antigenic stimulation.
    a. antigens
    b. antibodies
    c. antibiotics
    d. haptens

14. Progressive impairment of two or more organ systems resulting from an uncontrolled inflammatory response to a severe illness or injury is called:
    a. ALS.
    b. MODS.
    c. ARDS.
    d. AODS.

15. Advanced stages of shock when the body's compensatory mechanisms are no longer able to maintain normal perfusion are called:
    a. reversible shock.
    b. compensated shock.
    c. homeostatic shock.
    d. decompensated shock.

16. The most commonly used fluids in prehospital care are:
    a. D_5W
    b. normal saline.
    c. lactated Ringer's.
    d. all of the above.

17. Every human somatic cell contains _____ chromosomes.
    a. 48
    b. 46
    c. 24
    d. 23

18. The amount of blood ejected by the heart in one contraction is referred to as the:
    a. preload.
    b. afterload.
    c. stroke volume.
    d. cardiac force.

19. The energy that is produced during glucose breakdown is in the form of the chemical:
    a. ATP.
    b. APT.
    c. TAP.
    d. PTA.

20. Obstructive shock is caused by an obstruction that interferes with the return of blood to the heart, such as:
    a. cardiac tamponade.
    b. pulmonary embolism.
    c. tension pneumothorax.
    d. all of the above.

21. Prehospital care for hypovolemic shock should include either lactated Ringer's or normal saline, administered in small boluses to maintain the systolic blood pressure between _____ and _____ mmHg.
    a. 70, 90
    b. 70, 85
    c. 80, 90
    d. 85, 95

22. With a mortality rate of _____ – _____ percent, MODS is the major cause of death following sepsis, trauma, and burn injuries.
    a. 40–50
    b. 50–60
    c. 60–90
    d. 80–90

23. People with type _____ blood are known as universal donors, because this type of blood has no antigens that will trigger an immune response in any other group.
    a. A
    b. B
    c. O
    d. AB

24. _____ cells are the chief activators of the inflammatory response.
    a. T
    b. mast
    c. immune
    d. histamine

25. _____ occurs when a mother has developed antibodies that attack and severely reduce the level of neutrophils in her blood.
   a. myasthenia gravis
   b. rheumatoid arthritis
   c. isoimmune neutropenia
   d. systemic lupus erythematosus

See Answers to Review Questions at the back of this book.

Further Reading

Cotran, Ramzi, Vinay Kumar, Tucker Collins, and Stanley Robbins. *Robbins Pathological Basis of Disease.* 6th ed. Philadelphia: W. B. Saunders, 1999.

Guyton, Arthur, and John Hall. *Textbook of Medical Physiology.* 10th ed. Philadelphia: W. B. Saunders, 2000.

McCance, Kathryn, and Sue Huether. *Pathophysiology: The Biological Basis for Disease in Adults and Children.* 4th ed. St. Louis: Mosby, 2002.

On the Web

Visit Brady's Paramedic Website at **www.bradybooks.com/paramedic.**

General Principles of Pharmacology

Objectives

After reading this chapter, you should be able to:

Part 1: Basic Pharmacology (begins on p. 278)

1. Describe important historical trends in pharmacology. (p. 278)
2. Differentiate among the chemical, generic (nonproprietary), official (USP), and trade (proprietary) names of a drug. (pp. 278–279)
3. List the four main sources of drug products. (p. 279)
4. Describe how drugs are classified. (pp. 284-285)
5. List the authoritative sources for drug information. (p. 279)
6. List legislative acts controlling drug use and abuse in the United States. (pp. 280–282)
7. Differentiate among Schedule I, II, III, IV, and V substances and list examples of substances in each schedule. (p. 281)
8. Discuss standardization of drugs. (p. 282)
9. Discuss investigational drugs, including the Food and Drug Administration (FDA) approval process and the FDA classifications for newly approved drugs. (pp. 282–285)
10. Discuss special considerations in drug treatment with regard to pregnant, pediatric, and geriatric patients. (p. 286–289)
11. Discuss the paramedic's responsibilities and scope of management pertinent to the administration of medications. (pp. 285–286)

Please refer to the *Drug Guide for Paramedics* that accompanies this program as a special supplement.

12. Review the specific anatomy and physiology pertinent to pharmacology. (pp. 289–300)
13. List and describe general properties of drugs. (pp. 295–297)
14. List and describe liquid and solid drug forms. (pp. 294–295)
15. List and differentiate routes of drug administration. (pp. 293–294)
16. Differentiate between enteral and parenteral routes of drug administration. (pp. 293–294)
17. Describe mechanisms of drug action. (pp. 295–297)
18. List and differentiate the phases of drug activity, including the pharmaceutical, pharmacokinetic, and pharmacodynamic phases. (pp. 289–300)
19. Describe the processes called pharmacokinetics pharmocodynamics, including theories of drug action, drug-response relationship, factors altering drug responses, predictable drug responses, iatrogenic drug responses, and unpredictable adverse drug responses. (pp. 289–300)
20. Differentiate among drug interactions. (p. 300)
21. Discuss considerations for storing and securing medications. (p. 295)
22. List the components of a drug profile by classification. (p. 280)

Part 2: Drug Classifications (begins on p. 300)

1. Review the specific anatomy and physiology pertinent to pharmacology with additional attention to autonomic pharmacology. (pp. 301–364)
2. Review autonomic pharmacology. (pp. 310–325)
3. List and describe common prehospital medications, including indications, contraindications, side effects, routes of administration, and dosages. (pp. 301–364)
4. Given several patient scenarios, identify medications likely to be prescribed and those that are likely a part of the prehospital treatment regimen. (pp. 301–364)
5. Given various patient medications, assess the pathophysiology of a patient's condition by identifying classifications of drugs. (pp. 300–364)

Key Terms

active transport, p. 289
adjunct medication, p. 302
adrenergic, p. 311
affinity, p. 295
agonist, p. 296
agonist-antagonist, p. 296
analgesia, p. 302
analgesic, p. 302
anesthesia, p. 302
anesthetic, p. 303
antacid, p. 347

antagonist, p. 296
antibiotic, p. 358
anticoagulant, p. 339
antidysrhythmic, p. 329
antiemetic, p. 348
antihistamine, p. 344
antihyperlipidemic, p. 341
antihypertensive, p. 332
antineoplastic, p. 358
antiplatelet, p. 339
antitussive, p. 345

assay, p. 282
autonomic ganglia, p. 311
autonomic nervous
    system, p. 310
bioassay, p. 282
bioavailability, p. 291
bioequivalence, p. 282
biologic half-life, p. 299
biotransformation, p. 292
blood-brain barrier,
    p. 291

Case Study

Paramedics Jo Henderson and her partner, Scott Parker, are dispatched to a rural residence just outside of town on a "chest pain" call. The response time is approximately 8 minutes. First Responders from the Ferris Fire Department are already on the scene. As they pull up to the well-kept brick home, a woman waves to them from the front porch. She tells them she is the patient's wife and shows them through the house to the den, where her husband is seated in an overstuffed recliner. The patient is Reverend Charles Allen, a 54-year-old Methodist minister, who is well known to the paramedics. He is conscious and alert, but in obvious distress. He is breathing at a rate of 24 breaths per minute with some difficulty. His skin is pale and diaphoretic. While Jo is getting a brief history from him, she checks his radial pulse and finds that it is strong and regular at a rate of 84 beats per minute. Scott is busy attaching ECG electrodes and a pulse oximeter. The First Responders have already started oxygen administration with a nonrebreather mask. They inform Jo and Scott that the patient's blood pressure is 150/90 mm/Hg.

Reverend Allen tells Jo he is experiencing a "heaviness" in his chest, which is making it difficult for him to breathe. He says it feels as though "an elephant is sitting on it." He rates the discomfort as an 8 out of 10 and says it began about 15 minutes ago while he was watching television. He denies any other complaints and has no relevant medical history, takes no medications, and has no allergies. Per system standing orders, Jo administers 325 milligrams of chewable aspirin to her patient while she listens to his lungs. He has clear breath sounds in all fields. Jo asks Scott to start an IV of normal saline at a TKO rate while she administers 0.4 milligram (1/150 grain) of nitroglycerin (NitroStat) sublingually. The patient's pain has decreased somewhat, but he is still very uncomfortable and is now complaining of nausea. Jo has him place another nitroglycerin under his tongue while she administers 12.5 milligrams of promethezine (Phenergan) intravenously. She asks him to hold still while she runs a 12-lead ECG, and then she moves him to the ambulance for transport to the nearest cardiac center.

Jo anticipates an approximately 75-minute transport time to Our Lady of the Sea Hospital. The local community hospital closed several years ago due to financial reasons, forcing patients to drive 60 miles to a neighboring town for health care needs. Because of this, EMS has become even more important to the small community. Jo reassesses her patient and finds that he is still having chest discomfort, but he now rates it as a 6 out of 10. She administers another 2 milligrams of morphine sulfate intravenously. She notices that the ECG shows ST elevation in leads V_2 through V_6, indicating an anterolateral injury. Jo confirms the key findings of the history in order to determine if her patient is a candidate for prehospital fibrinolytic therapy. Finding no contraindications for fibrinolytic therapy, she contacts the hospital to notify them. The medical direction physician reviews the patient's risk factors and confirms that there are no contraindications to fibrinolytic therapy. Jo faxes him a copy of the 12-lead. He agrees with the paramedics' assessment of anterolateral myocardial ischemia and authorizes her to administer 10 units of retaplase (Retavase) intravenously over 2 minutes. Jo carefully documents the time the retaplase was administered. In addition, they are to continue titrating the morphine sulfate with the goal of eliminating all discomfort.

Jo continues to administer morphine incrementally until Reverend Allen reports he is free of discomfort. She carefully monitors his blood pressure and pulse rate throughout transport. Per the fibrinolytic protocol, the patient receives a second dose of 10 units of retaplase (Retavase) intravenously over 2 minutes, exactly 30 minutes after the first dose. Upon arrival at the hospital, the patient is moved to the chest pain unit of the emergency department. Initial laboratory studies and a chest x-ray are obtained. The patient is placed on a 12-lead ECG monitor. The paramedics note marked improvement in the ST segment elevation seen earlier in leads V_2 through V_6. The patient remains pain-free. Shortly thereafter, he is taken to the coronary care unit and has an uneventful night.

The next morning he undergoes cardiac catheterization and coronary angiography. Unfortunately, Reverend Allen has rather severe coronary artery disease with several high-grade blockages. The cardiologists determine that he has too much disease for balloon angioplasty. The patient is referred to cardiovascular surgery. The next day he undergoes four-vessel coronary artery bypass grafting (CABG). He does well in surgery and afterward. Thanks to the efforts of the paramedics, he has no permanent myocardial injury from the heart attack.

Reverend Allen is discharged from the hospital 4 days later and begins an aggressive cardiac rehabilitation program. Six weeks later he is able to resume his usual activities and returns to the pulpit, much to the satisfaction of his parishioners.

INTRODUCTION

The use of herbs and minerals to treat the sick and injured has been documented as long ago as 2000 B.C. Ancient Egyptians, Arabs, and Greeks probably passed formulations down through generations by word of mouth for centuries until they were finally recorded in pharmacopeias. By the end of the Renaissance, pharmacology was a distinct and growing discipline, separate from medicine. During the seventeenth and eighteenth centuries, tinctures of opium, coca, and digitalis were available. The related concept of vaccination with biologic extracts began in 1796 with Edward Jenner's smallpox inoculations. By the nineteenth century, atropine, chloroform, codeine, ether, and morphine were in use. The discoveries of animal insulin and penicillin in the early twentieth century dramatically changed the treatment of endocrine/metabolic and infectious diseases. Now, at the start of the twenty-first century, recombinant DNA technology has produced human insulin and tissue plasminogen activator (tPA). These drugs have markedly changed the treatment of diabetes and cardiovascular disease.

Presently in the United States, the Food and Drug Administration (FDA) is allowing many previously prescription-only drugs to become available over the counter. This is due in part to a growing consumer awareness in health care and also in part to consumer marketing by the pharmaceutical industry. The industry is actively seeking drugs that appeal widely to the consumer for treatments and cures. Pharmaceutical research to limit aging or increase the life span is growing rapidly. The federal government also offers incentives to pharmaceutical companies to research drugs for rare diseases. These so-called "orphan drugs" are often expensive to investigate and have a limited sales potential, making them less profitable to develop and manufacture than others.

General principles of pharmacology are presented in this chapter, which is divided into two parts:

Part 1: Basic Pharmacology
Part 2: Drug Classifications

Part 1: Basic Pharmacology

GENERAL ASPECTS

NAMES

drug *chemical used to diagnose, treat, or prevent disease.*

pharmacology *the study of drugs and their interactions with the body.*

Drugs are chemicals used to diagnose, treat, or prevent disease. **Pharmacology** is the study of drugs and their actions on the body. To study and converse about pharmacology, health care professionals must have a systematic method for naming drugs. The most detailed name for any drug is its chemical description, which states its chemical composition and molecular structure. Ethyl-1-methyl-4-phenylisonipecotate hydrochloride, for example, is a chemical name. A generic name is usually suggested by the manufacturer and confirmed by the United States Adopted Name Council. It becomes the Federal Drug Administration's (FDA) official name when listed in the *United States Pharmacopeia* (USP), the official standard for information about pharmaceuticals in the United States. In the case of ethyl-1-methyl-4-phenylisonipecotate hydrochloride, the generic name is meperidine hydrochloride, USP. To foster brand loyalty among its customers, the manufacturer gives the drug a brand name (sometimes called a trade name or proprietary name)—in our example, Demerol. The brand name is a proper name and should be capitalized. Most manufacturers also register the name as a trademark, so the stylized ® or ™ may follow the name, as in Demerol®. Another example is the widely prescribed sedative Valium:

- ★ *Chemical Name:* 7-chloro-1, 3-dihydro-1-methyl-5-phenyl-2H-1, 4-benzodiazepin-2-one
- ★ *Generic Name:* diazepam
- ★ *Official Name:* diazepam, USP
- ★ *Brand Name:* Valium®

Review

Drug Names

- Chemical name
- Generic name
- Official name
- Brand name

SOURCES

The four main sources of drugs are plants, animals, minerals, and the laboratory (synthetic). Plants may be the oldest source of medications; primitive people probably used them directly as "herbal" medicines. Indirectly, plant extracts such as gums and oils have long been a source of medications. Examples include the purple foxglove, a source of digitalis (a glycoside), and deadly nightshade, a source of atropine (an alkaloid). Animal extracts are another important source of drugs. For many years the primary sources of insulin for treating diabetes mellitus were the extracts of bovine (cow) and porcine (pig) pancreas. Minerals are inorganic sources of drugs such as calcium chloride and magnesium sulfate. Synthetic drugs are created in the laboratory. They may provide alternative sources of medications for those found in nature, or they may be entirely new medications not found in nature.

REFERENCE MATERIALS

Obtaining information on drugs can be difficult. Using multiple sources of information about drugs is usually a good idea. Every book about drugs, including this one, has a disclaimer regarding doses and current uses, referring the reader to local medical direction for the final word. Using multiple sources and comparing the authors' statements about a drug may lead you to the best available information. EMS providers generally like small, short guides that they can carry in a shirt pocket. These usually include important details about drugs that out-of-hospital providers administer along with a long list of commonly prescribed drugs and their classes. These EMS guides will be useful if you clearly understand the drugs used in your system and have a working knowledge of commonly prescribed drug classes.

Drug inserts, the printed fact sheets that drug manufacturers supply with most medications, contain information prescribed by the United States Food and Drug Administration. The *Physician's Desk Reference,* a compilation of these drug inserts, also includes three indices and a section containing photographs of drugs. It is among the most popular references, but it contains only factual information and must be interpreted by informed readers. The American Hospital Formulary Service annually publishes *Drug Information* as a service to the American Society of Health System Pharmacists. It contains an authoritative listing of monographs on virtually every drug used in the United States. A less bulky reference to keep in an ambulance might be one of the many drug guides for nurses. They contain information on hundreds of drugs in a format much like the EMS drug guides, but they also offer information on commonly prescribed drugs rather than only on emergency drugs. Also popular is the *Monthly Prescribing Reference.* Designed to assist physicians in prescribing medications, it can also help them determine which medications are available for treating specific diseases. Its information about new medications is especially useful. Most hospitals also maintain a listing of drugs, or formulary, that profiles the particular drugs they have available. The American Medical Association also publishes a useful reference, the *AMA Drug Evaluation.* The World Wide Web (WWW) provides an enormous amount of information, but you must be especially cautious when using it as a source, because it allows anyone with a computer to be a publisher, with no requirement for accuracy.

Review

Sources of Drug Information

- *United States Pharmacopeia* (USP)
- *Physician's Desk Reference*
- *Drug Information*
- *Monthly Prescribing Reference*
- *AMA Drug Evaluation*

It is helpful to carry a pharmaceutical reference in paramedic response vehicles.

Cultural Considerations

Folk Remedies Many cultures place great trust in herbal and folk remedies. Some have been proven beneficial by modern research. It is important to ask about them when you obtain your patient's history. Some folk medications can contain potentially toxic compounds such as lead or arsenic.

COMPONENTS OF A DRUG PROFILE

A drug's profile describes its various properties. As a paramedic student, you will become familiar with drug profiles as you study specific medications. A typical drug profile will contain the following information:

★ *Names.* These most frequently include the generic and trade names, although the occasional reference will include chemical names.

★ *Classification.* This is the broad group to which the drug belongs. Knowing classifications is essential to understanding the properties of drugs.

★ *Mechanism of Action.* The way in which a drug causes its effects; its pharmacodynamics.

★ *Indications.* Conditions that make administration of the drug appropriate (as approved by the Food and Drug Administration).

★ *Pharmacokinetics.* How the drug is absorbed, distributed, and eliminated; typically includes onset and duration of action.

★ *Side Effects/Adverse Reactions.* The drug's untoward or undesired effects.

★ *Routes of Administration.* How the drug is given.

★ *Contraindications.* Conditions that make it inappropriate to give the drug. Unlike when the drug is simply not indicated, a contraindication means that a predictable harmful event will occur if the drug is given in this situation.

★ *Dosage.* The amount of the drug that should be given.

★ *How Supplied.* This typically includes the common concentrations of the available preparations; many drugs come in different concentrations.

★ *Special Considerations.* How the drug may affect pediatric, geriatric, or pregnant patients.

Drug profiles may also include other components, such as its interactions with other drugs or with foods, when appropriate.

LEGAL ASPECTS

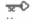
Know and obey the laws and regulations governing medications and their administration.

Knowing and obeying the laws and regulations governing medications and their administration will be an important part of your career. These laws and regulations come from three distinct authorities: federal law, state laws and regulations, and individual agency regulations.

FEDERAL

Drug legislation in the United States has been aimed primarily at protecting the public from adulterated or mislabeled drugs. The *Pure Food and Drug Act of 1906,* enacted to improve the quality and labeling of drugs, named the *United States Pharmacopeia* as this country's official source for drug information. The *Harrison Narcotic Act of 1914* limited the indiscriminate use of addicting drugs by regulating the importation, manufacture, sale, and use of opium, cocaine, and their compounds or derivatives. *The Federal*

Follow Orders of the Medical Director The administration of medications by a paramedic is allowed only by express physician order. This can be either verbal or through approved written standing orders. Always follow your medical director's orders in regard to medication administration.

Food, Drug and Cosmetic Act of 1938 empowered the Food and Drug Administration (FDA) to enforce and set premarket safety standards for drugs. In 1951, the *Durham-Humphrey Amendments* to the 1938 act (also known as the prescription drug amendments) required pharmacists to have either a written or verbal prescription from a physician to dispense certain drugs. It also created the category of over-the-counter medications. The *Comprehensive Drug Abuse Prevention and Control Act* (also known as the Controlled Substances Act) of 1970 is the most recent major federal legislation affecting drug sales and use. It repealed and replaced the Harrison Narcotic Act.

The federal government strictly regulates controlled substances because of their high potential for abuse. Since not all drugs cause the same level of physical or psychological dependence, they do not all need to be regulated in the same way. To accommodate their differences, the Controlled Substance Act of 1970 created five schedules of controlled substances, each with its own level of control and record keeping requirements (Table 9–1). Most emergency medical services administer only a few controlled substances, usually a narcotic analgesic such as morphine sulfate and a benzodiazepine anticonvulsant such as diazepam.

The majority of the remaining drugs provided by an EMS are prescription drugs—those whose use the FDA has designated sufficiently dangerous to require the supervision of a health care practitioner (physician, dentist, and in some states, nurse practitioner or certified physician's assistant). For emergency medical services this means the physician medical director is in effect prescribing the drugs in advance, based on the assessments and judgments of EMS providers in the field.

Over-the-counter (OTC) medications are generally available in small doses and, when taken as recommended, present a low risk to patients. Of the few OTC drugs that

✓ **Review**

Drug Laws and Regulations

- Federal law
- State laws and regulations
- Individual agency regulations

Table 9–1	Schedules of Drugs According to the Controlled Substances Act of 1970	
Schedule	**Description**	**Examples**
Schedule I	High abuse potential; may lead to severe dependence; no accepted medical indications; used for research, analysis, or instruction only	Heroin, LSD, mescaline
Schedule II	High abuse potential; may lead to severe dependence; accepted medical indications	Opium, cocaine, morphine, codeine, oxycodone, methadone, secobarbital
Schedule III	Less abuse potential than Schedule I and II; may lead to moderate or low physical dependence or high psychological dependence; accepted medical indications	Limited opioid amounts or combined with noncontrolled substances: Vicodin, Tylenol with codeine
Schedule IV	Low abuse potential compared to Schedule III; limited psychological and/or physical dependence; accepted medical indications	Diazepam, lorazepam, phenobarbital
Schedule V	Lower abuse potential compared to Schedule IV; may lead to limited physical or psychological dependence; accepted medical indications	Limited amounts of opioids; often for cough or diarrhea

EMS providers administer, acetaminophen and aspirin are probably the most common. Although laws vary from state to state, they still require most EMS providers to obtain a physician's order (either written, verbal, or standing) to administer OTC drugs.

Federal drug laws require that certain substances be appropriately secured, distributed, and accounted for. Because of the complexity of this issue and the large variability of drugs used in EMS systems across the country, specific answers to these concerns are not practical here. Consult your local protocols, laws, and most importantly, medical director for guidance in this area.

STATE

State laws vary widely. Some states have legislated which medications are appropriate for paramedics to give, while others have left those decisions to local control. Local control varies as well. In some areas, regional EMS authorities set the local standards; in others the individual medical directors and department directors do. In all cases, however, the physician medical director can delegate to paramedics the authority to administer medications, either by written, verbal, or standing order. You must know the laws of the state where you practice.

LOCAL

In each community, local leaders are responsible for ensuring public safety. Local EMS agencies have the responsibility to create local policies and procedures to ensure the public well-being. An excellent example of a local procedure protecting the patient (and thereby the individual EMS provider and agency) would be a requirement to use a pulse oximeter whenever a patient is sedated or paralyzed. While this requirement would not have the force of law, it would locally help to ensure that local EMS providers do not overlook hypoxia in these patients.

STANDARDS

Because some generic drugs affect patients differently than their brand name counterparts, standardization of drugs is a necessity. Despite FDA standards, drugs sold or distributed by various manufacturers may have biological or therapeutic differences. An **assay** determines the amount and purity of a given chemical in a preparation in the laboratory (in vitro). While two generically equivalent preparations may contain the same amount of a given chemical (drug), they may have different therapeutic effects. This relative therapeutic effectiveness of chemically equivalent drugs is their **bioequivalence.** Bioequivalence is determined by a **bioassay,** which attempts to ascertain the drug's availability in a biological model (in vivo). Again, the *United States Pharmacopeia* (USP) is the official standard for the United States.

assay *test that determines the amount and purity of a given chemical in a preparation in the laboratory.*

bioequivalence *relative therapeutic effectiveness of chemically equivalent drugs.*

bioassay *test to ascertain a drug's availability in a biological model.*

DRUG RESEARCH AND BRINGING A DRUG TO MARKET

The pharmaceutical industry is highly motivated to bring profitable new drugs to market. Proving the safety and reliability of these new drugs, however, requires extensive research. While better understanding of biology is shortening the time needed to bring a new drug to market, the process still takes many years. To assure the safety of new medications, the FDA has developed a process for evaluating their safety and efficacy. This process, illustrated in Figure 9-1 ■, adds even more time to the development cycle. Initial drug testing begins with the study of both male and female mammals. After testing

New Drug Development Timeline

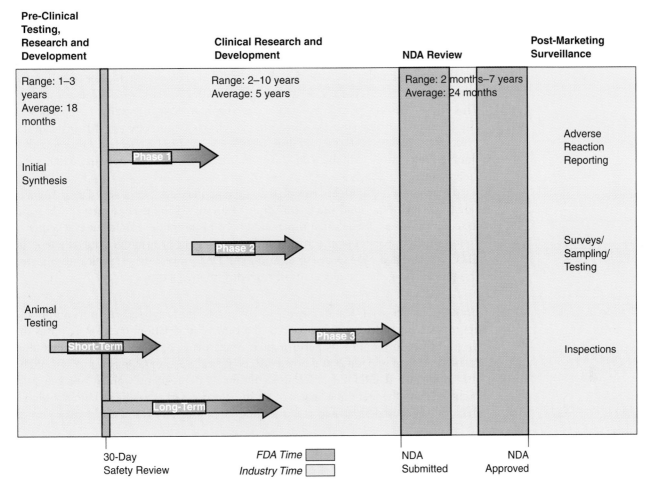

■ Figure 9-1   New drug development timeline.
(*United States Food and Drug Administration website,*
http://www.fda.gov/fdac/special/newdrug/testing.html.)

a drug's toxicity, researchers evaluate its pharmacokinetics—how it is absorbed, distributed, metabolized (biotransformed), and excreted—in animals. These animal studies also help determine the drug's therapeutic index (the ratio of its lethal dose to its effective dose). If the results of animal testing are satisfactory, the FDA designates the drug as an investigational new drug (IND) and researchers can then test it in humans.

PHASES OF HUMAN STUDIES

Human studies take place in four phases.

Phase 1   The primary purposes of phase 1 testing are to determine the drug's pharmacokinetics, toxicity, and safe dose in humans. These studies are usually carried out on limited populations of healthy human volunteers; some drugs with a high risk of untoward effects will not be tested on healthy individuals.

Phase 2   When phase 1 studies prove that the drug is safe, it is tested on a limited population of patients who have the disease it is intended to treat. The primary purposes of phase 2 studies are to find the therapeutic drug level and watch carefully for toxic and side effects.

Phase 3   The main purposes of phase 3 testing are to refine the usual therapeutic dose and to collect relevant data on side effects. Gathering the significant amounts of data needed for these goals requires a large patient population. Phase 3 studies are usually *double-blind*. That is, neither the patient nor the researcher knows whether the patient is receiving a placebo or the drug until after the study has been completed. This keeps personal biases from affecting the reporting of results. Some phase 3 studies are controlled studies, which are like placebo studies except that instead of a placebo the patient receives a treatment that is known to be effective. Occasionally a double-blind study will be ended sooner than planned if the early results are convincing.

Once phase 3 studies are completed, the manufacturer files a New Drug Application (NDA) with the Food and Drug Administration, which then evaluates the data collected in the investigation's first three phases. At this point the FDA decides whether to conditionally approve manufacturing and marketing the drug in the United States. The FDA's Abbreviated New Drug Application (ANDA) process may significantly shorten this process for generic equivalents of currently approved drugs.

Phase 4   Phase 4 testing involves postmarketing analysis during conditional approval. Once a drug is being used in the general population, the FDA requires the drug's maker to monitor its performance. Many drugs have been discontinued after marketing when previously unknown effects became apparent. One example would be the antiemetic thalidomide. Because children and pregnant women are generally excluded from the first three phases of testing, the premarket testing did not reveal that thalidomide caused birth defects in the children of pregnant women.

FDA CLASSIFICATION OF NEWLY APPROVED DRUGS

The FDA has developed a method for immediately classifying new drugs. This method of drug classification utilizes a number and a letter for each new drug in the IND phase or upon NDA review by the FDA. The manufacturer has a right to contest this classification and have it changed before the final classification is established.

Numerical Classification (Chemical)

1. A new molecular drug
2. A new salt of a marketed drug
3. A new formulation or dosage form not previously marketed
4. A new combination not previously marketed
5. A drug that is already on the market, a generic duplication
6. A product already marketed by the same company (This designation is used for new indications for a marketed drug.)
7. A drug product on the market without an approval NDA (drug was marketed prior to 1938)

Letter Classification (Treatment or Therapeutic Potential)

A. Drug offers an important therapeutic gain (P-priority)
B. Drug that is similar to drugs already on the market (S-similar)

Other Classifications

A. Drugs indicated for AIDS and HIV-related disease

B. Drugs developed to treat life-threatening or severely debilitating illness

C. An orphan drug

PATIENT CARE USING MEDICATIONS

Paramedics are responsible for the standard of care for patients in their charge. They are, therefore, personally responsible—legally, morally, and ethically—for the safe and effective administration of medications. The following guidelines will help you to meet that responsibility:

★ Know the precautions and contraindications for all medications you administer.

★ Practice proper techniques.

★ Know how to observe and document drug effects.

★ Maintain a current knowledge in pharmacology.

★ Establish and maintain professional relationships with other health care providers.

★ Understand the pharmacokinetics and pharmacodynamics.

★ Have current medication references available.

★ Take careful drug histories including:

 –Name, strength, and daily dose of prescribed drugs

 –Over-the-counter drugs

 –Vitamins

 –Herbal medications

 –Folk-medicine or folk-remedies

 –Allergies

★ Evaluate the compliance, dosage, and adverse reactions.

★ Consult with medical direction when appropriate.

SIX RIGHTS OF MEDICATION ADMINISTRATION

No pharmacology chapter would be complete without discussing the six rights of medication administration. They include the right medication, the right dose, the right time, the right route, the right patient, and the right documentation.

Right Medication   When following a physician's verbal medication order, repeat the order back to him to confirm that you both intend the same thing for the patient. Inspect the label on the drug at least three times before giving the medication to the patient: first, as you remove the medication from the drug box or cabinet; second, as you draw the medication into the syringe or dole the tablet into a cup; and third, immediately before you administer the medication. Failure to confirm the medication name is one of the most common medication administration errors. If you have any question about a drug, do not administer it without confirmation. Showing the medication container to your partner and asking for confirmation is an easy way to further ensure that you are giving the right drug.

 Review

Content

Six Rights of Medication Administration

- Right medication
- Right dose
- Right time
- Right route
- Right patient
- Right documentation

dose packaging *medication packages contain a single dose for a single patient.*

Right Dose   To reduce medication errors, many drugs come in unit **dose packaging.** That is, the package contains a single dose for a single patient. Dosages of many emergency drugs, however, are based on patient weight, so a prefilled syringe may not contain the exact amount a patient needs. You will have to calculate the correct dose. One good practice for identifying potential medication errors is to consider the number of unit dose packages needed for a single dose. If your calculations tell you to open 10 vials for one dose of medication, prudence requires you to check the calculation and dose carefully. The package may contain a unit dose of the wrong medication, or you may have miscalculated.

Right Time   While paramedics usually give medications in urgent and emergent situations rather than on a schedule, timing can still be very important. Giving nitroglycerin tablets too soon may precipitate hypotension; if epinephrine is not repeated on time during cardiac arrest it may not help to lower the threshold for defibrillation. Take care to give medications punctually and to document their administration promptly.

Right Route   You often will have to choose from among several treatments for a particular problem. In these cases, knowing the principles of pharmacokinetics can help greatly in giving your patient the medication via the right route. For example, your knowledge that you should administer epinephrine intravenously rather than subcutaneously to the patient in anaphylactic shock because his blood is being shunted away from the skin will guide you to the proper administration route.

Right Patient   As the paramedic's role in health care expands, you will find yourself caring for more people than just "the patient in the back of the truck." You will deal with multiple patients, and the potential for giving medication to the wrong patient will be real. You will have to identify patients by name before administering medications.

Right Documentation   The drugs you administer in the field do not stop affecting your patients when they enter the hospital. As a result, you must completely document all of your care, especially any drugs you have administered, so that long after you have gone on to your next call, other providers will know what drugs your patient has had.

Review

Special Considerations

- Pregnant patients
- Pediatric patients
- Geriatric patients

Content

SPECIAL CONSIDERATIONS

Pregnant Patients   Any time you administer drugs to a woman of childbearing years, you must consider the possibility that she is pregnant. Treating pregnant patients clearly means treating two patients. Although emphasis appropriately seems to center on the mother during care, you must understand that many drugs that affect the mother also affect the fetus. A drug's possible benefits to the mother must clearly outweigh its potential risks to the fetus. For example, some situations such as cardiac arrest justify giving the mother medications that may harm the fetus because the drug's possible harm to the fetus is clearly outweighed by the fetus's certain death if the mother dies.

Patho Pearls

Medications That Cross the Placenta   Some medications cross the placenta and affect the fetus. Because of this, it is prudent to ask whether a female patient might be pregnant before administering a medication.

Pregnancy presents two particular pharmacological problems: changes in the mother's anatomy and physiology, and the potential for drugs to harm the fetus. Because the mother is supporting the fetus entirely, her heart rate, cardiac output, and blood volume will increase. This altered maternal physiology can affect the onset and duration of action of many medications. During the first trimester of pregnancy the ingestion of some drugs (**teratogenic drugs**) may potentially deform, injure, or kill the fetus. During the last trimester, drugs administered to the mother may pass through the placenta to the fetus. Some of these drugs will have unwanted effects on the fetus. Others may not be metabolized and/or excreted, possibly resulting in toxic accumulations. Additionally, a breast-feeding mother's milk may pass some drugs to her infant.

teratogenic drug *medication that may deform or kill the fetus.*

Under some conditions, of course, the health and safety of mother and fetus demand the use of drugs during the pregnancy. Examples include pregnancy-induced diabetes, hypertension, and seizure disorders. To help health care providers determine when drugs are needed during pregnancy, the FDA has developed the classification system shown in Table 9–2. Always consult medical direction for any questions about drug safety in pregnancy.

Pediatric Patients Several physiological factors affect pharmacokinetics in newborns and young children. These patients' absorption of oral medications is less than an adult's due to various differences in gastric pH, gastric emptying time, and low enzyme levels. A newborn's skin is thinner than an older patient's and is therefore more permeable to topically administered drugs. This can result in unexpected toxicity. Older children still have less gastric acid than adults do, but their gastric emptying times reach an adult's around the sixth to eighth month of life. Because children up to a year old have diminished plasma protein concentrations, drugs that bind to proteins have higher **free drug availability.** That is, a greater proportion of the drug will be available in the body to cause either desired or undesired effects. Water distribution is different in the neonate as well. Neonates have a much higher proportion of extracellular fluid (nearly 80 percent) than adults (50 to 55 percent). This higher amount of water means

Children are not "small adults." Drug dosages must consider the various physiological differences.

free drug availability *proportion of a drug available in the body to cause either desired or undesired effects.*

Table 9–2	FDA Pregnancy Categories
Category	**Description**
A	Adequate studies in pregnant women have not demonstrated a risk to the fetus in the first trimester or later trimesters.
B	Animal studies have not demonstrated a risk to the fetus, *but* there are no adequate studies in pregnant women.
	OR
	Adequate studies in pregnant women have not demonstrated a risk to the fetus in the first trimester and there is no risk in the last trimester, *but* animal studies have demonstrated adverse effects.
C	Animal studies have demonstrated adverse effects, *but* there are no adequate studies in pregnant women; however, benefits may be acceptable despite the potential risks.
	OR
	No adequate animal studies or adequate studies of pregnant women have been done.
D	Fetal risk has been demonstrated. In certain circumstances, benefits could outweigh the risks.
X	Fetal risk has been demonstrated. This risk outweighs any possible benefit to the mother. Avoid using in pregnant or potentially pregnant patients.

a greater volume and, with less than expected protein binding, may require higher drug doses. The premature infant is especially susceptible to drugs penetrating the *blood-brain barrier* because his immature connective tissues form a weaker obstacle.

The newborn's metabolic rates may be much lower than an adult's, but they rise rapidly and by a few years of age may triple an adult's. These metabolic rates then decline steadily until early adolescence, when they reach adult levels. A newborn's low metabolic rate and incompletely developed hepatic system put him at higher risk for toxic interactions. Neonates' metabolic pathways also are different from an adult's, meaning that some drugs will not have the expected effect or may have other, unexpected effects. Finally, the neonatal renal and hepatic systems' immaturity delays elimination of many drugs and their metabolites. Dosing schedules may have to be adjusted to accommodate longer half-lives until these systems mature at about 6 months to 1 year of age.

With all of these factors, a pediatric patient's drug function can differ radically from an adult's. Pediatric drug dosages must be individualized to minimize the risks of toxicity. Body surface area and weight are the two most common factors in calculating dosages. The Broselow tape gives a good approximation for children of average height/weight ratio. It bases its calculations on the child's height (length), and assumes the child's weight is at the fiftieth percentile for his height (Figure 9-2 ■). The Broselow tape primarily addresses drugs administered in the critical care setting.

Geriatric Patients   Significant changes in pharmacokinetics may also occur in patients older than about 60 years. They may absorb oral medications slower due to decreased gastrointestinal motility. Decreased plasma protein concentration may alter distribution of drugs in their systems, leaving drugs free that would otherwise have been protein bound. Body fat increases and muscle mass decreases with age; therefore, lipid-soluble drugs may have greater deposition, thereby lowering the amount of available drug. Absorption and distribution of intramuscular injections may change if volumes are inappropriate for the remaining muscle mass. Because the liver primarily handles biotransformation, depressed liver function in an aging patient may delay or prolong drug action. The aging process may also slow elimination by the renal system.

Older patients are also more likely to be on multiple medications or to have multiple underlying disease processes. Various medication interactions can have a severe impact on patients. For example, sildenafil (Viagra) and nitroglycerin given together may

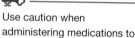
Since dosing for pediatric patients is based on their size and age, dosage ranges vary significantly. It is best to carry a reference containing the various common pediatric dosages.

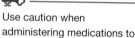
Use caution when administering medications to older patients because they are apt to be on multiple medications.

■ Figure 9-2   A Broselow tape is useful for calculating drug dosages for pediatric patients. (*Courtesy Broselow Corporation*)

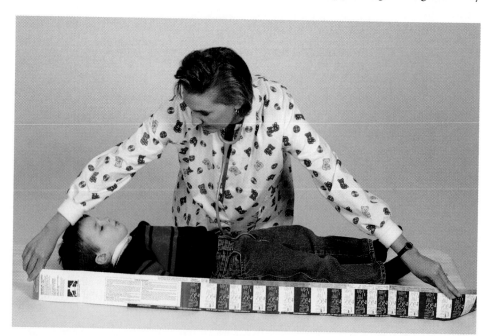

cause severe hypotension. Underlying diseases may affect therapeutics in unexpected ways. Congestive heart failure, for instance, may cause congestion of the gastrointestinal tract's vasculature, delaying the absorption of oral medications. The congestive heart failure patient may also have compromised renal function, delaying his elimination of drugs.

PHARMACOLOGY

Pharmacology is the study of drugs and their interactions with the body. Drugs do not confer any new properties on cells or tissues; they only modify or exploit existing functions. They may be given for their local action (in which case systemic absorption of the drug is discouraged) or for systemic action. Although generally given for a specific effect, drugs tend to have multiple actions at multiple sites, so they must be thought of in terms of their systemic effects rather than in terms of an isolated single effect. Pharmacology's two major divisions are pharmacokinetics and pharmacodynamics. You have already learned that **pharmacokinetics** addresses how drugs are transported into and out of the body. **Pharmacodynamics** deals with their effects once they reach the target tissues.

pharmacokinetics *how a drug is absorbed, distributed, metabolized (biotransformed), and excreted; how drugs are transported into and out of the body.*

pharmacodynamics *how a drug interacts with the body to cause its effects.*

PHARMACOKINETICS

Strictly defined, pharmacokinetics is the study of the basic processes that determine the duration and intensity of a drug's effect. These four processes are absorption, distribution, biotransformation, and elimination.

Review of Physiology of Transport

Pharmacokinetics is dependent upon the body's various physiological mechanisms that move substances across the body's compartments. These mechanisms can be broken down into two broad categories based on their energy requirements and then further classified. A mechanism is referred to as **active transport** if it requires the use of energy to move a substance. This energy is achieved by the breakdown of high-energy chemical bonds found in chemicals such as ATP (adenosine triphosphate). ATP is broken down into ADP (adenosine diphosphate) liberating a considerable amount of biochemical energy. A common example of an active transport mechanism is the sodium-potassium (Na^+-K^+) pump. This is a protein pump that actively moves potassium ions into the cell and sodium ions out of the cell. Because this movement goes *against* the ions' concentration gradients, it must use energy.

active transport *requires the use of energy to move a substance.*

Large molecules, such as glucose and most of the amino acids, do not readily pass through the cell membrane because of their size. These molecules are moved across the cell membrane with the help of special "carrier" proteins found on the surface of the target cells. These large molecules are "carried" across the cell membrane in a special transport process called **carrier-mediated diffusion** or **facilitated diffusion.** Once the molecule to be transported binds with the carrier protein, the configuration of the cell membrane changes, allowing the large molecule to enter the target cell. Insulin, an important hormone secreted by the endocrine pancreas, can increase the rate of carrier-mediated glucose transport from 10- to 20-fold. This is the principal mechanism by which insulin controls glucose use in the body.

carrier-mediated diffusion *or* **facilitated diffusion** *process in which carrier proteins transport large molecules across the cell membrane.*

Most drugs travel through the body by means of **passive transport,** the movement of a substance without the use of energy. This requires the presence of concentration gradients in a solution. Diffusion and osmosis are forms of passive transport. **Diffusion** involves the movement of solute in the solution, while **osmosis** involves the movement of the solvent (usually water). In diffusion, the solute's molecules or ions move *down*

passive transport *movement of a substance without the use of energy.*

diffusion *movement of solute in a solution from an area of higher concentration to an area of lower concentration.*

osmosis *movement of solvent in a solution from an area of lower solute concentration to an area of higher solute concentration.*

ionize *to become electrically charged or polar.*

their concentration gradients from an area of higher concentration to an area of lower concentration. Conversely, in osmosis the solvent's molecules move *up* the concentration gradient from an area of low solute concentration to an area of higher solute concentration. Another way of looking at this is to think of osmosis as simply the diffusion of solvent from an area of high *solvent* concentration to an area of low *solvent* concentration. A final type of passive transport is **filtration.** This is simply the movement of molecules across a membrane down a *pressure* gradient, from an area of high pressure to an area of lower pressure. This pressure typically results from the hydrostatic force of blood pressure.

Absorption

When a drug is administered to a patient it must find its way to the site of action. If a drug is given orally or injected into any place except the bloodstream, its absorption into the bloodstream is the first step in this process. (Since drugs given intravenously or intraarterially enter directly into the bloodstream no absorption needs to occur.) Several factors affect a drug's absorption. The body absorbs most drugs faster when they are given intramuscularly than when they are given subcutaneously. This is because muscles are more vascular than subcutaneous tissue. Of course, anything that slows blood flow will delay absorption. Shock and hypothermia are just two examples. Conversely, processes such as fever and hyperthermia increase peripheral blood flow and speed absorption.

Drugs given orally (enterally) must first survive the digestive processes before being absorbed across the mucosa of the gastrointestinal system. If a drug is not soluble in water, it will have difficulty being absorbed. Time-released medications take advantage of this with an enteric coating that slowly releases the medication. Some drugs have an enteric coating that will not dissolve in the more acidic environment of the stomach, but will dissolve in the alkaline environment of the duodenum. This allows a drug that would irritate the stomach or be destroyed by stomach acid to be passed through the stomach into the duodenum and absorbed there. Besides being able to survive stomach acid, a drug must also be somewhat lipid (fat) soluble in order to cross the cells' lipid two-layered (bilayered) membranes. Many drugs **ionize,** or become electrically charged or polar following administration. Generally speaking, ionized drugs do not absorb across the membranes of cells (lipid bilayers), but fortunately, most drugs do not fully ionize. Instead they reach an equilibrium between their ionized and nonionized forms, and the nonionized form can be absorbed. A drug's pH also affects the extent to which it ionizes. A drug that is a weak acid will ionize much more substantially in an alkaline environment than in an acidic environment; conversely, an alkaline drug will ionize more readily in an acidic environment than in an alkaline environment. For example, aspirin (an acidic drug) does not dissociate well in the stomach (an acidic environment) and is therefore readily absorbed there.

The nature of the absorbing surface and the blood flow to the administration site also affect drug absorption. The rate of absorption is directly related to the amount of surface area available for absorption. The greater the area, the faster the absorption. Much of the gastrointestinal system has multiple invaginations, or folds, that increase its surface area. Also, the greater the blood flow is to an area, the faster will be the rate of absorption. Again, the GI tract has a rich vascular system with many capillaries that perfuse its absorbing surfaces, allowing nutrients (and drugs) to diffuse into the bloodstream.

Finally, the drug's concentration affects its absorption. Because drugs diffuse in the body, the higher their concentration, the more rapidly the body will absorb them. This principle is frequently used when giving a "loading dose" of a drug and following it with a "maintenance infusion." The loading dose is typically a larger dose of the same concentration of the drug. On occasion, a more concentrated solution of the drug is used as the loading dose. Regardless, the desired effect is to rapidly raise the amount of the drug in the system to a therapeutic level. This is typically followed by a continuous infusion of the drug at a lower concentration, or slower administration rate, to keep it at the therapeutic level.

Bioavailability is the measure of the amount of a drug that is still active after it reaches its target tissue. This is the bottom line as far as absorption is concerned. The goal of administering a drug is to assure sufficient bioavailability of the drug at the target tissue in order to produce the desired effect, after considering all of the absorption factors.

bioavailability   amount of a drug that is still active after it reaches its target tissue.

Distribution

Once a drug has entered the bloodstream, it must be distributed throughout the body. Most drugs will pass easily from the bloodstream, through the interstitial spaces, into the target cells. Some drugs, however, will bind to proteins found in the blood, most commonly albumin, and remain in the body for a prolonged time. They thus have a sustained release from the bloodstream and a prolonged period of action. The therapeutic effects of a drug are primarily due to the unbound portion of the drug in the blood. A drug that is bound to plasma proteins cannot cross membranes and reach the target cells. Thus, only the unbound drug is in equilibrium with the target cells and can cross the cell membranes.

Changing the bloodstream's pH can affect the protein-binding action of a drug. Tricyclic antidepressants (TCAs), for instance, are strongly bound to plasma proteins. Making the blood more alkaline increases protein-binding of the TCA molecules. Therefore, in addition to supportive therapy, serious overdoses of TCAs are treated by administering sodium bicarbonate. Sodium bicarbonate makes the blood more alkaline (raises the pH) causing increased binding of the TCA to serum proteins. Cumulatively, this decreases the amount of free drug in the blood, thus decreasing the adverse effects. Sodium bicarbonate administration also facilitates elimination of the drug through the urine.

The presence of other serum protein-binding drugs can also affect drug-protein binding. For example, the drug warfarin (Coumadin) is highly protein-bound (99 percent). Its therapeutic effects are due to the 1 percent of the drug that is unbound and circulating in the bloodstream. Aspirin molecules bind to the same binding site on the serum proteins as do warfarin molecules. Thus, when aspirin is administered to a patient on warfarin, it displaces some of the protein-bound warfarin, increasing the amount of free (unbound) warfarin in the blood. Even if it displaces only 1 percent of the total warfarin, it effectively doubles the available warfarin. This can lead to unwanted side effects such as hemorrhage.

Albumin is one of the chief proteins in the blood that is available for binding with drugs. When albumin levels are low (hypoalbuminemia), as occurs in malnutrition, drugs that are normally protein bound rise to much greater blood levels than anticipated. For example, consider a patient who has been taking warfarin without difficulty. If he develops hypoalbuminemia, his normal dose of warfarin will result in much more of the drug being available in the body, possibly leading to dangerous bleeding.

Certain organs exclude some drugs from distribution. For example, the tight junctions of the capillary endothelial cells in the central nervous system (CNS) vasculature form a **blood–brain barrier.** These cells are packed together so tightly that only non-protein-bound, highly lipid-soluble drugs can cross into the CNS. The so-called **placental barrier** can likewise prevent drugs from reaching a fetus, although it is not the solid barrier that its name implies. The fetus is exposed to almost every drug that the mother takes. But because any drug must traverse the maternal blood supply and cross the capillary membranes into the placenta (fetal) circulation, delivering drugs to a fetus requires them to be lipid soluble, nonionized, and non-protein-bound. This may slow some drugs or reduce their placental transfer to benign levels.

blood–brain barrier   tight junctions of the capillary endothelial cells in the central nervous system vasculature through which only non-protein-bound, highly lipid-soluble drugs can pass.

placental barrier   biochemical barrier at the maternal/fetal interface that restricts certain molecules.

Other drugs are deposited in specific tissues. Fatty tissue, for example, can serve as a drug depot, or reservoir. Because blood flow is lower in fatty areas than in muscular areas, fatty tissue is a relatively stable depot; it can neither absorb nor release a large amount of drug in a short time. Similarly, bones and teeth can accumulate high amounts of drugs that bind to calcium, especially tetracycline antibiotics.

Biotransformation

metabolism *the body's breaking down chemicals into different chemicals.*

biotransformation *special name given to the metabolism of drugs.*

prodrug (parent drug) *medication that is not active when administered, but whose biotransformation converts it into active metabolites.*

Like other chemicals that enter the body, drugs are metabolized, or broken down into different chemicals (metabolites). The special name given to the **metabolism** of drugs is **biotransformation.** Biotransformation has one of two effects on most drugs: (1) it can transform the drug into a more or less active metabolite, or (2) it can make the drug more water soluble (or less lipid soluble) to facilitate elimination. Some drugs, such as lidocaine, are totally metabolized before elimination, others only partially, and still others not at all. The body will transform some molecules of most drugs and eliminate others without transformation. Protein-bound drugs are not available for biotransformation. Some so-called **prodrugs** (or parent drugs) are not active when administered, but biotransformation converts them into active metabolites.

first-pass effect *the liver's partial or complete inactivation of a drug before it reaches the systemic circulation.*

Many biotransformation processes occur in the liver. The endoplasmic reticula of hepatocytes (liver cells) contain microsomal enzymes that perform much of the metabolizing. (Smaller quantities of these enzymes are also found in the kidney, lung, and GI tract.) Because the blood supply from the GI tract passes through the liver via the portal vein, all drugs absorbed in the GI tract pass through the liver before moving on through the systemic circulation. The first pass through the liver may partially or completely inactivate many drugs. This **first-pass effect** is why some drugs cannot be given orally but instead must be given intravenously to bypass the GI tract and prevent first-pass hepatic metabolism. It also is why drugs that can be given either orally or intravenously may require a much higher oral dose than IV. Because we can observe the extent of first-pass metabolism, we can predict how much to increase a dose of an oral medication to deliver an effective amount of the drug into the general circulation.

oxidation *the loss of hydrogen atoms or the acceptance of an oxygen atom. This increases the positive charge (or lessens the negative charge) on the molecule.*

hydrolysis *the breakage of a chemical bond by adding water, or by incorporating a hydroxyl (OH^-) group into one fragment and a hydrogen ion (H^+) into the other.*

The liver's microsomal enzymes react with drugs in two ways: phase I, or nonsynthetic reactions; and phase II, or synthetic reactions. *Phase I reactions* most often **oxidize** the parent drug, although they may reduce it or **hydrolyze** it. These nonsynthetic reactions make the drug more water soluble to ease excretion. A number of drugs and chemicals increase the activity of, or induce, the microsomal enzyme that causes phase I reactions. This means that more enzyme is produced and drugs will be metabolized more rapidly. Because the microsomal enzymes are nonspecific, they can be induced by one drug or chemical and then biotransform other drugs or chemicals. *Phase II reactions,* which are also called conjugation reactions, combine the prodrug or its metabolites with an endogenous (naturally occurring) chemical, usually making the drug more polar and easier to excrete.

Elimination

Whether they are unchanged or metabolized before elimination, most drugs (toxins and metabolites) are excreted in the urine. Some are excreted in the feces or in expired air.

Renal excretion occurs through two major processes: glomerular filtration and tubular secretion. Glomerular filtration is a function of glomerular filtration pressure, which in turn results from blood pressure and blood flow through the kidneys. Conditions that affect blood pressure and blood flow can affect renal elimination. Specialized transport systems in the walls of the proximal kidney tubules secrete drugs into the urine. These "pumps" are active transport systems and require energy in the form of adenosine triphosphate (ATP) to function. Some are specialized and transport only specific chemicals, while others can transport a range of similar chemicals. When drugs compete for the same pump, toxicity or other unwanted effects can result; however, combinations of some drugs can take advantage of this specialization to prolong their circulation. For example, probenecid blocks renal tubular pumps and competes for them with many antibiotics, among them penicillin, ampicillin, and oxacillin. Probenecid thus is sometimes given with those antibiotics to increase and prolong their blood levels.

The same factors that affect absorption at any other site also affect reabsorption in the renal tubules. Of particular concern is the urine pH. Lipid soluble and nonionized molecules are readily reabsorbed. Changing the urine pH (usually by administering sodium bicarbonate to make it more alkaline) can affect the reabsorption in the renal tubules. For example, if a drug becomes ionized in a more alkaline environment, then making the urine more alkaline will interfere with reabsorption and cause more of the drug to be excreted. Some drugs and their metabolites can be eliminated in the expired air. This is the basis of the breath test that police use to determine a driver's blood alcohol level. Ethanol is released in the expired air in proportion to its concentration in the bloodstream. Although the liver degrades most ingested ethanol, exhalation releases a measurable quantity. Drugs also can be excreted in the feces. In enterohepatic circulation, if a drug (or its metabolites) is excreted into the intestines from bile, the body may reabsorb the drug and experience a sustained effect. Additionally, drugs may be excreted through sweat, saliva, and breast milk. Excretion through sweat glands is rarely a significant mechanism for elimination. Excretion through mammary glands becomes a concern when nursing mothers take medications.

Drug Routes

The route of a drug's administration clearly has an impact on the drug's absorption and distribution. The route's impact on biotransformation and elimination may not be so clear. The bloodstream will more quickly absorb and distribute water-soluble drugs if given in more vascular compartments than if given in less vascular compartments. Oral or nasogastric administration of alkaline drugs may allow the gastric acids to neutralize the drug and prevent its absorption. The liver's first-pass effect may biotransform some orally administered drugs and degrade them almost immediately.

Enteral Routes   Enteral routes deliver medications by absorption through the gastrointestinal tract, which goes from the mouth to the stomach and on through the intestines to the rectum. They may be oral, orogastric/nasogastric, sublingual, buccal, or rectal.

- ★ *Oral (PO).* The oral route is good for self-administered drugs. Most home medications are administered by this route. The drug must be able to tolerate the acidic gastric environment and be absorbed. Few emergency drugs are administered through this route.
- ★ *Orogastric/nasogastric tube (OG/NG).* This route is generally used for oral medications when the patient already has the tube in place for other reasons.
- ★ *Sublingual (SL).* This is a good route for self-administration and excellent absorption from the sublingual capillary bed without the problems of gastric acidity or absorption.
- ★ *Buccal.* Absorption through this route between the cheek and gum is similar to sublingual absorption.
- ★ *Rectal (PR).* This route is usually reserved for unconscious or vomiting patients or patients who cannot cooperate with oral or IV administration (small children).

Parenteral Routes   Broadly defined, parenteral denotes any area outside of the gastrointestinal tract; however, additional, specific criteria apply to parenteral drug administration. **Parenteral routes** typically use needles to inject medications into the

Make sure you know the correct route for a specific medication. Some medications that are therapeutic when given by the correct route can be dangerous when given by the wrong route.

 Review

Drug Routes

- Enteral
- Parenteral

enteral route   *delivery of a medication through the gastrointestinal tract.*

parenteral route   *delivery of a medication outside of the gastrointestinal tract, typically using needles to inject medications into the circulatory system or tissues.*

circulatory system or tissues. Consequently, some forms of parenteral drug delivery afford the most rapid drug delivery and absorption.

* *Intravenous (IV).* With its rapid onset, this is the preferred route in most emergencies.
* *Endotracheal (ET).* This is an alternative route for *selected* medications in an emergency.
* *Intraosseous (IO).* The intraosseous route delivers drugs to the medullary space of bones. Most often used as an alternative to IV administration in pediatric emergencies, it also sees limited use in adults.
* *Umbilical.* Both the umbilical vein and umbilical artery can provide an alternative to IV administration in newborns.
* *Intramuscular (IM).* The intramuscular route allows a slower absorption than IV administration, as the drug passes into the capillaries.
* *Subcutaneous (SC, SQ, SubQ).* This route is slower than the IM route, because the subcutaneous tissue is less vascular than the muscular tissue.
* *Inhalation/Nebulized.* This route, which offers very rapid absorption, is especially useful for delivering drugs whose target tissues are in the lungs.
* *Topical.* Topical administration delivers drugs directly to the skin.
* *Transdermal.* For drugs that can be absorbed through the skin, the transdermal route allows slow, continuous release.
* *Nasal.* Useful for delivering drugs directly to the nasal mucosa, the nasal route has an expanding role in delivering systemically acting drugs.
* *Instillation.* Instillation is similar to topical administration, but places the drug directly into a wound or an eye.
* *Intradermal.* For allergy testing, intradermal administration delivers a drug or biologic agent between the dermal layers.

Drug Forms

Drugs come in many forms. Solid forms, generally given orally, include:

* *Pills.* Drugs shaped spherically to be easy to swallow.
* *Powders.* Although they are not as popular as they once were, some powdered drugs are still in use.
* *Tablets.* Powders compressed into a disklike form.
* *Suppositories.* Drugs mixed with a waxlike base that melts at body temperature, allowing absorption by rectal or vaginal tissue.
* *Capsules.* Gelatin containers filled with powders or tiny pills; the gelatin dissolves, releasing the drug into the gastrointestinal tract.

Liquid drugs are usually solutions of a solid drug dissolved in a solvent. Some can be given parenterally, while others must be given enterally.

* *Solutions.* The most common liquid preparations. Generally water based; some may be oil based.
* *Tinctures.* Prepared using an alcohol extraction process; some alcohol usually remains in the final drug preparation.
* *Suspensions.* Preparations in which the solid does not dissolve in the solvent; if left alone, the solid portion will precipitate out.
* *Emulsions.* Suspensions with an oily substance in the solvent; even when well mixed, globules of oil separate out of the solution.
* *Spirits.* Solution of a volatile drug in alcohol.

★ *Elixirs.* Alcohol and water solvent, often with flavorings added to improve the taste.

★ *Syrups.* Sugar, water, and drug solutions.

Some drugs come in a gaseous form. The most common drug supplied this way is oxygen. Paramedics may also find nitrous oxide (N_2O) used as an inhaled analgesic in ambulances and emergency departments.

Drug Storage

Certain guidelines should dictate the manner in which drugs are stored; their properties may be altered by the environment in which they are stored. While some EMS units are parked in heated stations, others are kept outdoors and exposed to the elements. EMS systems must consider the storage requirements of all drugs and diluents when deciding operational issues such as vehicle design and posting policies (as occurs in system status management). This rapidly becomes a clinical issue because the actual potency of most medications is altered if they are not stored in proper conditions. Examples of variables to consider when determining the proper method of drug storage include temperature, light, moisture and shelf life.

PHARMACODYNAMICS

When we consider a drug's pharmacodynamics, or effects on the body, we are specifically interested in its mechanisms of action and the relationship between its concentration and its effect.

Actions of Drugs

Drugs can act in four different ways. They may bind to a receptor site, change the physical properties of cells, chemically combine with other chemicals, or alter a normal metabolic pathway. Each of these actions involves a physiochemical interaction between the drug and a functionally important molecule in the body.

Drugs That Act by Binding to a Receptor Site   Most drugs operate by binding to a **receptor.** Almost all drug receptors are protein molecules on the surfaces of cells. They are part of the body's normal regulatory stimulation/inhibition function, and can be stimulated or inhibited by chemicals. Each different receptor's name generally corresponds to the drug that stimulates it. For example, if an opiate stimulates the receptor, then the receptor is an opioid receptor. When multiple drugs stimulate the same receptor, standard practice is to use the generic name.

The force of attraction between a drug and a receptor is their **affinity.** The greater the affinity, the stronger the bond. Different drugs may bind to the same type of receptor site, but the strength of their bond may vary. The binding site's shape determines its receptivity to other chemicals, whether they are drugs or endogenous substances. These binding sites are relatively specific—a nonopiate drug generally will not affect an opiate binding site, although occasionally a drug with a similar receptor binding site will unexpectedly cross react. Receptors can also have subtypes. At least five subtypes of adrenergic receptors, for example, are important to paramedic practice.

A drug's pharmacodynamics also involve its ability to cause the expected response, or **efficacy.** Just as different drugs may have different affinities for a site, they may also have different efficacies; that is, drug A may cause a stronger response than drug B. Affinity and efficacy are not directly related. Drug A may cause a stronger response than drug B, even though drug B binds to the receptor site more strongly than drug A.

When a drug binds with its specific type of receptor, a chemical change occurs that ultimately leads to the drug's effect. In most cases, drugs will either stimulate or inhibit the cell's normal biochemical actions. In fact, a drug cannot impart a new function to a

Medications are vulnerable to extremes in temperature. It is important that they be stored in conditions where temperature fluctuation is minimized.

✓ Review

Content

Types of Drug Actions

- Binding to a receptor site
- Changing the physical properties of cells
- Chemically combining with other chemicals
- Altering a normal metabolic pathway

receptor *specialized protein that combines with a drug resulting in a biochemical effect.*

affinity *force of attraction between a drug and a receptor.*

efficacy *a drug's ability to cause the expected response.*

second messenger *chemical that participates in complex cascading reactions that eventually cause a drug's desired effect.*

cell. Some drugs may interact with a receptor and directly result in the desired effect. Other drugs, however, may interact with a receptor and cause the release or production of a second compound. This secondary compound, or **second messenger,** includes such compounds as calcium or cyclic adenosine monophosphate (cAMP). Cyclic AMP is the most common second messenger. It has a multitude of effects inside the cell. These secondary messengers are particularly important in the endocrine system, as they principally occur in endocrine glands. Once cAMP is formed inside the cell, it activates still other enzymes, usually in a cascading action. That is, the first enzyme activates another enzyme, which activates a third enzyme, and so forth. This is important in that it amplifies the action so that even a small amount of a drug (or hormone) acting on the cell surface can initiate a powerful, cascading, activating force for the entire cell.

The number of receptors on a target cell usually does not remain constant on a daily basis, or even from minute to minute. This is because the receptor proteins are often destroyed during the course of their function. At other times, they are either reactivated or remanufactured by the protein-manufacturing mechanism of the cell. Binding of a drug (or hormone) to a target cell receptor causes the number of receptors to decrease. This process is **down-regulation** of the receptors. It results in a decreased responsiveness of the target cell to the drug or hormone as the number of available active receptors decreases. In other cases, but less commonly, a drug (or hormone) can cause the formation of more receptors than normal. This process, **up-regulation,** increases the target tissue's sensitivity to the particular drug or hormone.

down-regulation *binding of a drug or hormone to a target cell receptor that causes the number of receptors to decrease.*

up-regulation *a drug causes the formation of more receptors than normal.*

Chemicals that stimulate a receptor site generally fall into two broad categories, agonists and antagonists. **Agonists** bind to the receptor and cause it to initiate the expected response. **Antagonists** bind to a site but do not cause the receptor to initiate the expected response. Some drugs, **agonist-antagonists** (also called **partial agonists**), may do both. Nalbuphine (Nubain), for instance, stimulates some of the opioid agonists' analgesic properties but partially blocks others such as respiratory depression.

agonist *drug that binds to a receptor and causes it to initiate the expected response.*

antagonist *drug that binds to a receptor but does not cause it to initiate the expected response.*

Receptor-mediated drug actions work like a lock (the receptor) and key (the agonist). If you put the key in the lock and turn it, the lock will open. An antagonist is like a key that fits into the lock but will not turn and cannot open the lock. Target tissues generally have many receptors, so to take the analogy another step, imagine that to get maximal effect a single key (agonist) must move around and open many doors (trigger many biochemical responses). An agonist-antagonist would be a key that unlocks and opens a door but gets stuck in the lock. That is, the drug will cause the expected effect, but that drug will also block another drug from triggering the same receptor. This **competitive antagonism** is considered *surmountable* because a sufficiently large dose of the agonist can overcome the antagonism.

agonist-antagonist (partial agonist) *drug that binds to a receptor and stimulates some of its effects but blocks others.*

competitive antagonism *one drug binds to a receptor and causes the expected effect while also blocking another drug from triggering the same receptor.*

Noncompetitive antagonism can also occur. Continuing the lock, key, and door analogy, imagine the door is barred. This antagonism would be *insurmountable;* no amount of agonist could overcome it. Noncompetitive antagonism occurs because the binding of the antagonist at a different site causes a deformity of the binding site that actually prevents the agonist from fitting and binding. **Irreversible antagonism** may also occur when a competitive antagonist permanently binds with a receptor site. When this occurs, no amount of agonist will stimulate the receptor. For the effects of such an antagonist to wear off, the body must create new receptors.

noncompetitive antagonism *the binding of an antagonist causes a deformity of the binding site that prevents an agonist from fitting and binding.*

irreversible antagonism *a competitive antagonist permanently binds with a receptor site.*

Two drugs may appear to be antagonists while actually acting independently. This physiologic antagonism can occur when one drug's effects counteract another's. While neither agent chemically affects the other, their net effect is antagonistic. An example of a receptor, agonist, antagonist, and agonist-antagonist can be described using an opiate receptor. These receptors occur naturally in the brain and respond to natural endorphins. Morphine sulfate acts as an agonist. It binds to the opiate receptor and causes the expected response of pain relief. Naloxone (Narcan) acts as an antagonist. It will bind to the opiate receptor, but will not initiate the pain relief. It will prevent morphine sulfate from binding to the site and thus effectively blocks the morphine and its response.

If the patient is given nalbuphine (Nubain), an agonist-antagonist, it will bind to the opiate receptor and relieve pain, but it is less efficacious than morphine. The nalbuphine blocks morphine from the receptor like an antagonist, but stimulates the receptor on its own like an agonist, although to a lesser extent.

Drugs That Act by Changing Physical Properties   Some drugs change the physical properties of a part of the body. Drugs that change the osmotic balance across membranes are good examples of this type of drug action. The osmotic diuretic mannitol (Osmotrol), for instance, increases urine output by increasing the blood's osmolarity, or osmotic "pull." This increased osmolarity triggers the normal regulatory systems to decrease water reabsorption in the renal tubules, thereby reducing the total amount of water in the body.

Drugs That Act by Chemically Combining with Other Substances   Drugs that participate in chemical reactions that change the chemical nature of their substrates (the chemical or substance on which a drug acts) play a large role in paramedic practice. For example, isopropyl alcohol, which is often used to disinfect skin before percutaneous needle insertion for phlebotomy or IV cannulation, denatures the proteins on the surface of bacterial cells. This ruptures the cells, destroying the bacteria. The antacids are another example. They act by chemically neutralizing the hydrochloric acid in the stomach. Sodium bicarbonate given intravenously chemically neutralizes some of the acids in the bloodstream, effectively making the blood more alkalotic.

Drugs That Act by Altering a Normal Metabolic Pathway   Some anticancer and antiviral drugs are chemical analogs of normal metabolic substrates. In a process that has been dubbed a counterfeit incorporation mechanism, these drugs can be incorporated into the products of metabolism of cancer cells. Since these drugs are not really the expected substrate, the anticipated product either will not form or, if formed, will be substantially or completely inactive.

Responses to Drug Administration

When a drug is administered, a response is obviously anticipated. The actual response may be the one desired, or it may be an unintended **side effect.** Most, if not all, drugs have at least some minor side effects. Because our knowledge of pharmacology and physiology has not yet arrived at the point where we can engineer the perfect drug, we

side effect   unintended response to a drug.

Legal Notes

Safety First Administration of medications is one area where a paramedic or EMT-Intermediate differs from the EMT-Basic. EMT-Basic skills, even if performed incorrectly, rarely have the potential to harm the patient. However, many advanced skills, if performed improperly, can severely harm or even kill the patient. Prehospital administration of emergency medications has saved countless lives. However, there have been instances where patients have been given the wrong medication or an incorrect dose of the correct medication, resulting in harm to the patient. Because of this, you must be extremely vigilant regarding medication administration. Be certain always to confirm orders and write them down. Follow the six "rights" of medication administration. Double check your drugs and expiration dates, the doses, the timing of administration, and the intended route of administration. Make sure the medication is being given to the right patient. Following administration, constantly monitor your patient for the desired effects as well as any possible side effects. Accurately document your findings, including any untoward effects. It is essential that you make prehospital medication administration as safe as possible for both the patient and you.

Always weigh the need for a drug's desired response against the dangers of its side effects.

must weigh the need for the desired response against the dangers of side effects. In essence, every time we give a medication, we must carefully weigh the risks against the benefits. Although undesirable, side effects are predictable. Iatrogenic responses, however, are not predicted. In general, the term *iatrogenic* refers to a disease or response induced by the actions of a care provider. Derived from the Greek *iatros* (physician) and *gennan* (to produce), it literally means *physician produced*. Negligence is not the only cause of iatrogenic responses. Some common unintended adverse responses to drugs include:

★ *Allergic Reaction.* Also known as hypersensitivity; this effect occurs as the drug is antigenic and activates the immune system, causing effects that are normally more profound than seen in the general population.

★ *Idiosyncrasy.* A drug effect that is unique to the individual; different than seen or expected in the population in general.

★ *Tolerance.* Decreased response to the same amount of drug after repeated administrations.

★ *Cross Tolerance.* Tolerance for a drug that develops after administration of a different drug. Morphine and other opioid agents are common examples. Tolerance for one agent implies tolerance for others as well.

★ *Tachyphylaxis.* Rapidly occurring tolerance to a drug. May occur after a single dose. This typically occurs with sympathetic agonists, specifically decongestant and bronchodilation agents.

★ *Cumulative Effect.* Increased effectiveness when a drug is given in several doses.

★ *Drug Dependence.* The patient becomes accustomed to the drug's presence in his body and will suffer from withdrawal symptoms upon its absence. The dependence may be physical or psychological.

★ *Drug Interaction.* The effects of one drug alter the response to another drug.

★ *Drug Antagonism.* The effects of one drug block the response to another drug.

★ *Summation.* Also known as an additive effect. Two drugs that both have the same effect are given together, analogous to $1+1=2$.

★ *Synergism.* Two drugs that both have the same effect are given together and produce a response greater than the sum of their individual responses, analogous to $1+1=3$.

★ *Potentiation.* One drug enhances the effect of another. A common example is promethazine (Phenergan) enhancing the effects of morphine.

★ *Interference.* The direct biochemical interaction between two drugs; one drug affects the pharmacology of another drug.

Drug-Response Relationship

To have its optimal desired or therapeutic effects, a drug must reach appropriate concentrations at its site of action. The magnitude of the response therefore depends on the dosage and the drug's course through the body over time. Factors that can affect the drug's concentration may be pharmaceutical (the dosage form's disintegration and the drug's dissolution), pharmacokinetic (the drug's absorption, distribution, metabolism, and excretion), or pharmacodynamic (drug-receptor interaction). To predict how the drug will affect different people, a **drug-response relationship** thus correlates different amounts of drug to the resultant clinical response.

Most of the information needed to describe drug-response relationships comes from **plasma-level profiles,** which describe the lengths of onset, duration, and termi-

drug-response relationship *correlation of different amounts of a drug to clinical response.*

plasma-level profile *describes the lengths of onset, duration, and termination of action, as well as the drug's minimum effective concentration and toxic levels.*

nation of action, as well as the drug's minimum effective concentration and toxic levels. The **onset of action** is the time from administration until a medication reaches its **minimum effective concentration** (the minimum level of drug necessary to cause a given effect). The length of time the amount of drug remains above this level is its **duration of action. Termination of action** is measured from when the drug's level drops below the minimum effective concentration until it is eliminated from the body.

The ratio of a drug's lethal dose for 50 percent of the population (LD_{50}) to its effective dose for 50 percent of the population (ED_{50}) is its **therapeutic index** (TI) or LD_{50}/ED_{50}. The therapeutic index represents the drug's margin of safety. As the range between effective dose and lethal dose decreases, the value of TI decreases; that is, it becomes closer to one. TI values of close to one indicate a very small margin of safety. In other words, the effective dose and lethal dose of a drug whose TI value is close to one are nearly the same. This drug would be very difficult to effectively dose without causing toxicity.

The last component of the drug-response relationship, the **biologic half-life,** is the time the body takes to clear one half of the drug. Although the rates of metabolism and excretion both affect it, a drug's half-life ($t_{1/2}$) is independent of its concentration. For example, if the concentration of a drug were 500 mcg/dL after administration and 250 mcg/dL in 10 minutes, then its half-life would be 10 minutes. After another 10 minutes, 125 mcg/dL would remain.

Factors Altering Drug Response

Different individuals may have different responses to the same drug given. Factors that alter the standard drug-response relationship include the following:

★ *Age.* The liver and kidney functions of infants are not yet fully developed, so the response to drugs may be altered. Likewise, as we age, the functions of these organs begin to deteriorate. As a result, infants and the elderly are most susceptible to having an altered response to a drug.

★ *Body Mass.* The more body mass a person has, the more fluid is potentially available to dilute a drug. A given amount of drug will cause a higher concentration in a person with little body mass than in a much larger person. Thus, most drug dosages are stated in terms of body mass. For example, the standard dose of lidocaine for a patient in cardiac arrest is 1.5 mg/kg. A 100-kg patient will receive 150 mg of lidocaine, while a 50-kg patient will receive only 75 mg.

★ *Sex.* Most differences in drug response due to sex result from the relative body masses of men and women. The different distribution and amounts of body fat also affect the amounts of drug available at any given time.

★ *Environmental Milieu.* Various stimuli in a patient's environment affect his response to a given drug. This is most clearly seen with drugs affecting mood or behavior. The same dose of an antianxiety medication such as diazepam (Valium) will have different effects, depending on the patient's mood or surroundings. For example, if the patient were afraid of heights, his usual dose of diazepam would not be likely to help him remain calm while rappelling from the top of a tall building. Surrounding conditions may also affect the distribution or elimination of a drug. Heat, for example, causes vasodilation and increases perspiration, both of which may alter the rate at which the body distributes and eliminates a drug.

★ *Time of Administration.* If a patient takes a drug immediately after eating, its absorption will be different than if he took the same drug before breakfast in the morning. Some drugs may cause nausea if taken on an empty stomach and must therefore be taken only after eating.

 Review

Content

Factors Affecting Drug-Response Relationship

- Age
- Body mass
- Sex
- Environment
- Time of administration
- Pathology
- Genetics
- Psychology

★ *Pathologic State.* Several disease states alter the drug-response relationship. Most notable are renal and hepatic dysfunctions, both of which may lead to excess accumulation of a drug in the body. Renal failure is likely to decrease elimination of drugs, while hepatic failure may decrease or inhibit their metabolism, prolonging their duration of action. Acid-base disturbances may alter a drug's solubility or the extent to which it ionizes, thus changing its absorption rate.

★ *Genetic Factors.* Genetic traits such as the lack of specific enzymes or lowered basal metabolic rate alter drug absorption or biotransformation and thus modify the patient's response.

★ *Psychological Factors.* A patient's mental state can also affect his response to a drug. The best-known example of this is the placebo effect. Essentially, if a patient believes that a drug will have a given effect, then he is much more likely to perceive that the effect has occurred.

The chance of a medication interaction increases significantly the greater the number of medications a patient is taking. Thus, proceed with caution when administering an emergency medication to a patient who routinely takes more than two.

Drug Interactions

Drug interactions occur whenever two or more drugs are available in the same patient. The interaction can increase, decrease, or have no effect on their combined actions. Any number of variables may cause these drug-drug interactions, including:

★ One drug could alter the rate of intestinal absorption.

★ The two drugs could compete for plasma protein binding, resulting in one's accumulation at the other's expense.

★ One drug could alter the other's metabolism, thus increasing or decreasing either's bioavailability.

★ One drug's action at a receptor site may be antagonistic or synergistic to another's.

★ One drug could alter the other's rate of excretion through the kidneys.

★ One drug could alter the balance of electrolytes necessary for the other drug's expected result.

In addition to drug-drug interactions, other types of interactions are possible. They include a drug's effects on the rate of absorption of food and nutrients, alteration of enzymes, and food-initiated alteration of drug excretion. Alcohol consumption and smoking may also cause interactions with drugs. Finally, some drugs are incompatible with each other. As an example, catecholamines such as epinephrine will precipitate in an alkaline solution such as sodium bicarbonate.

Part 2: Drug Classifications

CLASSIFYING DRUGS

The enormous amount of material that you must learn about pharmacology can easily become overwhelming. The best way to surmount this challenge is to break the information into manageable groups. Drugs can be classified many ways. You will often find them listed by the body system they affect, by their mechanism of action, or by their indications. Drugs also can be classified by source or by chemical class. Understanding the properties of drug classes (or the model drug of a class) can increase your understanding of drugs and quicken your learning of new drugs.

Grouping medications according to their uses is a very practical way of classifying them. For example, one class of drugs is used to treat heart dysrhythmias, while another treats hypertension. While the specific dosing regimens and contraindications vary among medications within any class, their general properties are consistent. If you understand those general principles, learning the specific information about individual medications becomes much easier. Thinking in terms of prototypical medications usually helps to describe each classification. A **prototype** is a drug that best demonstrates the class's common properties and illustrates its particular characteristics.

In the rest of this chapter we will look at specific classifications of medications that as a paramedic you will commonly either administer or encounter. Even though you may not frequently administer medications from every classification, knowing how they work remains important. It will help you to understand the implications of medications your patients may be taking themselves or getting from another caregiver. An example often cited to demonstrate the importance of understanding the classes of medications, even those that you will rarely administer, is the patient who has taken an overdose of tricyclic antidepressants. Based on your knowledge of this classification, you will know to increase your index of suspicion for hypotension and abnormal cardiac rhythms.

DRUGS USED TO AFFECT THE NERVOUS SYSTEM

The two major divisions of the nervous system are the central nervous system and the peripheral nervous system (Figure 9-3 ■). The *central nervous system* includes the brain and spinal cord; all nerves that originate and terminate within either the brain or the spinal cord are considered central. The *peripheral nervous system* comprises everything else. If a neuron originates within the brain and terminates outside of the spinal cord, it is part of the peripheral nervous system, which in turn consists of the somatic nervous system and the autonomic nervous system. The *somatic nervous system* controls voluntary, or motor, functions. The *autonomic nervous system*, which controls involuntary, or automatic, functions, is further divided into the sympathetic and parasympathetic nervous systems. The two major groupings of medications used to affect the

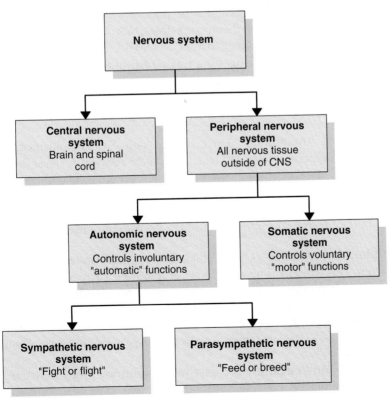

■ Figure 9-3 Functional organization of the autonomic nervous system within the overall nervous system.

nervous system are those that affect the central nervous system and those that affect the autonomic nervous system.

CENTRAL NERVOUS SYSTEM MEDICATIONS

Many pathologic conditions involve the central nervous system (CNS). As a result, a great number of drugs have been developed to affect the CNS, including analgesics, anesthetics, drugs to treat anxiety and insomnia, anticonvulsants, stimulants, psychotherapeutic agents (antidepressants and antimanic agents), and drugs used to treat specific nervous system disorders such as Parkinson's disease. Obviously, this is a very broad classification with many different types of agents. Having a firm grasp on the basic physiology involved will help you to understand the various drugs you encounter.

Analgesics and Antagonists

analgesic *medication that relieves the sensation of pain.*

analgesia *the absence of the sensation of pain.*

anesthesia *the absence of all sensations.*

adjunct medication *agent that enhances the effects of other drugs.*

Analgesics are medications that relieve the sensation of pain. The distinction between **analgesia,** the absence of the sensation of *pain,* and **anesthesia,** the absence of *all* sensation, is important. Where an analgesic decreases the specific sensation of pain, an anesthetic prevents all sensation, often impairing consciousness in the process. A frequently used class of medications, analgesics are available by prescription or over the counter. The two basic subclasses of analgesics are opioid agonists and their derivatives and nonopioid derivatives. Opioid antagonists, which we also discuss in this section, reverse the effects of opioid analgesics; **adjunct medications** enhance the effects of other analgesics.

Opioid Agonists An opioid is chemically similar to opium, which is extracted from the poppy plant and has been used for centuries for its analgesic and hallucinatory effects. Opium and all of its derivatives effectively treat pain because of their similarity to natural pain-reducing peptides called *endorphins.* Endorphins and, by extension, opioid drugs work by decreasing the sensory neurons' ability to propagate pain impulses to the spinal cord and brain.

The prototype opioid drug is morphine. Several of morphine's effects make it useful for clinical practice. At therapeutic doses, morphine causes analgesia, euphoria, sedation, and miosis (pupil constriction). It also decreases cardiac preload and afterload, which makes it useful in treating myocardial infarction and pulmonary edema. At higher doses, it may cause respiratory depression and hypotension. Give morphine with caution to patients at high risk for respiratory failure (COPD and asthma) and hypotension (trauma patients with hypovolemia).

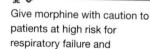

Give morphine with caution to patients at high risk for respiratory failure and hypotension.

Nonopioid Analgesics Three broad types of nonopioid medications also have analgesic properties, several of which also share antipyretic (fever fighting) properties. These are *salicylates* such as aspirin, *nonsteroidal anti-inflammatory drugs (NSAIDS)* such as ibuprofen, and *para-aminophenol derivates* such as acetaminophen. The drugs in each of these classes affect the production of prostaglandins and cyclooxygenase, important neurotransmitters involved in the pain response.

Opioid Antagonists Opioid antagonists are useful in reversing the effects of opioid drugs. This typically is necessary to treat respiratory depression. Naloxone (Narcan) is the prototype opioid antagonist. It competitively binds with opioid receptors but without causing the effects of opioid bonding. It is commonly used to treat overdoses of heroin and other opioid derivatives; however, it has a shorter half-life than most opioid drugs so repeated doses may be necessary to prevent its unwanted side effects.

Adjunct Medications Adjunct medications are given concurrently with other drugs to enhance their effects. While they may have only limited or no analgesic properties by themselves, combined with a true analgesic they either prolong or intensify its effect. Examples of adjunct medications are benzodiazepines (diazepam [Valium], lorazepam (Ativan), midazolam [Versed]), antihistamines (promethazine [Phenergan]), and caffeine. We will discuss many of these agents in separate sections.

Opioid Agonist-Antagonists   An opioid agonist-antagonist displays both agonistic and antagonistic properties. Pentazocine (Talwin) is the prototype for this class. Nalbuphine (Nubain) is commonly used in field care. It is an agonist because, like opioids, it decreases pain response, and it is an antagonist because it has fewer respiratory depressant and addictive side effects. Butorphanol (Stadol) is another common opioid agonist-antagonist.

Anesthetics

Unlike analgesics, an **anesthetic** induces a state of anesthesia, or loss of sensation to touch or pain. Anesthetics are useful during unpleasant procedures such as surgery or electrical cardioversion. At low levels of anesthesia, patients may have a decreased sensation of pain but remain conscious. **Neuroleptanesthesia,** a type of anesthesia that combines this effect with amnesia, is useful in procedures that require the patient to remain alert and responsive.

Anesthetics as a group tend to cause respiratory, central nervous system (CNS), and cardiovascular depression. Different agents affect these systems to different degrees and are typically chosen for their ability to produce the desired effect with minimal side effects. Anesthetic agents are rarely used singly; rather, several different agents are typically given together to achieve a balanced anesthetic result. For example, intubating a conscious patient requires his natural gag reflex to be inhibited. Neuromuscular blocking agents such as succinylcholine are used to induce paralysis. Because this would be a terribly frightening and potentially painful procedure, antianxiety, amnesic, and analgesic agents are also given to produce the desired anesthetic effect.

Anesthetics are given either by inhalation or injection. The gaseous anesthetics given by inhalation include halothane, enflurane, and nitrous oxide. The first clinically useful anesthetic was ether, a gas. Its discovery marked a new generation in surgical care, but it is very flammable. The modern gaseous anesthetics are much less volatile, while still decreasing consciousness and sensation as required. These drugs, by some as yet unidentified mechanism, hyperpolarize neural membranes, making depolarization more difficult. This decreases the firing rates of neural impulses and, therefore, the propagation of action potentials through the nervous system, thus reducing sensation. These effects appear to depend upon the gases' solubility. The rate of onset of anesthesia further depends on several additional factors including cardiac output, inhaled concentration of gas, pulmonary minute volume, and end organ perfusion. Because these gases clear mostly through the lungs, respiratory rate and depth affect the duration of their effect. While halothane is the prototype of inhaled anesthetics, nitrous oxide is the only medication in this class with which you are likely to have much involvement.

Most anesthetics used outside the operating room are given intravenously. This gives them a considerably faster onset and shorter duration, making them much more useful in emergency care. Paramedics primarily use these agents to assist with intubation in rapid sequence intubation. They include several pharmacologic classes including ultra-short acting barbiturates (thiopental [Pentothal] and methohexital [Brevital]), benzodiazepines (diazepam [Valium] and midazolam [Versed]), and opioids (fentanyl [Sublimaze], remifentanyl [Ultiva]). We discuss barbiturates' and benzodiazepines' mechanisms of action in the section on antianxiety and sedative-hypnotics.

Anesthetics are also given locally to block sensation for procedures such as suturing and most dentistry. These agents are injected into the skin around the nerves that

anesthetic *medication that induces a loss of sensation to touch or pain.*

neuroleptanesthesia *anesthesia that combines decreased sensation of pain with amnesia while the patient remains conscious.*

innervate the area of the procedure. They decrease the nerve's ability to depolarize and propagate the impulse from this area to the brain. Cocaine's first clinical use was as a topical anesthetic of the eye in 1884. The current prototype of this class is lidocaine (Xylocaine). It is frequently mixed with epinephrine. The epinephrine causes local vasoconstriction, decreasing bleeding and systemic absorption of the drug.

Antianxiety and Sedative-Hypnotic Drugs

sedation *state of decreased anxiety and inhibitions.*

hypnosis *instigation of sleep.*

Antianxiety and sedative-hypnotic drugs are generally used to decrease anxiety, induce amnesia, and assist sleeping and as part of a balanced approach to anesthesia. **Sedation** refers to a state of decreased anxiety and inhibitions. **Hypnosis** in this context refers to the instigation of sleep. Sleep may be categorized as either rapid-eye-movement (REM) or non-rapid-eye-movement (non-REM). REM sleep is characterized by rapid eye movements and lack of motor control. Most dreaming is thought to occur during REM sleep. Insomnia, or difficulty sleeping, typically presents with increased latency (the period of time between lying down and going to sleep) or awakening during sleep.

The two main pharmacologic classes within this functional class are benzodiazepines and barbiturates. Alcohol is also in this functional class. Benzodiazepines and barbiturates work in similar ways. Benzodiazepines are frequently prescribed for oral use and are relatively safe and effective for treating general anxiety and insomnia. Barbiturates, which have broader general depressant activities and a higher potential for abuse, are used much less frequently than benzodiazepines. Before the release of benzodiazepines in the 1960s, however, barbiturates were the drug of choice for treating anxiety and insomnia.

Both benzodiazepines and barbiturates hyperpolarize the membrane of central nervous system neurons, which decreases their response to stimuli. Gamma-aminobutyric acid (GABA) is the chief inhibitory neurotransmitter in the central nervous system. GABA receptors are dispersed widely throughout the CNS on proteins that make up chloride ion channels in the cell membrane. When GABA combines with these receptors, the channel "opens" and chloride, which is more prevalent outside of the cell, diffuses through the channel. As chloride is an anion, or negative ion, it makes the inside of the cell more negative than the outside. This hyperpolarizes the membrane and makes it more difficult to depolarize. Depolarization therefore requires a larger stimulus to cause the cell to fire. Both benzodiazepines and barbiturates increase the GABA receptor-chloride ion channel complexes' potential for binding with GABA, and both are dose dependent. At low doses, they decrease anxiety and cause sedation. As the dose increases, they induce sleep (hypnosis) and, at higher doses, anesthesia. Because benzodiazepines only increase the effectiveness of GABA, the amount of GABA present limits their effects. This actually makes benzodiazepines much safer than barbiturates, which at high doses can actually mimic GABA's effects and thus can have unlimited effects. Benzodiazepines and barbiturates are also useful in treating convulsions.

Just as opiates have an antagonist in naloxone (Narcan), benzodiazepines have an antagonist in flumazenil (Romazicon). Flumazenil competitively binds with the benzodiazepine receptors in the GABA receptor-chloride ion channel complex without causing the effects of benzodiazepines. This reverses the sedation from benzodiazepines, but it can occasionally have untoward consequences, specifically if a patient depends upon benzodiazepines for seizure control, is withdrawing from alcohol, or is taking tricyclic antidepressants. In these cases, the patient may develop seizures following the administration of flumazenil.

Antiseizure or Antiepileptic Drugs

Seizures are a state of hyperactivity of either a section of the brain (partial seizure) or all of the brain (generalized seizure). They may or may not be accompanied by convulsions. Therefore, although the medications in this functional class may be called anticonvulsants, they are more appropriately referred to as antiseizure or antiepileptic drugs. The goal of seizure management is to balance eliminating the seizures against the side effects of the medications used to treat them. Controlling seizures is a lifelong process for most patients and requires diligent compliance with medication dosing regimens.

Partial (or focal) seizures erupt from a specific focus and are described in terms of alterations in consciousness or behavior. These may be further divided into simple or complex partial seizures based upon the specific area of the brain in which the focus is located. Complex partial seizures are also known as psychomotor seizures and are characterized by repetitive motions.

Generalized seizures involve both hemispheres of the brain and are described in terms of visible motor activity. Generalized tonic-clonic seizures involve periods of muscle rigidity (tonic stage) followed by spasmodic twitching (clonic stage) and then flaccidity and a gradual return to consciousness (postictal stage). Absence seizures are also generalized but do not have obvious convulsions. They involve brief losses of consciousness that may occur hundreds of times a day. They are also called absence seizures and are treated differently than other types of seizures. Finally, status epilepticus is a life-threatening condition characterized by uninterrupted tonic-clonic seizures lasting more than 30 minutes or by two or more tonic-clonic seizures without an intervening lucid interval. The preferred therapy for each type of seizure differs.

Seizures are treated through several general mechanisms. The most common is direct action on the sodium and calcium ion channels in the neural membranes. Phenytoin (Dilantin) and carbamazepine (Tegretol) both inhibit the influx of sodium into the cell, thus decreasing the cell's ability to depolarize and propagate seizures. Valproic acid and ethosuximide act similarly, but they interact with calcium channels in the hypothalamus, where absence seizures typically begin. These two drugs are particularly useful because they are specific to hyperactive neurons and therefore have few side effects. Other medications such as benzodiazepines and barbiturates interact with the GABA receptor-chloride ion channel complex, as explained in the section on antianxiety and sedative-hypnotic drugs.

Antiseizure medications comprise several pharmacologic classes, including benzodiazepines (diazepam [Valium] and lorazepam (Ativan]), barbiturates (phenobarbitol [Luminal]), hydantoins (phenytoin [Dilantin], fosphenytoin [Cerebyx]), succinimides (ethosuximide [Zarontin]), and miscellaneous medications such as valproic acid (Depakote). Table 9–3 lists the preferred medication for treating each type of seizure.

Central Nervous System Stimulants

Stimulating the central nervous system is desirable in certain circumstances such as fatigue, drowsiness, narcolepsy, obesity, and attention deficit hyperactivity disorder. Broadly, two techniques may accomplish this:

★ Increasing the release or effectiveness of excitatory neurotransmitters

★ Decreasing the release or effectiveness of inhibitory neurotransmitters

The goal of seizure management is to balance eliminating the seizures against the side effects of the medications used to treat them.

Table 9–3	Antiseizure Medications
Type of Seizure	**Drug of Choice**
Partial Seizures	Phenytoin Carbamazepine
Grand Mal	Carbamazepine Phenytoin Phenobarbitol
Absence	Valproic acid Ethosuximide

Within the functional class of CNS stimulants are three pharmacologic classes: amphetamines, methylphenidates, and methylxanthines.

The amphetamines also include methamphetamine and dextroamphetamine. These drugs all increase the release of excitatory neurotransmitters including norepinephrine and dopamine. Norepinephrine is the primary cause of these drugs' effects, which include an increased wakefulness and awareness as well as a decreased appetite. Amphetamines' most common uses, therefore, are treating drowsiness and fatigue and suppressing the appetite. Most of amphetamines' side effects result from overstimulation; they include tachycardia and other dysrhythmias, hypertension, convulsions, insomnia, and occasionally psychoses with hallucinations and agitation. Examples of this class include amphetamine sulfate (the prototype) and Dexedrine.

Methylphenidate, marketed as Ritalin, is the most commonly prescribed drug for attention deficit hyperactivity disorder (ADHD). While it is chemically different than the amphetamines, its pharmacologic mechanism of action is similar. Also, like the amphetamines, it has a high abuse potential and is therefore listed as a Class II controlled substance. While treating hyperactivity with a stimulant may seem odd, it is quite effective. Frequently, the cause of inappropriate behavior in a child with ADHD is his inability to concentrate or focus. Ritalin's stimulant effects increase this ability, and the unwanted behavior often diminishes.

The methylxanthines include caffeine, aminophylline, and theophylline. While caffeine, the prototype drug in this class, has few clinical uses, it is frequently ingested in coffee, colas, and chocolates. Theophylline's relaxing effects on bronchial smooth muscle make it helpful in treating asthma. The methylxanthines' mechanism of action is unclear, but it seems to block adenosine receptors. Adenosine is an endogenous neurotransmitter which is used clinically for certain types of tachycardias. Because methylxanthines block the adenosine receptors, larger than normal doses may be needed to achieve the desired result. This class's side effects are similar to the amphetamines', but they have a much lower potential for abuse and are not controlled drugs.

Psychotherapeutic Medications

Psychotherapeutic medications treat mental dysfunction. Unlike other disease states, we do not thoroughly understand the pathophysiology of mental dysfunction; therefore, we base much of our pharmacologic treatment of these conditions on our limited knowledge and on clinical correlation (scientific observation that these medications are indeed effective, even if we do not fully understand their mechanism). Medications are typically only one tactic in a balanced strategy for treating mental illness. Depending on the specific disorder, physicians will use other treatments such as psychotherapy and electroconvulsive therapy in conjunction with pharmaceutical interventions.

While we do not completely understand these diseases' specific pathologies, they seem to involve the monoamine neurotransmitters in the central nervous system. These neurotransmitters (norepinephrine, dopamine, serotonin) have been implicated in the control and regulation of emotions. Imbalances in these neurotransmitters, especially dopamine, appear to be at least involved with, if not responsible for, most mental disease. Regulating these and other excitatory and inhibitory neurotransmitters forms the basis for psychopharmaceutical therapy. Schizophrenia appears to be related to an increased release of dopamine, so treatment is aimed at blocking dopamine receptors. Depression seems to be related to inadequate amounts of these neurotransmitters, so treatment is aimed at increasing their release or duration.

The major diseases treated with psychotherapeutic medications are schizophrenia, depression, and bipolar disorder. *The Diagnostic and Statistical Manual,* fourth edition (DSM-IV), published by the American Psychiatric Association, gives schizophrenia's chief characteristics as a lack of contact with reality and disorganized thinking. Its

psychotherapeutic medication *drug used to treat mental dysfunction.*

 Review

Major Diseases Treated with Psychotherapeutic Medications

- Schizophrenia
- Depression
- Bipolar disorder

Content

many different manifestations include delusions, hallucinations (auditory more frequently than visual), disorganized and incoherent speech, and grossly disorganized or catatonic behavior. Schizophrenia is typically treated with antipsychotic medications, frequently in conjunction with medications from other classes such as antianxiety drugs or antidepressants. **Extrapyramidal symptoms** (EPS), a common side effect of antipsychotic medications, include muscle tremors and parkinsonism-like effects. As a result, antipsychotic medications are also known as **neuroleptic** (literally, *affecting the nerves*) drugs.

The two chief pharmaceutical classes of antipsychotics and neuroleptics are phenothiazines and butyrophenones. Both have been mainstays of psychiatry since the mid-1950s and are considered traditional antipsychotic drugs. Medications in this group block dopamine, muscarinic acetylcholine, histamine, and alpha₁ adrenergic receptors in the central nervous system. These medications' therapeutic effects appear to come from blocking the dopamine receptors; their side effects are fairly well understood to originate in blocking the other receptors. The phenothiazines' and butyrophenones' mechanisms of action are the same; they differ only in potency and pharmacokinetics. The distinction between potency and strength is important. Strength refers to the drug's concentration, while potency is the amount of drug necessary to produce the desired effect. While the phenothiazines are considered low-potency and the butyrophenones are considered high-potency, they both produce the same effect. The differences in potency and pharmacokinetics determine which class of medication will be prescribed. Chlorpromazine (Thorazine) is the prototype phenothiazine; haloperidol (Haldol) is the prototype of the butyrophenones.

Since the phenothiazines' and the butyrophenones' mechanisms of action are identical, their common side effects are also similar: extrapyramidal symptoms from cholinergic blockade in the basal ganglia of the cerebral hemispheres; orthostatic hypotension from blockage of alpha₁ adrenergic receptors; sedation; and sexual dysfunction. Treatment for these side effects typically involves modifying the drug dose. Diphenhydramine (Benadryl), an antihistamine with anticholinergic properties, is indicated for treating acute dystonic reactions (manifestations of EPS), which often present with tongue and neck spasm. Patients with a newly prescribed antipsychotic may experience these effects and contact EMS. Fortunately, treatment with diphenhydramine is effective and rapid. Orthostatic hypotension is treated in the usual fashion described in the chapter on hemorrhage and shock, Volume 4, Chapter 4.

Other medications used to treat psychotic conditions are considered atypical antipsychotics. While their mechanisms of action are similar to those of the traditional antipsychotics, the atypical antipsychotics block more specific receptors. This specificity allows them to function much like traditional antipsychotics, but without causing the prominent extrapyramidal symptoms. These drugs include clozapine (Clozaril), risperidone (Risperdal), ziprasidone (Geodon), and olanzapine (Zyprexa).

Another functional class of psychotherapeutic medications includes the antidepressants. The DSM-IV characterizes major depressive episodes as causing significantly depressed mood, loss of interest in things that normally give the patient pleasure, weight loss or gain, sleeping disturbances, suicide attempts, feelings of hopelessness and helplessness, loss of energy, agitation or withdrawal, and an inability to concentrate. While the specific pathology of this disease is not yet known, it appears to be related to an insufficiency of monoamine neurotransmitters (norepinephrine and serotonin). Thus, the pharmaceutical interventions for this disease appear to increase the number of neurotransmitters released in the brain. The several ways of doing this include increasing the amount of neurotransmitter produced in the presynaptic terminal, increasing the amount of neurotransmitter released from the presynaptic terminal, and blocking the neurotransmitter's reuptake (reabsorption by the presynaptic terminal). This results in a net increase in the neurotransmitter. The antidepressants comprise

extrapyramidal symptoms (EPS) *common side effects of antipsychotic medications, including muscle tremors and parkinsonism-like effects.*

neuroleptic *antipsychotic (literally, affecting the nerves).*

 Review

Content

Major Classes of Antipsychotic Medications

- Phenothiazines
- Butyrophenones
- Atypicals

Be alert for the development of extrapyramidal symptoms any time you administer a phenothiazine.

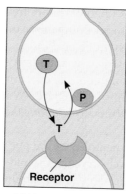
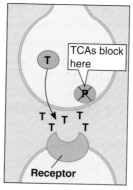

(a) Neurotransmission
without TCA

(b) Neurotransmission
with TCA

three pharmacologic classes: tricyclic antidepressants, selective serotonin reuptake inhibitors, and monoamine oxidase inhibitors.

Tricyclic antidepressants (TCAs) are frequently used in treating depression because they are effective, relatively safe, and have few significant side effects when taken in therapeutic dosages. TCAs act by blocking the reuptake of norepinephrine and serotonin, thus extending the duration of their action (Figure 9-4 ■). Unfortunately, they also have anticholinergic properties that cause many side effects including blurred vision, dry mouth, urinary retention, and tachycardia. Another frequent side effect, orthostatic hypotension, is likely due to the alpha$_1$ adrenergic blockade. This is commonly seen when patients try to stand up too quickly and become dizzy. Additionally, because TCAs can lower the seizure threshold, patients with existing seizure disorders are at risk for convulsions. Unfortunately, when taken in overdose, TCAs can have very significant cardiotoxic effects that make them a favored means of attempting suicide among depressed patients. These effects include myocardial infarction and dysrhythmias. Partly because of this potential for overdose, TCAs have fallen behind the newer selective serotonin reuptake inhibitors as the drug of choice for depression. Overdoses of these medications also frequently cause marked hypotension. Treatment of TCA overdoses is primarily supportive, with sodium bicarbonate given to increase the excretion of TCAs by alkalanizing the urine. The prototype tricyclic antidepressant, imipramine (Tofranil), was also the first one on the market. Other common examples include amitriptyline (Elavil), desipramine (Norpramin), and nortriptyline (Pamelor).

Selective serotonin reuptake inhibitors (SSRIs) are a recent addition to the antidepressants. The prototype, fluoxetine (Prozac), is the most widely prescribed antidepressant in the United States. These drugs' antidepressant effects are comparable to the TCAs', but because the SSRIs selectively block the reuptake of serotonin, they do not affect dopamine or norepinephrine. Nor do they block histaminic or cholinergic receptors, thus avoiding many of the TCAs' side effects. The primary adverse reactions to SSRIs are sexual dysfunction, headache, and nausea. Other selective serotonin reuptake inhibitors include sertraline (Zoloft) and paroxetine (Paxil).

A third pharmacologic class of psychotherapeutic medications includes the monoamine oxidase inhibitors (MAOIs). The monoamine neurotransmitters are thought to be insufficient in depression. Monoamine oxidase, an enzyme, metabolizes monoamines into inactive metabolites. MAOIs inhibit monoamine oxidase and block the monoamines' breakdown, thus increasing their availability. Monoamine oxidase is also present in the liver and has a significant role in metabolizing foods that contain tyramine, a substance that increases the release of norepinephrine. The MAOIs' major side effect is hypertensive crisis brought on by the consumption of foods rich in tyramine such as cheese and red wine. By inhibiting monoamine oxidase, these drugs also decrease the body's ability to inactivate tyramine; they therefore promote the release of norepinephrine, a potent vasopressor. Because of this and other unwanted side effects, MAOIs are not commonly used anymore; rather, they are reserved for treating depression that is refractory to TCAs and SSRIs. The prototype of this class is phenelzine (Nardil).

Patients with bipolar disorder (manic depression) exhibit cyclic swings from mania to depression with periods of normalcy in between. According to the DSM-IV the manic phases of this disease are characterized by hyperactivity, thoughts of grandeur or inflated self-esteem, decreased need for sleep, increased goal-oriented behavior, increased productivity, flight of ideas (moving from thought to thought with little connection between them), distractibility, and increased risk taking. Lithium is the drug of choice for the management of bipolar disorder. It is frequently given in conjunction with benzodiazepines or antipsychotics. Lithium's mechanism of action is unknown, but it effectively decreases the signs of mania without causing sedation. Adverse reactions include headache, dizziness, fatigue, nausea, and vomiting. Recently, two anti-seizure medications—carbamazepine (Tegretol) and valproic acid (Depakote)—have proven successful in treating bipolar disorder.

Lithium, widely used in the treatment of bipolar disorder, has a very low therapeutic index.

Drugs Used to Treat Parkinson's Disease

Parkinson's disease is a nervous disorder caused by the destruction of dopamine-releasing neurons in the *substantia nigra*, a part of the basal ganglia, which is a specialized area of the brain involved in controlling fine movements. Dysfunction of parts of the basal ganglia causes the extrapyramidal symptoms (EPS) often seen as a side effect of antipsychotic medications.

Parkinson's disease is characterized by dyskinesia (dysfunctional movements) such as involuntary tremors, unsteady gait, and postural instability. Severe cases also involve bradykinesia (slow movements) and akinesia (the absence of movement). In the later stages, patients frequently present with psychological impairment including dementia, depression, and impaired memory. Parkinson's is a progressive disease that usually begins in middle age with subtle signs and progresses to a state of incapacitation. While no treatments can cure Parkinson's or even slow its progression, treating the symptoms can return some function to the patient. The goal in treating these patients is to restore their ability to function without causing unacceptable side effects. Some remarkably effective drugs are available. Unfortunately, they usually are effective for only several years. After that, signs and symptoms return and often are more severe than before treatment began.

The medications that are effective in treating Parkinson's disease are also effective in treating the extrapyramidal side effects (EPS) of antipsychotics. This is because fine motor control is based in part on a balance between inhibitory and excitatory neurotransmitters. In the basal ganglia, dopamine, an inhibitory transmitter, opposes acetylcholine, an excitatory neurotransmitter. Parkinson's disease and the medications that cause EPS both decrease the number of presynaptic terminals that release dopamine in the basal ganglia. This allows the excitatory stimulus of acetylcholine to dominate, ultimately impeding fine motor control.

Pharmacologic therapy for Parkinson's disease seeks to restore the balance of dopamine and acetylcholine. This may be done either by increasing the stimulation of dopamine receptors or by decreasing the stimulation of acetylcholine receptors. Drugs can do this either through dopaminergic effects or through anticholinergic effects. Dopaminergic effects increase the release of dopamine from the neuron, directly stimulate the dopamine receptors, or decrease the breakdown of however much dopamine is being released. Anticholinergic effects prevent acetylcholine's effects either by reducing the amount of the neurotransmitter released or by directly blocking the acetylcholine receptors.

Dopamine cannot be given directly to Parkinson's disease patients because it cannot cross the blood–brain barrier and consequently would be ineffective in treating the disease while still causing many side effects. The drug of choice in treating Parkinson's disease, therefore, is levodopa, an inactive drug that readily crosses the blood–brain barrier. Levodopa is absorbed by the dopamine-releasing neuron terminals, where the enzyme decarboxylase metabolizes it into dopamine, thus increasing the amount of dopamine available for release. Levodopa is very effective and reduces symptoms in the vast majority of patients. As previously mentioned, however, symptoms will return within a period of years as the disease progresses. Levodopa's side effects include nausea, vomiting, and ironically, for unknown reasons, dyskinesias. Because it is converted to dopamine, levodopa may also have cardiovascular effects, including tachycardias and hypertension.

When given alone, levodopa is metabolized primarily outside of the brain, where it is ineffective. To prevent this, Sinemet, the most popular anti-Parkinson preparation available, combines levodopa with an inactive ingredient, carbidopa. While carbidopa by itself produces no effects, it prevents levodopa's conversion into dopamine in the periphery. Because carbidopa does not cross the blood–brain barrier, however, levodopa can still be metabolized in the CNS. This decreases the incidence of cardiovascular side effects and enables lower doses of levodopa to be effective. Sinemet's side effects are essentially those of levodopa by itself. Nausea and vomiting, stimulated from within the CNS, remain problematic.

Another dopaminergic medication, amantadine (Symmetrel), promotes the release of dopamine from those dopamine-releasing neurons that remain unaffected by the disease. It has a rapid onset but generally becomes ineffective in less than a year. While it can be effective alone, it is usually given in conjunction with Sinemet or levodopa. Several other medications such as bromocriptine directly stimulate the dopamine receptors instead of attempting to increase the amount of dopamine released.

One additional dopaminergic approach is to decrease the breakdown of dopamine after it has been released. The enzyme responsible for breaking down monoamines such as norepinephrine, dopamine, and serotonin is monoamine oxidase. (We have previously described monoamine oxidase inhibitors in our discussion of their role in depression.) One monoamine oxidase inhibitor, selegiline (Carbex), is specific for monoamine oxidase type B. This MAO-B enzyme is involved only in the breakdown of dopamine. (MAO-A is responsible for breaking down norepinephrine and serotonin.) By selectively inhibiting the breakdown of dopamine, selegiline increases the amount available for binding with dopamine receptors, thus promoting the dopamine-acetylcholine balance. This selective blockage avoids increased norepinephrine levels that can lead to undesired tachycardia and hypertension.

As opposed to dopaminergic medications, which act on the dopamine side of the dopamine-acetylcholine balance, anticholinergic medications act on the acetylcholine side to block the acetylcholine receptors. The prototype anticholinergic, atropine, was initially used in this context with success, but it also had the typical peripheral anticholinergic side effects of blurred vision, dry mouth, and urinary hesitancy. More recently developed medications affect the CNS more than they do the peripheral nervous system. The prototype centrally acting anticholinergic medication is benztropine (Cogentin). Another example is diphenhydramine (Benadryl), which is more frequently administered for its antihistaminic properties.

AUTONOMIC NERVOUS SYSTEM MEDICATIONS

autonomic nervous system
the part of the nervous system that controls involuntary actions.

The **autonomic nervous system** is the part of the nervous system that controls involuntary (automatic) actions. Many medications used in prehospital care directly affect the autonomic nervous system. It is essential that you have a good understanding of this aspect of the nervous system and the ways in which emergency medications affect it.

The two functional divisions of the autonomic nervous system are the sympathetic nervous system and the parasympathetic nervous system. The sympathetic nervous system allows the body to function under stress. It is often referred to as the fight-or-flight aspect of the nervous system. The parasympathetic nervous system, however, primarily controls vegetative functions such as digestion of food. It is often referred to as the feed-or-breed or the rest-and-repose aspect of the nervous system. The parasympathetic nervous system and the sympathetic nervous system work in constant opposition to control organ responses. For example, the sympathetic nervous system stimulates specific receptors in the heart that increase the heart rate. At the same time, the parasympathetic nervous system stimulates specific receptors that decrease the heart rate. The net result is the resting heart rate. When the body's physiologic needs dictate an increased heart rate, the sympathetic stimuli dominate the parasympathetic effects. Conversely, when the body needs to rest (with a decreased heart rate), the parasympathetic stimuli predominate.

Basic Anatomy and Physiology

The autonomic nervous system arises from the central nervous system. The nerves of the autonomic nervous system exit the central nervous system and subsequently enter specialized structures called **autonomic ganglia.** In the autonomic ganglia, the nerve fibers from the central nervous system interact with nerve fibers that extend from the ganglia to the various target organs. Autonomic nerve fibers that exit the central nervous system and terminate in the autonomic ganglia are called **preganglionic nerves.** Autonomic nerve fibers that exit the ganglia and terminate in the various target tissues are called **postganglionic nerves.** The ganglia of the sympathetic nervous system are located close to the spinal cord, while the ganglia of the parasympathetic nervous system are located close to the target organs (Figure 9-5).

No actual physical connection exists between two nerve cells or between a nerve cell and the organ it innervates. Instead, there is a space, or **synapse,** between nerve cells. The space between a nerve cell and the target organ is a **neuroeffector junction.** Specialized chemicals called **neurotransmitters** conduct the nervous impulse between nerve cells or between a nerve cell and its target organ.

Neurotransmitters are released from presynaptic **neurons** and subsequently act on postsynaptic neurons or on the designated target organ. When released by the nerve ending, the neurotransmitter travels across the synapse and activates membrane receptors on the adjoining nerve or target tissue. The neurotransmitter is then either deactivated or taken back up into the presynaptic neuron.

The two neurotransmitters of the autonomic nervous system are acetylcholine and norepinephrine. Acetylcholine is utilized in the preganglionic nerves of the sympathetic nervous system and in both the preganglionic and postganglionic nerves of the parasympathetic nervous system. Norepinephrine is the postganglionic neurotransmitter of the sympathetic nervous system. Synapses that use acetylcholine as the neurotransmitter are **cholinergic** synapses. Synapses that use norepinephrine as the neurotransmitter are **adrenergic** synapses.

Drugs Used to Affect the Parasympathetic Nervous System

The parasympathetic nervous system arises from the brain stem and the sacral segments of the spinal cord. The preganglionic neurons of the parasympathetic nervous system are typically much longer than those of the sympathetic nervous system, because the ganglia are located close to the target tissues. Parasympathetic nerve fibers that leave the brain stem travel within four of the cranial nerves including the oculomotor nerve (III), the facial nerve (VII), the glosso-pharyngeal nerve (IX), and the vagus nerve (X). These fibers synapse in the parasympathetic ganglia with short postganglionic fibers that then continue to their target tissues. Postsynaptic fibers innervate much of the body, including the intrinsic eye muscles, the salivary glands, the

autonomic ganglia *groups of autonomic nerve cells located outside the central nervous system.*

preganglionic nerves *nerve fibers that extend from the central nervous system to the autonomic ganglia.*

postganglionic nerves *nerve fibers that extend from the autonomic ganglia to the target tissues.*

synapse *space between nerve cells.*

neuroeffector junction *specialized synapse between a nerve cell and the organ or tissue it innervates.*

neurotransmitter *chemical messenger that conducts a nervous impulse across a synapse.*

neuron *nerve cell.*

cholinergic *pertaining to the neurotransmitter acetylcholine.*

adrenergic *pertaining to the neurotransmitter norepinephrine.*

✓ Review

Content

Cranial Nerves Carrying Parasympathetic Fibers

- III
- VII
- IX
- X

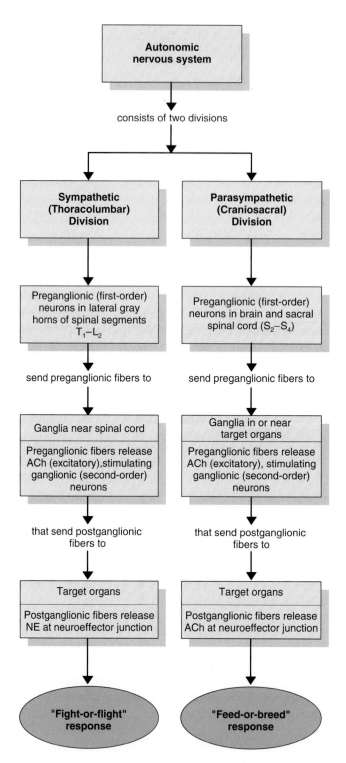

heart, the lungs, and most of the organs of the abdominal cavity. The sacral segment of
the parasympathetic nervous system forms distinct pelvic nerves that innervate ganglia
in the kidneys, bladder, sex organs, and the terminal portions of the large intestine
(Figure 9-6 ■). Stimulation of the parasympathetic nervous system results in the following conditions:

★ Pupillary constriction
★ Secretion by digestive glands

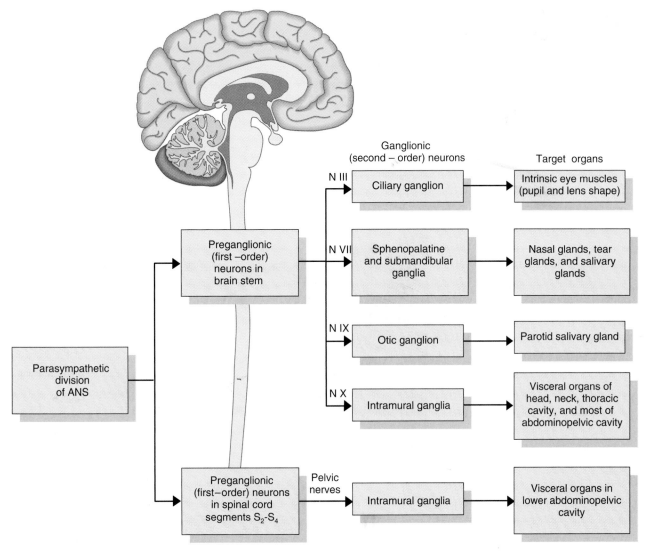

Ganglionic (second – order) neurons

Target organs

N III — Ciliary ganglion → Intrinsic eye muscles (pupil and lens shape)

Preganglionic (first –order) neurons in brain stem

N VII — Sphenopalatine and submandibular ganglia → Nasal glands, tear glands, and salivary glands

N IX — Otic ganglion → Parotid salivary gland

N X — Intramural ganglia → Visceral organs of head, neck, thoracic cavity, and most of abdominopelvic cavity

Parasympathetic division of ANS

Preganglionic (first–order) neurons in spinal cord segments S_2-S_4

Pelvic nerves — Intramural ganglia → Visceral organs in lower abdominopelvic cavity

■ **Figure 9-6** Organization of the parasympathetic division of the autonomic nervous system.

- ★ Reduction in heart rate and cardiac contractile force
- ★ Bronchoconstriction
- ★ Increased smooth muscle activity along the digestive tract

These and other functions facilitate the processing of food, energy absorption, relaxation, and reproduction (Figure 9-7 ■).

All preganglionic and postganglionic parasympathetic nerve fibers use acetylcholine as a neurotransmitter. Acetylcholine, when released by presynaptic neurons, crosses the synaptic cleft and activates receptors on the postsynaptic neurons or on the neuroeffector junction. Acetylcholine is also the neurotransmitter for the somatic nervous system and is present in the neuromuscular junction. Acetylcholine is very short-lived. Within a fraction of a second after its release, it is deactivated by another chemical called acetylcholinesterase. Acetic acid and choline, which are produced when acetylcholine is deactivated, are taken back up by the presynaptic neuron (Figure 9-8 ■).

The parasympathetic system has two main types of ACh receptors, nicotinic and muscarinic. Knowing these receptors' locations and functions will greatly simplify learning the functions of drugs in this class. Nicotinic$_N$ (neuron) receptors are found in

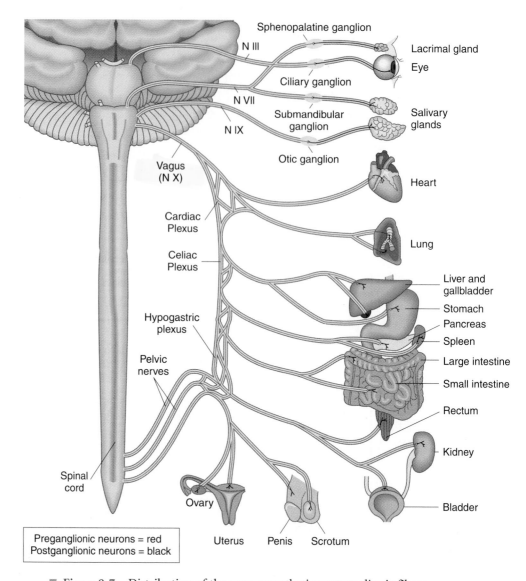

■ Figure 9-7   Distribution of the parasympathetic postganglionic fibers.

all autonomic ganglia, where acetylcholine serves as the presynaptic neurotransmitter of both the parasympathetic and sympathetic nervous systems. Nicotinic$_M$ (muscle) receptors are found at the neuromuscular junction and initiate muscular contraction as part of the somatic nervous system. Muscarinic receptors are found in many organs throughout the body and are primarily responsible for promoting the parasympathetic response. Table 9–4 summarizes the locations and actions of the muscarinic receptors.

Because both nicotinic and muscarinic receptors are specialized for acetylcholine, they are termed cholinergic receptors. Medications that stimulate them are known as cholinergics (**parasympathomimetics**), and those that block them are known as anticholinergics or cholinergic blockers (**parasympatholytics**).

Cholinergics   Cholinergic drugs act either directly or indirectly. Direct-acting cholinergics (also called cholinergic esters) simulate the effects of ACh by directly binding with the cholinergic receptors. Drugs in this class generally produce the same effects as cholinergic stimulation, mostly focused on the muscarinic receptors. Their adverse effects are related primarily to decreased heart rate, decreased peripheral

parasympathomimetic *drug or other substance that causes effects like those of the parasympathetic nervous system (also called* cholinergic).

parasympatholytic *drug or other substance that blocks or inhibits the actions of the parasympathetic nervous system (also called* anticholinergic).

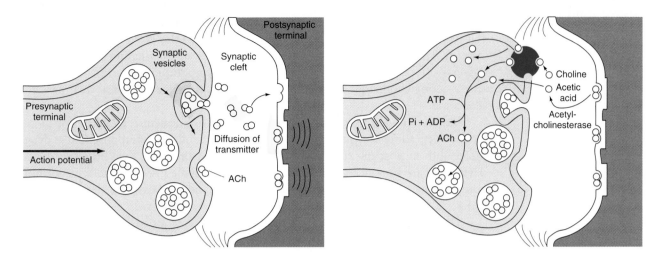

■ Figure 9-8   Physiology of a cholinergic synapse. Acetylcholine is released from the presynaptic nerve and stimulates receptors on the postsynaptic nerve. Subsequently, acetylcholinesterase breaks down the acetylcholine and the presynaptic nerve fiber takes up the products.

Table 9–4	Location and Effect of Muscarinic Receptors	
Organ	**Functions**	**Location**
Heart	Decreased heart rate	Sinoatrial node
	Decreased conduction rate	Atrioventricular node
Arterioles	Dilation	Coronary
	Dilation	Skin and mucosa
	Dilation	Cerebral
GI tract	Relaxed	Sphincters
	Increased motility	
	Increased salivation	Salivary glands
	Increased secretion	Exocrine glands
Lungs	Bronchoconstriction	Bronchiole smooth muscle
	Increased mucus production	Bronchial glands
Gallbladder	Contraction	
Urinary bladder	Relaxation	Urinary sphincter
	Contraction	Detrusor muscle
Liver	Glycogen synthesis	
Lacrimal glands	Secretion (increased tearing)	Eye
Eye	Contraction for near vision	Ciliary muscle
	Constriction	Pupil
Penis	Erection	

vascular resistance resulting in hypotension and excessive salivation, urination, defecation, and sweating. Vomiting and abdominal cramps may also occur. The acronym SLUDGE (*s*alivation, *l*acrimation, *u*rination, *d*efecation, *g*astric motility, *e*mesis) is helpful for remembering these effects.

The prototype direct-acting cholinergic is bethanechol (Urecholine). Its pharmacokinetics make it a good clinical substitute for acetylcholine. It is not broken down by cholinesterase, the enzyme responsible for destroying acetylcholine, and therefore

 Review

Sludge Effects of Cholinergic Medications

- Salivation
- Lacrimation
- Urination
- Defecation
- Gastric motility
- Emesis

Content

it has a longer duration of action. Most of its effects are on muscarinic receptors in the urinary bladder and gastrointestinal tract. It may be given orally or subcutaneously. Thus, it is used primarily to increase micturition (urination) and peristalsis. Adverse effects are rare but related to its parasympathomimetic effects. Another direct-acting cholinergic medication, pilocarpine, is used as a topical treatment for glaucoma.

Indirect-acting cholinergic drugs affect acetylcholinesterase. By inhibiting its actions in degrading acetylcholine, they prolong the cholinergic response. These drugs affect both muscarinic and nicotinic receptors and therefore have little specificity. Their uses are limited primarily to treating myasthenia gravis, some types of poisoning, and glaucoma as well as for reversing nondepolarizing neuromuscular blockade.

The two basic types of indirect-acting cholinergic drugs are reversible inhibitors and irreversible inhibitors. Both types bind with cholinesterase (ChE), acting as a substitute for ACh. In doing so, they prevent ChE from destroying ACh. The difference between the reversible and irreversible inhibitors is how long they remain bound with cholinesterase. The reversible inhibitors remain bound with cholinesterase much longer than acetylcholine but eventually release it. The irreversible inhibitors, too, will eventually release cholinesterase, but they remain bound for so long that, from a practical standpoint, they can be considered irreversible.

Neostigmine (Prostigmin) is the prototype reversible cholinesterase inhibitor. It is used to treat myasthenia gravis, an illness characterized by muscle weakness and progressive fatigue. This illness is an autoimmune disease that destroys the nicotinic$_M$ receptors at the neuromuscular junction. With fewer of these receptors, muscles cannot be stimulated as well and weakness occurs. Neostigmine treats the symptoms of myasthenia gravis by blocking the degradation of ACh, thereby prolonging its effects and increasing motor strength. Its primary side effects are due to the stimulation of muscarinic receptors and include the SLUDGE responses. Fortunately, these responses may be treated effectively with a cholinergic blocker. Neostigmine can also reverse a nondepolarizing neuromuscular blockade. This use is fairly uncommon, however, because such blockades typically are administered only intentionally as part of anesthesia or before intubation.

Physostigmine (Antilirium) is another reversible cholinesterase inhibitor. Its mechanism is similar to neostigmine's, with their primary difference being in their pharmacokinetics. While neostigmine is poorly absorbed across the cell membrane, physostigmine crosses rapidly and therefore has a shorter onset and may be given in lower doses. Physostigmine's chief use is for reversing overdoses of atropine, an anticholinergic drug that blocks muscarinic receptors.

Irreversible cholinesterase inhibitors have only one clinical function, the treatment of glaucoma, and only one drug, echothiophate (Phospholine Iodide), has been approved for that purpose. Cholinesterase inhibitors, however, are very useful as insecticides (organophosphates), and unfortunately, their mechanism of action is also very attractive for makers of chemical weapons. They are the chief component in nerve gases such as VX and sarin. They cause extensive stimulation of cholinergic receptors, ultimately resulting in the SLUDGE response. Toxic levels may also affect nicotinic$_M$ receptors, leading to paralysis. Treatment for such toxic exposures involves drugs such as high doses of atropine or pralidoxime (Protopam, 2-PAM) to block the effects of the accumulating acetylcholine. Pralidoxime can encourage irreversible cholinesterase inhibitors to release cholinesterase.

Anticholinergics Anticholinergic agents oppose the parasympathetic (cholinergic) nervous system. Just as there are multiple types of cholinergic receptors, there are multiple classes of cholinergic receptor antagonists. We will discuss agents that selectively block muscarinic and nicotinic receptors as well as nonselective blockers (ganglionic blockers). A special subclass of nicotinic receptors is neuromuscular blocking drugs.

Muscarinic Cholinergic Antagonists Cholinergic antagonists block the effects of acetylcholine almost exclusively at the muscarinic receptors. They are often called anticholinergics or parasympatholytics. They work by competitively binding with muscarinic receptors without stimulating them. As a result, these receptors cannot bind with acetylcholine.

The prototype anticholinergic drug is atropine, which is widely used to block muscarinic receptors and is commonly administered in the field. Found in the plant *Atropa belladonna*, atropine is one of several drugs classified as belladonna alkaloids (scopolamine is also in this classification). Readily absorbed through both enteral and parenteral routes, it has therapeutic effects at dose dependent levels at most sites with muscarinic receptors. At low doses, atropine decreases secretion from salivary and bronchial glands as well as from the sympathetically innervated sweat glands. At moderate doses, it increases heart rate and causes mydriasis (dilated pupils) and blurry vision. At higher doses, it decreases gastric motility and stomach acid secretion. Atropine is also useful in reversing overdoses of muscarinic agonists (cholinergics or cholinesterase inhibitors). Its side effects, which are predictable, include dry mouth, blurred vision and photophobia, urinary retention, increased intraocular pressure, tachycardia, constipation, and anhidrosis (decreased sweating), which may cause hyperthermia. A helpful mnemonic for remembering the effects of atropine overdose is "hot as hell, blind as a bat, dry as a bone, red as a beet, mad as a hatter."

Scopolamine is another belladonna anticholinergic. Its actions are similar to atropine's, but unlike atropine, scopolamine causes sedation and antiemesis. Thus, its primary purpose is to prevent motion sickness. It is available as a transdermal patch.

Several synthetic medications mimic the effects of the belladonna alkaloids while minimizing their side effects. Ipratropium bromide (Atrovent), an inhaled anticholinergic, is effective in treating asthma because it relaxes the bronchial smooth muscle and causes bronchodilation. It is frequently administered along with an inhaled beta-adrenergic agonist. Because it is inhaled and has little systemic effect, ipratropium bromide avoids many of atropine's side effects.

Other anticholinergic drugs include dicyclomine (Bentyl) and benztropine (Cogentin).

Nicotinic Cholinergic Antagonists Nicotinic cholinergic antagonists block acetylcholine only at nicotinic sites. They include ganglionic blocking agents that block the nicotinic$_N$ receptors in the autonomic ganglia and neuromuscular blocking agents that block nicotinic$_M$ receptors at the neuromuscular junction.

Ganglionic Blocking Agents Ganglionic blockade is produced by competitive antagonism with acetylcholine at the nicotinic$_N$ receptors in the autonomic ganglia. This can, in effect, turn off the entire autonomic nervous system. The two drugs in this class are trimethaphan (Arfonad) and mecamylamine (Inversine). Both are used to treat hypertension. The adverse effects of ganglionic blockade include signs associated with antimuscarinic drugs like atropine—dry mouth, blurred vision, urinary retention, and tachycardia. Other adverse effects arising from the vasodilation and decreased preload caused by sympathetic blockage include profound hypotension, with orthostatic hypotension even more evident. Trimethaphan is administered primarily for hypertensive crisis when other treatments are ineffective. These agents are almost never used anymore because they are not selective and many superior agents are available.

Neuromuscular Blocking Agents Neuromuscular blockade produces a state of paralysis without affecting consciousness. Imagine how terrifying it would be to be fully

Review

Types of Parasympathetic Acetylcholine Receptors

Content

- Muscarinic
- Nicotinic
  –Nicotinic$_N$ (neuron)
  –Nicotinic$_M$ (muscle)

Review

Effects of Atropine Overdose

Content

- Hot as hell
- Blind as a bat
- Dry as a bone
- Red as a beet
- Mad as a hatter

conscious and aware but completely paralyzed, unable to move or breathe. Neuromuscular blockade is caused by competitive antagonism of nicotinic$_M$ receptors at the neuromuscular junction. This is useful during surgery as part of anesthesia and during electroconvulsive therapy for depression. These agents are most often used in the field to facilitate intubation.

Neuromuscular blocking agents are either depolarizing or nondepolarizing, depending on their mechanism of action. Most are nondepolarizing; only one depolarizing drug, succinylcholine (Anectine), is commonly used in the clinical setting. Tubocurarine, while not frequently used clinically, is the oldest neuromuscular blocker and the prototype nondepolarizing agent. It produces neuromuscular blockade by binding with the nicotinic$_M$ receptor sites without causing muscle depolarization. Succinylcholine acts in the same manner, but like acetylcholine, it does cause muscle depolarization when it binds with the nicotinic$_M$ receptor. It is useful as a neuromuscular blocker because, in contrast to ACh, which rapidly separates from the receptor, it remains bound, preventing the muscle's repolarization. Several nondepolarizing agents are available; the specific agent chosen depends on its rate of onset and duration of action. Succinylcholine has the shortest onset and duration of action because it has a naturally occurring enzyme, pseudocholinesterase, which degrades it.

Ganglionic Stimulating Agents   Nicotinic$_N$ receptors reside at the ganglia of both the parasympathetic and sympathetic nervous systems. The alkaloid nicotine stimulates these receptors. Nicotine is found in tobacco and, although it has no therapeutic uses, is of interest for two reasons. Historically, nicotine, along with muscarine, led to a much better understanding of the autonomic nervous system's specific receptors. Also it is one of the most abused drugs in the world.

Nicotine may cause a variety of responses, most of which are dose related. At low doses, like those from smoking, nicotine causes excitation at the autonomic ganglia. This affects both the parasympathetic and sympathetic nervous systems. The parasympathetic response causes increased salivation, peristalsis, and secretion of gastric acid. The sympathetic response causes the release of norepinephrine and epinephrine. These lead to increases in heart rate, myocardial contractility, vasoconstriction, and blood pressure, all of which increase the heart's workload. Sympathetic stimulation also increases awareness and suppresses fatigue and appetite.

Nicotine administration devices such as gum and transdermal patches are available for use in smoking cessation. Their actions are similar to the actions of nicotine inhaled in smoke.

Drugs Used to Affect the Sympathetic Nervous System

The sympathetic nervous system arises from the thoracic and lumbar regions of the spinal cord. Preganglionic nerves leave the spinal cord through the spinal nerves and end in the sympathetic ganglia. There are two types of sympathetic ganglia: sympathetic chain ganglia and collateral ganglia (Figure 9-9 ■). In addition, special preganglionic sympathetic nerve fibers innervate the adrenal medulla. Postganglionic nerves that exit the sympathetic chain ganglia extend to several peripheral target tissues of the sympathetic nervous system. When stimulated, these fibers have several effects. They include:

★ Stimulation of secretion by sweat glands

★ Constriction of blood vessels in the skin

★ Increase in blood flow to skeletal muscles

★ Increase in the heart rate and force of cardiac contractions

★ Bronchodilation

★ Stimulation of energy production

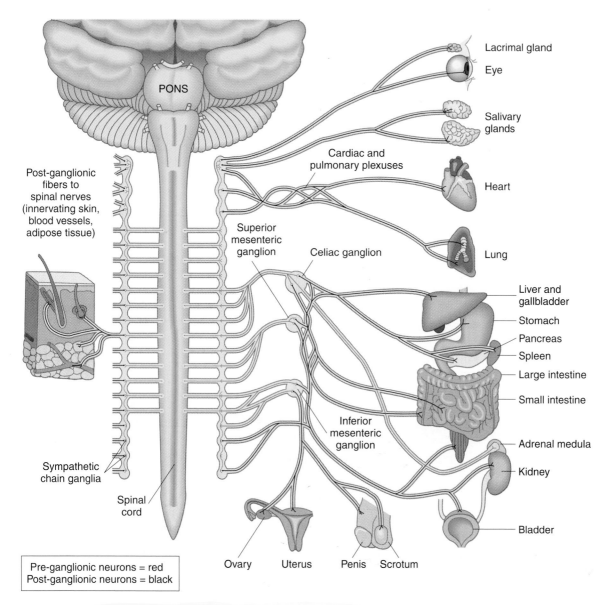

Lacrimal gland

Eye

Salivary glands

Cardiac and pulmonary plexuses

Heart

Lung

Superior mesenteric ganglion

Celiac ganglion

Liver and gallbladder

Stomach

Pancreas

Spleen

Large intestine

Small intestine

Inferior mesenteric ganglion

Adrenal medulla

Kidney

Bladder

Ovary   Uterus   Penis   Scrotum

PONS

Post-ganglionic fibers to spinal nerves (innervating skin, blood vessels, adipose tissue)

Sympathetic chain ganglia

Spinal cord

Pre-ganglionic neurons = red
Post-ganglionic neurons = black

■ Figure 9-9   Distribution of sympathetic postganglionic fibers.

The collateral ganglia are located in the abdominal cavity. Nerves leaving the collateral ganglia innervate many of the organs of the abdomen. Stimulation of these fibers causes several conditions. They include:

★ Reduction of blood flow to abdominal organs
★ Decreased digestive activity
★ Relaxation of smooth muscle in the wall of the urinary bladder
★ Release of glucose stores from the liver

Sympathetic nervous system stimulation also results in direct stimulation of the adrenal medulla, the inner portion of the adrenal gland (Figure 9-10 ■). The adrenal medulla in turn releases the hormones norepinephrine (noradrenalin) and epinephrine (adrenalin) into the circulatory system. Approximately 80 percent of the hormones released by the adrenal medulla are epinephrine, while norepinephrine constitutes the remaining 20 percent. Once released, these hormones are carried throughout the body where

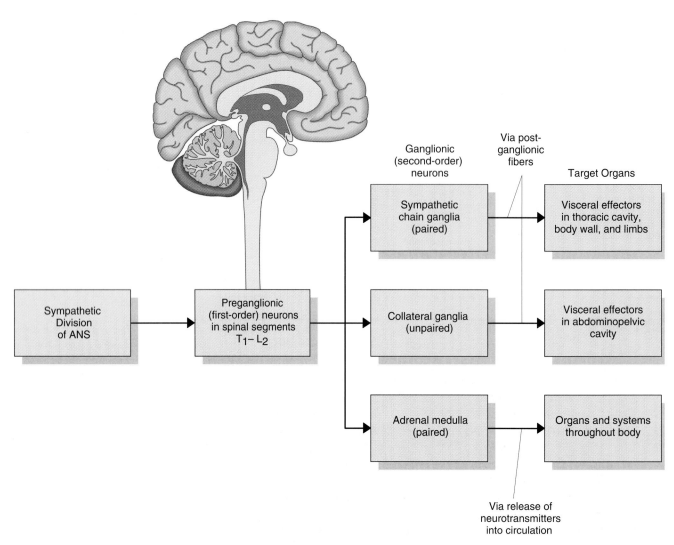

Via post-
ganglionic
fibers

Ganglionic
(second-order)
neurons

Target Organs

Sympathetic
chain ganglia
(paired)

Visceral effectors
in thoracic cavity,
body wall, and limbs

Sympathetic
Division
of ANS

Preganglionic
(first-order) neurons
in spinal segments
$T_1 - L_2$

Collateral ganglia
(unpaired)

Visceral effectors
in abdominopelvic
cavity

Adrenal medulla
(paired)

Organs and systems
throughout body

Via release of
neurotransmitters
into circulation

■ Figure 9-10   Organization of the sympathetic division of the autonomic nervous system.

they cause their intended effects by acting on hormone receptors. The release of norepinephrine and epinephrine by the adrenal medulla stimulates tissues that are not innervated by sympathetic nerves. In addition, it prolongs the effects of direct sympathetic stimulation. All of these effects serve to prepare the body to deal with stressful and potentially dangerous situations.

Adrenergic Receptors   Sympathetic stimulation ultimately results in the release of the hormone norepinephrine from postganglionic nerves. The norepinephrine subsequently crosses the synaptic cleft and interacts with adrenergic receptors on the postsynaptic nerves. Shortly thereafter, the norepinephrine is either taken up by the presynaptic neuron for reuse or broken down by enzymes present within the synapse (Figure 9-11 ■). Sympathetic stimulation also results in the release of the hormones epinephrine and norepinephrine from the adrenal medulla. In addition, both epinephrine and norepinephrine interact with specialized adrenergic receptors on the membranes of the target organs. These receptors are located throughout the body. Once stimulated by the appropriate hormone, they cause a response in the organ or organs they control.

 Review

Content

Types of Sympathetic Receptors

- Adrenergic
  –alpha$_1$ (α_1)
  –alpha$_2$ (α_2)
  –beta$_1$ (β_1)
  –beta$_2$ (β_2)
- Dopaminergic

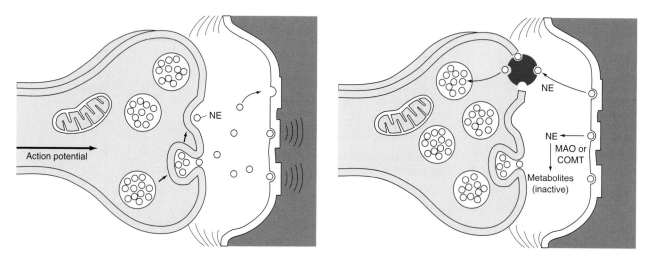

■ Figure 9-11   Physiology of an adrenergic synapse. Norepinephrine is released from the presynaptic nerve and stimulates receptors on the postsynaptic nerve. Subsequently, the norepinephrine is either taken up by the presynaptic nerve or deactivated by enzymes in the synapse.

The two known types of sympathetic receptors are the adrenergic receptors and the dopaminergic receptors. The adrenergic receptors are generally divided into four types. These four receptors are designated alpha 1 (α_1), alpha 2 (α_2), beta 1 (β_1), and beta 2 (β_2). The alpha$_1$ receptors cause peripheral vasoconstriction, mild bronchoconstriction, and stimulation of metabolism. The alpha$_2$ receptors are found on the presynaptic surfaces of sympathetic neuroeffector junctions. Stimulation of alpha$_2$ receptors is inhibitory. These receptors serve to prevent overrelease of norepinephrine in the synapse. When the level of norepinephrine in the synapse gets high enough, the alpha$_2$ receptors are stimulated and norepinephrine release is inhibited. Stimulation of beta$_1$ receptors causes increases in heart rate, cardiac contractile force, and cardiac automaticity and conduction. Stimulation of beta$_2$ receptors causes vasodilation and bronchodilation. Dopaminergic receptors, although not fully understood, evidently cause dilation of the renal, coronary, and cerebral arteries.

Medications that stimulate the sympathetic nervous system are **sympathomimetics.** Medications that inhibit the sympathetic nervous system are called **sympatholytics.** Some medications are pure alpha agonists, while others are pure alpha antagonists. Some medications are pure beta agonists, while others are pure beta antagonists. Medications such as epinephrine stimulate both alpha and beta receptors. Other medications, such as the bronchodilators, are termed beta selective, since they act more on beta$_2$ receptors than on beta$_1$ receptors.

The sympathetic nervous system releases norepinephrine from postganglionic end terminals and epinephrine from the adrenal medulla. These neurotransmitters bind with adrenergic receptors. (Epinephrine is also called adrenalin because of its release from the adrenal medulla; hence the term *adren*-ergic). There are two main types of adrenergic receptors, each with two subtypes. These receptors' effects depend primarily on their locations. Table 9–5 describes the chief locations and primary actions of each receptor.

The primary clinical purpose for medications that stimulate alpha$_1$ receptors is peripheral vasoconstriction. Constriction of the arterioles increases afterload, while constriction of venules increases preload (decreasing venous capacitance or "pooling"). Both of these effects increase systolic and diastolic blood pressure and represent the chief therapeutic indication for alpha$_1$ agonists. Stimulation of alpha$_1$ receptors locally

sympathomimetic *drug or other substance that causes effects like those of the sympathetic nervous system (also called* adrenergic).

sympatholytic *drug or other substance that blocks the actions of the sympathetic nervous system (also called* antiadrenergic).

Table 9–5	Location of Adrenergic Receptors and Effects of Stimulation	
Receptor	**Response to Stimulation**	**Location**
Alpha 1 (α_1)	Constriction	Arterioles
	Constriction	Veins
	Mydriasis	Eye
	Ejaculation	Penis
Alpha 2 (α_2)	Presynaptic terminals inhibition*	
Beta 1 (β_1)	Increased heart rate	Heart
	Increased conductivity	
	Increased automaticity	
	Increased contractility	
	Renin release	Kidney
Beta 2 (β_2)	Bronchodilation	Lungs
	Dilation	Arterioles
	Inhibition of contractions	Uterus
	Tremors	Skeletal muscle
Dopaminergic	Vasodilation (increased blood flow)	Kidney

*Stimulation of α_2 adrenergic receptors inhibits the continued release of norepinephrine from the presynaptic terminal. It is a feedback mechanism that limits the adrenergic response at that synapse. These receptors have no other identified peripheral effects.

may be useful in combination with local anesthetics. The main reason to add the alpha$_1$ agonist in this context is to cause local vasoconstriction so that the systemic absorption of the anesthetic will decrease, and its duration will increase. Alpha$_1$ agonists are also useful topically to decrease nasal congestion caused by dilation and engorgement of nasal blood vessels. The primary adverse responses to alpha$_1$ agonist agents are hypertension and local tissue necrosis. If a medication with significant alpha$_1$ properties infiltrates the surrounding tissue or distal body parts such as fingers, toes, earlobes, or nose, inadequate local blood flow due to profound vasoconstriction will likely kill the tissue. Also, alpha$_1$ stimulation may cause reflex bradycardia due to the feedback mechanism that regulates blood pressure. As baroreceptors detect a rise in blood pressure, heart rate decreases to compensate.

Alpha$_1$ antagonism is indicated almost exclusively for controlling hypertension. By preventing the peripheral vasoconstriction of alpha$_1$ stimulation, these agents decrease blood pressure. They are also useful in treating local tissue necrosis caused by infiltration of alpha$_1$ agonists. Injecting alpha$_1$ antagonists into the area surrounding the infiltration prevents tissue death from excessive vasoconstriction. The effects of pheochromocytoma, a tumor of the adrenal medulla that causes the release of large amounts of catecholamine, may be treated with an alpha$_1$ blocker. The most common adverse effects of alpha$_1$ antagonism are orthostatic hypotension and reflex tachycardia. Just as alpha$_1$ stimulation may increase blood pressure and cause a baroreceptor-mediated bradycardia, the hypotension from alpha$_1$ blockage may lead to reflex tachycardia from the same mechanism. Other side effects include nasal congestion and inhibition of ejaculation. These agents may also increase blood volume. This is ironic, since their primary indication is hypertension. As another feedback mechanism detects hypotension, the kidneys begin to reabsorb sodium and water to increase blood volume. This is typically addressed by use of a diuretic concomitant with the alpha$_1$ antagonist.

Beta$_1$ stimulation increases heart rate, contractility, and conduction. Its primary indications are cardiac arrest and hypotension resulting from inadequate pumping. During cardiac arrest, beta$_1$ activation may stimulate contractions or increase the force of any existing contractions. Even if the heart is only fibrillating, these agents may increase the effectiveness of electrical defibrillation. In cardiogenic shock, when the heart is not

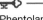

Phentolamine (Regitine), an alpha antagonist, can be used to help minimize tissue necrosis following extravasation of an alpha$_1$ agonist such as dopamine or norepinephrine.

pumping with enough force to overcome the afterload created by peripheral vascular resistance, beta$_1$ agonists can adequately increase the contractions' force. The chief adverse effects of beta$_1$ agonists include tachycardia, dysrhythmias, and chest pain from increasing workload.

Beta$_1$ antagonists are among the most frequently prescribed medications in the United States. Their most common use is to control blood pressure. By blocking the effects of beta$_1$ stimulation, they decrease heart rate (chronotropy) and contractility (inotropy). These agents are also effective in treating supraventricular tachycardias because they decrease the rate of impulse generation at the SA node (negative chronotropic effects) while also slowing conductivity through the AV node (negative dromotropic effects). Blocking beta$_1$ stimulation also helps treat angina pectoris and reduces the recurrence of myocardial infarction. Its main adverse effects are symptomatic bradycardia, hypotension, and AV block.

Beta$_2$ agonists are used to treat asthma and other conditions with excessive narrowing of the bronchioles. By stimulating beta$_2$ receptors in the lungs, these agents relax the bronchial smooth muscle and cause bronchodilation. Beta$_2$ agonists can also cause uterine smooth muscle relaxation, which may help to suppress preterm labor. Their primary adverse effects are muscle tremors and "bleed over" effects on unintended beta$_1$ stimulation such as tachycardias.

While beta$_2$ blockade serves no clinically useful purpose, nonselective beta-blockers have side effects of beta$_2$ blockade. Chief among these is bronchoconstriction and inhibition of glycogenolysis, the release of stored glycogen by the liver and skeletal muscles. Beta$_2$ stimulation causes glycogenesis. Antagonizing the beta$_2$ receptors can inhibit this release. While this is not typically a problem for most people, it can be very problematic for diabetics. It not only makes hypoglycemia more likely but also masks one of its common early warning signs, tachycardia.

Adrenergic Agonists   Drugs that stimulate the effects of adrenergic receptors work either directly, indirectly, or through a combination of the two. The direct-acting agents bind with the receptor and cause the same response as the normal neurotransmitter. In fact, most of the drugs in this category either are synthetically produced versions of the naturally occurring neurotransmitter or are derivatives of those synthetically produced versions. The indirect-acting agents stimulate the release of epinephrine from the adrenal medulla and of norepinephrine from the presynaptic terminals. In turn, the epinephrine and norepinephrine stimulate the adrenergic receptors. The mixed actions of direct-indirect-acting medications combine these mechanisms.

The most frequently used adrenergic agents are chemically and functionally similar to the endogenous neurotransmitters. These drugs, which are called catecholamines, include norepinephrine, epinephrine, and dopamine. Synthetic catecholamines are also available. They include dobutamine and isoproterenol. Noncatecholamine adrenergic agents, including ephedrine, phenylephrine, and terbutaline, also affect the adrenergic receptors and have useful clinical applications.

⊘ **Content** **Review**

Common Catecholamines

- Natural
  - Epinephrine
  - Norepinephrine
  - Dopamine
- Synthetic
  - Isoproterenol
  - Dobutamine

Patho Pearls

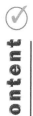

Adrenergic Agonists: Effects of Repeated Doses   Many adrenergic agonists, particularly decongestants and respiratory drugs, can result in tachyphylaxis. That is, repeated doses of the same drug have decreasing effects. In these cases, it may be prudent to change to a similar drug in the same family. The effects of a different drug can often be significantly better.

Table 9–6	Adrenergic Receptor Specificity				
Medication	*Receptor*				
	Alpha$_1$	**Alpha$_2$**	**Beta$_1$**	**Beta$_2$**	**Dopaminergic**
Phenylephrine	✔				
Norepinephrine	✔	✔	✔		
Ephedrine	✔	✔	✔	✔	
Epinephrine	✔	✔	✔	✔	
Dobutamine			✔		
Dopamine*			✔		✔
Isoproterenol			✔	✔	
Terbutaline				✔	

*Receptor specificity is dose dependent. The higher the dose, the less dopaminergic effects are seen.

Almost all of the drugs in this section act on more than one type of receptor. Their specificity varies and is important in determining their uses. Table 9–6 lists their actions on various receptors.

Adrenergic Antagonists   Unlike most adrenergic agonists, the majority of available adrenergic antagonists are remarkably selective in which receptor they affect. This selectivity, however, occurs only at therapeutic doses. At higher doses, most agents lose their selectivity and begin affecting other receptors as well.

The two basic subcategories of alpha adrenergic antagonists are "noncompetitive, long-acting" and "competitive, short-acting." They differ chiefly in the stability of their bond with the receptor. The prototype noncompetitive, long-acting alpha antagonist is phenoxybenzamine (Dibenzyline). The prototype competitive, short-acting antagonist is prazosin (Minipress). Prazosin also is the prototype for all alpha adrenergic antagonists. Phentolamine (Regitine) is an important nonselective alpha antagonist because of its effects in reversing tissue necrosis caused by catecholamine infiltration.

Beta adrenergic antagonists are more commonly referred to as beta-blockers. Propranolol (Inderal) is the prototype beta-blocker. It is a nonselective antagonist, which means that it blocks both beta$_1$ and beta$_2$ receptors. It is used to treat tachycardia, hypertension, and angina, all results of beta$_1$ blockade. Because it is nonselective, it also has the side effects of beta$_2$ blockade—bronchoconstriction and inhibited glycogenolysis. Propranolol was the first clinically employed beta-blocker, but its use has declined since the development of more selective beta$_1$ antagonists. The prototype of these cardioselective beta-blockers is metoprolol (Lopressor). At normal doses, metoprolol is selective for only beta$_1$ receptors; therefore, it does not cause propranolol's problematic side effects for asthmatics and diabetics. Atenolol (Tenormin) is another commonly used cardioselective beta-blocker.

Skeletal Muscle Relaxants   Skeletal muscle relaxants are used to treat muscle spasm from injury and muscle spasticity from CNS injuries or diseases such as multiple sclerosis. Treatment can involve centrally acting agents or direct-acting agents.

The centrally acting muscle relaxants' mechanism is not clear, but it appears to be associated with general sedation. The prototype centrally acting skeletal muscle relaxant is baclofen (Lioresal), which is indicated in the treatment of spasticity. While baclofen is effective in the treatment of muscle spasticity, it is generally ineffective in muscle spasm. Several drugs are effective in treating muscle spasm, including cyclobenzaprine (Flexeril) and carisoprodol (Soma).

The prototype of the direct-acting muscle relaxants is dantrolene (Dantrium). Unlike the centrally acting agents, dantrolene's mechanism is well understood. It decreases the release of calcium from the sarcoplasmic reticulum in response to action potentials propagated from the neuromuscular junction. This calcium is required for the cross-bridge binding of the actin and myosin filaments in the muscle fibers responsible for contraction. Dantrolene is indicated for treating the spasticity associated with multiple sclerosis and cerebral palsy. It is also indicated for treating malignant hyperthermia, which is on rare occasion seen with some anesthetics and succinylcholine. This hyperthermia results from muscular contractions. Since dantrolene decreases these contractions, the heat that they generate also decreases. Dantrolene is not effective in treating muscle spasm.

DRUGS USED TO AFFECT THE CARDIOVASCULAR SYSTEM

Cardiovascular drugs have traditionally comprised one of the largest parts of the paramedic's pharmacologic "tool box." While this is changing with the expansion of paramedic practice, cardiovascular care (and agents used in that care) remains an important and integral part of a paramedic's knowledge base.

CARDIOVASCULAR PHYSIOLOGY REVIEW

To understand cardiovascular pharmacology, you must first understand how electrical conduction and mechanical contraction work together to produce an organized and effective pumping action. We will briefly review the anatomy and physiology of the heart and then discuss the generation of electrical impulses and the creation of dysrhythmias. Then we will discuss how each classification acts on dysrhythmias.

The heart is essentially a two-sided pump. The right side is a low-pressure pump responsible for pulmonary circulation, and the left side is a high-pressure pump responsible for systemic circulation. The human heart has four chambers, two atria and two ventricles. The atria receive blood from the pulmonary and systemic circulation and pass it on to the ventricles, where most of the pumping pressure originates (Figure 9-12 ■). Because the left side of the heart has to generate substantially higher pressures than the right, the left ventricle's muscular wall is much larger than those of the other chambers. The atria accept blood and allow it to pour passively into the ventricles. Just before the ventricles contract, the atria contract to "top off" the volume of blood in the ventricles. After this atrial "kick" fills the ventricles, they contract, forcing blood out of the heart. The myocardial muscle contraction depends upon three factors: (1) electrical stimulation from the conduction system, (2) adequate amounts of ATP (energy), and (3) adequate amounts of the ion calcium. ATP and calcium are both needed for the thin and thick filaments to combine and shorten the muscle. To pump blood effectively, the entire heart must contract in a precise sequence. Both atria contract at the same time from the top down (towards the AV valves). A slight delay allows the ventricles to fill completely with blood, and then both ventricles contract simultaneously from the bottom up (towards the semilunar valves). This entire cycle must repeat itself continually.

Impulse Generation and Conduction

The key to the precise cardiac cycle is the electrical conduction system (Figure 9-13 ■). This system is composed of specialized cardiac tissue that generates electrical impulses and conducts them rapidly throughout the heart to assure the chambers contract in proper sequence. The sinoatrial (SA) node is the heart's dominant pacemaker. It spontaneously generates electrical impulses (action potentials) that are propagated through

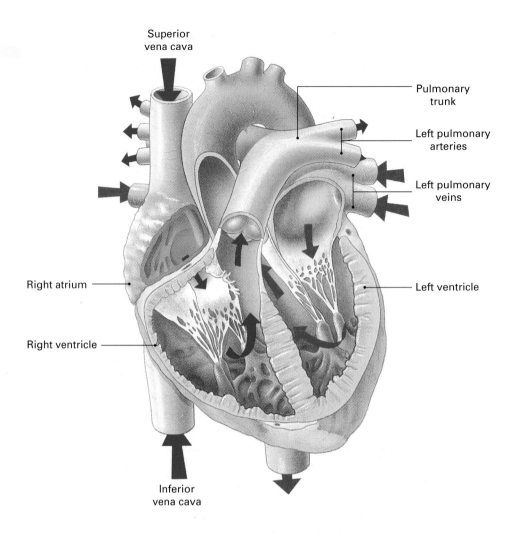

Superior vena cava

Pulmonary trunk

Left pulmonary arteries

Left pulmonary veins

Right atrium

Left ventricle

Right ventricle

Inferior vena cava

■ Figure 9-13   Cardiac conductive system.

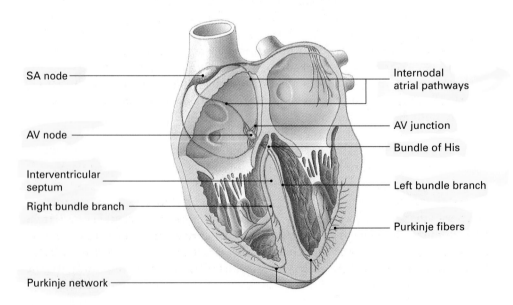

SA node

Internodal atrial pathways

AV node

AV junction

Bundle of His

Interventricular septum

Left bundle branch

Right bundle branch

Purkinje fibers

Purkinje network

intraatrial pathways to the atrioventricular (AV) node, where conduction is delayed momentarily. This delay gives the ventricles time to fill completely. The impulse then travels from the AV node throughout the ventricles via the bundle of His and the Purkinje network.

All myocardial tissue, both contractile and conductive, has the ability to self-generate electrical impulses (automaticity) and to propagate those impulses to surrounding tissue. It does this through the movement of ions across the cell membrane. At rest (when not stimulated), the cell membrane is polarized with a slight electrical charge. This charge is present because there are more positive ions outside the cell than inside, resulting in a slight negative charge on the inside. The primary ions involved are sodium (Na^+) on the outside of the cell and potassium (K^+) on the inside. Calcium (Ca^{++}), which is responsible for muscle contraction, is present in storage vesicles surrounding the cell. These vesicles are called the sarcoplasmic reticulum. The cell membrane is said to depolarize when this charge is eliminated or reversed. When an impulse is generated and conducted to the muscle cells, the process of depolarization and repolarization begins. Figure 9-14 ■ depicts the sequence of ion movements in the depolarization and repolarization of both slow and fast potentials. Fast potentials occur in cardiac muscle tissue as well as in the ventricular conduction system; slow potentials occur in the pacemaker cells of the SA and AV nodes.

Cyclic activity in the fast potentials has five phases. Phase 0, which represents depolarization, results from a rapid influx of Na^+ ions into the cell. This makes the inside of the cell more positive than the outside and is normally caused by the arrival of an impulse generated elsewhere in the heart, such as the SA node. Sodium stops entering the cell once the inside has become positive. Phases 1 through 3 represent repolarization. In phase 1, K^+ begins to leave the cell, slowly returning the cell to its normal negative charge. Phase 2 interrupts with an influx of Ca^{++} into the cell. Remember, the muscles are using calcium inside the cell for contraction. This plateau phase delays repolarization and is important for medications that affect the strength of contraction. Phase 3 is marked by a cessation of calcium influx and the rapid efflux of potassium. Phase 4 is normally a flat stage representing the resting membrane potential. However, in pathologic states, phase 4 may include a slow influx of sodium that will gradually make the inside of the cell more positive. When the interior of the cell reaches a point called its threshold potential, the cell will depolarize without waiting for an impulse. Many antidysrhythmics have their mechanism of action during this phase 4 depolarization.

The slow potentials, while similar to the fast ones, have several important distinctions. First, they are located in the dominant pacemakers of the heart. Second, they depolarize differently. Notice in Figure 9-14 how phase 4 normally exhibits a gradually increasing slope towards threshold potential. While sodium causes depolarization (phase 0) of the fast potentials, a gradual influx of calcium causes it in the slow potentials. The slow potentials normally undergo a gradual, phase 4 depolarization. While we do not know the exact mechanism, this gradual depolarization clearly is responsible for the spontaneous generation of impulses in the SA and AV nodes. While the AV node also has these slow potentials, the SA node's rate of depolarization is faster, making it the heart's dominant pacemaker.

Dysrhythmia Generation

Dysrhythmias are generated at various places in the heart through either abnormal impulse formation (automaticity) or abnormal conductivity. The most prevalent types of dysrhythmias are tachycardia (too fast) and bradycardia (too slow). An imbalance between the sympathetic and parasympathetic nervous systems most often causes these dysrhythmias. Typically, excessive parasympathetic stimulation through muscarinic receptors causes bradycardias, which are treated with anticholinergic medications. Tachycardias, however, have a variety of causes and are treated with the antidysrhythmics we discuss in this section.

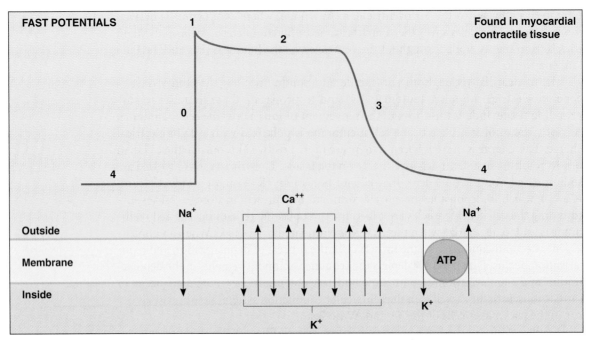

Action potential of cardiac contractile (muscle) tissue depends upon activation of fast sodium channels (opening the gates) via stimulus from pacing cells.

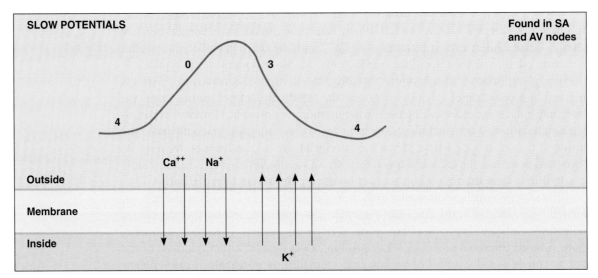

Action potential of cardiac pacing cells slows influx of Ca^{++} (leaking) and, to a lesser extent, Na$^+$ is responsible for automaticity or spontaneous depolarization. Class IV antidysrhythmics inhibit these calcium channels and decrease heart rate.

■ Figure 9-14 Ion movements in the depolarization and repolarization of slow and fast potentials.

As mentioned earlier, fast-potential means of depolarization dominate most of the heart, including the muscle cells and the ventricular conduction system. This process normally does not include a phase 4 depolarization; rather, depolarization most often happens in response to an impulse generated in the SA node and propagated to the cell. In pathologic conditions such as ischemia, myocardial infarction, and excessive sympathetic stimulation, these tissues will develop phase 4 depolarization and generate an impulse abnormally. This abnormal impulse will then be propagated throughout the

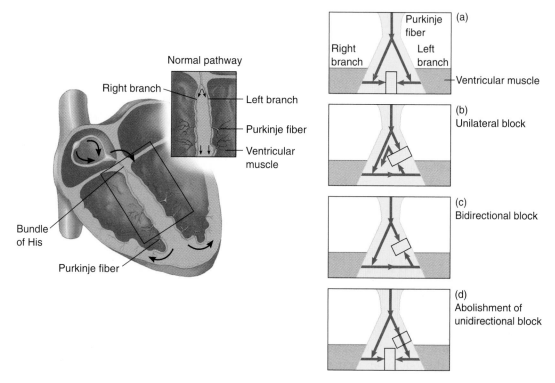

Normal pathway

Right branch
Left branch
Purkinje fiber
Ventricular muscle

Bundle of His

Purkinje fiber

(a) Purkinje fiber — Right branch — Left branch — Ventricular muscle

(b) Unilateral block

(c) Bidirectional block

(d) Abolishment of unidirectional block

■ Figure 9-15   Reentrant pathways.

heart. These are considered ectopic foci, meaning the focus for the electrical impulse generation originated someplace other than where it normally should.

Another cause of both abnormal beats and abnormal rhythms is abnormal conduction. Figure 9-15 ■ shows how an irregularity in the conduction system can generate dysrhythmias. The inverted Y in that diagram represents the Purkinje network attaching to a single muscle fiber (represented by the horizontal bar under the Y). Impulses normally travel down both legs of the Y and begin depolarizing the muscle tissue. The muscle tissue depolarizes in both directions and meets in the middle of the Y, where it ends because the tissue is now refractory in both directions. In pathologic conditions, a section of one of the Purkinje fibers has what amounts to a one-way valve that allows impulses to travel in only one direction. The impulse travels down the good leg and depolarizes the muscle fiber, which then propagates the impulse in both directions, unhindered by a refractory period in the opposing direction. Then the impulse will travel up the other leg of the Y, through the one-way valve. If the tissue of the other leg is no longer in the absolute refractory phase, the impulse will continue back down the first leg. This can create either an early beat or, if circumstances are just right, a very rapid reentrant rhythm (a so-called "circus rhythm").

CLASSES OF CARDIOVASCULAR DRUGS

The drugs used to treat cardiovascular disease generally fall into the two broad functional classifications of antidysrhythmics and antihypertensives.

Antidysrhythmics

Antidysrhythmic drugs are used to treat and prevent abnormal cardiac rhythms. Table 9–7 describes the pharmacological classes of antidysrhythmics. While these medications are useful in treating dysrhythmias, they can also cause them or deterioration in existing rhythms when used inappropriately.

antidysrhythmic *drug used to treat and prevent abnormal cardiac rhythms.*

Table 9-7 | Antidysrhythmic Classifications and Examples

General Action	Class	Prototype	ECG Effects
Sodium Channel Blockers	IA	Quinidine, procainamide*, disopyramide	Widened QRS, prolonged QT
	IB	Lidocaine*, phenytoin, tocainide, mexiletine	Widened QRS, prolonged QT
	IC	Flecainide*, propafenone	Prolonged PR, widened QRS
	I (Miscellaneous)	Moricizine*	Prolonged PR, widened QRS
Beta-Blockers	II	Propranolol*, acebutolol, esmolol	Prolonged PR, bradycardias
Potassium Channel Blockers	III	Bretylium*, amiodarone	Prolonged QT
Calcium Channel Blockers	IV	Verapamil*, diltiazem	Prolonged PR, bradycardias
Miscellaneous		Adenosine, digoxin	Prolonged PR, bradycardias

* Prototype.

Review

Antidysrhythmics

Antidysrhythmics are routinely classified in the Vaughn-Williams and Singh Classification System.

- I: Na$^+$ channel blockers
  - 1A
  - 1B
  - 1C
- II: Beta-blockers
- III: K$^+$ channel blockers
- IV: Ca^{++} channel blockers
- Miscellaneous

Sodium Channel Blockers (Class I)　All of the medications in this general class affect the sodium influx in phases 0 and 4 of fast potentials. This slows the propagation of impulses down the specialized conduction system of the atria and ventricles, although it does not affect the SA or AV node.

Class IA drugs include quinidine (Quinidex), procainamide (Pronestyl), and disopyramide (Norpace). In addition to slowing conduction, these drugs also decrease the repolarization rate. This widens the QRS complex and prolongs the QT interval. While quinidine is usually considered the prototype for this class, we will use procainamide here because it is administered more frequently in emergency medicine. Procainamide is indicated in the treatment of atrial fibrillation with rapid ventricular response and ventricular dysrhythmias. Quinidine has a similar mechanism of action, but it also has anticholinergic properties that may induce unintended tachycardias.

Class IB drugs include lidocaine (Xylocaine), phenytoin (Dilantin), tocainide (Tonocard), and mexiletine (Mexitil). Unlike Class IA drugs, Class IB drugs increase the rate of repolarization. They also reduce automaticity in ventricular cells, which makes them effective in treating rhythms originating from ectopic ventricular foci. Several of the drugs in this class are also used for other purposes. Lidocaine, the prototype, is frequently used with epinephrine as a local anesthetic, and phenytoin (Dilantin) is most commonly used as an antiseizure medication. Lidocaine is the drug of choice for treating ventricular tachycardia and ventricular fibrillation. While prophylactic administration of lidocaine was once thought to benefit patients with myocardial infarction, its use is now limited to life-threatening dysrhythmias. When given in overdose, lidocaine has significant CNS side effects including tinnitus, confusion, and convulsions.

Class IC drugs include flecainide (Tambocor) and propafenone (Rythmol). They decrease conduction velocity through the atria and ventricles as well as through the bundle of His and the Purkinje network. Like the Class IA drugs, they delay ventricular repolarization. Both of these medications, which are administered orally, are given to prevent recurrence of ventricular dysrhythmias, but both also have prodysrhythmic properties; that is, they are likely to cause dysrhythmias as well as treat them. They also depress myocardial contractility and are therefore reserved for potentially lethal ventricular dysrhythmias that do not respond to any other conventional therapy.

Moricizine (Ethmozine) is similar to the other Class I drugs but has additional properties that exclude it from the other subclasses. Like the other drugs in this class, it blocks sodium influx during fast potential depolarization, thereby decreasing conduction velocity, but it can also depress myocardial contractility. Like the Class IC drugs, it is reserved for the treatment of ventricular dysrhythmias refractory to other conventional therapy.

Beta-Blockers (Class II) The drugs in this class, propranolol (Inderal), acebutolol (Sectral), and esmolol (Brevibloc), are all beta adrenergic antagonists. Propranolol is nonselective, while acebutolol and esmolol are both selective for the $beta_1$ receptors in the heart. (The mechanism of action at the $beta_1$ receptor is described in the section on adrenergic antagonists.) Of the many beta-blockers, these are the only ones approved for the treatment of dysrhythmias. They are indicated in the treatment of tachycardias resulting from excessive sympathetic stimulation. The $beta_1$ receptor in the heart is attached to the calcium channels. Blocking the $beta_1$ receptors thus blocks the calcium channel and prevents the gradual influx of calcium in phase 0 of the slow potential. As a result, the effects of beta-blocker therapy on dysrhythmias are almost identical to those of calcium channel blockers. Propranolol is the prototype Class II drug. Because it is nonselective, it also blocks the effect of $beta_2$ receptors, which leads to many of its side effects. Other side effects are consistent with those discussed in the section on drugs that affect the sympathetic nervous system.

Potassium Channel Blockers (Class III) Potassium channel blocking drugs are also known as antiadrenergic medications because of their complex actions on sympathetic terminals. They include bretylium (Bretylol) and amiodarone (Cordarone); bretylium is the prototype. Their mechanism of action is on the potassium channels in the fast potentials. By blocking the efflux of potassium, bretylium prolongs repolarization and the effective refractory period. It is indicated in the treatment of ventricular fibrillation and refractory ventricular tachycardia. It causes an initial release of norepinephrine at the sympathetic end terminals, followed by an inhibition of that neurotransmitter's release. This delayed repolarization prolongs the QT interval; consequently, bretylium's primary and frequent side effect is hypotension.

Calcium Channel Blockers (Class IV) Calcium channel blockers' effect on the heart is almost identical to that of beta-blockers. They decrease SA and AV node automaticity, but most of their usefulness arises from decreasing conductivity through the AV node. They effectively slow the ventricular conduction of atrial fibrillation and flutter, and they can terminate supraventricular tachycardias originating from a reentrant circuit. Verapamil (Calan) and diltiazem (Cardizem) are the only two calcium channel blockers that affect the heart. Verapamil is the prototype. Their chief side effect is hypotension and bradycardia. The section on antihypertensives discusses calcium channel blockers in more detail.

Miscellaneous Antidysrhythmics Adenosine (Adenocard) and digoxin (Lanoxin) are both effective antidysrhythmics. Magnesium is the drug of choice in *torsades de pointes,* a type of polymorphic ventricular tachycardia. We will briefly discuss each.

Adenosine does not fit any of the previous categories. It is an endogenous nucleoside with a very short half-life (about 10 seconds). It acts on both potassium and calcium channels, increasing potassium efflux and inhibiting calcium influx. This results in a hyperpolarization that effectively slows the conduction of slow potentials such as those found in the SA and AV nodes. It has little effect on the fast potentials in the ventricles and is not particularly effective on ventricular tachycardias or atrial fibrillation or flutter. Because of its short half-life its side effects are short lived, but they can be alarming. They include facial flushing, shortness of breath, chest pain, and marked bradycardias. Adenosine must be given as a rapid IV push, as the drug is rapidly metabolized. Doses should be increased in patients taking adenosine blockers such as aminophylline or caffeine. They should be decreased in patients taking adenosine uptake inhibitors like dipyridamole (Persantine) and carbamazepine (Tegretol).

Digoxin (Lanoxin) is a paradoxical drug. Its many effects on the heart make it both an effective antidysrhythmic and a potent prodysrhythmic (generator of dysrhythmias). While we do not clearly understand its specific actions on the heart's electrical activity, we do understand its effects. Digoxin decreases the intrinsic firing rate in the SA node, whereas it decreases conduction velocity in the AV node. Both of these effects are due to its increasing the strength of the parasympathetic effects on the heart. In the Purkinje fibers and ventricular myocardial cells, it decreases the effective refractory period and increases automaticity, both of which may explain its ability to increase ventricular dysrhythmias. To compound this, by depressing SA node activity, digoxin makes ectopic ventricular beats more likely to assume the pacing activity of the heart. Its side effects include bradycardias, AV blocks, PVCs, ventricular tachycardia, ventricular fibrillation, and atrial fibrillation. Actually, there are few dysrhythmias that digoxin does not produce. In addition, digoxin has a very narrow therapeutic index, meaning that it is difficult to find a patient's effective dose without producing side effects. Digoxin also increases cardiac contractility. It is indicated for atrial fibrillation with rapid ventricular conduction and chronic treatment of congestive heart failure.

Magnesium is the drug of choice in *torsades de pointes,* a polymorphic ventricular tachycardia, and in other ventricular dysrhythmias refractory to other therapy. Its mechanism of action is not known, but it may act on the sodium or potassium channels or on Na^+K^+ATPase.

Antihypertensives

Hypertension affects more than 50 million people in the United States alone and is a major contributor to coronary artery disease, stroke, and blindness. Fortunately, available drugs can effectively manage blood pressure with limited side effects in the vast majority of patients. Multiple studies have shown conclusively that controlling blood pressure decreases both morbidity and mortality.

Blood pressure is the force of blood against the arteries' walls as the heart contracts and relaxes. It is equal to cardiac output times the peripheral vascular resistance:

$$\text{Blood pressure} = \text{Cardiac output} \times \text{Peripheral vascular resistance}$$

Cardiac output is equal to the heart rate times the stroke volume:

$$\text{Cardiac output} = \text{Heart rate} \times \text{Stroke volume}$$

antihypertensive *drug used to treat hypertension.*

Antihypertensive agents can manipulate each of these factors. The primary determinant of peripheral vascular resistance is the diameter of peripheral arterioles, which are affected by alpha$_1$ receptors. Heart rate is affected by both muscarinic receptors of the parasympathetic nervous system and beta$_1$ receptors of the sympathetic nervous system; however, hypertension control typically manipulates only beta$_1$ receptors. Stroke volume is affected by contractility and volume. Recall that Starling's law says that preload and stroke volume are proportionate; that is, as preload increases stroke volume increases (up to a point) and as preload decreases stroke volume decreases. Drugs that affect blood volume control hypertension by manipulating preload.

Several pharmacologic classes of medications are used to control blood pressure. The major approaches to dealing with hypertension are diuretics, beta-blockers and other antiadrenergic drugs, angiotensin converting enzyme (ACE) inhibitors, calcium channel blockers, and direct vasodilators. Of these, diuretics and beta-blockers are the most frequently prescribed, and they are effective in many patients. The remaining agents are used when diuretics or beta-blockers are contraindicated or when those approaches are not effective, although ACE inhibitors are gaining increasing popularity. Often, physicians must prescribe multiple drugs to manage hypertension effectively. In these cases, they will pick one drug from two or more classes that complement each other. For example, a physician might prescribe a diuretic with a beta-blocker.

Diuretics   Diuretics reduce circulating blood volume by increasing the amount of urine. This reduces preload to the heart, which in turn reduces cardiac output. The main categories of diuretics include loop diuretics (high ceiling diuretics), thiazides, and potassium sparing diuretics. They all affect the reabsorption of sodium and chloride and create an osmotic gradient that decreases the reabsorption of water. These classes differ according to which area of the nephron they affect. In general, the earlier in the nephron the drug works, the more sodium and water will be affected. Almost all electrolytes and other small particles in the blood are filtered through the glomerulus. Most sodium and water (approximately 65 percent) is reabsorbed in the proximal convoluted tubule. Another 20 percent is reabsorbed in the thick portion of the ascending loop of Henle, while only about 1 to 5 percent is recaptured in the distal convoluted tubule and collecting duct. Therefore, a drug that decreases sodium reabsorption in the proximal convoluted tubule will cause the kidneys to excrete more water than will a drug that works on the distal convoluted tubule.

Loop diuretics profoundly affect circulating blood volume. In fact, they decrease blood volume so well that they are typically considered excessive for treating moderate hypertension. They are, however, one of the primary tools in treating left ventricular heart failure (congestive heart failure). Their use for hypertension is typically because other diuretics have failed. Furosemide (Lasix) is the prototype of this class. Furosemide blocks sodium reabsorption in the thick portion of the ascending loop of Henle (hence, the name *loop diuretic*). In doing so, it decreases the pull of water from the tubule and into the capillary bed, thus decreasing fluid volume. Furosemide's main side effects are hyponatremia, hypovolemia, hypokalemia, and dehydration. Because the decrease in volume is most noticeable as decreased preload, orthostatic hypotension is a problem. Reflex tachycardia may also occur as the baroreceptors detect a decreased blood pressure and attempt to compensate by increasing heart rate. This happens in individuals with hypertension because the homeostatic "thermostat" has been set too high. In other words, the body believes that what is actually hypertension is normal and tries to maintain a higher blood pressure than is healthy. This reflex tachycardia is frequently treated with concurrent administration of a loop diuretic with a beta$_1$ blocker. Hypokalemia is frequently treated by increasing dietary potassium intake (bananas are rich in potassium) or by prescribing potassium supplements. An unexplained side effect of loop diuretics is ototoxicity (tinnitus and deafness). Administering loop diuretics slowly can decrease ototoxicity.

Thiazides have a mechanism similar to loop diuretics. The main difference is that the thiazides' mechanism affects the early part of the distal convoluted tubules and therefore cannot block as much sodium from reabsorption. Thiazides are often the drugs of choice in hypertension treatment because they can decrease fluid volume sufficiently to prevent hypertension but not so much that they promote hypotension. The prototype thiazide is hydrochlorothiazide (HydroDIURIL). This class has essentially the same side effects as loop diuretics. One important distinction is that thiazides depend on the glomerular filtration rate, while loop diuretics do not. Thus, loop diuretics may be preferred for patients with renal disease.

Review

Pharmacological Classes of Antihypertensives

- Diuretics
- Beta-blockers and antiadrenergic drugs
- ACE inhibitors
- Calcium channel blockers
- Direct vasodilators

diuretic   *drug used to reduce circulating blood volume by increasing the amount of urine.*

Loop diuretics, particularly furosemide (Lasix), play a major role in the emergency treatment of CHF and acute pulmonary edema.

Potassium sparing diuretics have a slightly different mechanism than other diuretics. Although they still affect sodium absorption, they do so by inhibiting either the effects of aldosterone on the distal tubules (as does spironolactone) or the specific sodium-potassium exchange mechanism (as does triamterene). Acting so late in the nephritic loop, these agents are not very potent diuretics. In fact, they are rarely used alone but instead are typically administered in conjunction with either a loop diuretic or a thiazide diuretic. They are useful as adjuncts to other diuretics because they not only decrease sodium reabsorption (although in small volumes) but also increase potassium reabsorption. This helps to limit the other diuretics' hypokalemic effects. Spironolactone (Aldactone) is the prototype potassium sparing diuretic.

While not used in the treatment of hypertension, osmotic diuretics are important because they alter the reabsorption of water in the proximal convoluted tubule. To do this, they use an osmotically large sugar molecule that is freely filtered through the glomerulus and pulls water after it. Mannitol (Osmitrol), the prototype osmotic diuretic, is used to treat increased intracranial and intraocular pressure.

Adrenergic Inhibiting Agents   Inhibiting the effects of adrenergic stimulation can also control hypertension. Several broad mechanisms accomplish this: beta adrenergic antagonism, centrally acting alpha adrenergic antagonism, adrenergic neuron blockade, alpha$_1$ blockade, and alpha/beta blockade.

Beta Adrenergic Antagonists   From Table 9–5 in our earlier discussion of beta$_1$ blockers, you will recall that most beta$_1$ receptors are in the heart but some also exist in the juxtaglomerular cells of the kidney. Selective beta$_1$ blockade is useful in treating hypertension for several reasons. It decreases contractility, thereby directly decreasing cardiac output. It also reduces reflex tachycardia by inhibiting sympathetically induced compensatory increases in heart rate. Finally, it represses renin release from the kidneys, which in turn inhibits the vasoconstriction activated by the renin-angiotensin-aldosterone system. The prototype selective beta$_1$ blocker is metropolol (Lopressor); the prototype nonselective beta-blocker is propranolol (Inderal). The section on beta$_1$ blockers discussed these agents' side effects.

Centrally Acting Adrenergic Inhibitors   Centrally acting adrenergic inhibitors reduce hypertension by inhibiting CNS stimulation of adrenergic receptors. In effect, they are CNS alpha$_2$ agonists. Recall that alpha$_2$ receptors are located on the presynaptic end terminals in the sympathetic nervous system. When stimulated, they inhibit the release of norepinephrine to counterbalance sympathetic stimulation. By increasing the stimulation of alpha$_2$ receptors in the section of the CNS responsible for cardiovascular regulation, centrally acting adrenergic inhibitors decrease the sympathetic stimulation of both alpha$_1$ and beta$_2$ receptors. The net effect is to decrease heart rate and contractility by decreasing release of norepinephrine at beta$_1$ receptors and to promote vasodilation by decreasing norepinephrine release at alpha$_1$ receptors at vascular smooth muscle. The prototype drug in this category is clonidine (Catapres). While it does have some side effects, notably drowsiness and dry mouth, clonidine is a relatively safe and frequently prescribed antihypertensive agent. Methyldopa (Aldomet) is another centrally acting antihypertensive with a mechanism similar to clonidine.

Peripheral Adrenergic Neuron Blocking Agents   Like the centrally acting adrenergic inhibitors, peripheral adrenergic neuron blocking agents work indirectly to decrease stimulation of adrenergic receptors. They do this by decreasing the amount of norepinephrine released from sympathetic presynaptic terminals. These agents are no longer commonly used.

The prototype of this class is reserpine (Serpalan). Reserpine has two actions that decrease the amount of norepinephrine released. First, it decreases the synthesis of norepinephrine. Second, it exposes norepinephrine in the terminal vesicles to monoamine

Beta-blockers have proven to decrease both short-term and long-term mortality associated with acute MI.

oxidase, an enzyme that destroys it. This decreases stimulation of $alpha_1$ receptors, resulting in peripheral vasodilation, and of $beta_1$ receptors, resulting in decreased heart rate and contractility. The decreased peripheral vascular resistance and cardiac output in turn lower blood pressure.

Reserpine also decreases synthesis of several CNS neurotransmitters (serotonin and other catecholamines). This causes reserpine's primary adverse effect, depression. Reserpine, therefore, is not frequently used as an antihypertensive. Additional side effects include gastrointestinal cramps and increased stomach acid production. Other drugs with similar actions include guanethidine (Ismeline) and guanadrel (Hylorel).

Alpha$_1$ Antagonists This chapter's section on drugs affecting the sympathetic nervous system discusses the $alpha_1$ receptor antagonists in detail. Only their specific action will be repeated here. The prototype selective $alpha_1$ antagonist is prazosin (Minipress). It decreases blood pressure by competitively blocking the $alpha_1$ receptors, thereby inhibiting the sympathetically mediated increases in peripheral vascular resistance. By causing the arterioles to dilate, prazosine directly decreases afterload. By causing the venules to dilate, it promotes venous pooling, which decreases preload. The decreased afterload and preload help to lower blood pressure. Terazosin (Hytrin) is another drug with similar properties.

Combined Alpha/Beta Antagonists Labetalol (Normodyne) and carvedilol (Coreg) competitively bind with both $alpha_1$ and $beta_1$ receptors, increasing their antihypertensive actions. Hypertension is treated by decreasing $alpha_1$ mediated vasoconstriction, which, again, decreases both preload and afterload. $Beta_1$ blockade decreases heart rate, contractility, and renin release from kidneys. By blocking the release of renin, which promotes vasoconstriction, these agents decrease peripheral vascular resistance even further. Labetalol is commonly used to treat hypertensive crisis and is rapidly replacing the use of sublingual nifedipine (Procardia) for this purpose.

Angiotensin Converting Enzyme (ACE) Inhibitors

Agents in this class interrupt the renin-angiotensin-aldosterone system (RAAS) by preventing the conversion of angiotensin I to angiotensin II. Angiotensin II is one of the most potent vasoconstrictors yet discovered. By decreasing the amount of circulating angiotensin II, peripheral vascular resistance can be decreased, which leads to a decrease in blood pressure.

The juxtaglomerular apparatus in the kidneys releases renin in response to decreases in blood volume, sodium concentration, and blood pressure. Renin acts as an enzyme to convert the inactive protein angiotensinogen into angiotensin I. Neither angiotensinogen nor angiotensin I has much pharmaceutical effect, but angiotensin-converting enzyme (ACE) almost immediately converts angiotensin I in the blood into angiotensin II. (ACE is found in the lumen of almost all vessels and is found in the lungs in very high concentrations.) Angiotensin II causes both systemic and local vasoconstriction, with more pronounced effects on arterioles than on venules. It also lessens water loss by decreasing renal filtration secondary to renal vasoconstriction. Finally, angiotensin II also increases the release of aldosterone, a corticosteroid produced in the adrenal cortex. Aldosterone in turn increases sodium and water reabsorption in the distal convoluted tubule of the nephrons.

Angiotensin-converting enzyme inhibitors are very effective in treating hypertension and have also seen success in managing heart failure and renal failure. ACE inhibitors block the conversion of angiotensin I to angiotensin II, thereby providing a host of beneficial effects for patients with hypertension. These include a rapid decrease in arteriolar constriction, which lowers peripheral vascular resistance and afterload. While it does cause some dilation of the venules, this effect is limited. Because of the limited decrease in preload, orthostatic hypotension, common in other antihypertensives, is not a significant concern with ACE inhibitors. These agents also appear to be effective in preventing some of the untoward structural changes in the heart and blood vessels that angiotensin II causes over time.

In addition to their role in the treatment of hypertension, ACE inhibitors play an important role in the treatment of CHF by decreasing afterload.

The prototype ACE inhibitor is captopril (Capoten). Captopril acts like all ACE inhibitors to prevent hypertension. Its main advantage is the absence of side effects common to other antihypertensives. It does not interfere with beta receptors, so it does not decrease the ability to exercise or respond to hemorrhage. It does not cause potassium loss like many diuretics, and it does not cause depression or drowsiness. Because it has no effect on sexual desire or performance, it is much more attractive to many patients who might not comply with other medications. Other common ACE inhibitors include enalapril (Vasotec) and lisinopril (Zestril). These medications are all taken orally. For intravenous use in hypertensive crisis, enalaprilat (Vasotec I.V.) is available.

The most dangerous side effect of ACE inhibitors is pronounced hypotension after the first dose. This can be minimized by reducing initial doses, and it does not reoccur. The main adverse effects of continual use are a persistent cough and angioedema.

Angiotensin II Receptor Antagonists

This recently developed classification of antihypertensive drugs also acts on the renin-angiotensin-aldosterone system. Angiotensin II receptor antagonists achieve the same effects as the ACE inhibitors without the side effects of cough or angioedema. The prototype of this new class is losartan (Cozaar).

Calcium Channel Blocking Agents

We have already discussed two calcium channel blockers, verapamil and diltiazem, in the section on antidysrhythmics. Another structural subclass of calcium channel blockers is the dihydropyridines. The prototype dihydropyridine is nifedipine (Procardia, Adalat). Nifedipine, as well as the other members of the dihydropyridines, differs from verapamil and diltiazem in that it does not affect the calcium channels of the heart at therapeutic doses. Rather, it acts only on the vascular smooth muscle of the arterioles. These agents act by blocking the calcium channels in the arterioles. Calcium, which is required for muscle contraction, is released from sarcoplasmic reticulum upon activation by an action potential. When it enters the muscle cell through calcium channels, muscle contraction ensues. Blocking the calcium channels prevents the arterioles' smooth muscle from contracting and therefore dilates these vessels. When this occurs, peripheral vascular resistance decreases and blood pressure falls as a result of lower afterload. Because nifedipine has little effect on veins, it does not cause a corresponding drop in preload and consequently avoids orthostatic hypotension. While nifedipine does not affect the cardiac electrical conduction system, it is effective in dilating the coronary arteries and arterioles and thereby helps to increase coronary perfusion. The primary indications for nifedipine are angina pectoris and chronic treatment of hypertension. Its primary side effects include reflex tachycardia (responding to baroreceptor response to decreased blood pressure), facial flushing, dizziness, headache, and peripheral edema. It has been used commonly for the emergent reduction of blood pressure in the field; however, labetalol is replacing it.

Direct Vasodilators

We have already discussed several drugs that cause vasodilation. Two specific classes of vasodilators are those that dilate arterioles and those that dilate both arterioles and veins. All of these drugs are used to decrease blood pressure.

Selective dilation of arterioles causes a decrease in peripheral vascular resistance or afterload. This is the resistance that the heart must overcome in order to eject blood. Decreasing peripheral vascular resistance lowers blood pressure, increases cardiac output, and reduces cardiac workload. However, dilating the veins increases capacitance and decreases preload, the amount of blood in the heart prior to contraction. Starling's law tells us that as preload increases, so do stroke volume and cardiac output (up to a point). By decreasing preload, venodilators decrease both blood pressure and cardiac output.

Hydralizine (Apresoline) is the prototype for the selective arteriole dilators. It is effective in decreasing peripheral vascular resistance and afterload and thus lowering

Nifedipine was used extensively for emergent reduction of blood pressure. Now, other agents, such as labetalol, are preferred.

Hydralizine (Apresoline) is the preferred antihypertensive for the management of pregnancy-induced hypertension.

blood pressure. Its primary side effects are reflex tachycardia and increased blood volume. Both occur as a compensatory mechanism to lowered blood pressure, and both have the effect of increasing cardiac workload. As a result, hydralazine is almost always prescribed in conjunction with a beta-blocker and a diuretic. It is frequently used in the treatment of pregnancy-induced hypertension.

Minoxidil (Loniten) is another selective arteriole dilator with properties similar to those of hydralazine. One side effect deserves comment. It produces hypertrichosis (excessive hair growth) in about 80 percent of those taking it. While this is particularly irritating when it occurs all over a patient's body, it can become a therapeutic effect when the drug is applied as a topical ointment. Minoxidil is marketed in this form as Rogaine for promoting hair growth in men.

Unlike hydralazine, sodium nitroprusside (Nipride) acts on both arterioles and veins. It is the fastest acting antihypertensive available and is the drug of choice in hypertensive emergencies. It is very potent and is given via controlled IV infusion. Its effects are almost immediate and end within minutes of drug cessation; therefore, blood pressure must be carefully and continuously monitored during infusion, preferably in the ICU. Sodium nitroprusside has several significant side effects. Obviously, hypotension can be a problem when this medication is not carefully administered. Because cyanide and thyocyanate are byproducts of nitroprusside metabolism, other adverse effects include cyanide poisoning and thyocyanate toxicity.

Ganglionic Blocking Agents Ganglionic blocking agents are nicotinic$_N$ antagonists. The prototype is trimethaphan (Arfonad). Since nicotinic$_N$ receptors exist at the ganglia of both the sympathetic and the parasympathetic nervous systems, competitive antagonism of these receptors turns off the entire autonomic nervous system, which is obviously not a very selective approach. When this happens, the effects on each organ system are determined by the predominant autonomic tone (the division of the ANS that normally has the greater influence on that organ). Because the arteries and veins have predominant sympathetic control, they dilate in response to trimethaphan administration. This reduces both preload and afterload, and blood pressure drops. Trimethaphan also directly affects vascular smooth muscle, causing dilation and the release of histamine, which is also a vasodilator. Mecamylamine (Inversine) is the other ganglionic blocking drug available in the United States, although it is not commonly used anymore.

Cardiac Glycosides The cardiac glycosides occur naturally in the foxglove plant. The two drugs in the class, digoxin (Lanoxin) and digitoxin (Crystodigin), are chemically related. These drugs are also known as digitalis glycosides. Digoxin is the prototype. One of the 10 most frequently prescribed medications in the country, it is indicated for heart failure and some types of dysrhythmias. Digoxin's mechanism of action is complex. It blocks the effects of $Na^+K^+ATPase$, an enzyme responsible for returning ion flow to normal levels after muscle depolarization. By interfering with this sodium-potassium pump, digoxin increases the intracellular levels of sodium. Because sodium is also involved in a reciprocal exchange with calcium, a buildup of intracellular sodium leads to a similar buildup of intracellular calcium. These elevated levels of intracellular calcium increase the strength of muscle contraction and are the basis for digoxin's primary indication. Digoxin reduces the symptoms of congestive heart failure by increasing myocardial contractility and cardiac output. This diminishes the dilation of the heart's chambers frequently seen in left heart failure because it enables the heart to effectively pump blood out of its ventricles, thus decreasing the engorgement typical of this condition. Increasing cardiac output decreases the sympathetic discharge mediated by baroreceptor reflexes, resulting in reduced afterload. Furthermore, digoxin indirectly lessens preload by increasing renal blood flow, which results in higher glomerular filtration and decreased blood volume. Digoxin also has antidysrhythmic effects, which we discuss more thoroughly in the section on antidysrhythmic medications.

While digoxin effectively treats the symptoms of heart failure, it also is potentially dangerous. Its therapeutic index is very small, and the individual variability is large.

Digitalis (Lanoxin) is still frequently used to increase cardiac output in CHF and to control the rate of ventricular response in atrial fibrillation.

This leads to toxicity in some individuals even though they have normal digoxin levels. Digoxin's chief adverse effects are dysrhythmias. In fact, digoxin frequently induces some of the same dysrhythmias it is used to treat. Other side effects include fatigue, anorexia, nausea and vomiting, and blurred vision with a yellowish haze and halos around dark objects.

Other Vasodilators and Antianginals   The drugs discussed in this section have vasodilatory properties that are useful in reducing blood pressure, but they are most commonly used to treat angina. The three basic types of angina pectoris (chest pain) are stable (exertional) angina; unstable angina; and variant, or Prinzmetal's, angina. Stable and unstable angina have the same pathophysiology and differ only by causation: stable angina occurs after exercise as a result of increased myocardial oxygen demand; unstable angina occurs without exertion. Both result from an imbalance between myocardial supply and demand. A buildup of plaque (atherosclerosis) along the walls of coronary arteries decreases these vessels' diameter and, as a result, the amount of blood flow to the heart. The same imbalance causes Prinzmetal's angina but it results from vasospasm instead of plaque buildup. The medications discussed in this section all either increase oxygen supply or decrease oxygen demand.

In addition to their previously discussed use as antihypertensives and antidysrhythmics, calcium channel blockers have a role in the treatment of angina. The three calcium channel blockers most frequently used for this purpose are verapamil (Calan, Isoptin), diltiazem (Cardizem), and nifedipine (Procardia). Recall that calcium is an integral part of both depolarization and muscle contraction. The effects of blocking its entry into the cells are twofold. All of these agents directly affect vascular smooth muscle, leading to dilation of the arterioles and, to a lesser degree, of the venules. This arterial dilation decreases peripheral vascular resistance and, as a result, afterload, which in turn directly decreases the workload of the heart and myocardial oxygen demand. Verapamil and diltiazem also reduce SA and AV node conductivity, which can decrease reflex tachycardia and dysrhythmias. Nifedipine has relatively few effects on the heart and, thus, has limited antidysrhythmic properties. The calcium channel blockers are effective in all forms of angina. A primary side effect of these agents is hypotension.

Organic nitrates are potent vasodilators used to treat all forms of angina. First used clinically in 1879, nitroglycerin (Nitrostat) is the oldest of these drugs and is the category's prototype. Other agents include isosorbide (Isordil, Sorbitrate) and amyl nitrite. Nitroglycerin acts on vascular smooth muscle via a complex series of events to decrease intracellular calcium, thus causing vasodilation. Nitroglycerin primarily dilates veins rather than arterioles. This decreases preload and thus decreases myocardial workload, which is its primary antianginal effect. In Prinzmetal's angina, nitroglycerin reverses coronary artery spasm and increases oxygen supply.

Nitroglycerin is very lipid soluble, which allows it to cross membranes easily. Because of this, it is readily absorbed and can be administered via sublingual, buccal, and transdermal routes. The primary concern with nitroglycerin is orthostatic hypotension, a side effect more common in the presence of right ventricular failure. Other common side effects include headache and reflex tachycardia. Headache is frequently used as an indicator of the effectiveness of nitroglycerin, which rapidly loses its potency when exposed to light. While orthostatic hypotension is a serious concern with the administration of nitroglycerin, this condition typically responds well to fluid infusions.

Hemostatic Agents

Hemostasis is the stoppage of bleeding. It is a series of events in response to a tear in a blood vessel. Damage to the vessel's intima (innermost layer) exposes the underlying collagen and triggers a release of two naturally occurring substances, adenosine diphosphate (ADP) and thromboxane A_2 (TXA_2). Both ADP and TXA_2 stimulate the aggregation of platelets and vasoconstriction. The vasoconstriction decreases the flow of

Nitroglycerin is effective in the management of angina pectoris as it decreases cardiac work.

hemostasis   *the stoppage of bleeding.*

blood past the tear, thus allowing the newly "sticky" platelets to form a plug that temporarily occludes the bleeding.

While this plug effectively halts bleeding for the short term, it must be reinforced to continue the stoppage until the tear can be permanently repaired. Stabilizing the plug requires a complex cascade of events involving the activation of naturally occurring factors and ending with the conversion of prothrombin into thrombin. The thrombin then converts fibrinogen into fibrin, a strandlike substance that attaches to the vessel's surface and contracts in a mesh web over the platelet plug to form a blood clot. Several of the factors involved need vitamin K to carry out their functions. A vitamin K deficiency inhibits clotting and makes uncontrolled bleeding more likely. Conversely, limiting the clotting cascade to the immediate area of the vessel injury is important for obvious reasons. The protein antithrombin III is key in this process. Antithrombin III binds with several of the factors needed for clotting, thus inhibiting their ability to coagulate.

Once the vessel has been permanently repaired, the fibrin mesh must be broken down. This process, called fibrinolysis, involves another cascading system that ends with the activation of plasminogen into plasmin, which in turn breaks up the clot. Tissue plasminogen activator, a substance in the tissue, activates this last conversion.

Thrombi (blood clots that obstruct vessels or heart cavities) are the primary pathology in several clinical conditions, including myocardial infarction, stroke, and pulmonary embolism. Drugs can effectively treat the causes of these conditions by decreasing platelet aggregation (antiplatelet drugs), by interfering with the clotting cascade (anticoagulants), or by directly breaking up the thrombus (fibrinolytics).

 Review

Drugs Used to Treat Thrombi

- Antiplatelets
- Anticoagulants
- Fibrinolytics

Antiplatelets Antiplatelet drugs decrease the formation of platelet plugs. The prototype antiplatelet drug is aspirin. Aspirin inhibits cyclooxygenase, an enzyme needed for the synthesis of thromboxane A_2 (TXA_2). Remember that TXA_2 causes platelets to aggregate and promotes local vasoconstriction. By inhibiting TXA_2, aspirin decreases the formation of platelet plugs and potential thrombi. Aspirin, as well as other antiplatelet and anticoagulant drugs, has no effect on existing thrombi; it only curbs the formation of new thrombi. Aspirin is indicated in the acute treatment of developing myocardial infarction. It is also useful in preventing the reoccurrence of MI and of ischemic stroke following transient ischemic attacks (TIAs).

One of aspirin's primary side effects is bleeding. Aspirin also may lead to an increase in gastric ulcers, which are a frequent source of gastrointestinal hemorrhage. By both stimulating the development of a potential source of bleeding as well as blocking an important mechanism for stopping that bleeding, aspirin can cause dangerous blood loss. Other antiplatelet drugs include dipyridamole (Persantine), abciximab (ReoPro), and ticlopidine (Ticlid).

antiplatelet *drug that decreases the formation of platelet plugs.*

Anticoagulants Anticoagulants interrupt the clotting cascade. The two main types of anticoagulants are parenteral and oral. The prototype parenteral anticoagulant is heparin, a substance derived from the lungs of cattle or the intestines of pigs. Its primary mechanism of action is to enhance antithrombin III's ability to inhibit the clotting cascade. Because heparin is very polar, it is very poorly absorbed and must be given parenterally. Heparin injections and infusions are indicated in treating and preventing deep vein thrombosis, pulmonary embolism, and some forms of stroke. Heparin also is used frequently in conjunction with fibrinolytics to treat myocardial infarction. Finally, it is used to keep rubber-capped IV catheters (Hep-Locks) free from clots. As you would expect, bleeding is heparin's primary side effect. Other untoward effects include thrombocytopenia (decreased platelet counts) and allergic reactions. Heparin is measured in units rather than milligrams. A unit is that amount of heparin necessary to keep 1 mL of sheep plasma from clotting for 1 hour. Using this

anticoagulant *drug that interrupts the clotting cascade.*

measurement is necessary because heparin's potency varies greatly when measured in milligrams.

Protamine sulfate is available as a heparin antagonist. Protamine can reverse the effects of heparin in the presence of dangerous and unintended bleeding by binding with heparin. This prevents heparin from binding with antithrombin III and enhancing its anticlotting abilities.

The prototype oral anticoagulant is warfarin (Coumadin). Warfarin's history serves as a useful reminder of its primary side effect. Warfarin was first developed as a rat poison that killed through uncontrolled bleeding. After noticing that a patient who attempted suicide by ingesting warfarin did not, in fact, die, its clinical use was investigated. Needless to say, this drug's primary side effect is bleeding.

Warfarin prevents coagulation by antagonizing the effects of vitamin K, which is needed for the synthesis of multiple factors involved in the clotting cascade. It is prescribed for chronic use to prevent thrombi in high-risk patients such as those who have hip replacements or artificial heart valves or those who are in atrial fibrillation. Because warfarin easily crosses the placental barrier and has dangerous *teratogenic* (capable of causing malformations) properties, it is contraindicated in pregnant patients. It also interacts adversely with many other medications. Like heparin, warfarin may lead to bleeding. In cases of overdose, you may give vitamin K as an antidote.

fibrinolytic *drug that acts directly on thrombi to break them down; also called* thrombolytic.

Fibrinolytics Fibrinolytics (also called *thrombolytics*) act directly on thrombi to break them up. The several available fibrinolytics share a similar mechanism of action. Through a chemical conversion, these drugs activate enzymes that dissolve thrombi or clots. The prototype drug of this class is streptokinase (Streptase). Other fibrinolytics include alteplase (tPA), reteplase (Retavase), and anistreplase (Eminase). These medications all dissolve clots effectively; they differ primarily in their administration and risk of bleeding side effects.

Streptokinase, which is derived from the streptococci bacterium, is the oldest available fibrinolytic. Its mechanism of action is to promote plasminogen's conversion to plasmin. Since plasmin dissolves the fibrin mesh of clots, it can directly treat the cause of most myocardial infarctions and some strokes, as opposed to antiplatelet agents and anticoagulants, which can only prevent potential future thrombi. Streptokinase also breaks down fibrinogen, the precursor to fibrin. While this action does not serve a clinical purpose (the problematic clot has already been formed), it does play an important role in streptokinase's chief side effect, bleeding. Other side effects include allergic reaction, hypotension, and fever.

Alteplase (Activase) is produced by recombinant DNA technology that is identical to the naturally occurring tissue plasminogen activator (hence its common name, tPA).

The window of opportunity for fibrinolytic therapy is limited. Because of this, some EMS systems administer fibrinolytics in the prehospital setting. Many have chosen to use reteplase (Retavase) because of its ease of administration (two 10-unit boluses administered 30 minutes apart).

Antihyperlipidemic Agents

Elevated levels of low-density lipoproteins (LDLs) have been clearly indicated as a causative factor in coronary artery disease. Lipoproteins are essentially transport mechanisms for lipids (triglycerides and cholesterol). Because lipids are insoluble in plasma, the body coats them in a plasma-soluble shell in order to transport them to their target destinations. Lipoproteins are categorized as very low-density (VLDL), low-density (LDL), intermediate-density (IDL), and high-density (HDL). Low-density lipoproteins contain most of the cholesterol in the blood and are required for transporting cholesterol from the liver to the peripheral tissues. Conversely, high-density lipoproteins (HDLs) carry cholesterol from the peripheral tissues to the liver, where it is broken down.

HDLs have been described as good cholesterol because they lower blood cholesterol levels and decrease the risk of coronary artery disease (CAD). LDLs are known as bad cholesterol because they increase blood cholesterol levels and the risk of CAD. As blood cholesterol levels increase, fatty plaque is deposited under the arteries' endothelial tissues. Atherosclerosis then develops, and coronary arteries decrease in diameter. Coronary vasoconstriction in turn reduces blood flow to the heart and, in times of increased myocardial oxygen demand, may lead to angina. Also, newly deposited plaque is often unstable. Typically, the plaque is under the endothelial tissues, which cap the plaque deposits. As the deposits age, the cap usually becomes fairly stable. In some cases, however, the cap breaks open and exposes the plaque to the blood. When this happens, platelet aggregation and coagulation begin. If the developing clot breaks free of the vessel, it becomes a thrombus and may completely occlude a coronary artery, leading to myocardial infarction.

The goal in lowering LDL levels is to prevent atherosclerosis and subsequent CAD. While raising HDL levels would help accomplish this, no pharmaceutical means of doing so currently exists. By far, the best way to lower LDL levels remains dietary modification. If this is not sufficient, several classifications of **antihyperlipidemic** medications may be used. The most common are drugs that inhibit hydroxymethylglutaryl coenzyme A (HMG CoA) reductase. The liver must have HMG CoA to synthesize cholesterol. By inhibiting this enzyme, HMG CoA agents lower LDL levels; however, they also increase the number of LDL receptors in the liver, causing a further uptake of LDL.

anithyperlipidemic *drug used to treat high blood cholesterol.*

Five HMG CoA reductase inhibitors are available. Because the names of all five end in *statin*, these agents are also known as statins. They include lovastatin (Mevacor) and simvastatin (Zocor). Lovastatin is the HMG CoA reductase inhibitors' prototype. Overall, these drugs are well tolerated. Their chief side effects are headache, rash, and flushing. In rare cases, they may cause hepatotoxicity and lead to liver failure.

Bile acid-binding resins can also reduce LDL levels. Inert substances that have no direct biologic activity, these agents pass straight through the GI system without being absorbed and are excreted in feces. They are useful, however, in that they indirectly increase the number of LDL receptors in the liver by binding with bile acids, thus decreasing their availability. Because the liver needs cholesterol to synthesize bile acids, it must have more cholesterol to compensate for the decrease in bile acids. The body therefore increases the LDL receptors on the liver. As more LDLs remain in the liver, their levels in the blood drop. Since the body does not absorb bile acid-binding agents, they have no systemic effects. Their chief untoward effect is constipation. Cholestyramine (Questran) is the prototype.

DRUGS USED TO AFFECT THE RESPIRATORY SYSTEM

Drugs that affect the respiratory system are useful for several purposes. The most obvious is the treatment of asthma, but this class also includes cough suppressants, nasal decongestants, and antihistamines.

ANTIASTHMATIC MEDICATIONS

Asthma is a common disease that decreases pulmonary function and may limit daily activities. It typically presents with shortness of breath, wheezing, and coughing. Its basic pathophysiology has two components, bronchoconstriction and inflammation. Typically a response to some sort of allergen sets both of these processes in motion. Common culprits include pet dander, mold, and dust. In patients with existing asthma, cold air, tobacco smoke, or other pollutants may bring on acute episodes of shortness of breath.

The response to asthma typically begins with an allergen's binding to an antibody on mast cells. This causes the mast cell membrane to rupture and release its contents, including histamine, leukotrines, and prostaglandins. These cause immediate bronchoconstriction followed by a slower inflammatory response that can lead to mucus plugs and a further decrease in airway size. The inflammation may in turn cause a hyperreactivity to stimuli, and allergens that might not normally produce dyspnea may lead to an acute attack.

Drug treatment of asthma aims to relieve bronchospasm and decrease inflammation. Specific approaches are categorized as beta$_2$ selective sympathomimetics, nonselective sympathomimetics, methylxanthines, anticholinergics, glucocorticoids, and leukotriene antagonists. Cromolyn (Intal), a frequently used anti-inflammatory agent, does not fit neatly into any of those categories. Table 9–8 summarizes these agents.

Drug treatment of asthma aims to relieve bronchospasm and decrease inflammation.

Beta$_2$ Specific Agents Drugs that are selective for beta$_2$ receptors are the mainstay in treating asthma-induced shortness of breath. Albuterol (Proventil, Ventolin) is the prototype of this class. In general, these agents relax bronchial smooth muscle, which results in bronchodilation and relief from bronchospasm. Agents from this class are first-line therapy for acute shortness of breath and may also be used daily for prophylaxis. Most are administered via metered dose inhaler or nebulizer. Albuterol and terbutaline may both be taken orally, and terbutaline may be given by injection. These medications' beta$_2$ specificity is not absolute; some patients may experience beta$_1$ effects such as tachycardia or dysrhythmias. Patients may also experience tremors resulting from the stimulation of beta$_2$ receptors in smooth muscles. Overall, these agents are very safe.

Table 9–8	Drugs Used in the Treatment of Asthma
Mechanism of Action	**Medication**
Bronchodilators	
Nonspecific agonists	Epinephrine
	Ephedrine
Beta$_2$ specific agonists	
Inhaled (short acting)	Albuterol (Ventolin, Proventil)
	Metaproterenol (Alupent)
	Terbutaline (Brethine)
	Bitolterol (Tornalate)
Inhaled (long-acting)	Salmeterol (Serevent)
Methylxanthines	Theophylline (Theo-Dur, Slo-Bid)
	Aminophylline
Anticholinergics	Atropine
	Ipratropium (Atrovent)
Anti-inflammatory agents	
Glucocorticoids	
Inhaled	Beclomethasone (Beclovent)
	Flucticasone (Flovent)
	Triamcinolone (Azmacort)
Oral	Prednisone (Deltasone)
Injected	Methyprednisolone (Solu-Medrol)
	Dexamethasone (Decadron)
Leukotriene Antagonists	Zafirlukast (Accolate)
	Zileuton (Zyflo)
Mast-Cell Membrane Stabilizer	Cromolyn (Intal)

Nonselective Sympathomimetics Medications that stimulate both beta$_1$ and beta$_2$ receptors, as well as alpha receptors, are rarely used to treat asthma because they have the undesired effects of increased peripheral vascular resistance and increased risks for tachycardias and other dysrhythmias. Nonselective drugs include epinephrine, ephedrine, and isoproterenol. Epinephrine is the only nonselective sympathomimetic in common use today, due to the availability of selective agents. It may be given subcutaneously for patients who have severe bronchospasm that does not respond to other treatments.

Methylxanthines The methylxanthines are CNS stimulants that have additional bronchodilatory properties. While they were once first-line therapy for asthma, now they are used only when other drugs such as beta$_2$ specific agents are ineffective. We do not know the methylxanthines' specific action, but they may block adenosine receptors. The prototype methylxanthine, theophylline, is taken orally. Aminophylline, an IV medication, is rapidly metabolized into theophylline and, therefore, has identical effects. These agents' chief side effects are nausea, vomiting, insomnia, restlessness, and dysrhythmias. Aminophylline is still used occasionally in the emergency treatment of acute asthma attacks.

Anticholinergics Ipratropium (Atrovent) is an atropine derivative given by nebulizer. Because stimulating the muscarinic receptors in the lungs results in constriction of bronchial smooth muscle, ipratropium, a muscarinic antagonist, causes bronchodilation. Ipratropium is inhaled and, therefore, has no systemic effects. Ipratropium and beta$_2$ agonists like albuterol act along different pathways, so their concurrent administration has an additive effect. Ipratropium's most common side effect is dry mouth. It results from the local effects of the drug that remains in the oropharynx after administration.

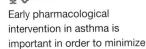

Glucocorticoids Glucocorticoids have anti-inflammatory properties. They lower the production and release of inflammatory substances such as histamine, prostaglandins, and leukotrienes, and they reduce mucus and edema secondary to decreasing vascular permeability. These drugs may be inhaled or taken orally, or they may be given intravenously in emergencies. The prototype inhaled glucocorticoid is beclomethasone; the prototype oral glucocorticoid is prednisone. Primarily preventive, they are taken on a regular schedule as opposed to the as-needed administration of the beta$_2$ agonists. An injectable glucocorticoid (methylprednisolone) is available for use secondary to beta$_2$ agonists in emergencies. When inhaled, glucocorticoids cause few side effects. Those are due mostly to direct exposure on the oropharynx, and gargling after taking the drug can decrease them. Likewise, side effects from the intravenous administrations of methylprednisolone in emergencies are not likely. Given orally or intravenously over long periods, however, glucocorticoids may have profound side effects, including adrenal suppression and hyperglycemia.

Another anti-inflammatory agent used to prevent asthma attacks is cromolyn (Intal), an inhaled powder. While it is not a glucocorticoid, its actions are similar. While the inhaled glucocorticoids are relatively safe, cromolyn is even safer. In fact, it is the safest of all antiasthma agents. Its only side effects are coughing or wheezing due to local irritation caused by the powder. Cromolyn is often used for preventing asthma in adults and children. It is also a useful prophylaxis before activities known to cause shortness of breath such as exercise or mowing grass.

Leukotriene Antagonists **Leukotrienes** are mediators released from mast cells upon contact with allergens. They contribute powerfully to both inflammation and bronchoconstriction. Consequently, agents that block their effects are useful in treating

Early pharmacological intervention in asthma is important in order to minimize inflammation.

leukotriene *mediator released from mast cells upon contact with allergens.*

asthma. Leukotriene antagonists can either block the synthesis of leukotrienes or block their receptors. Zileuton (Zyflo) is the prototype of those that block the synthesis of leukotrienes. Zafirlukast (Accolate) is the prototype of those that block their receptors.

DRUGS USED FOR RHINITIS AND COUGH

Rhinitis (inflammation of the nasal lining) comprises a group of symptoms including nasal congestion, itching, redness, sneezing, and rhinorrhea (runny nose). Either allergic reactions or viral infections such as the common cold may cause it. Drugs that treat the symptoms of rhinitis and cold are commonly found in over-the-counter remedies. In addition, nasal decongestants, antihistamines, and cough suppressants are available in prescription medications. Although manufacturers of cold medications often combine several drugs in one product intended to treat multiple symptoms, we will discuss each class separately.

Nasal Decongestants Nasal congestion is caused by dilated and engorged nasal capillaries. Drugs that constrict these capillaries are effective nasal decongestants. The main pharmacologic classification in this functional category is alpha$_1$ agonists. Alpha$_1$ agonists may be given either topically or orally. The chief examples of these agents, phenylephrine, pseudoephedrine, and phenylpropanolamine, can be administered either as a mist or in drops. Topical administration reduces systemic effects but has the undesired local effect of rebound congestion, a form of tolerance. Rebound congestion occurs after long-term use (greater than 7 consecutive days). As the drug wears off, congestion becomes progressively worse. This effect ends when the patient stops taking the drug; however, the longer the patient has been using the drug, the more unpleasant stopping becomes.

antihistamine *medication that arrests the effects of histamine by blocking its receptors.*

histamine *an endogenous substance that affects a wide variety of organ systems.*

Antihistamines Antihistamines arrest the effects of histamine by blocking its receptors. **Histamine** is an endogenous substance that affects a wide variety of organ systems. It is noted for its role in allergic reaction. In the vasculature, histamine binds with H$_1$ receptors to cause vasodilation and increased capillary permeability. In the lungs, H$_1$ receptors cause bronchoconstriction. In the gut, H$_2$ receptors cause an increase in gastric acid release. Histamine also acts as a neurotransmitter in the central nervous system. Histamine is synthesized and stored in two types of granulocytes: tissue-bound mast cells and plasma-bound basophils. Both types are full of secretory granules, which are vesicles containing inflammatory mediators such as histamine, leukotrienes, and prostaglandins, among others. When these cells are exposed to allergens, they develop antibodies on their surfaces. On subsequent exposures, the antibodies bind with their specific allergen. The secretory granules then migrate towards the cell's exterior and fuse with the cell membrane. This causes them to release their contents. While some available medications stabilize this membrane to prevent the release of these substances, the traditional antihistamines work by antagonizing the histamine receptors.

Commonly thought of as a nuisance, histamines are useful in our immune systems. Only when our immune systems overreact do allergies such as hay fever or cedar fever send us running for the antihistamines. The typical symptoms of allergic reaction include most of those associated with rhinitis. Severe allergic reactions (anaphylaxis) may cause hypotension. While histamines play a major role in mild and moderate allergic reactions, their part in anaphylaxis is minimal; therefore, antihistamines are at best only a secondary drug for treating anaphylaxis. (Epinephrine is the drug of choice.)

Just as there are H_1 and H_2 histamine receptors, there are H_1 and H_2 histamine receptor antagonists. When most people refer to antihistamines, they are thinking of H_1 receptor antagonists. These agents were in popular use long before the discovery of the H_2 receptors. (We discuss H_2 receptor antagonists in the section on drugs used to treat peptic ulcer disease.) The chief side effect of antihistamines is sedation, which the early antihistamines all caused to some degree. Now a second generation of antihistamines that do not cause sedation is available.

The first-generation antihistamines comprise several chemical subclasses. Examples include alkylamines (chlorpheniramine [Chlor-Trimeton]), ethanolamines (diphenhydramine [Benadryl], clemastine [Tavist]), and phenothiazines (promethazine [Phenergan]). While the different classes of agents have the same actions, they differ in the degree of sedation they cause and in their ability to block other, nonhistamine receptors. Several antihistamines also have significant anticholinergic properties. In fact, some are used specifically for their anticholinergic effects, notably promethazine and dimenhydrinate (Dramamine), which are used to reduce motion sickness. Other than the sedation that first-generation antihistamines cause, these agents' primary side effects are constipation and the effects of muscarinic blockade, such as dry mouth. Because they can thicken bronchial secretions, antihistamines should not be used in patients with asthma.

The second-generation antihistamines include terfenadine (Seldane), loratadine (Claritin), cetirizine (Zyrtec), and fexofenadine (Allegra). These agents' actions are similar to the first generation's, with the notable exception that they do not cross the blood–brain barrier and therefore do not cause sedation. In addition, their H_1 receptor antagonism is more pronounced, and their anticholinergic actions are greatly diminished. Terfenadine was used widely until the FDA removed it from the market because it had rare but significant side effects of cardiac dysrhythmias in patients with liver dysfunction or taking certain medications. Terfenadine's manufacturer is now marketing fexofenadine (Allegra) as a replacement.

Because they can thicken bronchial secretions, you should not use antihistamines in patients with asthma.

Cough Suppressants   Coughing is a complex reflex that depends on functions in the CNS, the PNS, and the respiratory muscles. It is a defense mechanism that aids the removal of foreign particles like smoke and dust. A productive cough is one in which these particles are actually being coughed up. In general, treating a productive cough is not appropriate, as it is performing a useful function. An unproductive cough, however, usually results from an irritated oropharynx and can be troublesome. The three classifications of cough suppressants include one that is supported by evidence and two that are not. **Antitussive** medications suppress the stimulus to cough in the central nervous system. This functional class includes two specific pharmacologic types, opioids and nonopioids. The two most common opioid antitussives are codeine and hydrocodone. Both inhibit the stimulus for coughing in the brain but also produce varying degrees of euphoria. The doses required for cough suppression are not high enough to cause euphoria, but these drugs still have the potential for abuse. The nonopioid antitussives, in contrast, do not have the potential for abuse. Dextromethoraphan is the leading drug in this class. While it is almost never given alone, it is the most common antitussive used in over-the-counter combination products for treating cold and flu symptoms. Diphenhydramine (Benadryl) is also used as a nonopioid antitussive, although its mechanism of action is not clear. Finally, the locally acting anesthetic benzonatate (Tessalon) depresses the cough stimulus by directly reducing oropharyngeal irritation. **Expectorants** are intended to increase the productivity of cough, and **mucolytics** make mucus more watery and, therefore, easier to cough up; however, little data supports the effectiveness of either of these approaches to cough suppression.

In general, treating a productive cough is not appropriate, as the cough is performing a useful function.

antitussive *medication that suppresses the stimulus to cough in the central nervous system.*

expectorant *medication intended to increase the productivity of cough.*

mucolytic *medication intended to make mucus more watery.*

DRUGS USED TO AFFECT THE GASTROINTESTINAL SYSTEM

The main purposes of drug therapy in the gastrointestinal system are to treat peptic ulcers, constipation, diarrhea, and emesis, and to aid digestion.

DRUGS USED TO TREAT PEPTIC ULCER DISEASE

Peptic ulcer disease (PUD) is characterized by an imbalance between factors in the gastrointestinal system that increase acidity and those that protect against acidity. PUD may manifest as indigestion, heartburn, or more seriously, as perforated ulcers. If the imbalance becomes too severe, parts of the lining of the GI system may be eaten away, exposing the tissue and vasculature underneath to the highly acidic environment of the stomach or duodenum. The GI system's structure fits its function. Many mucus-lined folds surround the GI lumen. The cells of these folds secrete acids needed to help break down foods; they secrete protective mucus that prevents the acid from injuring the underlying tissue; and finally, they secrete bicarbonates, which buffer the effects of acids on the GI system's absorbing surfaces. To absorb the digested nutrients and supply the mucus-producing cells of the lumen wall with oxygen, the entire GI system is very vascular. If the protective lining covering these vessels is removed, hemorrhage may occur.

Several pathologic factors oppose the GI system's defenses. Contrary to popular belief, the most common cause of peptic ulcer disease is not stress or alcohol, but the *Helicobacter pylori* bacterium. *H. pylori* infests the space between the endothelial cells and the mucus lining of the stomach and duodenum. It can remain there for decades, protected against the acid environment by the mucus layer. While we are still uncertain how this bacteria promotes ulcers, it apparently decreases the body's ability to produce the protective mucus lining. *H. pylori* by itself, however, does not cause ulcers. Many people remain infected for years and years without signs of PUD. Evidently, predisposing and contributing factors combine with *H. pylori* to cause ulceration. Some of these factors include smoking and long-term use of nonsteroidal anti-inflammatory drugs (NSAIDs) like aspirin and acetaminophen.

The approaches to treating PUD include antibiotics and drugs that block or decrease the secretion of gastric acid. Most often they are used in conjunction with each other. First, and most effective, are antibiotics. When the *H. pylori* infection is eliminated, the signs of PUD resolve and recurrence is low. Typically, three antibiotics will be utilized to assure elimination of the bacteria and prevent resistance. Common medications for this purpose include bismuth (Pepto-Bismol), metronidazole (Flagyl), amoxicillin (Amoxil), and tetracycline (Achromycin V).

Drugs that block or decrease the secretion of gastric acid include H_2 receptor antagonists (H_2RAs), proton pump inhibitors, and anticholinergic agents. Mucosal protectants and antacids are also used.

H_2 receptors occur throughout the gut on the membranes of the parietal cells lining the GI lumen. When stimulated with histamine, they increase the action of H^+K^+ATPase, an enzyme that exchanges potassium for hydrogen, leading to increased gastric acid secretion. Acetylcholine and prostaglandin receptors appear along with H_2 receptors. Stimulating the ACh receptors (muscarinic receptors) increases gastric acid secretion; stimulating the prostaglandin receptors inhibits it.

H_2 Receptor Antagonists H_2RA agents block the H_2 receptors in the gut. This inhibits gastric acid secretion and helps return the balance between protective and aggressive factors. Four approved H_2RAs are in use: cimetidine (Tagamet), ranitidine (Zantac), famotidine (Pepcid), and nizatidine (Axid Pulvules). Cimetidine is the oldest of these and serves as the prototype. These agents' primary therapeutic use is for ulcers, gastroesophageal reflux, heartburn or acid indigestion, and preventing aspiration pneumonia during anesthesia. Most of these agents have few significant side effects, with the exception of cimetidine, which may lead to decreased libido, impotence, and CNS effects in some patients. While these agents could technically be called antihistamines, that name by tradition is reserved for the H_1 antagonists. The H_2RAs have no effect on the H_1 receptors and are of no value in allergic reaction.

Proton Pump Inhibitors   Proton pump inhibitors act directly on the K^+H^+ATPase enzyme that secretes gastric acid. Omeprazole (Prilosec) and lansoprazole (Prevacid) are examples. Omeprazole is the prototype. These agents irreversibly block this enzyme, which means that the body must produce new enzyme in order to begin secreting acid again. This gives proton pump inhibitors a long duration of effect. Side effects are minor and rare, occurring in less than 1 percent of patients. They include diarrhea and headache.

Antacids   Antacids are alkalotic compounds used to increase the gastric environment's pH. Most available products are either aluminum, magnesium, calcium, or sodium compounds. They are used in conjunction with other approaches to PUD and are available over the counter for relief of acid indigestion and heartburn.

antacid alkalotic compound used to increase the gastric environment's pH.

Anticholinergics   While it might seem that all muscarinic blocking agents would be effective in decreasing gastric acid secretion, most atropinelike drugs produce too many unwanted effects and, therefore, are not used. The one exception is pirenzepine (Gastrozepine), because of its ability to selectively block the ACh receptors in the gut.

DRUGS USED TO TREAT CONSTIPATION

Laxatives decrease the firmness of stool and increase the water content. While an uninformed public frequently uses these agents unnecessarily, they are effective in some situations, specifically with patients for whom excessive strain is inappropriate. These patients include those with recent episiotomy, hemorrhoids, colostomies, or cardiovascular disease (for whom excessive straining may decrease heart rate).

laxative medication used to decrease stool's firmness and increase its water content.

Laxatives are traditionally grouped into four categories based on their mechanism of action: bulk-forming, surfactant, stimulant, and osmotic. The bulk-forming agents such as methylcellulose (Citrucel) and psyllium (Metamucil) produce a response almost identical to normal dietary fiber intake. Fiber is undigestible and unabsorbable; therefore, it remains in the lumen of the GI system and is passed more or less intact in stool. Most water absorption takes place in the colon. Fiber (or bulk-forming laxatives) in the colon absorbs water, leading to a softer, more bulky stool. Fiber can also provide nutrients for bacteria living in the colon. These bacteria feed and provide even more bulk. The enlarged stool stimulates stretch receptors in the colonic wall, which increases peristalsis. Softening the stool also lessens strain on defecation.

Review

Categories of Laxatives

- Bulk-forming
- Stimulant
- Osmotic
- Surfactant

The **surfactant** laxatives include docusate sodium (Colace). They decrease surface tension, which increases water absorption into the feces. They also increase water secretion and limit its reabsorption by the intestinal wall.

surfactant substance that decreases surface tension.

Stimulant laxatives increase motility. Like the surfactant laxatives, they also increase water secretion and decrease its absorption. The prototype stimulant laxative is phenolphthalein (Ex-Lax, Correctol). Bisacodyl (Bisacolax) is another example.

The osmotic laxatives are poorly absorbed salts that increase the feces' osmotic pull, thereby increasing their water content. Magnesium hydroxide, the active ingredient in Milk of Magnesia, is the prototype of this class.

DRUGS USED TO TREAT DIARRHEA

Diarrhea is the abnormally frequent passage of soft, liquid stool. It is a symptom of an underlying disease, usually a bacterial infection. It may be caused by an increased gastric motility (the stool does not stay in the colon long enough to have much water absorbed), increased water secretion, or decreased water absorption. While it is a nuisance, diarrhea is often a helpful process because it increases the expulsion of the offending agent. It is usually self-correcting and does not need to be treated. When treatment is necessary, either specific or nonspecific agents may be used. A specific agent directly treats the cause, usually a bacteria. As you would expect, antibiotics are a common specific antidiarrheal medication.

DRUGS USED TO TREAT EMESIS

Emesis is a complex process that involves different parts of the brain as well as receptors and muscles in the stomach and inner ear. The two involved parts of the brain include the vomiting center in the medulla and the chemoreceptor trigger zone (CTZ). The vomiting center stimulates vomiting directly, while the CTZ does so indirectly.

The vomiting center is stimulated by H_1 and ACh receptors in the pathway between itself and the inner ear, by sensory input from the eyes and nose (unpleasant or disturbing sights and smells), and by other parts of the brain in response to anxiety or fear. The CTZ stimulates the vomiting center in response to stimuli from serotonin receptors in the stomach and bloodborne substances such as opioids and ipecac.

Stimulating emesis is rarely desired, but it can be useful in treating certain types of overdoses or poisonings. Ipecac is the drug of choice when stimulating emesis is indicated. It stimulates the CTZ which, in turn, stimulates the vomiting center.

Ipecac is the drug of choice when stimulating emesis is indicated.

antiemetic *medication used to prevent vomiting.*

Many of the antiemetics used in emergency care can cause extrapyramidal symptoms. Always be alert for these.

Antiemetics Unlike causing emesis, preventing emesis is frequently desirable. **Antiemetics** are indicated in conjunction with chemotherapy, which may cause violent nausea and vomiting. Antiemetics are also indicated in the prophylactic treatment of motion sickness.

Multiple transmitters are involved in the vomiting reflex. They include serotonin, dopamine, acetylcholine, and histamine. Drugs that interfere with any of these transmitters can decrease or prevent nausea and vomiting. This functional class includes several pharmacologic subclasses: serotonin antagonists, dopamine antagonists, anticholinergics, and cannabinoids.

Serotonin Antagonists The prototype serotonin antagonist is ondansetron (Zofran). It blocks the serotonin receptors in the CTZ, the stomach, and the small intestines. It is very effective in the treatment of nausea and vomiting associated with chemotherapy, and unlike the dopamine antagonists, it does not cause extrapyramidal effects like dystonia and ataxia. Its most common side effects are headache and diarrhea.

Dopamine Antagonists Both phenothiazines and butyrophenones effectively block dopamine receptors in the CTZ. (This chapter's section on psychotherapeutic medications discusses both of these medications at length.) The phenothiazines include prochlorperazine (Compazine) and promethazine (Phenergan), while the butyrophenones include haloperidol (Haldol) and droperidol (Inapsine). Agents from both classes cause side effects of extrapyramidal effects and sedation. Another dopamine antagonist, metoclopramide (Reglan), is neither a phenothiazine nor a butyropenone. It is unique in that it blocks both serotonin and dopamine receptors in the CTZ.

Cannabinoids The cannabinoids are derivatives of tetrahydrocannabinol (THC) and are effective antiemetics used to treat chemotherapy-induced nausea and vomiting. The two available agents are dronabinol (Marinol) and nabilone (Cesamet). Because both agents are essentially the same as THC (the active ingredient in marijuana), their side effects include euphoria similar to that of marijuana. While those effects may be desirable for some, they may be intensely unpleasant for others.

DRUGS USED TO AID DIGESTION

Several drugs are available to aid the digestion of carbohydrates and fats. These agents are similar to endogenous digestive enzymes released into the duodenum in response to vagal stimulation. Occasionally, supplemental enzymes are necessary for patients whose vagal stimulus has been surgically severed or whose duodenum has been by-passed. Two of these drugs are pancreatin (Entozyme) and pancrelipase (Viokase). Their chief side effects are nausea, vomiting, and abdominal cramping.

DRUGS USED TO AFFECT THE EYES

Ophthalmic drugs are used to treat conditions involving the eyes, primarily glaucoma and trauma. In addition, some ophthalmic agents are used in diagnosing and examining the eyes.

Glaucoma is a degenerative disease that affects the optic nerve. Its causative factors are not clear; however, correlations are known between it and several risk factors including intraocular pressure, race (its rate is three times higher among African Americans than among whites), and age. The medications used to treat glaucoma are all aimed at reducing intraocular pressure (IOP). Beta-blockers and cholinergics are the most common. Beta-blockade decreases IOP by an unknown mechanism. Timolol (Timoptic) and betaxolol (Betoptic) are examples of this class. Pilocarpine (Isopto Carpine) is the prototype cholinergic drug for treating glaucoma. It stimulates muscarinic receptors in the eye to cause miosis (pupil constriction) and ciliary muscle contraction, which indirectly lowers IOP. Drugs from these classes are given topically. Beta-blockers have few side effects, while pilocarpine causes blurred vision and local irritation.

Some diagnostic procedures call for causing mydriasis (pupil dilation) and cycloplegia (paralysis of the ciliary muscles used to focus vision). The two pharmacologic approaches to doing this involve anticholinergics or adrenergic agonists. In this functional class, atropine solutions such as Atropisol and scopolamine solutions such as Isopto Hyoscine are typical anticholinergics; phenylephrine solution (AK-Dilate) is the class's principal adrenergic agonist. This chapter's sections on anticholinergics and adrenergic agonists discuss these pharmacologic classes in more detail.

Tetracaine (Pontocaine) is a local anesthetic of the ester class. (It is related to cocaine, another ester, but not to lidocaine, an amide.) It is used to decrease pain and sensation in the eye from trauma or during ophthalmic procedures.

If tetracaine is administered in the field, remind the patient not to rub his eyes, as he can worsen the injury.

DRUGS USED TO AFFECT THE EARS

Most drugs used to treat conditions involving the ear are aimed at eliminating underlying bacterial or fungal infections or at breaking up impacted ear wax. Chloramphenicol (Chloromycetin Otic) and gentamicin sulfate otic solution (Garamycin) are common antibiotics; carbamide peroxide (Auro Ear Drops) and carbamide peroxide and glycerin (Ear Wax Removal System) are both used to treat ear wax. Finally, several drugs are available to treat swimmer's ear, an inflammation/irritation of the external ear. They include isopropyl alcohol (Auro-Dri Ear Drops) and boric acid and isopropyl alcohol (Aurocaine 2).

Some drugs that are used for other purposes have ototoxic (harmful to the organs or nerves that produce hearing or balance) properties if taken in overdose or administered too quickly. The most common ototoxic symptom is tinnitus, or ringing in the ears. Drugs with ototoxic properties include aspirin and other NSAIDs, some antibiotics (including erythromycin and vancomycin), and the diuretic furosemide (Lasix).

DRUGS USED TO AFFECT THE ENDOCRINE SYSTEM

The endocrine system and nervous system together are chiefly responsible for the regulatory activities that maintain homeostasis. The nervous system, with its direct connections between nerves and organs, may be thought of as a "wired" system, while the endocrine system, which releases hormones directly into the bloodstream, may be thought of as "wireless." The endocrine system comprises the following glands: pituitary (anterior and posterior lobes), pineal, thyroid, parathyroid, thymus, adrenal, pancreas, ovaries, and testes. (Table 9–9 lists the specific hormones that each gland releases.) Of these, the pituitary is commonly referred to as the master gland because of its role in controlling the other endocrine glands. (The hypothalamus in turn controls many of the pituitary's functions.) Once in the bloodstream, the hormones from these glands circulate widely throughout the body. To be effective, however, they must bind with very specific receptors. This discussion will focus on the pharmacologic actions of drugs that affect the various endocrine glands.

DRUGS AFFECTING THE PITUITARY GLAND

The pituitary gland is made up of a posterior lobe and an anterior lobe. It sits in the sella turcica, a depression of the sphenoid bone, and is physically connected to the hypothalamus. The posterior pituitary hormones are actually synthesized in the hypothalamus and then migrate into the posterior pituitary, where they are released upon hypothalamic stimulation. In contrast, the hormones of the anterior pituitary are actually synthesized in that lobe. The hypothalamus secretes releasing hormones into a portal system that carries them into the anterior pituitary, where they stimulate the release of the anterior pituitary hormones. There are six main anterior pituitary hormones.

Table 9–9	Summary of Hormone Actions	
Gland	**Hormone**	**Action**
Posterior pituitary	Oxytocin	Uterine contraction, milk ejection
	Vasopressin (ADH)	Retains salt and water, increases ECF volume
Anterior pituitary	Thyroid-stimulating hormone (TSH)	Increases metabolic rate
	Growth hormone (GH)	Increases use of stored fats, decreases glucose use
	Adrenocorticotropic hormone (ACTH)	Stimulates adrenal cortex to release hormones
	Follicle-stimulating hormone (FSH)	Males: sperm production Females: stimulates growth and development of ovarian follicles
	Luteinizing hormone (LH)	Males: responsible for secretion of testosterone by testes Females: ovulation, secretion of estrogen and progesterone
	Prolactin (PRL)	Enhances breast development and milk production
Thyroid	Thyroid hormone	Increases metabolic rate
Parathyroid	Parathyroid hormone	Increases calcium in ECF
Pancreas	Insulin	Decreases blood glucose
	Glucagon	Increases blood glucose
Adrenal	Glucocorticoids	Increase blood glucose, prevent inflammation

Anterior Pituitary Drugs   The only conditions treated with anterior pituitary-like drugs are those associated with abnormal growth, specifically dwarfism, acromegaly, and gigantism. Dwarfism is caused by a deficiency of growth hormone, and therapy is aimed at hormone replacement. Somatrem (Protropin) and somatropin (Humatrope) are both essentially the same as the endogenous growth hormone, acting indirectly to increase skeletal growth as well as cell numbers by stimulating another hormone, insulinlike growth factor 1 (IGF-1), to cause its effects. These drugs' primary side effects are pain and redness at the injection site. Some cases of inadvertent gigantism have been reported, but this can be avoided with careful observation.

Acromegaly and gigantism are caused by excesses of growth hormone, usually resulting from a tumor. While the treatment of choice is surgical removal of the tumor, octreotide (Sandostatin) is available for pharmacologic intervention. Octreotide is a synthetic drug with actions similar to somatostatin, the endogenous growth hormone inhibiting hormone. Its main action inhibits the release of growth hormone. Octreotide's many side effects include bradycardia, diarrhea, and stomach distress.

Posterior Pituitary Drugs   The two posterior pituitary hormones are oxytocin and antidiuretic hormone. Oxytocin is discussed in the section on drugs affecting labor and delivery. Antidiuretic hormone (ADH) increases water reabsorption in the renal collecting tubules, thus promoting the retention of water and a more concentrated urine. Physiologically, ADH is a key component in regulating blood volume, blood pressure, and electrolyte balance. Clinically, ADH analogues are used to treat diabetes insipidus and nocturnal enuresis (bedwetting). Diabetes insipidus, unlike diabetes mellitus, is caused by inadequate amounts of centrally acting ADH. This causes a profound polyuria and polydipsia. At higher doses, ADH can cause vasoconstriction and increased blood pressure; hence its other name, vasopressin. Vasopressin (Pitressin), desmopressin (Stimate), and lypressin (Diapid) are all available to reverse this ADH deficiency. Desmopressin is also available for administration via intranasal spray for nocturnal enuresis.

DRUGS AFFECTING THE PARATHYROID AND THYROID GLANDS

The parathyroid glands are primarily responsible for regulating calcium levels. Hypoparathyroidism leads to decreased levels of calcium and Vitamin D. Treatment, therefore, is through calcium and Vitamin D supplements. Hyperparathyroidism leads to high levels of calcium. Because it usually results from tumors, the treatment of choice is surgical removal of all or part of the parathyroid glands.

The thyroid gland produces thyroid hormones, which play a vital role in regulating growth, maturation, and metabolism. Hypothyroidism can occur in children or adults. When it develops in children, it is known as cretinism and manifests itself as dwarfism and mental retardation with characteristic features. Because most growth and maturation in adults is complete, adult onset of hypothyroidism appears as decreased metabolic rate, weight gain, fatigue, and bradycardia. In some cases, myxedema (facial puffiness) may be present. Treatment is aimed at thyroid hormone replacement. The prototype drug, levothyroxine (Synthroid), is also the most commonly used. A synthetic analogue of T_4 (thyroxine), one of the thyroid hormones, levothyroxine generally has no significant side effects when taken in therapeutic doses. Overdose may lead to thyrotoxicosis or thyroid storm. Thyrotoxicosis is a condition in which hyperthyroidism causes an increase in thyroid hormones. Thyroid storm is a severe form of thyrotoxicosis where the manifestations of the disease increase to life-threatening proportions. Thyroid storm is characterized by tachycardic dysrhythmias, angina, hypertension, and hyperthermia.

Goiters are enlargements of the thyroid gland. They are typically caused by insufficient dietary iodine. In developed countries, goiter is much rarer than in undeveloped countries and is most commonly caused by Hashimoto's disease, a chronic autoimmune disease. Treatment of goiters is aimed at supplementing the inadequate iodine.

Hyperthyroidism is caused by excessive release of thyroid hormones, typically as a result of tumors. The most common cause of hyperthyroidism in the United States is Graves' disease. It presents with tachycardia, hypertension, hyperthermia, nervousness, insomnia, increased metabolic rate, and weight loss. In severe cases, exophthalmos (protrusion of the eyeballs) may occur. Treatment is typically surgical removal of all or part of the thyroid gland. Radioactive iodine (^{131}I) may also be given for radiation therapy. Propylthiouracil (PTU) may be given alone or as adjunct therapy to surgery or radiation in treating hyperthyroidism.

DRUGS AFFECTING THE ADRENAL CORTEX

The adrenal cortex synthesizes and secretes three classes of hormones: glucocorticoids, mineralocorticoids, and androgens. The glucocorticoids and mineralocorticoids are referred to collectively as corticosteroids, adrenocorticoids, or corticoids. As their name implies, glucocorticoids increase the production of glucose by enhancing carbohydrate metabolism, promoting gluconeogenesis, and reducing peripheral glucose utilization. The most important glucocorticoid is cortisol. The mineralocorticoids regulate salt and water balance. The primary mineralocorticoid is aldosterone. The androgens are important hormones in regulating sexual maturation and development.

Two diseases typify the disorders associated with the adrenal cortex: Cushing's disease and Addison's disease. Cushing's disease is characterized by hypersecretion of adrenocorticotropic hormone, an anterior pituitary tropic hormone that increases the synthesis of corticoids, leading to excessive glucocorticoid secretion. Common signs and symptoms include hyperglycemia, obesity, hypertension, and electrolyte imbalances. Addison's disease is characterized by hyposecretion of corticoids as a result of damage to the adrenal gland. Common signs and symptoms include hypoglycemia, emaciation, hypotension, hyperkalemia, and hyponatremia.

Treatment of Cushing's disease is typically surgical. Symptomatic pharmacologic intervention with an antihypertensive (potassium sparing diuretics such as spironolactone [Aldactone] or ACE inhibitors such as captopril [Capoten]) may be necessary. Drugs that may inhibit the synthesis of corticosteroids (antiadrenals) may also be used as an adjunct to surgery or radiation. In high doses, the antifungal agent ketoconazole (Nizoral) is an effective temporary antiadrenal drug. At such doses, however, it may cause liver dysfunction.

Treatment of Addison's disease is aimed at replacement therapy. Cortisone (Cortistan) and hydrocortisone (SoluCortef) are the drugs of choice. Occasionally, a specific mineralocorticoid is necessary. Fludrocortisone (Florinef Acetate) is the only mineralocorticoid available.

DRUGS AFFECTING THE PANCREAS

Diabetes mellitus is the most important disease involving the pancreas. Diabetes mellitus (as opposed to diabetes insipidus, which involves inadequate ADH secretion) involves inappropriate carbohydrate metabolism. Traditionally, the term *diabetes* used alone refers to diabetes mellitus, of which the two main types are, logically, type I and type II. Type I diabetes is also known as insulin-dependent diabetes mellitus, or IDDM. It results from an inadequate release of insulin from the beta cells of the pancreatic islets. Patients with type I diabetes rely on insulin replacement therapy to survive. Because IDDM typically manifests itself at an early age (usually before 30 years) it is also commonly called juvenile onset diabetes. Most diabetics have type II diabetes, which is also referred to as non-insulin-dependent diabetes mellitus (NIDDM) or adult onset diabetes. It results from a decreased responsiveness to insulin and a lack of synchronization between insulin release and blood glucose levels. Type II diabetes typically begins later in life (after 40 years) and almost always occurs in patients with obesity. Because they have functioning beta cells that release insulin, type II diabetics usually do not depend on insulin replacement. Gestational diabetes, a third type, occurs transitionally during pregnancy. Gestational diabetes is a form of stress-induced diabetes in which the mother cannot effectively manage her blood glucose levels during pregnancy without medical intervention. Gestational diabetes resolves itself within hours to days after delivery.

The two main substances involved with regulating blood glucose are insulin and glucagon. Both are secreted from the pancreas and both are used to manage diabetes. Secreted from the beta cells of the pancreatic islets of Langerhans in response to increased blood glucose levels, **insulin** increases cellular transport of glucose, potassium, and amino acids. It also converts glucose into glycogen for storage in the liver and in skeletal muscle. Finally, insulin promotes cell growth and division.

insulin *substance that decreases blood glucose level.*

Glucagon, too, is secreted from the pancreatic islets, but by alpha cells rather than by the insulin-producing beta cells. Glucagon's actions are the direct opposite of insulin's; it increases both glycogenolysis (glycogen breakdown into glucose) and gluconeogenesis (the synthesis of glucose from glycerol and amino acids). So, while insulin decreases blood glucose levels, glucagon increases them.

glucagon *substance that increases blood glucose level.*

Patients with either type I or type II diabetes may experience both hyperglycemia and hypoglycemia. While hyperglycemia more often results from the disease, hypoglycemia is a common side effect of treatment. The main intervention for patients with IDDM is insulin-replacement therapy. Several insulin preparations are available. The most effective therapy for patients with NIDDM is usually weight loss through diet modification and exercise. When this is not effective, oral hypoglycemic agents and, occasionally, insulin are used. Finally, glucagon and diazoxide (both can be considered hyperglycemic agents) are occasionally used for treating emergency hypoglycemia.

Always consider glucagon in the hypoglycemic patient when an IV cannot be started.

Insulin Preparations Insulin comes from one of three sources. Initially, it came from either beef or pork intestines. Now, recombinant DNA technology has made human insulin available (that is, insulin synthesized with a human RNA template, not harvested directly from humans). Insulin preparations differ primarily in their onset and duration of action and in their incidence of allergic reaction. Insulin preparations may be short acting, intermediate acting, or long acting, depending on their onset and duration of action. (Table 9–10 lists insulin preparations.)

Insulin is also classified as natural (regular) or modified. As their name suggests, the natural insulins are used as they occur in nature. The other insulin preparations have been modified to increase their duration of action and thus decrease the frequency of their administration. All insulin preparations are given subcutaneously, with the exception of regular insulin, which may also be given intravenously. Insulin is not available as an oral medication because the digestive enzymes would rapidly render it inactive; therefore, IDDM patients must take multiple injections every day of their lives. This may discourage compliance in some patients.

Diabetic ketoacidosis (DKA) is best treated by a continuous insulin infusion accompanied by frequent checks of the blood glucose levels.

The modified insulin preparations include NPH (neutral protamine Hagedorn) insulin, which is regular insulin attached to a large protein designed to delay absorption, and the lente series, which is attached to zinc. Two preparations of lente insulin are available by themselves, lente and ultralente. A third, semilente insulin, is available only in a combination product with other insulins.

Insulin preparations are used for lifelong replacement therapy in IDDM and for emergency treatment of hyperglycemia and hyperkalemia in nondiabetics. (Recall that

Table 9–10 | Insulin Preparations

Classification	Trade Name	Source	Onset (Hrs)	Peak (Hrs)	Duration (Hrs)
Rapid-Acting			0.25+	<0.75–2.5	3.5–5.0
Lispro Insulin	Humalog	Human			
Aspart Insulin	NovoRapid	Human			
Short-Acting or Regular			0.5–10	2.0–5.0	5.0–8.0
	Humulin R	Human			
	Novolin R	Human			
	Iletin II R	Pork			
Intermediate-Acting or NPH			1–2	4–12	14–18
	Humulin N	Human			
	Novolin N	Human			
	Iletin II NPH	Pork			
Premixed			0.5–1.0	2–12	14–18
	Humulin 70/30	Human			
	Humulin 50/50	Human			
	Novolin 70/30	Human			
	Novolin 50/50	Human			
Intermediate-Acting			2–4	7–15	12–24
	Humulin L	Human			
	Iletin II Lente	Pork			
Long-Acting			3–4	8–24	24–28
	Humulin U	Human			
	Ultralente				
Insulin Glargine			>1.5	No peak	>20
	Lantus	Human			

insulin also increases potassium uptake by cells and is therefore useful in lowering potassium levels.) These preparations' primary side effect is unintended hypoglycemia. Because $beta_2$ adrenergic blockers can hide the effects of hypoglycemia, patients may not recognize this condition's signs until they cannot care for themselves. Also, beta-blockers decrease the release of glucagon, so these patients' hypoglycemia may be even worse. Insulin preparations derived from beef or pork, as well as the lentes, may lead to allergic reactions. The natural human insulin preparations do not have this effect.

Oral Hypoglycemic Agents   Oral hypoglycemic agents are used to stimulate insulin secretion from the pancreas in patients with NIDDM. These agents are ineffective in people with type I diabetes since those patients cannot secrete insulin. This functional class comprises four pharmacologic classes: sulfonylureas, biguanides, alpha-glucosidase inhibitors, and thiazolidinediones. The sulfonylureas were the first class of oral hypoglycemics available and as such are also known as first-generation or second-generation oral hypoglycemics, depending on when they were released. Drugs in this class include tolbutamide (Orinase), chlorpropamide (Diabinese), glipizide (Glucotrol), and glyburide (Micronase). They work by increasing insulin secretion from the pancreas and may also increase tissue response to insulin. Their major side effect is hypoglycemia.

The only agent in the biguanide class is metformin (Glucophage). It decreases glucose synthesis and increases glucose uptake. It does not stimulate the release of insulin from the pancreas and therefore does not cause hypoglycemia. Its primary side effects are nausea, vomiting, and decreased appetite.

Alpha-glucosidase inhibitors include acarbose (Precose) and miglitol (Glyset). They work by delaying carbohydrate metabolism, which moderates the increase in blood glucose that occurs after meals. These agents' primary side effects are flatulence, cramps, diarrhea, and abdominal distention resulting from colonic bacteria feeding on the increased number of carbohydrates remaining in fecal matter.

Thiazolidinediones are a new class of oral hypoglycemic agents unrelated to the others. The only drug in this class is troglitazone (Rezulin). It works by promoting tissue response to insulin and thus making the available insulin more effective. Troglitazone has no major side effects.

Hyperglycemic Agents   Two hyperglycemic agents, glucagon and diazoxide (Proglycem), act to increase blood glucose levels. Glucagon is indicated for the emergency treatment of patients with hypoglycemia. It will frequently be given intramuscularly to hypoglycemic patients in whom an IV line is unobtainable. Occasional side effects are nausea and vomiting and, rarely, allergic reactions. Diazoxide (Proglycem) inhibits insulin release and is typically used only for patients with hyperinsulin secretion resulting from pancreatic tumors; it is more commonly used for hypertension. It is not indicated for treating diabetes-induced hypoglycemia.

$D_{50}W$ (50 percent dextrose in water) is a sugar solution given intravenously for acute hypoglycemia. Its primary side effect is local tissue necrosis if infiltration occurs.

Dilute $D_{50}W$ to $D_{25}W$ for administration to pediatric patients.

DRUGS AFFECTING THE FEMALE REPRODUCTIVE SYSTEM

The main groups of drugs affecting the female reproductive system are estrogens, progestins, oral contraceptives, drugs affecting uterine contraction, and those used to treat infertility.

Estrogens and Progestins   Estrogens are produced in females by the ovaries and the ovarian follicles, and in pregnancy, the placenta. Outside of pregnancy, the ovaries are the principal source of estrogens. The principal ovarian estrogen is estradiol, of which there are many commercial preparations. The principal indication for estrogen is replacement therapy in postmenopausal women. After menopause, estrogen levels drop significantly and have been indicated as the cause of menopausal symptoms such as hot flashes and vaginal dryness and as an increased risk factor for osteoporosis. Hormone replacement therapy (HRT) with estrogen has been shown to alleviate menopausal symptoms and reverse the increased risk for osteoporosis; however, it is not without its own risks. Recent studies have shown increased chances of breast cancer and stroke associated with hormone replacement therapy. Side effects include nausea, fluid retention, and breast tenderness. The nausea usually diminishes after several months of therapy. Estrogen is also administered in cases of delayed puberty in girls as a result of hypogonadism.

The progestins' principal noncontraceptive use is to counteract the untoward effects of estrogen on the endometrium in hormone replacement therapy for postmenopausal women. They are also used to treat amenorrhea, endometriosis, and dysfunctional uterine bleeding.

Oral Contraceptives Oral contraception is an effective means of preventing pregnancy. All oral contraceptives' primary mechanism of action is the prevention of ovulation, which makes the endometrium less favorable for implantation and promotes the development of a thick mucus plug that blocks access to sperm through the cervix. These contraceptives are either a combination of estrogen and progestin or, in the case of "mini-pills," progestin only. They may also be classified based on their administration cycle as monophasic, biphasic, or triphasic. These classes differ in how they alter the dose of estrogen or progestin throughout the menstrual cycle. Many different preparations are available, although they all work in similar fashion. In general, these drugs are well tolerated and have few side effects. The oral contraceptives' chief side effects are unintended pregnancy (in less than 3 percent of users), thromboembolism (this risk is much lower with the newer low-estrogen dose preparations), hypertension, and abnormal uterine bleeding. They are in wide use and are one of the most widely prescribed drug classes. They are the second most popular means of birth control after surgical sterilization (male and female combined).

Uterine Stimulants and Relaxants Drugs that increase uterine contraction (uterine stimulants) are oxytocics (oxytocin means rapid birth). Drugs that relax the uterus or inhibit uterine contraction are tocolytics.

The primary indications for administration of an oxytocic are to induce labor and to treat severe postpartum hemorrhage. Oxytocin is available commercially as Pitocin and Syntocinon. The uterus becomes increasingly sensitive to oxytocin throughout gestation, progressing from relatively insensitive before pregnancy to very sensitive around the time of labor. Oxytocin's chief side effect, water retention, is rarely significant and only so if large volumes of fluid have been administered without careful ongoing assessment. Ergonovine (Ergotrate), a derivative of a rye fungus, is a powerful uterine stimulant. It increases both the force and duration of contraction. Because of this increased duration, ergonovine is only used in the treatment of postpartum hemorrhage.

The tocolytics relax uterine smooth muscle by stimulating the beta$_2$ receptors in the uterus. The two beta$_2$ agonists commonly used for this purpose are terbutaline (Brethine) and ritodrine (Yutopar). Terbutaline's primary use is to treat asthma, but it is commonly used to delay labor even though the FDA does not currently approve it for that purpose. Both agents decrease both the force and frequency of contraction. Their chief side effects are the same as those of the other beta$_2$ agonists used to treat asthma: tremors and tachycardia. Occasionally, hyperglycemia may result from glycogenolysis in the liver.

Infertility Agents A number of conditions may cause infertility, which is the inability to become pregnant, and medications can treat only some of them. Most infertility drugs are developed for women and promote maturation of ovarian follicles. Clomiphene (Clomid), urofollitropin (Metrodin), and menotropins (Pergonal) are all within this class, although they each act by a different mechanism. These agents' side effects include ovarian enlargement or cysts, abdominal pain, and menstrual irregularities.

DRUGS AFFECTING THE MALE REPRODUCTIVE SYSTEM

Drugs that affect the male reproductive system include those that treat testosterone deficiency and benign prostatic hyperplasia. Testosterone replacement therapy may be indicated in testosterone deficiency caused by cryptorchidism (failure of one or both of the testes to descend during puberty), orchitis (testicular inflammation), or orchidectomy (testicular removal). It is also used in delayed puberty. Preparations include testosterone enanthate, methyltestosterone (Metandren), and fluoxymesterone (Halotestin).

Benign prostatic hyperplasia is an enlarged prostate. This is a common but problematic age-related disease. By the age of 70, close to 75 percent of men will have symptoms severe enough to seek therapy. These symptoms may include urinary hesitancy and retention. Treatment has traditionally been surgery, but several drugs are available, including finasteride (Proscar), which interferes with the production of an enzyme involved with prostate growth. Side effects may include rash, breast tenderness, headache, impotence, and decreased libido.

DRUGS AFFECTING SEXUAL BEHAVIOR

For centuries, cultures have searched for drugs that would increase libido and sexual potency. Ironically, the reverse has most commonly been found. The largest category of drugs affecting sexual behavior do so as a side effect of their intended purpose. Many drug classifications decrease libido in both sexes and inhibit erection and ejaculation. Examples include antihypertensives (beta-blockers, centrally acting alpha antagonists, and diuretics) and antianxiety/antipsychotic medications (benzodiazepines, phenothiazines, MAO inhibitors, and tricyclic antidepressants).

Many drugs are purported to increase libido. The most notable of these is cantharis (Spanish fly). Despite common belief, no evidence indicates that cantharis actually increases sexual appetite. Indeed, it can produce some very dangerous side effects. Hallucinogens such as LSD and marijuana, as well as alcohol, are also commonly believed to heighten sexuality. Any such effect from these agents is likely an indirect result of decreased inhibitions or anxiety. These drugs all have very different effects, depending on each individual's unique physiology, expectations before use, and surrounding circumstances. They have no proven direct physiologic effect on sexual gratification.

Levodopa (L-dopa), an anti-Parkinson's drug, has demonstrated increased libido and improved erectile ability as a side effect of treatment. Whether this results directly from increased autonomic stimulation or indirectly from improved self-esteem achieved in therapy, any improvement seems to be only temporary. Several drugs have been developed that aid in erectile dysfunction. Erectile dysfunction becomes more frequent with age or with certain diseases such as diabetes or cardiovascular disease. Drugs that aid in erectile dysfunction increase blood supply to the penis. These include sildenafil (Viagra), vardenafil (Levitra), and tadalafil (Cialis). These drugs act by relaxing vascular smooth muscle, which increases blood flow to the corpus cavernosum, the spongelike tissue on the sides of the penis responsible for erection. These drugs are unique in that they have no effect in the absence of sexual stimulation. Other drugs used to treat impotence have caused prolonged and painful erections (priapism). The chief side effect of sildenafil is seen when it is used in combination with nitrates. The combined effect of relaxing vascular smooth muscle may lead to a dangerously decreased preload, which may lower blood pressure and lead to myocardial infarction. Prehospital personnel should be aware of this important interaction. If you are called on to treat a patient with chest pain who has taken sildenafil, vardenafil, or tadalafil recently, do not give him nitroglycerin or any other nitrate.

DRUGS USED TO TREAT CANCER

antineoplastic agent *drug used to treat cancer.*

Drugs used to treat cancer are called **antineoplastic** agents. A detailed discussion of the many different antineoplastic agents is beyond the scope of this text; however, this section will briefly overview their main classes and prototype drugs.

Cancer involves the modification of cellular DNA leading to an abnormal growth of tissues. Of the many known types of cancer, only a few are successfully treated with chemotherapy. In fact, most cancers are best treated by surgical removal of the tumor. Unfortunately, many of the more lethal cancers do not involve a compact growth; rather, they affect the formed elements of the blood, especially leukocytes. Treating these widely dispersed cancers with surgery is not possible, as there is nothing for the surgeon to remove.

Chemotherapy is not nearly as safe or devoid of side effects as antibiotic therapy; however, scientists have yet to identify any unique characteristics of cancer cells that would allow them to develop drugs specific to those cells. Because cancer is the abnormal growth of normal cells, drugs that kill cancerous cells therefore also kill noncancerous cells. Chemotherapy is thus largely a balancing act aimed at maximizing the kill rate of cancer cells while minimizing the death of normal tissue. The one characteristic that most cancer cells share is rapid cell division and replication. Consequently, most antineoplastic agents have their greatest effect on cancer cells during mitosis and on young, small cancers that are undergoing rapid growth.

The agents used to kill cancer cells are grouped according to their mechanism of action. Antimetabolite drugs mimic some of the enzymes and proteins needed for DNA replication but do not have the same effects; therefore, they prevent cells from reproducing. Their prototype is fluorouracil (Adrucil). Alkylating agents that interfere with DNA splitting include cyclophosphamide (Cytoxan) and mechlorethamine (Mustargen). Mitotic inhibitors also interfere with cell division; they include vinblastine (Velban) and vincristine (Oncovin).

Chemotherapy's primary side effects include nausea, vomiting, and other gastrointestinal disturbances, as well as hair loss and weakness. Almost all antineoplastic agents cause severe side effects and are given in conjunction with antiemetics.

DRUGS USED TO TREAT INFECTIOUS DISEASES AND INFLAMMATION

Infectious diseases are typically caused by bacteria, viruses, or funguses and may be treated with antimicrobial drugs developed to fight those particular invaders. We will discuss each broad class.

antibiotic *agent that kills or decreases the growth of bacteria.*

Antibiotics An **antibiotic** agent may either kill the offending bacteria (bactericidal agents) or so decrease the bacteria's growth that the patient's immune system can effectively fight the infection (bacteriostatic agents). In general, all of these agents share one of several mechanisms. Drugs in the penicillin and cephalosporin classes, as well as vancomycin (Vancocin), are bactericidal and act by inhibiting cell wall synthesis. Unlike animal cells, bacteria have hypertonic cell cytoplasm and depend on the rigid and relatively impermeable cell wall to maintain integrity. When cell wall synthesis is inhibited, osmotic pressure pulls water into the cell, and the cell ruptures, killing the bacteria. The macrolide, aminoglycoside, and tetracycline antibiotics inhibit protein synthesis, preventing the bacterial cell from replicating and thus spreading infection. These agents are usually bacteriostatic but can be bactericidal at high doses. Typical side effects from antibiotics include gastrointestinal dysfunction, which commonly results from a decrease in the natural gastrointestinal bacteria that inhabit the colon.

Antifungal and Antiviral Agents Fungi are parasitic microorganisms that cannot synthesize their own food. Fungal infections (mycoses) may be treated with several drugs. The azole antifungals inhibit fungal growth. Their prototype is ketoconazole (Nizoral). Drugs used to treat viruses work by a variety of mechanisms and include acyclovir (Zovirax) and zidovudine (Retrovir), which is commonly known as AZT. Protease inhibitors are one of the more promising classes of drugs for treating viruses such as HIV. Indinavir (Crixivan) is the prototype of this class.

Other Antimicrobial and Antiparasitic Agents While most diseases treated with the medications discussed in this section are uncommon in developed countries, they are leading causes of death in third-world countries. They include malaria, tuberculosis, leprosy, amebiasis, and helminthiasis. Tuberculosis is increasingly appearing in the United States in patients with compromised immune systems.

Malaria is a parasitic infection common in the tropics. It is transmitted by certain types of mosquitoes or, less commonly, by blood transfusion. Drugs used to treat malaria are called schizonticides. They include chloroquine (Aralen), mefloquine (Lariam), and quinine. Treatment is aimed at either preventing infestation (prophylactic treatment for individuals traveling to high-risk areas) or killing the parasites in infected patients.

Tuberculosis is caused by bacteria that are transmitted through airborne droplets from the coughing and sneezing of infected patients. The bacteria can grow only in well-oxygenated areas. Because of the route of infection and the need for oxygen, most patients with tuberculosis have infestations in the lungs. Once in the lungs, the bacteria are typically "walled off," or enclosed in tubercules, and become dormant and non-infective. If the patient's immune system is compromised, the bacteria may become active again and begin to cause symptoms. Drugs commonly used to treat tuberculosis include isoniazid (Nydrazid, INH) and rifampin (Rifadin).

Amebiasis is a parasitic infection of the intestines common in tropical areas. Transmission most frequently occurs via the oral-fecal route from eating poorly cooked food contaminated by cooks who inadequately wash their hands. Drugs used to treat amebiasis include paromomycin (Humatin) and metronidazole (Flagyl).

Helminthiasis is caused by parasitic worms (helminths) including flatworms and roundworms. These worms usually invade the host's intestinal tract and attach themselves to the lumen wall with hooks or suckers. They cause symptoms by depriving the host of nutrients (especially in children); by obstructing the intestinal lumen, which leads to bowel obstruction; and by producing toxins. Treatment is aimed at either killing the organism outright or destroying its ability to latch onto the intestinal wall so it passes with the patient's feces. These drugs include mebendazole (Vermox) and niclosamide (Niclocide).

Leprosy, also known as Hansen's disease, is caused by bacteria. It leads to characteristic lesions, footdrop (plantar flexion), and plantar ulceration. Drugs used to treat it include dapsone (DDS, Avlosulfon) and clofazimine (Lamprene).

Nonsteroidal Anti-Inflammatory Drugs   NSAIDs (nonsteroidal anti-inflammatory drugs) are commonly used as analgesics and antipyretics (fever reducers). Many are available over the counter, including acetaminophen and ibuprofen. As a group, these agents interfere with the production of prostaglandins, thereby interrupting the inflammatory process. NSAIDs are indicated for the relief of pain, fever, and inflammation associated with common headache, arthritis, dysmenorrhea, and orthopedic injuries. They are also commonly prescribed to relieve pain following trauma and surgery. Other NSAIDs include ketorolac (Toradol), piroxicam (Feldene), and naproxen (Naprosyn).

Uricosuric Drugs   Uricosuric drugs are used to treat and prevent acute episodes of gout. Gout is an inflammatory disease caused by an altered metabolism of uric acid and marked by hyperuricemia (high levels of uric acid in the blood). It may present with acute episodes characterized by pain and swelling of joints. Left untreated, gout may lead to crystal deposits in various parts of the body that can cause kidney stones, nephritis, and atherosclerosis. Drugs used to treat gout include colchicine and allopurinol (Zyloprim).

Serums, Vaccines, and Other Immunizing Agents   The human body has a complex series of systems that help prevent disease. The most important of these are the anatomical barriers such as the skin and mucous membranes that block the entrance of **pathogens** (disease-causing organisms including viruses and bacteria). If pathogens get past these protective barriers, our immune system comes into play. This system consists of the spleen, lymph nodes, thymus, leukocytes, and proteins called antibodies in plasma. The ability to respond to pathogens is called **immunity.**

Immunity may be acquired passively or actively. It is passively acquired when antibodies pass directly into a person, either through artificial routes such as injection or through natural routes such as the placenta or breast milk. Immunity may also be actively acquired in response to the presence of a pathogen.

Actively acquired immunity occurs when T lymphocytes (a type of leukocyte that becomes specialized in the thymus gland) comes in contact with a new pathogen. The body produces an infinite variety of T cell configurations. When the pathogen comes into contact with a T cell that is specific to it, that T cell begins to rapidly reproduce. Some of these cells become involved in the immune response to the pathogen, while others act as "memory" cells. The cells involved in the immune response either directly attack the pathogen (cell-mediated immunity) or activate the complement system, a complex cascade of events that leads to the immune response. The memory cells remain in the body in higher numbers so that the next time this specific pathogen enters the body, a much faster response is possible. At the same time, B cells (lymphocytes that differentiate or become more specialized in the body, as opposed to the thymus) that are specific for the invading pathogen begin to produce antibodies for that antigen. This process is called humoral immunity or antibody immunity. When an antibody contacts its specific antigen, it forms a complex that triggers the complement system, leading to the immune response.

Serums and vaccines may augment the immune system. A **serum** is a solution containing whole antibodies for a specific pathogen. The antibodies give the recipient temporary, passive immunity. A **vaccine** contains a modified pathogen that does not actually cause disease but still stimulates the development of antibodies specific to it. These pathogens may be either dead or attenuated (having a decreased disease-causing ability).

The best age for vaccination against disease is within the first 2 years of life, as the immune system is fairly immature. Table 9–11 summarizes the recommended schedule for immunization.

Immune Suppressing and Enhancing Agents   Available drugs can either suppress the immune system (immunosuppressants) or enhance it (immunomodulators). Suppressing the immune system is indicated to prevent the rejection of transplanted

pathogen   *disease-causing organism.*

immunity   *the body's ability to respond to the presence of a pathogen.*

serum   *solution containing whole antibodies for a specific pathogen.*

vaccine   *solution containing a modified pathogen that does not actually cause disease but still stimulates the development of antibodies specific to it.*

This schedule indicates the recommended ages for routine administration of currently licensed childhood vaccines, as of April 1, 2004, for children through age 18 years. Any dose not given at the recommended age should be given at any subsequent visit when indicated and feasible. Additional vaccines may be licensed and recommended during the year. Licensed combination vaccines may be used whenever any components of the combination are indicated and the vaccine's other components are not contraindicated. Providers should consult the manufacturer's package inserts for detailed recommendations. Clinically significant adverse events that follow immunization should be reported to the Vaccine Adverse Event Reporting System (VAERS). Guidance about how to obtain and complete a VAERS form can be found on the Internet: **www.vaers.org** or by calling 800–822–7967.

1. Hepatitis B (HepB) Vaccine. All infants should receive the first dose of hepatitis B vaccine soon after birth and before hospital discharge; the first dose may also be given by age 2 months if the infant's mother is hepatitis B surface antigen (HBsAg) negative. Only monovalent HepB can be used for the birth dose. Monovalent or combination vaccine containing HepB may be used to complete the series. Four doses of vaccine may be administered when a birth dose is given. The second dose should be given at least 4 weeks after the first dose, except for combination vaccines which cannot be administered before age 6 weeks. The third dose should be given at least 16 weeks after the first dose and at least 8 weeks after the second dose. The last dose in the vaccination series (third or fourth dose) should not be administered before age 24 weeks.

Infants born to HBsAg-positive mothers should receive HepB and 0.5 mL of Hepatitis B Immune Globulin (HBIG) within 12 hours of birth at separate sites. The second dose is recommended at age 1 to 2 months. The last dose in the immunization series should not be administered before age 24 weeks. These infants should be tested for HBsAg and antibody to HBsAg (anti-HBs) at age 9 to 15 months.

Infants born to mothers whose HBsAg status is unknown should receive the first dose of the HepB series within 12 hours of birth. Maternal blood should be drawn as soon as possible to determine the mother's HBsAg status; if the HBsAg test is positive, the infant should receive HBIG as soon as possible (no later than age 1 week). The second dose is recommended at age 1 to 2 months. The last dose in the immunization series should not be administered before age 24 weeks.

2. Diphtheria and tetanus toxoids and acellular pertussis (DTaP) vaccine. The fourth dose of DTaP may be administered as early as age 12 months, provided 6 months have elapsed since the third dose and the child is unlikely to return at age 15 to 18 months. The final dose in the series should be given at age ≥4 years. **Tetanus and diphtheria toxoids (Td)** is recommended at age 11 to 12 years if at least 5 years have elapsed since the last dose of tetanus and diphtheria toxoid-containing vaccine. Subsequent routine Td boosters are recommended every 10 years.

3. Haemophilus influenzae type b (Hib) conjugate vaccine. Three Hib conjugate vaccines are licensed for infant use. If PRP-OMP (pedvaxHIB or ComVax [Merck]) is administered at ages 2 and 4 months, a dose at age 6 months is not required. DTaP/Hib combination products should not be used for primary immunization in infants at ages 2, 4, or 6 months but can be used as boosters following any Hib vaccine. The first dose in the series should be given at age ≥12 months.

4. Measles, mumps, and rubella vaccine (MMR). The second dose of MMR is recommended routinely at age 4 to 6 years but may be administered during any visit, provided at least 4 weeks have elapsed since the first dose and both doses are administered beginning at or after age 12 months. Those who have not previously received the second dose should complete the schedule by the visit at 11–12 years.

5. Varicella vaccine. Varicella vaccine is recommended at any visit at or after age 12 months for susceptible children (i.e., those who lack a reliable history of chicken pox). Susceptible persons age ≥13 years should receive 2 doses, given at least 4 weeks apart.

6. Pneumococcal vaccine. The heptavalent **pneumococcal conjugate vaccine (PCV)** is recommended for all children age 2 to 23 months. It is also recommended for certain children age 24 to 59 months. The final dose in the series should be given at age ≥12 months. **Pneumococcal polysaccharide vaccine (PPV)** is recommended in addition to PCV for certain high-risk groups. See *MMWR* 2000;49(RR-9);1–35.

7. Influenza vaccine. Influenza vaccine is recommended annually for children age ≥6 months with certain risk factors (including but not limited to children with asthma, cardiac disease, sickle cell disease, HIV, and diabetes), healthcare workers and other persons (including household members) in close contact with persons at high risk (see *MMWR* 2004;53[RR6]:1–40) and can be administered to all others wishing to obtain immunity. In addition, healthy children age 6 to 23 months and close contacts of healthy children age 0–23 months are recommended to receive influenza vaccine, because children in this age group are at substantially increased risk of influenza-related hospitalizations. For healthy persons age 5 to 49 years, the intranasally administered live-attenuated influenza vaccine (LAIV) is an acceptable alternative to the intramuscular trivalent inactivated influenza vaccine (TIV). See *MMWR* 2004;53[RR6]:1–40. Children receiving TIV

(continued)

Table 9–11 | (continued)

should be administered a dosage appropriate for their age (0.25 mL if age 6 to 35 months or 0.5 mL if age ≥3 years). Children age ≥8 years who are receiving influenza vaccine for the first time should receive two doses (separated by at least 4 weeks for TIV and at least 6 weeks for LAIV).

8. Hepatitis A vaccine. Hepatitis A vaccine is recommended for children and adolescents in selected states and regions and for certain high-risk groups; consult your local public health authority. Children and adolescents in these states, regions, and high-risk groups who have not been immunized against hepatitis A can begin the hepatitis A immunization series during any visit. The two doses in the series should be administered at least 6 months apart. See *MMWR*1999;48(RR-12);1–37.

For additional information about vaccines, including precautions and contraindications for immunization and vaccine shortages, please visit the National Immunization Program website at **www.cdc.gov/nip/** or call the National Immunization Information Hotline at 800–222–2522 (English) or 800–232–0233 (Spanish).

Approved by the Advisory Committee on Immunization Practices (**www.cdc.gov/nlp/acip**), the American Academy of Pediatrics (**www.aap.org**), and the American Academy of Family Physicians (**www.aafp.org**)

organs and grafted skin. Azathioprine (Imuran) is a commonly used immunosuppressant that acts by decreasing cell-mediated reactions and suppressing antibody production.

Immunomodulating agents enhance the natural immune reaction in immunosuppressed patients such as those with HIV. Zidovudine (Retrovir), commonly known as AZT, and several protease inhibitors such as ritonavir (Norvir) and saquinavir (Invirase) are examples of these agents.

DRUGS USED TO AFFECT THE SKIN

Dermatologic drugs are used to treat skin irritations. They are common over-the-counter medications. The many different general preparations include baths, soaps, solutions, cleansers, emollients (Lubriderm, Vaseline), skin protectants (Benzoin), wet dressings or soaks (Domeboro Powder), and rubs and liniments (Ben-Gay, Icy Hot). Prophylactic agents such as sunscreens are also available to help prevent skin disease and irritation.

DRUGS USED TO SUPPLEMENT THE DIET

Many disease processes affect the production, distribution, and utilization of essential dietary nutrients. Additionally, the body's intricate balance of fluid (including specific amounts of electrolytes) is a vital component of maintaining homeostasis. Dietary supplements can help to maintain needed levels of these essential nutrients and fluids.

VITAMINS AND MINERALS

Vitamins are organic compounds necessary for many different physiologic processes including metabolism, growth, development, and tissue repair. The body absorbs most vitamins through the gastrointestinal tract following dietary ingestion. Vitamins must be obtained from the diet, as the body cannot manufacture them. In developed countries, healthy adults usually receive adequate amounts of vitamins and do not need supplements. Vitamin supplements may, however, be indicated for special populations including pregnant and nursing women, patients with absorption disorders, the chronically ill, surgery patients, alcoholics, and the malnourished. Additionally, people on a strict vegetarian diet may need supplemental vitamins. Vitamins are either fat soluble or water soluble. The liver stores the fat-soluble vitamins (A, D, E, and K), so the patient will become deficient only after long periods of inadequate vitamin intake. Vitamin D is unique in that the skin produces it with exposure to sunlight. The water-soluble vitamins (C and those in the B complex) must be routinely ingested, as the body does not store them. Af-

Table 9-12	Vitamin Sources and Deficiencies	
Vitamin	**Problems Resulting from Deficiency**	**Source**
Fat Soluble		
A	Night blindness, skin lesions	Butter, yellow fruit, green leafy vegetables, milk
D	Bone and muscle pain, weakness, softening of bones	Fish, fortified milk, exposure to sunlight
E	Hyporeflexia, ataxia, anemia	Nuts, green leafy vegetables, wheat
K	Increased bleeding	Liver, green leafy vegetables
Water Soluble		
B_1 (thiamine)	Peripheral neuritis, depression, anorexia, poor memory	Whole grain, beef, pork, peas, beans, nuts
B_2 (riboflavin)	Sore throat, stomatitis, painful or swollen tongue, anemia	Milk, eggs, cheese, green leafy vegetables
B_2 (niacin)	Skin eruptions, diarrhea, enteritis, headache, dizziness, insomnia	Meat, eggs, milk
B_6 (pyridoxine)	Skin lesions, seizures, peripheral neuritis	Liver, meats, eggs, vegetables
B_9 (folic acid)	Megaloblastic anemia	Liver, fresh green vegetables, yeast
B_{12} (cyanocobalamin)	Irreversible nervous system damage, pernicious anemia	Fish, egg yolk, milk
C	Scurvy	Citrus fruits, tomatoes, strawberries

ter short periods of deprivation, patients may begin to experience vitamin deficiency. The B complex vitamins are grouped only because they occur together in foods; otherwise they share no significant characteristics. The individual B vitamins are named for the order in which they were discovered (B_1, B_2, B_3, and so forth). These vitamins also have specific names. For example, B_1 is also known as thiamine, a vitamin that plays a key role in carbohydrate metabolism. Table 9-12 details selected vitamins. Iron is an essential mineral necessary for oxygen transport and several metabolic processes. Iron supplements are the most common mineral supplement. They are indicated for iron deficiency.

FLUIDS AND ELECTROLYTES

Water comprises approximately 60 percent of a person's total body weight. The specific composition and amounts of this fluid are vital to a patient's well-being. The specific amounts of electrolytes such as calcium, potassium, sodium, and chlorine are similarly important. This book's chapter on pathophysiology reviews the physiology of fluids and electrolytes and discusses acid-base balance. The indications and contraindications for administering fluids and electrolytes, as well as these medications' interactions, are covered in the chapter on medication administration in this book and in the chapter on hemorrhage and shock, Volume 4, Chapter 4.

DRUGS USED TO TREAT POISONING AND OVERDOSES

The treatment for poisoning and overdose depends greatly on the substance involved. In general, therapy aims at eliminating the substance by emptying the gastric contents, by increasing gastric motility in order to decrease the time available for absorption, by alkalinizing the urine with sodium bicarbonate (for tricyclic antidepressant and salicylate overdose), or by filtering the substance from the blood with dialysis. When gastric emptying is indicated, syrup of ipecac is the drug of choice; otherwise, activated charcoal may be used as a gastric absorbent.

Actual antidotes are few; however, some medications are effective in treating certain overdoses or poisonings. General mechanisms for antidote action include receptor site antagonism, blocking enzyme actions involved with metabolism of the substance, and chelation (binding the substance with a stable compound such as iron so that it becomes inactive). Specific antidotes include acetylcysteine (Mucomyst) for acetaminophen overdose and deferoxamine for iron chelation. Organophosphates are a common ingredient in insecticides and herbicides as well as chemical weapons. They are aggressive acetylcholinesterase (AChE) inhibitors that prevent the breakdown of acetylcholine, leading to overstimulation of the parasympathetic nervous system as well as neuromuscular junctions. Signs and symptoms of this overstimulation may be remembered by the acronym SLUDGE (salivation, lacrimation, urination, defecation, gastric motility, and emesis). Other signs include bradycardia, hypotension, bronchospasm, muscle fasiculations, miosis (pupil constriction), and respiratory arrest. The antidotes for organophosphate poisoning are atropine and pralidoxamine (2-PAM, Protopam). Atropine antagonizes ACh, while pralidoxamine breaks the organophosphate-acetylcholinesterase bond, freeing AChE to break down the excess ACh.

Summary

Pharmacology is a cornerstone of paramedic practice. Paramedics must have a solid understanding of its foundations (legal issues, terminology, drug forms, and routes), pharmacokinetics, and pharmacodynamics if they are to practice their profession safely. Additionally, paramedics must understand not only the medications they personally administer, but also the medications that their patients are taking on an ongoing basis. While you are not likely to remember everything in this chapter after your first reading, with diligent study and practice you can master this information. This chapter has barely broken the surface of pharmacology. To continue your education, you should take the time to understand the mechanisms and interactions of the medications your patients are taking. If you do not already know them (you will not in the majority of cases as you begin your career), look them up. Many very useful drug references are available today. Most are small and can be easily carried with you on your unit or in your station.

Finally, pharmacology is a dynamic field with new discoveries being made every day. If you take your responsibilities as a paramedic seriously and remain current on the latest changes in this field, you can be sure that you can give your patients the care they deserve.

You Make the Call

You and your partner are caring for a 62-year-old male with acute pulmonary edema and cardiogenic shock. He is responsive only to painful stimuli, has ashen skin, and is very diaphoretic. He is in obvious respiratory distress with a rate of 36 per minute. You note bilateral crackles in all fields. His blood pressure is 82/50 and his heart rate is 108. The ECG shows atrial fibrillation. You immediately have your partner begin assisting the patient's ventilations with a bag-valve mask and 100 percent high-flow, high-concentration oxygen. You establish two IV lines at TKO and begin to administer a dopamine infusion through one of them at 6 mcg/kg/min and move the patient to your unit for transport to the hospital.

The dopamine appears to be helping, as your patient's blood pressure rises to 110/60; however, your partner is having an increasingly difficult time bagging the patient, whose oxygen saturation has not risen above 86 percent. You decide to perform a facilitated intubation and administer the following medications: 0.5 mg of atropine, 1.0 mg/kg of lidocaine, and 5.0 mg of midazolam (Versed). Your partner applies cricoid pressure, and you then administer 1.5 mg/kg of succinylcholine. After placing a size 8.0 ET tube, you confirm placement and secure the tube. Now that the patient is being successfully ventilated, you turn your attention back to the pulmonary edema. You administer furosemide and morphine, which decreases the edema. As you are delivering your patient to the ED staff, you note that his color and breath sounds have improved remarkably and the pulse oximeter now reads 96 percent.

1. What is dopamine and what is its mechanism of action?
2. What was the purpose of the dopamine infusion?
3. What classification of drug is furosemide? What is its mechanism of action?
4. Why was dopamine administered before furosemide?
5. What is atropine's mechanism of action?
6. What is the purpose of giving lidocaine to this patient?
7. Why was midazolam administered before succinylcholine?
8. What are succinylcholine's classification and mechanism of action?

See Suggested Responses at the back of this book.

Review Questions

1. The study of drugs and their interactions with the body is called:
   a. physiology.
   b. toxicology.
   c. pharmacology.
   d. pharmacopeia.

2. A drug or other substance that blocks the actions of the sympathetic nervous system is called:
   a. adrenergic.
   b. sympatholytic.
   c. sympathomimetic.
   d. anticholinergic.

3. _____ is the preferred antihypertensive for the management of pregnancy-induced hypertension.
   a. Coreg
   b. Apresoline
   c. Captopril
   d. Nifedipine

4. Because they can thicken bronchial secretions, you should not use _____ in patients with asthma.
   a. mucolytics
   b. antitussives
   c. antihistamines
   d. antidysrhythmics

5. The following describes a Schedule _____ drug: High abuse potential; may lead to severe dependence; accepted medical indications.
   a. I
   b. II
   c. III
   d. IV

6. An example of an anticholingeric drug used in the treatment of asthma is:
   a. atropine.
   b. ephedrine.
   c. proventil.
   d. beclovent.

7. The drug name found in the *United States Pharmacopeia* (USP) is its:
   a. official name.
   b. chemical name.
   c. generic name.
   d. trade name.

8. The drug name that is derived from its chemical composition is referred to as its:
   a. official name.
   b. chemical name.
   c. generic name.
   d. trade name.

9. The proprietary name of a drug, such as Valium, is the same as the:
   a. official name.
   b. chemical name.
   c. generic name.
   d. trade name.

10. Drug legislation was instituted in 1906 by the:
    a. Narcotics Act.
    b. Cosmetics Act.
    c. Pure Food and Drug Act.
    d. Pharmacology Act.

11. _____ drug sources may provide alternative sources of medications to those found in nature, or they may be entirely new medications not found in nature.
    a. plant
    b. animal
    c. synthetic
    d. mineral

12. The six rights of medication administration include the right:
    a. dose.
    b. time.
    c. route.
    d. all of the above.

13. Which of the following routes is the least appropriate for medication administration in the prehospital setting?
    a. oral
    b. sublingual
    c. subcutaneous
    d. intravenous

14. Drugs manufactured in gelatin containers are called:
    a. pills.
    b. tablets.
    c. capsules.
    d. extracts.

15. A drug's pharmacodynamics involve its ability to cause the expected response, or:
    a. affinity.
    b. efficacy.
    c. side effect.
    d. contraindication.

16. A type of anesthesia that combines decreased sensation of pain with amnesia, while the patient remains conscious, is a(n):
    a. opioid.
    b. nonopioid.
    c. anesthetic.
    d. neuroleptanesthesia.

17. _____ agents oppose the parasympathetic nervous system.
    a. cholinergic
    b. adrenergic
    c. antiadrenergic
    d. anticholinergic

18. In antidysrhythmic classifications, Class IA drugs include all of the following except:
    a. quinidine.
    b. lidocaine.
    c. procainamide.
    d. disopyramide.

19. One of aspirin's primary side effects is:
    a. stasis.
    b. bleeding.
    c. headache.
    d. seizures.

20. _____ are mediators released from mast cells upon contact with allergens.
    a. histamines
    b. leukotrienes
    c. glucocorticoids
    d. methylxanthines

See Answers to Review Questions at the back of this book.

Further Reading

Bledsoe, Bryan E. and Dwayne E. Clayden. *Prehospital Emergency Pharmacology.* 6th ed. Upper Saddle River, N.J.: Pearson/Prentice Hall, 2005.

Katzung, Bertram G. *Basic and Clinical Pharmacology.* 9th ed. Stamford, Conn.: Appleton & Lange, 2004.

Lehne, Richard A. *Pharmacology for Nursing Care.* 5th ed. Philadelphia: W. B. Saunders, 2004.

Salerno, Evelyn. *Pharmacology for Health Professionals.* St. Louis: Mosby, 1999.

Shannon, Margaret T., Billie Ann Wilson, and Carolyn L. Stang. *Prentice Hall's Health Professionals Drug Guide 2005–2006.* Upper Saddle River, N.J.: Pearson/Prentice Hall, 2005.

Sherwood, Lauralee. *Human Physiology: From Cells to Systems.* 5th ed. Belmont, Calif.: Wadsworth, 2004.

On the Web

Visit Brady's Paramedic Website at **www.bradybooks.com/paramedic**.

Intravenous Access and Medication Administration

Objectives

After reading this chapter, you should be able to:

Part 1: Principles and Routes of Medication Administration (begins on p. 372)

1. Review the specific anatomy and physiology pertinent to medication administration. (pp. 376–406)

2. Describe the indications, equipment needed, techniques used, precautions, and general principles for the following:

   a. inhalation routes of medication administration. (pp. 380–384)

   b. parenteral routes of medication administration. (pp. 390–406)

   c. percutaneous routes of medication administration. (pp. 376–380)

   d. enteral routes of medication administration, including gastric tube administration and rectal administration. (pp. 384–390)

3. Describe the indications, contraindications, side effects, dosages, and routes of administration for medications commonly administered by paramedics. (pp. 376–406)

4. Discuss legal aspects affecting medication administration. (pp. 372–373, 375–376)

5. Discuss the "six rights" of drug administration and correlate them with the principles of medication administration. (pp. 372–373)

6. Differentiate among the percutaneous routes of medication administration. (pp. 376–380)

7. Discuss medical asepsis and the differences between clean and sterile techniques. (p. 374)

8. Describe uses of antiseptics and disinfectants. (p. 374)

9. Describe the use of body substance isolation (BSI) procedures when administering a medication. (pp. 373–374)

10. Describe disposal of contaminated items and sharps. (p. 375)

11. Synthesize a pharmacologic management plan including medication administration. (pp. 372–406)

Part 2: Intravenous Access, Blood Sampling, and Intraosseous Infusion (begins on p. 407)

1. Review the specific anatomy and physiology pertinent to medication administration. (pp. 407–449)

2. Describe the indications, equipment needed, technique used, precautions, and general principles for the following:

   a. peripheral venous or external jugular cannulation. (pp. 407–437)

   b. intraosseous needle placement and infusion. (pp. 441–449)

   c. obtaining a blood sample. (pp. 437–441)

Part 3: Medical Mathematics (begins on p. 449)

1. Review mathematical equivalents. (pp. 449–452)

2. Differentiate temperature readings between the centigrade and Fahrenheit scales. (pp. 451–452)

3. Discuss formulas as a basis for performing drug calculations. (pp. 452–458)

4. Describe how to perform mathematical conversions from the household system to the metric system. (pp. 451–452)

Key Terms

administration tubing, p. 411
air embolism, p. 427
ampule, p. 392
angiocatheter, p. 416
anticoagulant, p. 427
antiseptic, p. 374
asepsis, p. 374
aural medication, p. 379
blood tube, p. 437
blood tubing, p. 414
body substance isolation (BSI), p. 373
bolus, p. 389
buccal, p. 377
burette chamber, p. 414

cannula, p. 411
cannulation, p. 407
catheter inserted through the needle, p. 416
central venous access, p. 408
circulatory overload, p. 427
colloid, p. 409
concentration, p. 453
crystalloid, p. 409
desired dose, p. 453
disinfectant, p. 374
dosage on hand, p. 453
drip chamber, p. 412
drip rate, p. 412
drop former, p. 412

drugs, p. 372
embolus, p. 426
enema, p. 389
enteral drug administration, p. 384
extension tubing, p. 413
extravasation, p. 425
extravascular, p. 436
gauge, p. 391
gtts, p. 412
hemoconcentration, p. 441
hemolysis, p. 441
heparin lock, p. 432
hepatic alteration, p. 387
hollow-needle catheter, p. 416

Case Study

It is early in February and clouds heavy with snow loom not far in the distance. Paramedic Susan Adams watches the sky and hopes that she will get off work on time, before the storm hits. Suddenly the tones drop, alerting her and her partner, EMT-Intermediate Todd Michaels, of a 28-year-old female patient with shortness of breath. After acknowledging the call and confirming the location in the map book, Susan and Todd get underway. In preparation, Susan dons gloves and eye protection. Additionally, she reviews the likely causes of shortness of breath in a 28-year-old patient.

As Susan and Todd pull up to the residence, they observe a well-kept house. A woman frantically waves them inside, shouting that her daughter cannot breathe. Quickly, they grab the airway kit, cardiac monitor, and drug bag and then cautiously enter the residence.

Once inside, Susan and Todd begin to size up the scene. Immediately to their left, they find the female patient seated on a chair in the tripod position. Quick observation reveals her to be in considerable respiratory distress and exhibiting cyanosis around the lips and in the extremities. Even without a stethoscope, Susan detects expiratory wheezing.

Promptly, Susan introduces herself and Todd to the patient and asks what is wrong. As the patient can barely talk, Susan cannot obtain a specific chief complaint. Recognizing a life-threatening situation, she gains consent for treatment and turns her attention to the initial assessment.

The patient is responsive but exhibits lethargy and fatigue from the increased work of breathing and hypoxia. Inspection of the oral cavity reveals no foreign bodies or other obstructions. Susan deems the patient able to maintain her airway and forgoes a nasopharyngeal airway adjunct.

The patient presents tachypneic at 36 breaths per minute. Tidal and minute volume are shallow. Todd obtains a pulse oximetry reading of 86 percent on room air. A quick 2-point auscultation reveals expiratory wheezing in the upper lobes of both the right and left lungs. As the patient will not tolerate the assistance of ventilations with a bag-valve mask, Susan applies a nonrebreathing face mask with 15 liters per minute of supplemental oxygen.

Without missing a beat, Susan proceeds to evaluate the circulatory system. The patient's radial pulse is weak and rapid, with accompanying cool, diaphoretic skin. Again Susan notes cyanosis.

Realizing the situation is critical, Susan turns to the patient's mother as Todd applies the cardiac monitor and obtains vital signs. When Susan asks about a history of asthma, the mother confirms it and adds that this particular episode has been occurring over the past day and a half. Her daughter's metered dose inhaler of Alupent has not provided any relief, as it has in the past. Aside from the Alupent and asthma, the patient has no other medical history. She has no allergies and has not eaten or drunk anything today.

Confident that she is dealing with an asthmatic patient, Susan performs the detailed physical exam. She accordingly notes bilateral distention of the jugular veins and retractions at the suprasternal notch and intercostal spaces, along with nasal flaring and pursed lips. Quickly she auscultates breath sounds from the posterior thorax in a 6-point pattern. She observes bilateral expiratory wheezing in the apices of the lungs with no net air movement in the bases.

Todd informs Susan of the patient's vital signs: pulse, 116 beats per minute; respirations, 56 per minute; and blood pressure, 152/94 mmHg. With the initial assessment and SAMPLE history obtained, Susan begins emergency interventions. The cardiac monitor displays sinus tachycardia with no ectopy.

As Todd obtains a venous blood sample and establishes an IV line, Susan assembles a nebulizer to administer 2.5 mg of albuterol. She gives the nebulizer complete with medication to the patient for self-administration. Following standing orders, she draws 0.5 mg of epinephrine 1:1,000 from a glass ampule with a syringe and hypodermic needle. Then she cleanses the site and delivers the subcutaneous injection into the tissue on the back of the patient's left arm. Susan proceeds to administer 125 mg of methylprednisolone (Solu-Medrol). Todd prepares the cot and loads the patient for transport.

En route to the hospital, Susan performs the ongoing assessment by evaluating the components of the initial assessment and the effects of all interventions. The patient now is more alert and breathes easier. Her pulse oximetry reads 92 percent, and her expiratory wheezing has subsided significantly. Susan now notes air movement in the bases of the lungs. Additionally, the cyanosis and diaphoresis have almost subsided and vital signs have returned to normal limits. Because the pulse oximeter reading is still low and some residual wheezing persists, Susan gives another nebulized treatment of 2.5 mg of albuterol. She alerts the receiving hospital by cellular telephone.

Once at the hospital, Susan and Todd turn over care to the emergency department staff. Later they find out that the woman was admitted for overnight observation with the diagnosis of acute exacerbation of asthma. She is doing fine and is expected to be released in the morning.

INTRODUCTION

medications/drugs *agents used in the diagnosis, treatment, or prevention of disease.*

Medications, or **drugs,** are foreign substances placed into the human body. They serve a variety of purposes such as controlling specific diseases like hypertension or helping the body cure diseases like cancer and infection.

Medication administration will be an important part of the medical care you provide as a paramedic. You may have to use medications to correct or prevent many life-threatening situations. You may also use them to stabilize or comfort a patient in distress. In addition to your knowledge of particular medications and their properties from the previous chapter on pharmacology, you must also be thoroughly skilled in drug administration. Specific drugs require specific routes and administration techniques. Their effectiveness depends directly upon their correct route of delivery. Incorrect or sloppy drug administration can have tremendous legal implications for the paramedic. More importantly, it equates to poor care that can harm or even kill the patient.

This chapter discusses the routes and techniques you will use to correctly deliver your patient's medications. It is divided into three parts:

Part 1: Principles and Routes of Medication Administration

Part 2: Intravenous Access, Blood Sampling, and Intraosseous Infusion

Part 3: Medical Mathematics

Part 1: Principles and Routes of Medication Administration

GENERAL PRINCIPLES

As a paramedic, you are responsible for ensuring that all emergency drugs are in place and ready for immediate use. Therefore, you must know your local drug distribution system. You will have to know where to obtain and replace each drug as it expires or is used, as another patient may require it at any time. You also will have to thoroughly document the administration and restocking of narcotics, as many local, state, and federal agencies mandate such record keeping.

Always be certain that you correctly give all drugs in the right dose. Medication errors may prove disastrous in terms of patient care and legal responsibility. Your knowledge of drug indications, contraindications, side effects, dosages, and routes of administration is crucial to effective patient care. (See Chapter 9.)

You can attain effective pharmacologic therapy and eliminate medication errors by following the six rights of drug administration:

★ *Right person.* Ensure that the patient receiving the drug is the right person. Generally, you will provide one-on-one attention. In a clinical setting, however, keeping track of multiple patients proves more challenging.

★ *Right drug.* Ensure that you administer the proper drug. Many drugs are contained in similar appearing packages. To avoid inadvertently delivering the incorrect drug, read the label! Administering the incorrect medication can have disastrous consequences.

★ *Right dose.* Be certain that you administer the exact dosage of any drug. The correct dose may be standardized or require calculation. Never underdose or overdose a patient.

Your knowledge of drug indications, dosages, and routes of administration is of paramount importance.

✓ **Review**

Six Rights of Drug Administration

Right person
Right drug
Right dose
Right time
Right route
Right documentation

★ *Right time.* Timing their administration is important for many drugs. Typically, in the emergent setting, you will quickly administer the necessary emergency drugs. During transfers and critical care transports, you may have to administer other drugs at preestablished intervals.

★ *Right route.* Specific drugs require specific delivery routes. You must not only be familiar with the properties of individual drugs but also with their different routes of administration.

★ *Right documentation.* Documenting drug administration is of paramount importance. You must record all appropriate information about every medication you administer. Pertinent information includes, but is not limited to, drug name(s), dose, route of delivery, person administering, time administered, and patient response to the drug—both good and bad.

In the field, you will be responsible for the safe and appropriate delivery of medications. If you ever doubt the use or dosage of a medication, contact medical direction immediately. You must repeat back, or echo, all drug orders issued by direct medical command. For example, if medical direction ordered you to administer 25 mg of diphenhydramine (Benadryl), you would echo, "Medic 101 copies the medication order for 25 mg of diphenhydramine to be administered slow IV push." By echoing, you confirm your reception and understanding of the order. If medical direction has issued an inappropriate medication or dosage, echoing may bring it to light and elicit an immediate correction. If you still find the order questionable after echoing, diplomatically request clarification or ask about the intent.

Pharmacologic therapy permits you to function as an extension of the physician. No room exists for medication errors, as once a drug is given it is difficult if not impossible to retrieve. In addition, withholding a needed medication can have catastrophic consequences. Concentration and knowledge are the keys to this component of paramedical care.

MEDICAL DIRECTION

Paramedics do not practice autonomously. You will operate under the license of a medical director who is responsible for all of your actions. This responsibility extends to the administration of medications.

The medical director determines which medications you will use and the routes by which you will deliver them. Some states have a "state drug list" whereby the medications a service carries are dictated by law or a legislative or regulatory agency. While some medications can be administered via off-line medical direction (written standing orders), you will need specific authorization for others after consulting on-line or direct medical direction. You must strictly abide by all of your medical director's guidelines.

Knowing all drug administration protocols is essential, especially which drugs to administer under standing orders and which to deliver only after getting authorization from medical direction. You can ill afford to waste valuable time looking up procedures and directives for the critical patient who requires immediate drug therapy. Furthermore, because inappropriate drug delivery can have serious consequences, you may face severe legal ramifications even if your patient suffers no harm.

BODY SUBSTANCE ISOLATION

Establishing routes for drug delivery presents the constant potential for exposure to blood and other body fluids. Always take appropriate **body substance isolation (BSI)** measures to decrease your risk of exposure. The type of BSI you use will vary according to the delivery route and your patient's condition. At a minimum, you should wear

If you ever doubt the use or dosage of a medication, contact medical direction immediately.

You can ill afford to waste valuable time looking up procedures and directives for the critical patient who requires immediate drug therapy.

body substance isolation (BSI) *measures to decrease your risk of exposure to blood and body fluids.*

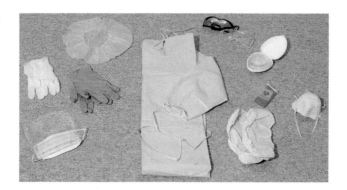

gloves. Optimally, you will also wear goggles and a mask (Figure 10-1 ■). Remarkably, the simplest form of BSI is often the most neglected: hand washing. Washing your hands before and after patient contact is one of the most effective ways to decrease your exposure to infectious material. This book's chapter on the well-being of the paramedic includes a thorough discussion of BSI measures.

⊸○
Always take appropriate body substance isolation measures to decrease your risk of exposure to infectious material.

MEDICAL ASEPSIS

asepsis *a condition free of pathogens.*

Medical **asepsis** (*a-*, without; *sepsis,* infection) describes a medical environment free of pathogens. Many paramedical procedures, especially those related to drug administration, place the patient at increased risk for infection. The external environment is full of microorganisms, many of them pathogenic. Techniques such as intravenous access or endotracheal intubation can allow pathogens to enter the patient's body, where they may cause **local** or **systemic** complications.

local *limited to one area of the body.*

Sterilization

systemic *throughout the body.*

sterile *free of all forms of life.*

medically clean *careful handling to prevent contamination.*

The most aseptic environment is a sterile one. A **sterile** environment is free of all forms of life. Generally, environments are sterilized with extensive heat or chemicals. A sterile environment is difficult to attain in the prehospital setting. Consequently, you must practice medically clean techniques to minimize your patient's risk of infection. **Medically clean** techniques involve the careful handling of sterile equipment to prevent contamination. For example, much of the equipment used for drug administration is packaged sterilely. Once you open the package, you must use a medically clean technique to keep the equipment clean and uncontaminated until you use it. If you drop a piece of equipment on a dirty surface, you should discard it and obtain a new piece. Other medically clean techniques, including hand washing, glove changing, and discarding equipment in opened packages, help to prevent equipment and patient contamination. Remember, too, that many patients have lowered immunity levels or carry infectious diseases. Thus, keeping the ambulance and equipment clean is another essential medically clean procedure.

Disinfectants and Antiseptics

disinfectant *cleansing agent that is toxic to living tissue.*

antiseptic *cleansing agent that is not toxic to living tissue.*

When administering medications, you must use disinfectants and antiseptics to assure local cleanliness. Do not confuse disinfectants and antiseptics; the distinction is important. **Disinfectants** are toxic to living tissue. You will therefore use them only on nonliving surfaces or objects such as the inside of an ambulance or laryngoscope blades after use. Never use disinfectants on living tissue. **Antiseptics** are not toxic to living tissue. They destroy or inhibit pathogenic microorganisms already on living surfaces and are generally used to cleanse the local area before needle puncture. Common antiseptics include alcohol and iodine preparations used either alone or together. Frequently, antiseptics are diluted disinfectants.

DISPOSAL OF CONTAMINATED EQUIPMENT AND SHARPS

Blood and body fluid can harbor infectious material that endangers the health care provider, family, bystanders, or the patient himself. Many times, the patient is infected with pathogenic organisms long before signs and symptoms appear. Therefore, you must treat all blood and body fluids as potentially infectious.

Drug administration commonly involves needles in direct contact with the patient's blood and body fluid. Once used, a needle presents a significant risk. Inadvertent needle sticks, the most common accident in health care as a whole, can transmit diseases between the patient and paramedic. Properly handling needles and other sharps before and after patient use can prevent many of these accidental needle sticks. To minimize or eliminate the risk of an accidental needle stick, take these precautions:

★ *Minimize the tasks you perform in a moving ambulance.* Use needles as sparingly as possible in the back of a moving ambulance. When appropriate, perform all interventions involving needles on scene. If en route, it may be occasionally necessary to have the driver pull the ambulance to the side of the road and stop briefly. Most paramedics become quite proficient at completing these procedures in a moving ambulance.

★ *Immediately dispose of used sharps in a sharps container.* A **sharps container** is a rigid, puncture-resistant container clearly marked as biohazardous. You can deposit whole needles and prefilled syringes in it, thus eliminating the need for bending or cutting. Some sharps containers have adapters that permit the easy removal of needles from blood draw equipment and syringes. You should also dispose of items such as used ampules in the sharps container. Avoid dropping sharps onto the floor for later disposal. In the heat of the moment, you may forget the sharp or mentally misplace it.

★ *Recap needles only as a last resort.* If you absolutely must recap a needle, never use two hands to do so. Place the sharp on a stationary surface and replace the cap with one hand. While the one-hand method is still hazardous, it at least reduces the chance for an accidental needle stick.

By law, every medical organization must have a biological hazard exposure plan. Be familiar with yours. If you are exposed to blood or other body substances, follow the plan and immediately notify the appropriate resources. Remember that prevention is the best medicine.

MEDICATION ADMINISTRATION AND DOCUMENTATION

When administering medications, proper and thorough documentation is extremely important. You must record all information concerning the patient and the medication including:

★ Indication for drug administration

★ Dosage and route delivered

★ Patient response to the medication—both positive and negative

You must also document the patient's condition and vital signs before medication administration as well as after. In addition to communicating all information to those to whom you transfer care, you must record it on a copy of the patient care report.

In emergent and nonemergent situations alike, you will administer a variety of medications through a variety of delivery routes. The routes of drug administration fall

Treat all blood and body fluids as potentially infectious.

 Review

Needle Handling Precautions

Minimize tasks in a moving ambulance.
Properly dispose of all sharps.
Recap needles only as a last resort.

sharps container *rigid, puncture-resistant container clearly marked as a biohazard.*

 Review

Routes of Drug Administration

Percutaneous
Pulmonary
Enteral
Parenteral

topical medications *material applied to and absorbed through the skin or mucous membranes.*

into four basic categories: percutaneous, pulmonary, enteral, and parenteral. Technically, drug deliveries through the rectum and pulmonary system are **topical** applications; however, accepted practice classifies these routes separately. Which route you use will depend on the drug you are administering and your patient's status.

 Review

PERCUTANEOUS DRUG ADMINISTRATION

Percutaneous medications are applied to and absorbed through the skin or mucous membranes. They are easy to administer and bypass the digestive tract, making their absorption more predictable.

TRANSDERMAL ADMINISTRATION

transdermal *absorbed through the skin.*

Medications given by the **transdermal** (*trans-,* across; *dermal,* skin) route promote slow, steady absorption. Nitroglycerin, hormones, and analgesics are commonly administered transdermally. Transdermal delivery can also produce localized effects, as with anti-inflammatories and other bacteriostatic and softening agents. Applying medication locally avoids passing larger quantities of the medication through the entire body, where it is not needed. Transdermal medications include lotions, ointments, creams, foams, wet dressings, adhesive-backed applications, and suppositories.

To administer a transdermal medication, use the following technique:

1. Use BSI. Gloves avoid contaminating the medication and inadvertently getting it on your skin.
2. Clean and dry your patient's skin at the administration site.
3. Apply medication to the site as specified by the manufacturer. Avoid overdosing or underdosing when using lotion, ointment, cream, or foam.
4. Leave the medication in place for the required time. Monitor the patient for desirable or adverse effects.

You may need to place a dressing over the medication to protect the site and quantity of drug. Carefully follow all recommendations. Administration may vary subtly, depending upon the form of medication and the specific manufacturer's instructions.

Several factors can affect how quickly the skin absorbs transdermal medications. Thin skin, overdose, or penetrating solvents can increase the absorption rate. Conversely, thick skin, scar tissue, or peripheral vascular disease can decrease the rate. If these factors are present, consider alternative sites or dosage adjustments.

 Review

MUCOUS MEMBRANES

The mucous membranes absorb medications at a moderate to rapid rate. Similar to transdermal administration, drug delivery through the mucous membranes avoids the digestive tract and complications associated with that route. You can deliver drugs through the mucous membranes at several sites. However, specific drugs are made for specific sites and generally are not interchangeable.

Sublingual

sublingual *beneath the tongue.*

Sublingual drugs are absorbed through the mucous membranes beneath the tongue (*sub-,* below; *lingual,* tongue). The sublingual region is extremely vascular and permits rapid absorption with systemic delivery. These medications are generally dissolvable tablets or sprays. One commonly administered sublingual medication is nitroglycerin.

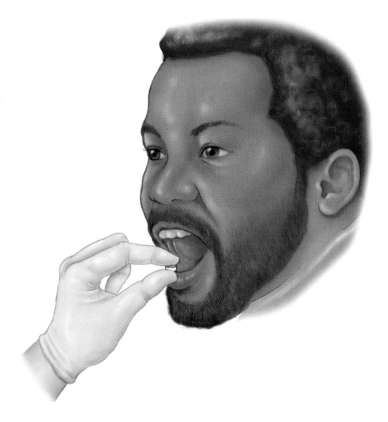

■ Figure 10-2 Sublingual medication administration. Place the pill or direct spray between the underside of the tongue and the floor of the oral cavity.

To administer a medication via the sublingual route, follow these steps (Figure 10-2 ■):

1. Use appropriate BSI.
2. Confirm the indication, medication, dose, sublingual route, and expiration date.
3. Have your patient lift his tongue toward the top and back of his oral cavity.
4. Place the pill or direct spray between the underside of the tongue and the floor of the oral cavity. Have your patient relax his tongue and mouth. If administering a pill, instruct the patient to let the pill dissolve and not to swallow.
5. Monitor the patient for desirable or adverse effects.

Buccal

The **buccal** region lies in the oral cavity between the cheek and gums. Buccal medications are generally tablets. Hormonal and enzyme preparations are typically given buccally.

To administer a medication buccally, follow these steps (Figure 10-3 ■):

1. Use appropriate BSI.
2. Confirm the indication, medication, dose, buccal route, and expiration date.
3. Place the medication between the patient's cheek and gum. Instruct the patient to allow the pill or other preparation to dissolve. Ensure that the patient does not swallow the medication.
4. Monitor the patient for desirable or adverse effects.

Ocular

Ocular medications are topical medications that are administered through the mucous membranes of the eye. These are typically local medications for alleviating eye pain, treating infection, decreasing intraocular pressure, or lubricating the eyelid. Medications

buccal *between the cheek and gums.*

ocular medication *drug administered through the mucous membranes of the eye.*

Eyedrops are for single patient use. Once administered, the container must be properly disposed of. Never reuse ophthalmic medications.

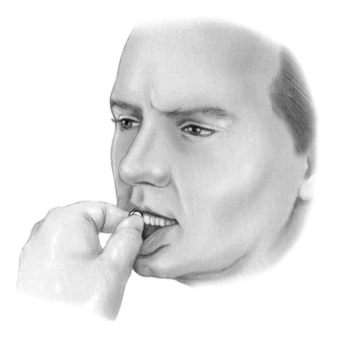

■ Figure 10-3   Buccal medication administration. Place the medication between the patient's cheek and gum.

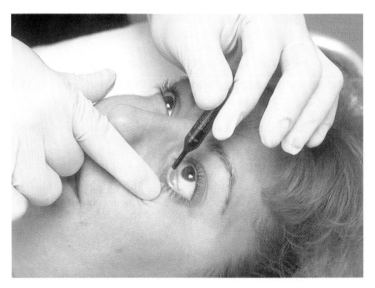

■ Figure 10-4   Eyedrop administration. Use a medicine dropper to place the prescribed dosage on the conjunctival sac.

delivered by way of the eye are labeled for ophthalmic use and packaged as drops or ointments.

If medication is to be administered only to one eye, be sure to medicate the correct eye. The following abbreviations designate right, left, or both eyes:

o.d.   right eye (*oculus dexter*)

o.s.   left eye (*oculus sinister*)

o.u.   both right and left eyes (*oculus uterque*)

To administer a medication via eyedrops, use the following technique (Figure 10-4 ■):

1. Use gloves and appropriate BSI.

2. Have your patient lie supine or lay his head back and look toward the ceiling.

3. Pull the lower eyelid downward to expose the conjunctival sac. Never touch the eye.

4. Use a medicine dropper to place the prescribed dosage on the conjunctival sac. Never administer medications directly on the eye unless specifically instructed.

5. Instruct the patient to hold his eye(s) shut for 1 to 2 minutes.

Ocular medications may also be packaged as ointments. To apply an ointment, follow the same procedure as above, but carefully squeeze the ointment onto the conjunctival sac. If you administer too much medication, carefully blot away the excess drops or ointment with sterile gauze. The ointment will melt as it warms to body temperature and will spread smoothly across the surface of the eye.

Nasal

The mucous membranes of the nose are another port for topical medication delivery. Given through the nares (nostrils), these **nasal medications** are usually drops or sprays intended for local effect. They commonly treat nasal congestion, hemorrhage, and infection.

nasal medication *drug administered through the mucous membranes of the nose.*

To administer a medication via the nose, use the following technique (Figure 10-5 ■):

1. Use gloves and appropriate BSI.

2. Have the patient blow his nose and tilt his head backwards.

3. Use a medicine dropper or squeezable nebulizer to administer the medication into the appropriate nare(s) according to the manufacturer's instructions.

4. Hold the nare(s) shut and/or tilt the head forward to distribute the medication.

5. Monitor the patient for desirable and undesirable effects.

Aural

Some medications are delivered to the mucous membranes of the ear and ear canal through drops or medicated gauze. These **aural medications** primarily treat local infections and ear pain. Use the following technique to administer medicated drops (Figure 10-6 ■):

aural medication *drug administered through the mucous membranes of the ear and ear canal.*

1. Use gloves and appropriate BSI.

2. Confirm the indication, medication, dose, and expiration date.

3. Determine the correct ear for administration.

4. Have the patient lie in the lateral recumbent position with the affected ear upward.

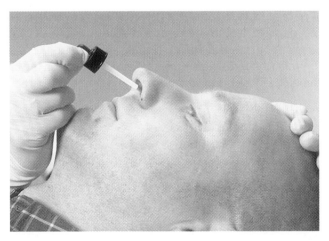

■ Figure 10-5 Nasal medication administration.

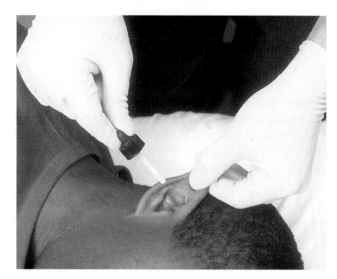

Figure 10-6 Aural medication administration. Manually open the ear canal and administer the appropriate dose.

5. Manually open the ear canal: for adult patients, pull the ear up and back; for pediatric patients, pull it down and back.

6. Administer the appropriate dose of medication with a medicine dropper.

7. Have the patient continue to lie with his ear up for 10 minutes.

8. Monitor the patient for desirable and undesirable effects.

Using medicated gauze or cotton is generally reserved for the hospital setting. If your local protocols permit you to administer these medications, follow the procedure previously outlined, gently inserting the gauze into the ear instead of instilling medicated drops. Avoid tightly packing the ear canal.

PULMONARY DRUG ADMINISTRATION

inhalation *drawing of medication into the lungs along with air during breathing.*

injection *placement of medication in or under the skin with a needle and syringe.*

Special medications can be administered into the pulmonary system via **inhalation** or **injection.** Generally gases, fine mists, or liquids, these drugs include those that promote bronchodilation for respiratory emergencies. Other inhaled drugs are mucolytics, antibiotics, and topical steroids. Inhalation can also be used for humidification and pulmonary decongestion.

NEBULIZER

Typically, drugs administered by inhalation are delivered with the aid of a small volume nebulizer. A **nebulizer** uses pressurized oxygen to disperse a liquid into a fine aerosol spray or mist. Inhalation carries the aerosol into the lungs. Figure 10-7 ■ illustrates a typical nebulizer. The specific design depends upon the manufacturer, but they all work on the same principle and typically have the same parts:

- ★ Mouthpiece
- ★ Medication reservoir
- ★ Oxygen port
- ★ Relief valve
- ★ Oxygen tubing
- ★ Oxygen source

 Review

Content

Pulmonary Medication Mechanisms

Nebulizer
Metered dose inhaler
Endotracheal tube

nebulizer *inhalation aid that disperses liquid into aerosol spray or mist.*

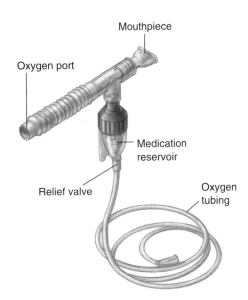

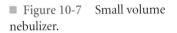

Figure 10-7   Small volume nebulizer.

To administer a drug with a nebulizer, follow these steps:

1. Put the medication in the medication reservoir. If the medication is not diluted, combine it with 3 to 5 cc sterile saline solution. This will allow adequate aerosolization. Screw the reservoir in place.

2. Assemble the nebulizer.

3. Attach oxygen tubing to the oxygen port and oxygen source.

4. Set the oxygen source regulator for 5 to 8 liters per minute.

    Note: Never set the oxygen pressure outside of this range. Less than 5 liters per minute will not create enough pressure to aerosolize the medication. More than 8 liters per minute will create too much pressure and destroy the oxygen tubing or nebulizer at its weakest point. Furthermore, because of pressure restrictions, do not attach the nebulizer to an oxygen humidifier.

5. Place the nebulizer in the patient's mouth. Instruct him to exhale and then seal his lips around the mouthpiece. Now have him hold the nebulizer and slowly inhale as deeply as possible. Upon maximum inhalation, instruct the patient to hold in the medication for 1 to 2 seconds before exhaling. This permits maximum deposition and absorption. Continue this process until the medication is completely gone. Typically, this takes 3 to 5 minutes.

Nebulizers also come preattached to an oxygen face mask in both pediatric and adult sizes (Figure 10-8). Use nebulization face masks for pediatric or adult patients who cannot hold the nebulizer. Nebulizers for those who require long-term therapy may be powered by a battery or other energy source.

For a nebulizer to be effective, the patient must have an adequate tidal volume and respiratory rate. If the tidal volume is shallow or respiratory rate low, the medication will not move from the nebulizer into the lungs. For patients with a poor tidal and/or respiratory rate who cannot pull the medication into their lungs, you can connect nebulizers to a bag-valve mask and/or endotracheal tube.

METERED DOSE INHALER

Inhaled medications are also delivered through **metered dose inhalers** (MDI). These small, handheld devices produce a medicated spray for inhalation. Patients with

metered dose inhaler
handheld device that produces a medicated spray for inhalation.

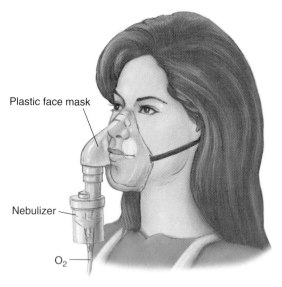

Plastic face mask

Nebulizer

O₂

(a) Nebulizer with attached face mask

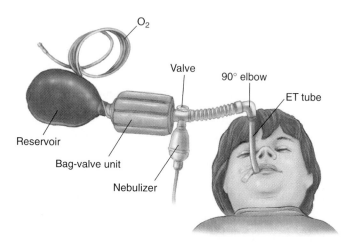

O₂

Valve

90° elbow

ET tube

Reservoir

Bag-valve unit

Nebulizer

(c) Nebulizer with bag-valve unit

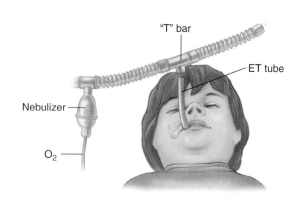

"T" bar

ET tube

Nebulizer

O₂

(b) Nebulizer with endotracheal tube

■ Figure 10-8   Nebulizer with attached face mask, endotracheal tube, and bag-valve mask.

Metered dose inhalers (MDIs) are for single patient use. Once administered, the container must be properly disposed of. Never reuse MDIs. Because of the cost, most EMS services use small-volume nebulizers instead of MDIs.

conditions such as asthma or COPD use metered dose inhalers to deliver a specific, or metered, dose of medication. A metered dose inhaler consists of two parts, a medication canister and a plastic shell and mouthpiece (Figure 10-9 ■). Some metered dose inhalers come equipped with a spacer. The spacer is a cylindrical canister between the inhaler and the mouthpiece. Prior to self-administration, the patient will depress the inhaler sending a measured dose of drug into the spacer. The patient will then breathe in and out of the spacer through the mouthpiece, thus inhaling the drug into the lungs. This system is particularly useful for patients who have a hard time operating and inhaling the metered dose inhaler. This is common in the elderly and in young children. The spacer, when used in conjunction with a metered dose inhaler, is very effective.

Metered dose inhalers are usually self-administered. However, if your patient is incapacitated, you may have to physically assist with the administration or educate the patient or his caregivers in its use. To assist a patient in the use of a metered dose inhaler, follow this technique:

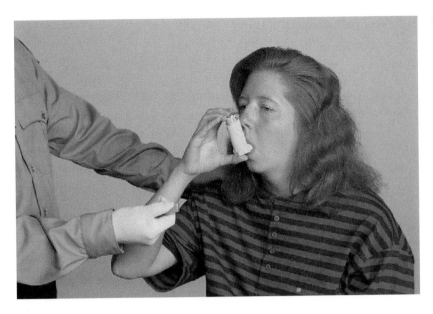

1. Insert the medication canister into the plastic shell.

2. Remove the cap from the mouthpiece.

3. Gently shake the MDI for 2 to 5 seconds.

4. Instruct the patient to maximally exhale.

5. Place the mouthpiece in the patient's mouth and have him form a seal with his lips.

6. As the patient inhales, press the canister's top downward to release the medication.

7. Have the patient hold his breath for several seconds.

8. Remove the inhaler from the patient's mouth and instruct him to breathe slowly.

9. If a second dose is necessary, wait according to the manufacturer's instructions. Then repeat.

10. In an acute respiratory emergency involving a patient with a metered dose inhaler, always use a nebulizer instead of the MDI. While the metered dose inhaler delivers a small amount of medication, the nebulizer delivers larger quantities of medication mixed with water and oxygen.

Nebulizers and metered dose inhalers offer several advantages. In respiratory emergencies, less medication is needed because it reaches its exact site of action. The lower dosage is less likely to promote side effects, and if the patient has an adverse reaction, implementing or discontinuing drug delivery is easy. Furthermore, because the patient can hold the nebulizer, he will benefit from feeling more in control of his overall therapy. Most importantly, if your patient is hypoxic you can administer inhaled medications with supplemental oxygen.

The nebulizer and metered dose inhaler also have disadvantages. Moving the aerosolized medication into the lungs depends on adequate ventilation. For the patient with a poor tidal and minute volume, nebulized medications are ineffective, as the drug cannot reach its site of action. In these cases, you should use the nebulizer in conjunction with a bag-valve mask and/or endotracheal tube. Additionally, the patient must exhibit an adequate level of consciousness and manual dexterity to hold the nebulizer and follow instructions correctly.

Review

Endotracheal Medications

- Lidocaine
- Epinephrine
- Atropine
- Naloxone

ENDOTRACHEAL TUBE

When you have not yet established an IV, you can administer certain medications such as lidocaine (Xylocaine), vasopressin epinephrine, atropine, and naloxone (Narcan) through an endotracheal tube. Delivering liquid medications into the lungs permits rapid absorption through the pulmonary capillaries. Recent research has shown the administration of medications via an endotracheal tube is not as effective as once thought.

When using an endotracheal tube, you must increase conventional IV dosages from two to two-and-one-half times. You also should dilute the medication in normal saline to create 10 mL of solution and then quickly inject it down the endotracheal tube. Several ventilations must follow to aerosolize the medication and enhance its absorption. Ideally, you can pass a commercially manufactured catheter through the endotracheal tube and inject the medication through it. If CPR is underway, stop compressions while you administer the medication and ventilate for aerosolization.

ENTERAL DRUG ADMINISTRATION

enteral drug administration *through the gastrointestinal tract.*

 Review

Enteral Routes

Oral
Gastric tube
Rectal

Enteral drug administration is the delivery of any medication that is absorbed through the gastrointestinal tract. The gastrointestinal tract, or alimentary canal, travels from the mouth to the stomach and on through the intestines to the rectum (Figure 10-10 ■). You can administer enteral medications orally, through a gastric tube, or rectally.

Several advantages make the gastrointestinal tract the most common route for medication delivery. Aside from sheer convenience, it is the least expensive route, and its use requires little equipment and minimal training. In some instances, after you have delivered a drug you may be able to retrieve it by inducing vomiting, by removing it from the rectum, or simply by having the patient spit it out.

Conversely, enteral drug administration poses several disadvantages. Physical activity, emotions, or food can significantly alter the gastrointestinal tract's chemical and physical environment, making absorption unreliable. In addition, as all blood from the stomach and small intestine must pass through the hepatic circulatory system (portal circulation), the liver's condition can reduce the medication's effectiveness. A dysfunctional liver can significantly alter drug distribution and, in extreme cases, metabolize therapeutic medications into inert or harmful substances. Furthermore, a patient resistant to or *noncompliant* in taking medications makes administration via the enteral route very difficult.

ORAL ADMINISTRATION

Oral drug administration denotes any medication taken by mouth (oral) and swallowed into the gastrointestinal (GI) tract. From the GI tract, the medication is absorbed and distributed throughout the body. When administering a medication by the oral route, you must be sure that the patient has an adequate level of consciousness to support his airway. Administering an oral medication to a patient who cannot support his airway may result in an airway occlusion or aspiration into the lungs. If aspiration into the lungs occurs, aspiration pneumonia and its deadly consequences may occur.

Medications for oral delivery come in a variety of forms, either solid or liquid.

- ★ *Capsules.* Capsules contain liquid, dry, or beaded medication in a soluble casing. For maximum effectiveness, the patient must swallow them whole.

- ★ *Tablets.* Tablets comprise medicated powder compressed into a small, solid disk. Typically, tablets may be scored to permit breaking in half or quarters when lesser dosages are required.

- ★ *Pills.* Pills, comprised of medicated powder compressed into a small disk, are the same as tablets. In the past, the term pill was used to denote a

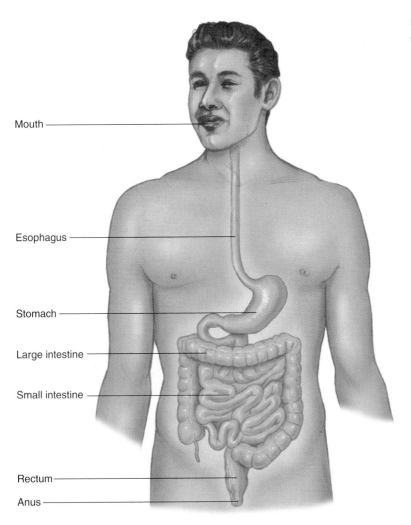

Mouth

Esophagus

Stomach

Large intestine

Small intestine

Rectum

Anus

solid medication taken by mouth. Over time, tablet has become the accepted term.

★ *Enteric coated/time-release capsules and tablets.* These forms of medication release the drug gradually as layers of the capsule or tablet slowly erode. Time-release capsules or tablets must be swallowed whole.

★ *Elixirs.* Elixirs are liquid medications combined with alcohol or placed in a sweetened fluid.

★ *Emulsions.* Emulsions are medications combined with a fat or oil emulsifier.

★ *Lozenges.* Lozenges are solid forms of medication that slowly dissolve in the mouth, thus permitting gradual swallowing.

★ *Suspensions.* A suspension is a liquid that contains small particles of solid medication.

★ *Syrups.* A syrup is a concentrated solution of sugar in water or another liquid to which a medication is added.

Equipment for Oral Administration

Administering oral medications is simple and easy. The basic equipment that you may need depends upon the medication and the patient's status:

★ *Soufflé cup.* A soufflé cup is a paper or plastic cup. Placing a solid medication in a soufflé cup makes it easy to see and minimizes contact with the provider's hands.

★ *Medicine cup.* A medicine cup is a plastic or glass cup with volumetric measurements on the side. It facilitates giving specific amounts of liquid medication. When you pour medication into the cup, the liquid does not form a flat surface but clings to the sides at a higher level, forming a *meniscus.* To compensate for the meniscus, measure the medication toward the center, at its lowest level.

★ *Medicine dropper.* A medicine dropper has markings for measuring liquid volumes. You will use it for special medications and to administer medications to children or patients who cannot tolerate other forms of oral medication.

★ *Teaspoon.* You will use these accurately sized measuring spoons to administer liquid medications. A teaspoon normally holds 5 milliliters of fluid; however, the volume of household teaspoons varies significantly. To ensure accurate medication administration, use a measured teaspoon or syringe.

★ *Oral syringe.* Oral syringes are calibrated plastic syringes without a hypodermic needle. They are considered the most accurate oral means of administering liquid-based medications. When administering a medication with the oral syringe, place the end of the syringe in the patient's mouth and deliver only as much medication as the patient can safely swallow. Several administrations may be necessary to deliver a complete dose.

★ *Nipple.* For the neonate or infant, liquid medication can be delivered with a plastic nipple.

General Principles of Oral Administration

To administer medications orally, use the following technique:

1. Use appropriate BSI measures.
2. Note whether to administer the medication with food or on an empty stomach.
3. Gather any necessary equipment such as a soufflé cup or teaspoon; mix liquids or suspensions, or otherwise prepare medications as needed.
4. Have your patient sit upright (when not contraindicated).
5. Place the medication into your patient's mouth. Allow self-administration when possible; assist when needed.
6. Follow administration with 4 to 8 ounces of water or other liquid. Swallowing a liquid pushes the medication into the stomach.
7. Ensure that the patient has swallowed the medication and it is not hidden in his mouth. For some pediatric and psychiatric patients, you may have to visually confirm that the patient has swallowed the medication by inspecting the oral cavity.

GASTRIC TUBE ADMINISTRATION

For patients who have difficulty swallowing or whose nutritional status is poor, you may place a *gastric tube* to support or completely supplement nutritional requirements. Gastric tubes are also used in instances of drug overdose, trauma, and upper gastrointestinal bleeding. They may be surgically inserted directly into the stomach through the abdomen or indirectly through the nose (nasogastric tube) or mouth (orogastric tube). Placing a gastric tube through the abdominal wall is reserved for the hospital setting. In some EMS systems, paramedics insert orogastric or nasogastric tubes in the field for emergencies. A properly placed gastric tube allows enteral medication delivery. Activated charcoal for toxic ingestion is commonly administered through a nasogastric or

Never use household teaspoons to measure medications, as they vary significantly in volume.

Many types of tubes and access devices are used in modern health care. Never assume that a tube exiting the abdomen is a gastric tube. Use only tubes that are clearly marked as gastric tubes. If you are uncertain, withhold medication or fluid administration.

orogastric tube. Other medications, many used in the nonacute setting, also are administered via the gastric tube. With modification, most oral medications can be administered this way. However, you should avoid administering time-release capsules and enteric-coated tablets through a gastric tube, as crushing them for delivery destroys their slow-release mechanism. Also, ensure that the medication has been sufficiently crushed so as not to become trapped and occlude the gastric tube.

To administer a medication via a gastric tube, use the following technique (Procedure 10-1):

1. Confirm proper tube placement. Disconnect the tube from the drainage or suction unit or clamping device. Clamp the tube from the drainage or suction unit to avoid gastric contents' spilling from either device. Attach a cone-tipped syringe to the proximal end of the gastric tube. Gently inject air while auscultating over the stomach. Following this, withdraw the plunger while observing for the presence of gastric fluid or contents, which indicates appropriate placement. Leave the tube disconnected from the drainage or suction unit.

2. Irrigate the gastric tube. To irrigate the gastric tube, draw up 50 to 100 mL of normal saline into a cone-tipped syringe. Insert the syringe into the open end of the gastric tube. With the syringe tip pointed at the floor, gently inject the saline into the tube. If the saline encounters resistance, look for problems such as tube kinking. Also, have the patient lie on his left side and reattempt injection. If the saline still meets resistance, reattach the tube to the drainage or suction unit and contact medical direction for further directives.

3. Prepare the medication(s) for delivery. Crush tablets or empty capsules into 30 cc of warm water. Ensure that all particles are small so that they will not occlude the tube. You may administer liquid medications without further preparation.

4. Draw the medication into a 30 to 50 mL cone-tipped syringe and place the tip into the open gastric tube. Gently administer the medication into the gastric tube. Forceful application may create considerable distention and patient discomfort.

5. Draw 50 to 100 mL of warm normal saline into a cone-tipped syringe and attach it to the open end of the gastric tube. Gently inject the saline. This facilitates the medication's passage into the stomach and rinses the tube, ensuring that the patient receives the entire dose. Repeated administrations may be necessary.

6. Clamp off the distal tube. Use a commercially manufactured device or hemostat to clamp shut the distal portion of the gastric tube for approximately 30 minutes after you administer the medication. Do not reattach to the drainage or suction unit. This will prevent the medication's inadvertent removal from the stomach.

If you must refill the syringe in order to administer the full dosage of medication, do not allow the syringe to empty completely before you detach it from the gastric tube. This prevents drawing air into the syringe and then introducing it into the stomach, which causes discomfort.

RECTAL ADMINISTRATION

The rectum's extreme vascularity promotes rapid drug absorption. Additionally, because medications given rectally do not pass through the liver, they are not subject to **hepatic alteration;** thus, their absorption is more predictable.

hepatic alteration *change in a medication's chemical composition that occurs in the liver.*

Medication Administration through a Nasogastric Tube

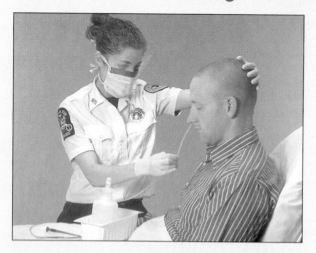

10-1a   Confirm proper tube placement.

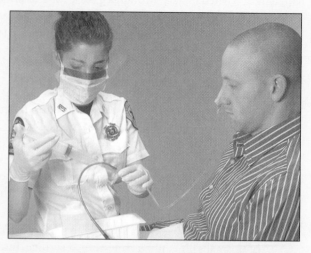

10-1b   Withdraw the plunger while observing for the presence of gastric fluid or contents.

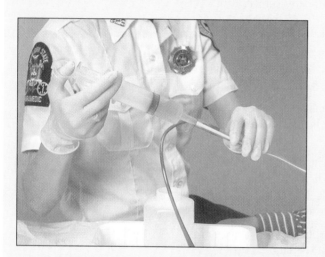

10-1c   Instill medication into the gastric tube.

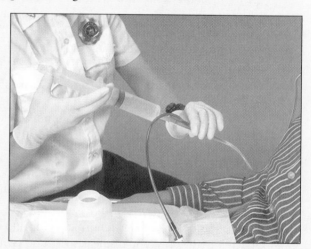

10-1d   Gently inject the saline.

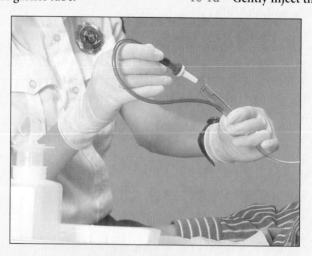

10-1e   Clamp off the distal tube.

In the emergency setting, you may give certain drugs rectally if you cannot establish an intravenous line or use the oral route. These include diazepam (Valium) for protracted seizures or aspirin for cardiac or neurologic emergencies. In the nonacute setting, you may administer sedatives, antiemetics, or other specially prepared medications rectally.

Rectal administration may prove advantageous with the unconscious or pediatric patient, or when administering drugs with an objectionable taste or odor. Unfortunately, drug absorption may be erratic if gross fecal matter exists. In addition, some drugs may cause considerable anal or rectal irritation.

Rectal medications come in a variety of forms. In the emergency setting, they are typically liquid, thus permitting easy administration and rapid absorption. To administer a rectal medication in the emergent setting follow this technique:

1. Confirm the indication for administration and dose, and draw the correct quantity of medication into a syringe.

2. Place the hub of a 14-gauge Teflon catheter (removed from the angiocatheter) on the end of a needleless syringe (Figure 10-11 ■).

3. Insert the Teflon catheter into the patient's rectum and inject the medication. Try to keep the medication in the lower part of the rectum. Administration higher in the rectum may result in the medication's being absorbed by veins that deliver the drug to the portal circulation.

4. Withdraw the catheter and hold the patient's buttocks together, thus permitting retention and absorption.

An alternative technique utilizes a small endotracheal tube instead of the Teflon angiocatheter. Remove the 15/22-mm BVM adapter and connect a syringe to the proximal end of the tube (Figure 10-12 ■). Lubricate the tube and insert it into the rectum. Inject the medication, remove the tube, and hold the buttocks together.

In the nonemergent setting, suppositories or enemas are common methods for rectal administration. Because your responsibilities as a paramedic may include nonemergent clinical settings, you should master these techniques. Additionally, the rectal route may prove beneficial for a pediatric patient who resists oral administration or for whom IV access proves impractical.

Suppositories are medications packaged in a soft, pliable form. Generally refrigerated until they are used, they begin to melt at body temperature in the rectum. Some are lubricated to ease insertion. Suppositories can be lubricated by running a small amount of lukewarm tap water over the suppository prior to insertion. To administer a suppository, manually insert it into the rectum. Hold the buttocks shut for 5 to 10 minutes to allow for retention and absorption.

An **enema** is typically a liquid **bolus** of medication that is injected into the rectum. Medications given via this route are typically referred to as small volume enemas. They are typically prepackaged in a squeezable container with a rectal tip (Figure 10-13 ■).

suppository *medication packaged in a soft, pliable form for insertion into the rectum.*

enema *a liquid bolus of medication that is injected into the rectum.*

bolus *concentrated mass of medication.*

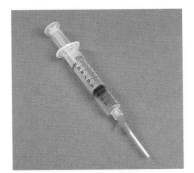

■ Figure 10-11 Catheter placement on needleless syringe.

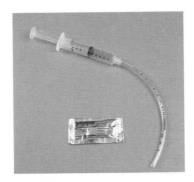

■ Figure 10-12 Syringe attached to endotracheal tube.

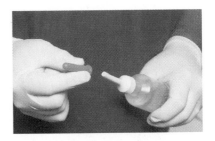

■ Figure 10-13 Prepackaged enema container.

To administer a medicated small volume enema, use the following technique:

1. Apply appropriate BSI and confirm the need for administration via a small volume enema.
2. Place the patient on his left side. Flex his right leg to expose the anus.
3. Insert the prelubricated rectal tip into the anus and advance 3 to 4 inches.
4. Gently squeeze the medicated solution of the bottle into the rectum and colon.
5. Hold the buttocks together to enhance absorption into the rectal and intestinal tissue.

Only those medications with specific guidelines for rectal administration should be delivered through this route. Do not administer rectal medications in the presence of diarrhea, rectal bleeding, hemorrhoids, or any other situation involving severe anal irritation.

Do not administer rectal medications in the presence of diarrhea, rectal bleeding, hemorrhoids, or any other situation involving severe anal irritation.

PARENTERAL DRUG ADMINISTRATION

parenteral *outside of the gastrointestinal tract.*

Parenteral denotes any drug administration outside of the gastrointestinal tract. Broadly, this encompasses pulmonary and some topical forms of medication delivery; however, additional, specific criteria apply to parenteral administration. Typically, the parenteral route involves the use of needles as medications are injected into the circulatory system or tissues. Consequently, some forms of parenteral drug delivery afford the most rapid drug delivery and absorption.

SYRINGES AND NEEDLES

Frequently, giving medications via the parenteral route requires a syringe and hypodermic needle.

Syringe

syringe *plastic tube with which liquid medications can be drawn up, stored, and injected.*

A **syringe** is a plastic tube with which liquid medications can be drawn up, stored, and injected. Syringes range in size from 1 to 100 cc and greater. Remember that while medication dosages are generally given by weight (g/mg/mcg), syringes represent volume. Therefore, you must be prepared to mathematically convert these measurements.

A syringe's two major components are a barrel and a plunger (Figure 10-14 ■). The tubelike barrel, or body, functions as a reservoir for medication. Markings on its side calibrate its overall volume. Smaller syringes are calibrated in 0.10-mL intervals, larger syringes in 1.0-mL intervals.

Legal Notes

Accidental Needle Sticks Administering medications in an emergency setting increases the chances of accidental needle-stick injuries for all involved. It is paramount that paramedics anticipate potential dangers and avoid them. For example, a natural reaction to pain (such as occurs with a medication injection) is to withdraw. This sudden movement can cause an accidental needle-stick injury. Similarly, the combative or agitated patient poses a significant risk. Always make sure that medication administration is safe. If it is not, defer administration until additional resources or personnel are available. Your safety and the safety of your partner come first.

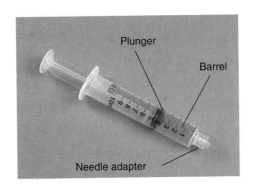

The plunger is a device that fits into the barrel. At one end it has a handle for pulling or pushing. At the opposite end, a rubber stopper fits snugly into the barrel. Pulling on the plunger draws material into the barrel; pushing on it expels material from the barrel. The rubber end forms a tight seal from which the fluid medication cannot escape.

The junction of the fluid and rubber stopper measures the total volume of liquid in the syringe. The barrel's maximum volume should correspond closely to the volume of medication needed. For example, to administer 2 mL of medication, a 3-mL syringe would prove most appropriate.

An adapter at the syringe's distal end is compatible with the hub of an IV catheter or, as many cases will require, a hypodermic needle.

Hypodermic Needle

The **hypodermic needle** is a hollow metal tube used with the syringe to administer medications. It is sharp enough to easily puncture tissues, blood vessels, or IV medication ports.

hypodermic needle *hollow metal tube used with the syringe to administer medications.*

The hypodermic needle's primary components include a hilt and shaft. The hilt is a threaded plastic tube that screws securely onto the syringe's distal adapter. The shaft is a thin metal tube through which medications can flow from the syringe into the delivery site. A bevel at the shaft's distal end accounts for its sharpness (Figure 10-15 ■).

Hypodermic needles come in a variety of gauges and lengths. A needle's **gauge** describes its diameter. Generally, hypodermic needle gauges range from 18 to 27. The gauge and actual diameter are inversely related: the higher the gauge, the smaller the diameter. Thus, a 25-gauge needle's diameter is smaller than an 18-gauge needle's. Conversely, a 20-gauge needle's diameter is larger than a 22-gauge needle's. Hypodermic needle lengths generally range from $\frac{3}{8}$ to $1\frac{1}{2}$ inch. The package label lists the size of the syringe and the gauge and length of the hypodermic needle.

gauge *the size of a needle's diameter.*

Because syringes and hypodermic needles frequently involve invasive procedures, they are packaged sterile. Never use either a syringe or a hypodermic needle from a package that has been opened or tampered with. Used hypodermic needles are sharp and present a biohazard. Dispose of them immediately after you complete any task involving their use.

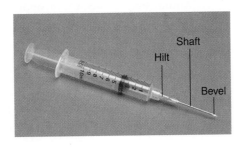

■ Figure 10-15   Hypodermic needle.

MEDICATION PACKAGING

All medications delivered by the parenteral route are liquids. They are packaged in a variety of containers with which you must be familiar, as obtaining medication from each type requires a different procedure. The kinds of parenteral drug containers include:

* Glass ampules
* Single and multidose vials
* Nonconstituted drug vials
* Prefilled syringes
* Intravenous medication fluids

You must also be thoroughly familiar with the information included on the labels of all medication containers:

* *Name of medication.* The label lists both the generic and trade name of the medication. Always ensure that you have selected the right medication.
* *Expiration date.* All medications have an expiration date after which they cannot be used. Never use an expired medication.
* *Total dose and concentration.* The total dose of drug is the total weight (g/mg/mcg) of medication in the container. The concentration represents the weight of the drug per volume of fluid. For example, if 10 mg of a drug were packaged in 10 mL of fluid, the total dose would be 10 mg, and the concentration would be 10 mg/10 mL or 1 mg/mL. Beware, identical drugs can be packaged in different dosages and concentrations.

These labels are printed directly on the vial, ampule, prefilled syringe, or IV medication bag. Always use them to confirm the correct medication.

Glass Ampules

An **ampule,** or amp, is a breakable glass vessel containing liquid medication. It has a cone-shaped top, thin neck, and circular tubular base for storing the medication (Figure 10-16 ■). The thin neck is a vulnerable point where you intentionally break the ampule to retrieve its contents. Ampules usually range in volume from 1 to 5 mL. The least-expensive form of drug packaging, they contain single doses of medication.

To obtain medication from a glass ampule you will need a syringe and needle. Use the following technique (Procedure 10-2):

1. Confirm medication indications and patient allergies.
2. Confirm the ampule label (medication name, dose, and expiration).
3. Hold the ampule upright and tap its top to dislodge any trapped solution.
4. Place gauze around the thin neck and snap it off with your thumb.
5. Place the tip of the hypodermic needle inside the ampule and withdraw the medication into the syringe.
6. Reconfirm the indication, drug, dose, and route of administration.
7. Administer the medication appropriately via the indicated route.
8. Properly dispose of the needle, syringe, and broken glass ampule.

Single and Multidose Vials

Vials are plastic or glass containers with a self-sealing rubber top (Figure 10-17 ■). Vials may contain single or multiple doses of medication; the self-sealing rubber top prevents leakage from punctures and permits multiple access with a syringe and hypodermic needle. The medication inside the vial is packaged in a vacuum.

Always use the label printed directly on the container to confirm the correct medication.

ampule *breakable glass vessel containing liquid medication.*

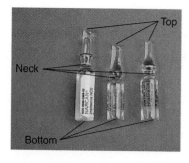

■ Figure 10-16   Ampules.

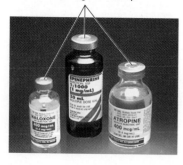

■ Figure 10-17   Vials.

vial *plastic or glass container with a self-sealing rubber top.*

Obtaining Medication from a Glass Ampule

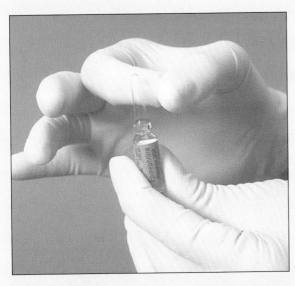

10-2a   Hold the ampule upright and tap its top to dislodge any trapped solution.

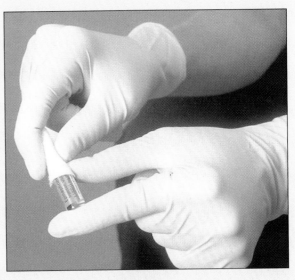

10-2b   Place gauze around the thin neck . . .

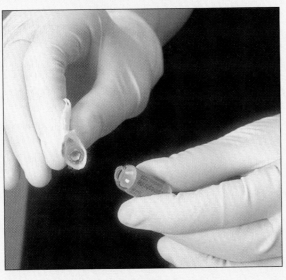

10-2c   . . . and snap it off with your thumb.

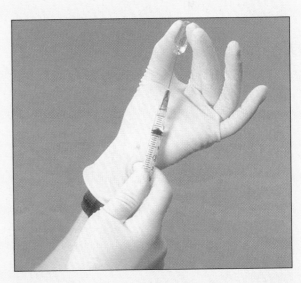

10-2d   Draw up the medication.

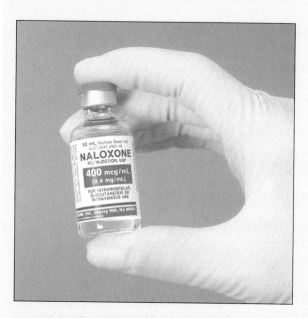

10-3a   Confirm the vial label.

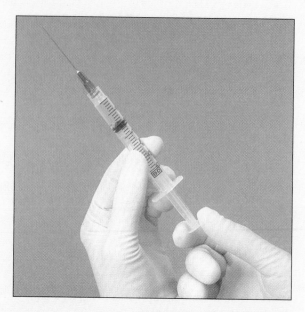

10-3b   Prepare the syringe and hypodermic needle.

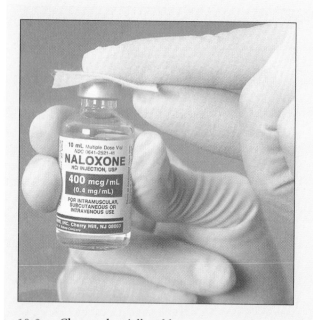

10-3c   Cleanse the vial's rubber top.

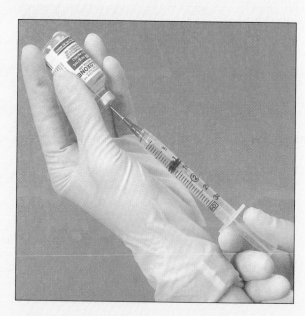

10-3d   Insert the hypodermic needle into the rubber top and inject the air from the syringe into the vial.

To obtain medication from a vial, follow these steps (Procedure 10-3):

1. Confirm medication indications and patient allergies.
2. Confirm the vial label (name, dose, and expiration).
3. Determine the volume of medication to be administered.
4. Prepare the syringe and hypodermic needle. Because the vial is vacuum packed, you will have to replace the volume of medication removed with air in order to maintain equilibrium in the vial. Withdraw the plunger to draw a volume of air into the syringe equal to the volume of medication to be administered. This technique permits easy medication retrieval from the vial.
5. Cleanse the vial's rubber top with an antiseptic alcohol preparation.
6. Insert the hypodermic needle into the rubber top and inject the air from the syringe into the vial. Then withdraw the appropriate volume of medication.
7. Reconfirm the indication, drug, dose, and route of administration.
8. Administer appropriately via the indicated route.
9. Properly dispose of the needle, syringe, and vial.

Nonconstituted Drug Vial

The **nonconstituted drug vial** extends the viability and storage time of drugs that have a short shelf life or are unstable in liquid form. The nonconstituted drug vial actually consists of two vials, one containing a powdered medication and one containing a liquid mixing solution (Figure 10-18 ■). To prepare the drug you must mix it, or reconstitute it, by withdrawing the liquid solution from its vial and placing it in the powdered medication's vial. In a **Mix-o-Vial** system, the two vials are joined and you must squeeze them together to break the seal and mix.

To prepare a medication from a nonconstituted drug vial, use the following technique (Procedure 10-4):

1. Confirm medication indications and patient allergies.
2. Confirm the vial's label (name, dose, expiration date).
3. Remove all solution from the vial containing the mixing solution, using the same procedure as you would to withdraw medication from a single or multidose vial.
4. With an alcohol preparation, cleanse the top of the vial containing the powdered drug and inject the mixing solution.
5. Gently agitate or shake the vial to ensure complete mixture.
6. Determine the volume of newly constituted medication to be administered.
7. Prepare the syringe and hypodermic needle. Because the vial is vacuum packed, you will have to replace the volume of medication removed with air in order to retain equilibrium in the vial. By withdrawing the plunger, place into the syringe a volume of air equal to the volume of medication that will be removed. This technique permits easy medication retrieval from the vial.
8. Cleanse the medication vial's rubber top with an antiseptic alcohol preparation.
9. Insert the hypodermic needle into the rubber top and withdraw the appropriate volume of medication.

nonconstituted drug vial/ Mix-o-Vial *vial with two containers, one holding a powdered medication and the other holding a liquid mixing solution.*

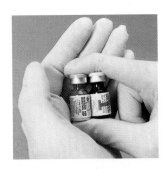

■ Figure 10-18 The nonconstituted drug vial actually consists of two vials, one containing a powdered medication and one containing a liquid mixing solution.

Preparing Medication from a Nonconstituted Drug Vial

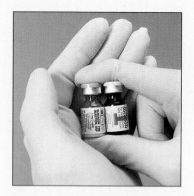

10-4a Nonconstituted drugs come in separate vials. Confirm the labels.

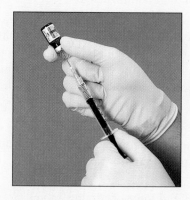

10-4b Remove all solution from the vial containing the mixing solution.

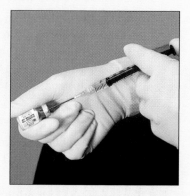

10-4c Cleanse the top of the vial containing the powdered drug and inject the solution.

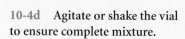

10-4d Agitate or shake the vial to ensure complete mixture.

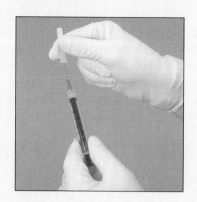

10-4e Prepare a new syringe and hypodermic needle.

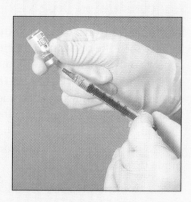

10-4f Withdraw the appropriate volume of medication.

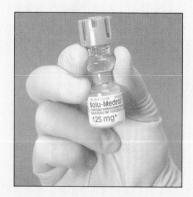

10-4g In the Mix-o-Vial system, the vials are joined at the neck. Confirm the labels.

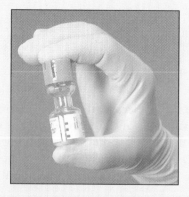

10-4h Squeeze the vials together to break the seal. Agitate or shake to mix completely.

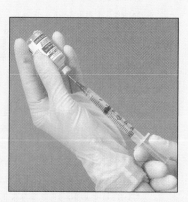

10-4i Withdraw the appropriate volume of medication.

10. Reconfirm the indication, drug, dose, and route of administration.

11. Administer appropriately via the indicated route.

12. Monitor the patient for the desired effects.

13. Properly dispose of the needle and syringe.

In some instances you may have to place multiple medications into one syringe for a single delivery. For example, meperidine (Demerol) and promethazine (Phenergan) may be delivered in this manner. Meperidine, an analgesic, can cause nausea and vomiting when administered. To decrease the incidence of nausea and vomiting, you can simultaneously administer promethazine, an antiemetic. To perform this task, draw all medications in the appropriate order according to the procedures discussed. Always anticipate total volume and select an appropriate syringe size. To avoid complications, you must always be aware of drug incompatibilities.

Prefilled or Preloaded Syringes

Prefilled or **preloaded syringes** are packaged in tamperproof containers with the medication already in the syringe. Because the syringe is prefilled, you do not need to draw the medication from another source. Generally, prefilled syringes contain standard dosages, thus decreasing the chance of dosage error.

The prefilled syringe consists of two parts, a syringe and a glass tube prefilled with liquid medication. The plastic syringe is similar to those described earlier; however, it does not have a plunger. Rather, you screw the prefilled glass tube into the syringe barrel and secure it (Figure 10-19 ■). Pushing the glass container into the syringe barrel expels the medication through the attached hypodermic needle.

Follow these steps to administer a medication from a prefilled syringe:

1. Confirm medication indications and patient allergies.

2. Confirm the prefilled syringe label (name, dose, and expiration date).

3. Assemble the prefilled syringe. Remove the pop-off caps and screw together.

4. Reconfirm the indication, drug, dose, and route of administration.

5. Administer appropriately via the indicated route.

6. Properly dispose of the needle and syringe.

Intravenous Medication Solutions

Medicated solutions are another form of parenteral medication. They are packaged in an IV bag and administered as an IV **infusion.** IV medication solutions may be premixed or you may have to mix them. The section on intravenous drug infusions later in this chapter discusses their actual preparation and administration.

medicated solution *parenteral medication packaged in an IV bag and administered as an IV infusion.*

infusion *liquid medication delivered through a vein.*

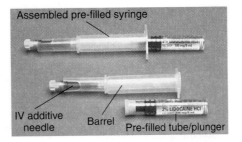

Assembled pre-filled syringe

IV additive needle
Barrel
Pre-filled tube/plunger

2% LIDOCAINE HCl

■ Figure 10-19 Prefilled syringes.

PARENTERAL ROUTES

Parenterally administered drugs can be absorbed locally or systemically. Additionally, depending on the route of administration, their absorption rate may be slow, sustained, or rapid. Parenteral delivery bypasses the digestive tract, thus making the drug's absorption, action, and onset more predictable. Because parenteral routes use hypodermic needles that contact body fluids, the risk of disease transmission is ever present.

Parenteral drug delivery employs the following routes:

★ Intradermal injection

★ Subcutaneous injection

★ Intramuscular injection

★ Intravenous access

★ Intraosseous infusion

Specific medications require specific routes of parenteral delivery; therefore, you must be competent with every route. In this section we will discuss the specialized equipment, medications, and routes for intradermal, subcutaneous, and intramuscular injections. Because of their complexity, we will discuss intravenous access and intraosseous infusions separately in the following sections.

Whether you are administering a parenteral injection or an IV bolus or infusion, you should explain the entire procedure to the patient to help alleviate his anxiety. Finally, remember that hypoperfusion (hypovolemia or peripheral vascular disease, for instance) may significantly reduce parenteral absorption.

Intradermal Injection

intradermal within the dermal layer of the skin.

Using a syringe and hypodermic needle, **intradermal** injections deposit medication into the dermal layer of the skin (*intra-,* within; *derma,* skin). The amount of medication placed in the dermal layer is quite small, typically less than 1 mL (Figure 10-20 ■).

Capillaries in the dermis afford a very slow rate of absorption, with little or no systemic distribution. Rather, the bulk of medication remains localized in the area of administration. Intradermal delivery proves useful for allergy testing and tuberculin skin testing and for administering local anesthetics during suturing, wound debridement, and IV establishment.

The forearm and upper back are preferred sites for intradermal injections. They have little hair and are highly visible. Additionally, you should look for sites free of superficial blood vessels, which increase the chance for systemic absorption.

To administer an intradermal injection, you will need the following equipment:

★ BSI protection

★ Alcohol or betadine antiseptic preparations

★ Packaged medication

Review

Parenteral Routes

Intradermal injection
Subcutaneous injection
Intramuscular injection
Intravenous access
Intraosseous infusion

Capillaries in the dermis afford a very slow rate of absorption, with little or no systemic distribution.

■ Figure 10-20   Intradermal injection.

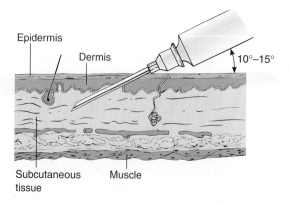

- ★ Tuberculin syringe (1 cc)
- ★ 25- to 27-gauge needle, $\frac{3}{8}$ to 1 inch long
- ★ Sterile gauze and adhesive bandage

To administer an intradermal injection, follow these steps (Procedure 10-5):

1. Assemble and prepare the needed equipment.
2. Apply BSI and confirm the drug, indication, dosage, and need for intradermal injection.
3. Draw up medication as appropriate.
4. Prepare the site with alcohol or betadine. The intended site must be cleansed of pathogens, therein decreasing the likelihood of infection. Generally, you will use alcohol or betadine antiseptics. To appropriately cleanse the site, start at the site itself and work outward with an expanding circular motion. This motion will push pathogens away from the intended site of puncture.
5. Pull the patient's skin taut with your nondominant hand.
6. Insert the needle, bevel up, just under the skin, at a 10° to 15° angle.
7. Slowly inject the medication; look for a small bump or wheal to form as medication is deposited and collects in the intradermal tissue.
8. Remove the needle and dispose of it in the sharps container.
9. Place the adhesive bandage over the site; use the gauze for hemorrhage control if needed.

Do not rub or massage the injection site. This promotes systemic absorption and nullifies the advantage of localized effect.

Subcutaneous Injection

Subcutaneous injections place medication into the subcutaneous tissue (*sub-*, below; *cutaneous*, skin). The subcutaneous layer consists of loose connective tissue between the skin and muscle (Figure 10-21). The subcutaneous tissue has few blood vessels and thus promotes slow, sustained absorption, which prolongs a drug's effect on the body. Like intradermal injections, no more than 1.0 mL of medication is administered subcutaneously. Administering more than 1.0 mL of medication can cause irritation and, possibly, an abscess.

Administer subcutaneous injections where you can easily pinch the skin on the upper arms, thighs, or occasionally, the abdomen (Figure 10-22 ■). Easily pinched skin

subcutaneous *the layer of loose connective tissue between the skin and muscle.*

The subcutaneous tissue has few blood vessels and thus promotes slow, sustained absorption, which prolongs a drug's effect on the body.

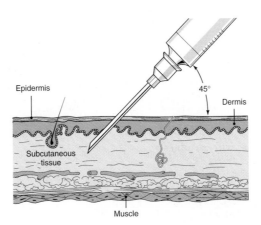

■ Figure 10-21   Subcutaneous injection.

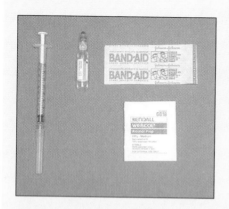

10-5a   Assemble and prepare the needed equipment.

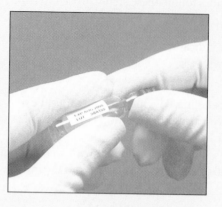

10-5b   Check the medication.

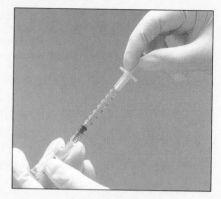

10-5c   Draw up the medication.

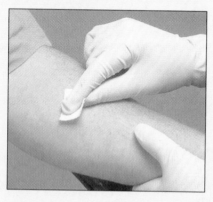

10-5d   Prepare the administration site.

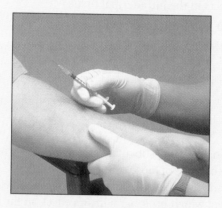

10-5e   Pull the patient's skin taut.

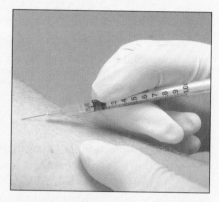

10-5f   Insert the needle, bevel up, at a 10° to 15° angle.

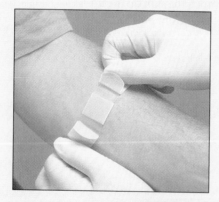

10-5g   Remove the needle and cover the puncture site with an adhesive bandage.

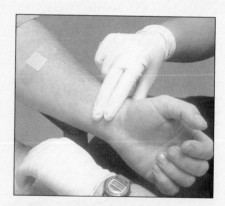

10-5h   Monitor the patient.

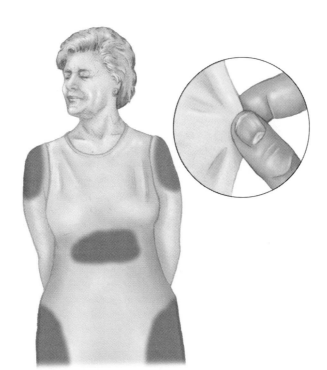

contains more subcutaneous tissue and readily separates from the muscle. All sites should be free of superficial blood vessels, nerves, and tendons. Additionally, avoid areas with tattoos or bruising.

To perform a subcutaneous injection, you will need the following equipment:

★ BSI protection

★ Alcohol or betadine antiseptic preparations

★ Packaged medication

★ Syringe (1 to 3 cc)

★ 24- to 26-gauge hypodermic needle, $\frac{3}{8}$ to 1 inch long

★ Sterile gauze and adhesive bandage

To administer a subcutaneous injection, use the following technique (Procedure 10-6):

1. Assemble and prepare equipment.

2. Apply BSI and confirm the drug, indication, dosage, and need for subcutaneous injection.

3. Draw up the medication as appropriate.

4. Prepare the site with alcohol or betadine as described for an intradermal injection.

5. Gently pinch a 1-inch fold of skin.

6. Insert the needle just into the skin at a 45° angle with the bevel up.

7. Pull the plunger back to aspirate tissue fluid.

8. If blood appears, the hypodermic needle is in a blood vessel and absorption will be too rapid. Start the procedure over with a new syringe.

9. If no blood appears, proceed with step 10.

10. Slowly inject the medication.

11. Remove the needle and dispose of it in a sharps container.

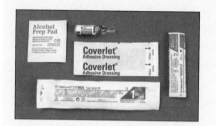

10-6a   Prepare the equipment.

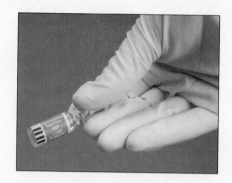

10-6b   Check the medication.

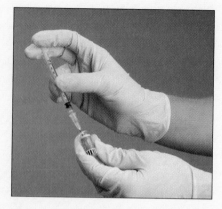

10-6c   Draw up the medication.

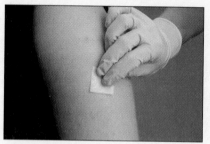

10-6d   Prep the site.

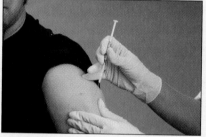

10-6e   Insert the needle at a 45° angle.

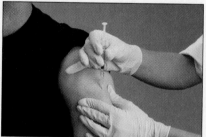

10-6f   Remove the needle and cover the puncture site.

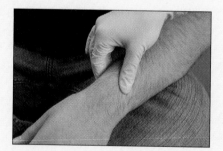

10-6g   Monitor the patient.

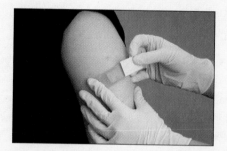

10-6h   Apply an adhesive bandage to the injection site.

(Photos © Scott Metcalfe)

12. Place an adhesive bandage over the site; use the gauze for hemorrhage control if needed.

13. Monitor the patient.

After you give the injection, gently rubbing or massaging the site will help initiate systemic absorption.

Some authorities recommend using an air plug in the syringe. This is approximately 0.1 mL of air that follows the injection and pushes the medication further into the subcutaneous tissue, thus preventing leakage or medication loss. To place an air plug in the syringe, aspirate approximately 0.1 mL of air into the barrel after you have drawn up the medication. Pointing the needle downward and perpendicular to the ground, tap the syringe with your finger to dislodge the air pocket. It will float to the top of the plunger, and from there it will follow the medication into the subcutaneous tissue.

You can also deliver a subcutaneous injection into the sublingual region, or fleshy tissue below the tongue. To administer a subcutaneous injection, you place the hypodermic needle of a small, medication-filled syringe into the sublingual tissue and then inject the medication as appropriate. Epinephrine in severe cases of asthma or anaphylaxis can be administered in this manner.

Intramuscular Injection

Intramuscular injections deposit medication into muscle (*intra-*, within; *muscular*, muscle). Muscle is extremely vascular and permits systemic delivery at a moderate absorption rate. Drug absorption through muscle is also relatively predictable. To reach the muscle, a needle must penetrate the dermal and subcutaneous tissue (Figure 10-23).

Several sites are used for intramuscular injections (Figure 10-24). Depending upon the site, varying quantities of medication can be delivered. These sites and their correlating volumes of medication include:

★ *Deltoid.* The deltoid muscle is 3 to 4 finger breadths below the acromial process (the bony bump on the shoulder). It is highly vascular and permits easy access. You can deliver up to 2.0 mL into this muscle.

★ *Dorsal gluteal.* The dorsal gluteal muscle, or buttock, is a common administration point for intramuscular injections. Injections here can deliver 5.0 mL of medication or more. They cause little discomfort, but you must avoid the large sciatic nerve, which is the leg's major motor nerve. Damage to the sciatic nerve can decrease mobility or totally paralyze the leg. To help prevent neurological complication, envision an imaginary quadrant over the buttock; administer all injections in the upper and outer quadrant.

★ *Vastus lateralis.* The vastus lateralis muscle of the thigh is another common site for intramuscular injection, especially for pediatric patients.

intramuscular *within the muscle.*

✓ **Review**

Intramuscular Injection Sites

Deltoid
Dorsal gluteal
Vastus lateralis
Rectus femoris

Muscle is extremely vascular and permits systemic delivery at a moderate absorption rate.

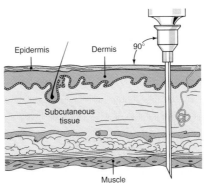

Figure 10-23 Intramuscular injection.

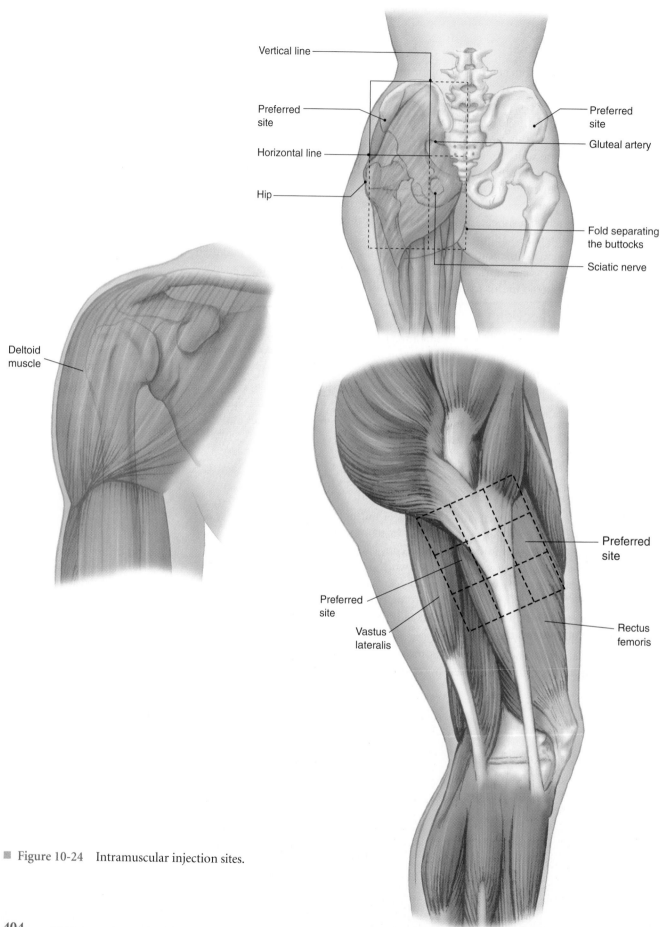

Vertical line

Preferred site

Horizontal line

Hip

Deltoid muscle

Preferred site

Gluteal artery

Fold separating the buttocks

Sciatic nerve

Preferred site

Preferred site

Vastus lateralis

Rectus femoris

■ Figure 10-24   Intramuscular injection sites.

As at the dorsal gluteal muscle, injections here can deliver 5 mL of medication or more. To deliver medication at this site, imagine a grid of nine boxes. Administer injections in the middle, outer box, or anterolateral part of the muscle.

★ *Rectus femoris.* The rectus femoris lies over the femur and is closely associated with the vastus lateralis muscle. When utilizing the rectus femoris for intramuscular injection, place the medication into the center of the muscle at approximately midshaft of the femur. Up to 5 mL of drug volume can be administered into the rectus femoris.

When choosing a site, avoid bruised or scarred areas. Areas free of superficial blood vessels are most desirable.

To perform an intramuscular injection, you will need the following equipment:

★ BSI protection
★ Alcohol or betadine antiseptic preparation
★ Packaged medication
★ Syringe (1 to 5 mL, depending on dosage)
★ 21- to 23-gauge hypodermic needle, $\frac{3}{8}$ to 1 inch long
★ Sterile gauze and adhesive bandage

Follow these steps to administer an intramuscular injection (Procedure 10-7):

1. Assemble and prepare the needed equipment.
2. Apply BSI and confirm the drug, indication, dosage, and need for intramuscular injection.
3. Draw up medication as appropriate.
4. Prepare the site with alcohol or betadine as described for an intradermal injection.
5. Stretch the skin taut over the injection site with your nondominant hand.
6. Insert the needle just into the skin at a 90° angle with the bevel up.
7. Pull back the plunger to aspirate tissue fluid.
   — If blood appears, the hypodermic needle is in a blood vessel, and absorption of the medication will be too rapid. Start the procedure over with a new syringe.
   — If no blood appears proceed with step 8.
8. Slowly inject the medication.
9. Remove the needle and dispose of it in the sharps container.
10. Place an adhesive bandage over the site; use gauze for hemorrhage control if needed.
11. Monitor the patient.

After administration, gently rubbing or massaging the site helps to initiate systemic absorption. Do not massage the site, however, if you have administered heparin or another anticoagulant. Again, some authorities recommend a 0.1-mL air plug as described under subcutaneous injection.

Intravenous and Intraosseous Routes

Two important parenteral drug administration routes—intravenous access and intraosseous infusion—are discussed in detail in Part 2.

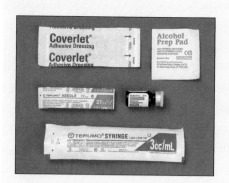

10-7a Prepare the equipment.

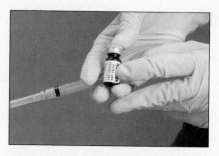

10-7b Check the medication.

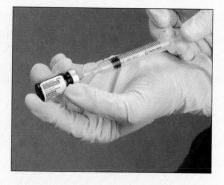

10-7c Draw up the medication.

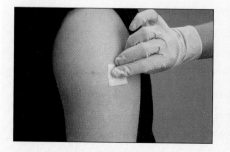

10-7d Prepare the site.

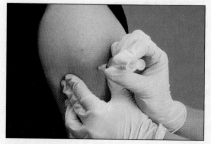

10-7e Insert the needle at a 90° angle.

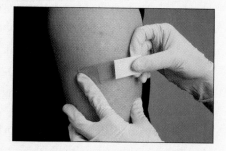

10-7f Remove the needle and cover the puncture site.

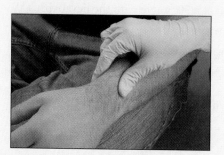

10-7g Monitor the patient.

(Photos © Scott Metcalfe)

Part 2: Intravenous Access, Blood Sampling, and Intraosseous Infusion

INTRAVENOUS ACCESS

Intravenous (IV) access (*intra-*, within; *venous*, vein), or **cannulation,** is a routine paramedic procedure. Circulating blood transports chemicals, proteins, and fluids throughout the body. Venous circulation can likewise deliver medications and fluids into the body and provides an invaluable tool for treating the sick and injured.

The following situations indicate intravenous access:

★ Fluid and blood replacement

★ Drug administration

★ Obtaining venous blood specimens for laboratory analysis

Since veins are easier to locate and penetrate, venous access is preferable to arterial access. Additionally, venous circulation pressure is lower than arterial and presents fewer hemorrhage control complications.

intravenous (IV) access
surgical puncture of a vein to deliver medication or withdraw blood. Also called **cannulation.**

TYPES OF INTRAVENOUS ACCESS

Medical care providers use two types of intravenous access, peripheral and central. As a paramedic, you will most often perform peripheral intravenous access. Central venous access is rarely, if ever, performed in the prehospital setting.

Peripheral Venous Access

Although challenging, **peripheral venous access** is relatively easy to master. As its name implies, it uses peripheral veins. Common sites include the arms and legs and, when necessary, the neck. Figure 10-25 ■ illustrates the specific veins commonly accessed on the hand, forearm, and leg.

As some patients' veins may not be readily visible, you must know venous topography. In these cases, you will have to locate veins based on anatomical layout and palpation. Exhaust all possibilities on the arms before trying to locate the veins of the legs. Leg veins are more difficult to access and present complications more frequently. For neonates and infants, you may access veins in the scalp. Volume 5, Chapter 2 explains that technique.

When establishing a peripheral IV, start at the distal end of the extremity and work proximally. Once you have attempted cannulation, the disruption in blood flow hinders using veins distal to that site. However, the purpose of access also determines site selection. For example, rapid fluid administration requires larger veins like the antecubital fossa, as opposed to the smaller veins of the hand. The external jugular vein is considered a peripheral vein and can be accessed when other peripheral sites are not available.

The major advantage of peripheral venous access is that it is relatively simple to perform because visualizing and accessing the veins is usually easy. Additionally, you can access peripheral veins while simultaneously doing other life-sustaining procedures such as CPR or endotracheal intubation. Conversely, peripheral veins collapse in hypovolemia or circulatory failure, thus becoming difficult to locate and access. Furthermore, the peripheral veins of geriatric patients, pediatric patients, or those with peripheral vascular disease may be fragile and difficult to cannulate. Finally, peripheral veins may roll and elude IV placement.

peripheral venous access
surgical puncture of a vein in the arm, leg, or neck.

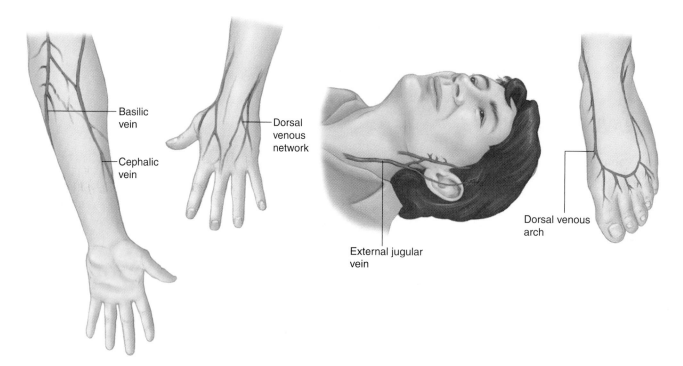

■ Figure 10-25   Peripheral IV access sites: veins of the arm, hand, neck, and foot.

Central Venous Access

central venous access surgical puncture of the internal jugular, subclavian, or femoral vein.

Central venous access utilizes veins located deep within the body. These include the internal jugular, subclavian, and femoral veins. They are larger than peripheral veins and will not collapse in shock. Central IV lines are placed near the heart for long-term use. Typically, they are used when medical conditions require repeated access for medication and/or fluid delivery. They also are used for transvenous pacing or for monitoring central venous pressure.

peripherally inserted central catheter (PICC) line threaded into the central circulation via a peripheral site.

A special type of central line is the **peripherally inserted central catheter,** or **PICC,** line. PICC lines are smaller than those routinely used for central access and are threaded into the central circulation via a peripheral site. PICC lines are most often used in infants and children requiring long-term care.

Central venous access is typically restricted to the hospital setting because of its invasive nature and high risk of complications such as arterial puncture, pneumothorax, and air embolism. Central veins cannot be accessed during procedures such as CPR, and they often require a chest x-ray for placement confirmation. You may nonetheless encounter a central line during interfacility transports or in a chronically ill homebound patient. Protocols in some EMS systems allow paramedics to access existing central lines during emergency care. Still other systems allow their paramedics to place certain central lines. Always follow local protocols regarding central line access and insertion. For more information about central venous access, consult a text on advanced venipuncture techniques.

Do not attempt to access an indwelling central venous access port unless you have been trained in its use and have the correct type of access needles.

EQUIPMENT AND SUPPLIES FOR VENOUS ACCESS

To establish intravenous access, you will need the following specialized equipment and supplies.

Intravenous Fluids

Intravenous fluids are chemically prepared solutions tailored to the body's specific needs. They replace the body's lost fluids and/or aid the delivery of IV medications. They also can keep a vein patent when no fluid or drug therapy is required.

Intravenous fluids come in four different forms: colloids, crystalloids, blood, and oxygen-carrying fluids.

Colloids   **Colloidal** solutions contain large proteins that cannot pass through the capillary membrane. Consequently, they remain in the circulatory system for a long time. In addition, colloids have osmotic properties that attract water into the circulatory system. A small quantity of colloid can significantly increase intravascular volume (volume of blood and fluid contained within the blood vessels). Common colloids include:

★ *Plasma protein fraction (plasmanate).* Plasmanate is a protein-containing colloid. Its principal protein, albumin, is suspended with other proteins in a saline solvent.

★ *Salt poor albumin.* Salt poor albumin contains only human albumin. Each gram of albumin will retain approximately 18 milliliters of water in the bloodstream.

★ *Dextran.* Dextran is not a protein but a large sugar molecule with osmotic properties similar to albumin's. It comes in two molecular weights: 40,000 and 70,000 daltons. Dextran 40 has from two to two-and-a-half times the colloidal osmotic pressure of albumin. Anaphylactic reaction is a possible side effect.

★ *Hetastarch (Hespan).* Like Dextran, hetastarch is a sugar molecule with osmotic properties similar to protein's. Hetastarch does not appear to share Dextran's side effects.

Although colloids help maintain vascular volume, using them in the field is not practical. Their high cost, short shelf life, and specific storage requirements suit them better to the hospital setting. However, the paramedic who works in an emergency department, aeromedical service, or at a mass casualty incident may have to administer colloidal solutions.

Crystalloids   **Crystalloids** are the primary prehospital IV solution. Crystalloids contain electrolytes and water but lack colloids' larger proteins and larger molecules. The many preparations of crystalloid solutions are classified by their tonicity (number of particles per unit volume) relative to that of body plasma:

★ *Isotonic solutions.* **Isotonic** solutions have a tonicity equal to blood plasma's. In a normally hydrated patient, they will not cause a significant fluid or electrolyte shift.

★ *Hypertonic solutions.* **Hypertonic** solutions have a higher solute concentration than do the cells. When administered to the normally hydrated patient, they cause fluid to shift out of the intracellular compartment and into the extracellular compartment. Later, solute will diffuse in the opposite direction.

★ *Hypotonic solutions.* **Hypotonic** solutions have a lower solute concentration than do the cells. When administered to a normally hydrated patient, they cause fluid to move from the extracellular

intravenous fluid *chemically prepared solution tailored to the body's specific needs.*

colloid *intravenous solutions containing large proteins that cannot pass through capillary membranes.*

crystalloid *intravenous solutions that contain electrolytes but lack the larger proteins associated with colloids.*

 Review

Crystalloid Classes

Isotonic
Hypertonic
Hypotonic

isotonic *state in which solutions on opposite sides of a semipermeable membrane are in equal concentration.*

hypertonic *state in which a solution has a higher solute concentration on one side of a semipermeable membrane than on the other side.*

hypotonic *state in which a solution has a lower solute concentration on one side of a semipermeable membrane than on the other side.*

compartment and into the intracellular compartment. Later, the solutes will move in the opposite direction.

The particular type of IV solution you select depends on your patient's needs. The three most commonly used IV fluids in prehospital care are:

★ *Lactated Ringer's.* Lactated Ringer's solution is an isotonic electrolyte solution. It contains sodium chloride, potassium chloride, calcium chloride, and sodium lactate in water.

★ *Normal saline solution.* Normal saline is an isotonic electrolyte solution containing 0.90 percent sodium chloride in water.

★ *5 percent dextrose in water (D_5W).* D_5W is a hypotonic glucose solution used to keep a vein patent and to supply calories needed for cellular metabolism. While D_5W initially increases circulatory volume, glucose molecules rapidly diffuse across the vascular membrane and increase the free water.

Both lactated Ringer's and normal saline solution are used for fluid replacement because of their immediate ability to expand the circulating volume. However, due to the movement of electrolytes and water, two thirds of either solution will be lost to the extravascular space within 1 hour. Crystalloids such as normal saline mixed with D_5W or half-strength normal saline (0.45 percent) are combinations or modifications of the previous solutions.

Occasionally, you will have to warm or cool the IV fluid. A hypothermic patient may benefit from having a crystalloid warmed before and during fluid administration. Warm fluids assist in elevating the patient's core temperature. Conversely, cool fluids may benefit the patient with an increased core temperature. You can cool or warm fluids by storing them in a special temperature-controlled compartment or by using the heater or air conditioner in the ambulance, helicopter, or mobile intensive care unit. Commercial fluid heaters are available. Their use is detailed later in this chapter. Some fluids, such as blood and some colloids, require constant storage in a cool environment.

Blood   The most desirable fluid for replacement is whole blood. Unlike colloids and crystalloids, the hemoglobin in blood carries oxygen. Blood, however, is a precious commodity and must be conserved so that it can be of benefit to the most people. Its use in the field is generally limited to aeromedical services or mass casualty incidents. O-negative blood's universal compatibility makes it ideal for administration in the field. Volume 3, Chapter 9 discusses blood in detail.

Oxygen-Carrying Solutions   Considerable research has been devoted to the development of solutions that carry oxygen. There are two general classes of oxygen-carrying solutions: perfluorocarbons and hemoglobin-based oxygen-carrying solutions (HBOCs). These agents provide a significant advantage over standard colloids and crystalloids because, as their name indicates, in addition to replacing volume they can transport oxygen.

★ *Perfluorocarbons.* Perfluorocarbon compounds are in various stages of research and testing. These agents are denser than water and have a high capacity to dissolve large quantities of gases such as oxygen. Products in development include LiquiVent and Oxygent.

★ *Hemoglobin-based oxygen-carrying solutions (HBOCs).* HBOCs represent a major development in the field of emergency and critical care. These products differ from other intravenous fluids in that they have the capability to transport oxygen. HBOCs contain long chains of *polymerized hemoglobin.* This hemoglobin is obtained from either expired donated human blood or bovine (cow) blood. The hemoglobin is removed from the red blood cells and then repeatedly filtered to remove any infectious substances or antigenic proteins. Finally, the individual hemoglobin molecules are joined together in a large chain through a chemical process known as polymerization. HBOCs are compatible with all blood types and do not require blood typing, testing, or cross-matching.

–*PolyHeme* is an HBOCs derived from expired donated human blood. PolyHeme contains 50 grams of hemoglobin per unit, which is the same as human blood. PolyHeme must be refrigerated and the shelf life is 1 year.

–*Hemopure* is an HBOCs derived from bovine (cow) blood. It has been widely used in South Africa. Hemopure does not require refrigeration and has a shelf life of 3 years.

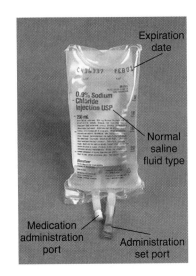

■ Figure 10-26   IV solution container.

Packaging of Intravenous Fluids   Most intravenous fluids and blood are packaged in soft plastic or vinyl bags of various sizes (50, 100, 250, 500, 1,000, 2,000, and 3,000 mL) (Figure 10-26 ■). Some contain medication that is incompatible with plastic or vinyl and must be packaged in glass bottles.

The IV-fluid container provides important information.

★ *Label.* A label on every IV bottle or bag lists the fluid type and expiration date. Like any other medication, intravenous solutions have a shelf life; do not use them after their expiration date. Discard any fluid that appears cloudy, discolored, or laced with particulate. Additionally, avoid using any fluid whose sealed packaging has been opened or tampered with.

★ *Medication administration port.* A medication port on IV-solution bags or bottles permits you to inject medication into the fluid for infusion.

★ *Administration set port.* The administration set port is where you place the spike from the IV administration tubing.

Do not use any IV fluids after their expiration date; any fluids that appear cloudy, discolored, or laced with particulate; or any fluid whose sealed packaging has been opened or tampered with.

Administration Tubing

Intravenous **administration tubing** connects the solution bag to the IV **cannula** that is inserted into the patient's vein. Administration tubing is made of very flexible clear plastic. You must select from several types of administration tubing according to your patient's need. All tubing is packaged in a sterile container. If the container is opened or appears damaged, select another administration set. Any pathogens on the tubing will enter the patient, possibly causing long-term complications.

Microdrip and Macrodrip Tubing   **Microdrip** administration tubing delivers relatively small amounts of fluid to the patient. It is more appropriate when you need to restrict the overall fluid volume a patient will receive. **Macrodrip** administration tubing delivers relatively large amounts of fluid. It is more appropriate when volume replacement is necessary, as in shock, fluid replacement, or hypotension.

To effectively deliver intravenous fluids, you must be thoroughly familiar with the microdrip and macrodrip administration sets, their components, and their subtle differences (Figure 10-27 ■).

★ *Spike.* The **spike** is a sharp-pointed plastic device that you insert into the administration set port on the IV solution bag. A plastic sheath covering the spike keeps it sterile. When the sheath is removed, you must use a medically clean technique to avoid contaminating the spike. If the spike becomes contaminated, discard the administration set and start over with new tubing.

administration tubing
flexible, clear plastic tubing that connects the solution bag to the IV cannula.

cannula   *hollow needle used to puncture a vein.*

microdrip tubing
administration tubing that delivers a relatively small amount of fluid.

macrodrip tubing
administration tubing that delivers a relatively large amount of fluid.

spike   *sharp-pointed device inserted into the IV solution bag's administration set port.*

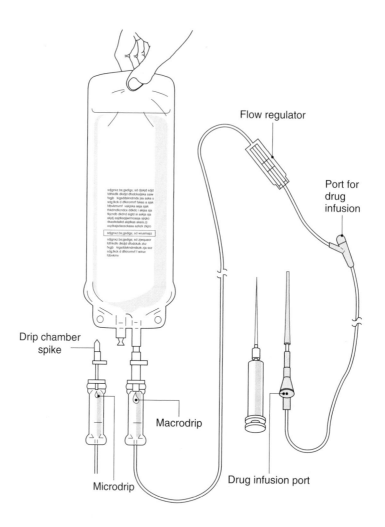

drip chamber *clear plastic chamber that allows visualization of the drip rate.*

drip rate *pace at which the fluid moves from the bag into the patient.*

drop former *device that regulates the size of drops.*

gtts *drops (Latin guttae, drops [gutta, drop]).*

★ *Drip chamber.* The **drip chamber** is a clear plastic chamber that allows you to view the **drip rate.** The drip chamber is squeezable; when compressed, it collects fluid from the IV solution bag and acts as a reservoir for administration. For optimal fluid delivery, the drip chamber should be about one-third full; a line on the chamber marks the correct fluid level.

★ *Drop former.* Inside the drip chamber is a **drop former.** In microdrip administration tubing, the drop former is a hollow metal stylet. In macrodrip tubing, it is a large circular opening at the top of the drip chamber. The drop former regulates each drop's size. The narrow metal stylet in the microdrip tubing creates smaller drops; the wider opening in the macrodrip tubing creates larger drops. In either case, the drop former's precise calibration allows you to calculate fluid volumes by counting drops, or **gtts:**

• Microdrip   60 gtts = 1 mL
• Macrodrip   10 gtts = 1 mL

Depending upon the manufacturer, macrodrip sets may equate 15 or 20 gtts to 1 mL. You must know drops per milliliter to calculate flow rates or medicated infusion dosages.

★ *Tubing.* Intravenous administration tubing is clear and very flexible. Thus, you can watch the solution flow through the administration set, and you can manipulate the tubing in tight situations. Some medications such as intravenous nitroglycerin are chemically incompatible with regular tubing and require special tubing.

★ *Clamp.* IV administration tubing has a simple plastic clamp. When slid over the tubing, the clamp completely stops the flow of solution from the IV bag to the patient. It prevents both the entrainment of air into the tubing when changing IV bags and the backflow of medication when administering medications. You can also use it to stop infusion without disturbing the flow-regulator setting.

★ *Flow regulator.* The flow regulator is a dial enclosed in a triangular plastic casing. It allows infinite control of flow rates ranging from a continuous stream to completely stopped. Rolling the dial towards the IV solution bag increases the drip frequency; rolling the dial towards the patient decreases the drip frequency.

★ *Medication injection ports.* The **medication injection ports** have a self-sealing membrane into which you can insert a hypodermic needle for drug administration. Their design varies, depending upon the manufacturer. When possible, use the medication port nearest the patient.

★ *Needle adapter.* The **needle adapter** is a rigid plastic device at the administration tubing's distal end. It is specifically constructed to fit into the hub of an intravenous cannula. Similar to the spike, the needle adapter is sterile and covered by a protective cap. If it becomes contaminated at any time, start over with a new administration set.

IV Extension Tubing   Extension tubing is IV tubing used to extend the original macrodrip or microdrip setup (Figure 10-28 ■). Its packaging clearly marks it as such. Like administration sets, extension tubing is sterile and must be handled accordingly.

Extension tubing also permits the paramedic to change the original administration tubing or the IV solution bag with little difficulty. For example, if you have to switch from a macrodrip set to a microdrip set, you can close the clamp on the extension and detach the primary tubing. Once you have flushed the new tubing with fluid, you place the needle adapter into the receiving port on the extension tubing and release the clamp. You can now resume fluid therapy without risking complications or having to painfully reinitiate a second IV line.

medication injection port *self-sealing membrane into which a hypodermic needle is inserted for drug administration.*

needle adapter *rigid plastic device specifically constructed to fit into the hub of an intravenous cannula.*

extension tubing *IV tubing used to extend a macrodrip or microdrip setup.*

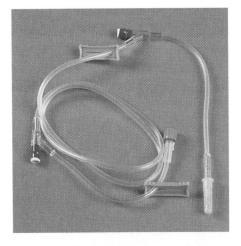

■ Figure 10-28   Extension tubing.

Electromechanical Pump Tubing Mechanical infusion devices may require specially manufactured pump tubing. Typically, pump tubing has special components that attach directly to the pump. Additionally, bladders and relief points permit you to void possible air bubbles. Many specific models of electromechanical infusion pumps require specific pump tubing. When using a mechanical infusion pump, be sure to have the appropriate tubing on hand. Consult the section on electromechanical infusion pumps for more information.

measured volume administration set *IV setup that delivers specific volumes of fluid.*

burette chamber *calibrated chamber of Berutrol IV administration tubing that enables precise measurement and delivery of fluids and medicated solutions.*

Measured Volume Administration Set The **measured volume administration set** can deliver specific volumes of fluid with or without medication. It works well for patients who need specific or limited volumes of fluid, and it is especially advantageous for pediatrics, renal failure, or other patients who cannot tolerate fluid overload.

The measured volume administration set consists of either micro- or macrodrip tubing, with the addition of a large **burette chamber** marked in 1.0-mL increments (Figure 10-29 ■). The burette chamber holds between 120 and 150 mL of fluid. The component of the measured volume administration set include:

★ Flanged spike
★ Clamp
★ Airway handle
★ Medication injection port
★ Burette chamber
★ Float valve
★ Drip chamber
★ Flow regulator
★ Medication injection port
★ Needle adapter

When opened, the airway handle on top of the burette chamber permits air to be displaced or replaced as fluid enters or exits the chamber. If a medication must be mixed in a specific amount of IV solution, you can add it through the medication administration port after correctly filling the chamber.

blood tubing *administration tubing that contains a filter to prevent clots or other debris from entering the patient*

Blood Tubing Administering whole blood or blood components requires **blood tubing,** which contains a filter that prevents clots and other debris from entering the patient. Without exception, all blood must be filtered. Blood that is stored or delivered over an extended period is prone to form fibrin clots or to accumulate other debris. If these clots or debris enter the circulatory system, they can travel in the form of an embolus. Remember, once an embolus encounters a blood vessel too small for its passage, it will lodge and effectively block all blood flow distal to the point of occlusion.

Many aeromedical and facility-based paramedics administer blood and must be familiar with blood tubing. Although most ambulances do not carry blood, paramedics

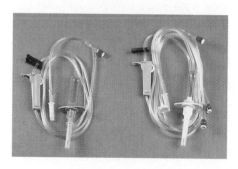

■ Figure 10-29 Measured volume administration set.

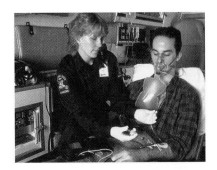

may initiate normal saline with blood tubing in anticipation that whole blood or blood products will be required immediately in the emergency department (Figure 10-30 ■).

Blood tubing comes in two configurations, straight and Y. Y tubing has two administration ports, one for blood and one for IV normal saline solution. Typically, blood is administered with normal saline. Fluids like lactated Ringer's increase the potential for blood coagulation. The two-port design permits immediate access to normal saline if the blood supply is exhausted or must be shut down, as for a transfusion reaction. When you use Y blood tubing, establish a traditional IV by connecting a bag of normal saline to the tubing. Attach the blood to the second port when needed, while maintaining strict medical asepsis. Using the flow regulator, discontinue the normal saline while opening the clamp regulating the flow of blood. Straight blood tubing has only one reservoir. Therefore, only blood is attached to the tubing. A medication administration port close to the needle adapter allows you to piggyback a secondary line of normal saline into the tubing.

Miscellaneous Administration Sets Some tubing now has a manual dial that can set drops per minute or specific flow rates. Some manufacturers have created a single drip chamber that can create either microdrips or macrodrips, depending upon the patient's need.

In-Line Intravenous Fluid Heaters

Technology now makes it possible to heat IV fluids to near body temperature in the field. Most EMS units store their IV fluids in the unit. These fluids, when opened, are at the same temperature as the ambient air. Thus, the temperature of IV fluids can vary significantly depending on where in the country (or world) you work. Many patients are very prone to the development of hypothermia following fluid administration. These include the elderly, children, the frail, and those suffering from fever or similar conditions. When indicated, it is prudent to use an in-line IV fluid heater to warm the IV fluid to body temperature. These devices are designed to shut down if the IV fluid temperature exceeds body temperature. Likewise, different devices are available in order to meet the various flow requirements of, for example, trauma patients, pediatrics, or geriatrics.

Always follow BSI precautions. Open the unit and test the battery. Attach the in-line intravenous fluid heater between the end of the IV tubing and the extension tubing supplied with the unit. Turn the device on and monitor the indicator lights. The unit should remain with the patient upon arrival at the hospital and throughout his hospital stay. It is switched to a direct current (DC) adapter upon the patient's arrival at the floor.

Intravenous Cannulas

The intravenous cannula permits actual puncture and access into a patient's vein. The distal portion of the administration tubing connects to the IV cannula, thus

■ Figure 10-31 Over-the-needle catheter.

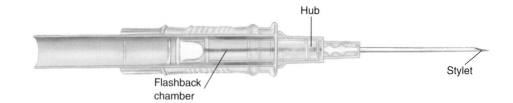

■ Figure 10-31 Over-the-needle catheter.

completing the bridge between the solution bag and patient. The three basic types of IV cannulas are:

★ Over-the-needle catheter

★ Hollow-needle catheter

★ Plastic catheter inserted through a hollow needle

over-the-needle catheter/angiocatheter *semiflexible catheter enclosing a sharp metal stylet.*

Over-the-Needle Catheter Often called an **angiocatheter,** an **over-the-needle catheter** comprises a semiflexible catheter enclosing a sharp metal stylet (needle) that is hollow and beveled at the distal end (Figure 10-31 ■).

★ *Metal stylet (needle).* The metal stylet permits easy puncturing of the skin and blood vessel. Blood from the vein flows through the hollow stylet to the flashback chamber.

★ *Flashback chamber.* The clear plastic flashback chamber allows you to see the blood after the metal stylet has punctured the vein. Blood in the flashback chamber confirms placement of the stylet in the vein.

★ *Teflon catheter.* The Teflon catheter slides over the metal stylet into a successfully punctured vein.

★ *Hub.* Located on the back of the Teflon catheter, the hub receives the needle adapter of the administration tubing once removed from the metal stylet.

For peripheral venous access, the over-the-needle catheter is preferred since it is easy to place and anchor and permits freer movement of the patient.

hollow-needle catheter *stylet that does not have a Teflon tube but is itself inserted into the vein and secured there.*

catheter inserted through the needle/intracatheter *Teflon catheter inserted through a large metal stylet.*

Hollow-Needle Catheter For pediatrics or other patients with tiny, delicate veins, use **hollow-needle catheters** (Figure 10-32 ■). These catheters do not have a Teflon tube; rather, the metal stylet itself is inserted into the vein and secured there. Because the sharp metal stylet can easily damage the vein, you must insert it very carefully. Some hollow-needle catheters have wings for guidance and securing into a vein. These hollow-needle catheters are referred to as winged catheters or butterfly catheters.

Catheter Inserted through the Needle The **catheter inserted through the needle** is also called an **intracatheter.** It consists of a Teflon catheter inserted through a

■ Figure 10-32 Hollow-needle catheter.

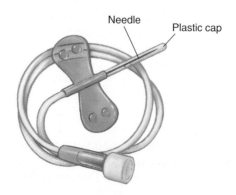

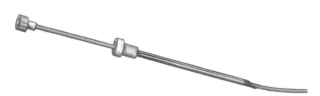

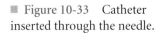

large metal stylet (Figure 10-33 ■). Used in the hospital setting to implement central lines, its proper placement requires great skill, as discussed previously.

The size of an intravenous cannula is expressed as its gauge. The *larger* the gauge, the *smaller* the diameter of the stylet and catheter. For example, a 22-gauge cannula is smaller than a 14-gauge cannula. The larger diameter, 14-gauge catheter allows greater flow rates than the smaller diameter 22-gauge cannula. When establishing venous access, choose the cannula size most appropriate for the patient condition. Typical uses for the various sizes of cannulas are:

★ *22-gauge.* Small gauges are used for *fragile* veins such as those of the elderly or children.

★ *20-gauge.* Moderate gauges are used for the average adult who does not need fluid replacement.

★ *18-gauge, 16-gauge, or 14-gauge.* Larger gauge cannulas are used to increase volume or to administer viscous medications such as dextrose. Blood can be administered only through a cannula that is 16 gauge or larger.

The largest gauge cannula that will fit into a vein is not always appropriate. A cardiac patient with large veins should not receive a 14-gauge cannula for medication administration, just as a multisystems trauma patient with good veins should not receive a 22-gauge cannula for fluid administration. Remember that intravenous access is painful and causes discomfort not only to those receiving it but also to family members watching a loved one in distress.

Miscellaneous Equipment

The **venous constricting band** is a flat rubber band applied proximal to the intended puncture site. It impedes venous return, thereby engorging veins and making them easier to see. This helps you to select the best site and makes venipuncture easier. Never restrict arterial blood flow with the constricting band, and never leave it in place longer than 2 minutes.

Intravenous access is an invasive procedure; therefore, you must use medically clean techniques, including antiseptic preparations, to prevent infection. Applying alcohol and betadine before and after venipuncture decreases the chance of infection.

Once you have established an IV, you must secure it to avoid losing the access. Medical tape and an adhesive bandage are inexpensive and easy to apply. You can also apply clear membranes over the site. Commercial devices manufactured specifically for this task are also available. Have gauze on hand for hemorrhage control if IV cannulation is unsuccessful or if blood leaks from around the site.

Obtaining a venous blood specimen at the time of venipuncture will save the patient from being stuck with a needle again later. This chapter's section on venous blood sampling discusses this technique in detail.

INTRAVENOUS ACCESS IN THE HAND, ARM, AND LEG

As a paramedic you will most often establish peripheral IVs in the hand, arm, or leg. The veins in these places are relatively easy to locate and accessing them causes the patient less pain. In addition, the likelihood of complications is less with these veins than

Intravenous access is painful and causes discomfort not only to those receiving it but also to family members watching a loved one in distress.

venous constricting band
flat rubber band used to impede venous return and make veins easier to see.

To minimize the chances of a catheter shear reaching the patient's central circulation, always leave the venous constricting band in place until you have completely removed the needle from the catheter. However, never leave the constricting band in place more than 2 minutes.

with the external jugular vein (discussed later) or central IV initiation. Therefore, the veins of the hand, arm, and leg are the primary sites for IV initiation.

To establish a peripheral IV in the hand, arm, or leg, use the following technique (Procedure 10-8):

1. Confirm indication and type of IV setup needed. Gather and arrange all supplies and equipment beforehand to make the process easy and accessible.
   — IV fluid
   — Administration set
   — Intravenous cannula
   — Tape or commercial securing device
   — Venous blood drawing equipment
   — Venous constricting band
   — Antiseptic swab (betadine/alcohol)

   When appropriate, explain the entire process to the patient. Apply the proper BSI—gloves and goggles, as IV access is invasive and presents the potential for blood exposure.

2. Prepare all needed equipment. Examine the IV fluid for clarity and expiration date. Insert the administration tubing spike in the IV solution bag's administration set port. Squeeze fluid from the IV fluid container into the drip chamber until it reaches the fill line. Open the clamp and/or flow regulator to flush the solution through the administration tubing and expel trapped air bubbles. Shut down the flow regulator and replace the cap over the needle adapter. Remember that the IV administration set is sterile; if any contamination occurs you must replace the set with a new one.

3. Select the venipuncture site. Acceptable sites have clearly visible veins and are free of bruising or scarring. Straight veins are easier to cannulate than crooked ones.

4. Place the constricting band proximal to the intended site of puncture. Tighten it enough to impede venous blood flow without restricting arterial blood passage. Never leave the constricting band in place more than 2 minutes, as intrinsic changes will occur in the slowed venous blood.

5. Cleanse the venipuncture site. You must cleanse the intended site of pathogens to decrease the likelihood of infection. Alcohol and betadine are the most commonly used antiseptics. Start at the site itself and work outward in an expanding circle. This pushes pathogens away from the puncture site.

6. Insert the intravenous cannula into the vein. With your nondominant hand, pull all local skin taut to stabilize the vein and prevent it from rolling. With the distal bevel of the metal stylet up, insert the cannula into the vein at a 10° to 30° angle. Continue until you feel the cannula "pop" into the vein or see blood in the flashback chamber. The metal stylet is now in the vein; however, the Teflon catheter is not. To place the catheter into the vein, carefully advance the cannula approximately 0.5 cm further. (If you are using a butterfly cannula, it has no Teflon catheter, and you must carefully advance the needle itself.)

7. Holding the metal stylet stationary, slide the Teflon catheter over the needle into the vein. Place a finger over the vein at the catheter tip and tamponade (press gently downward to occlude the vein), thus preventing blood from flowing from the catheter and/or air from entraining into the

Peripheral Intravenous Access

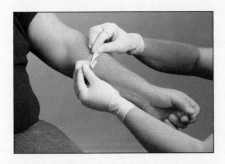

10-8a   Place the constricting band.

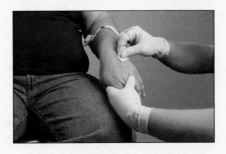

10-8b   Cleanse the venipuncture site.

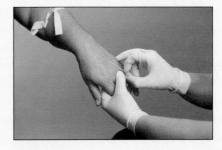

10-8c   Insert the intravenous cannula into the vein.

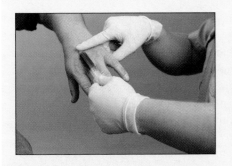

10-8d   Withdraw any blood samples needed.

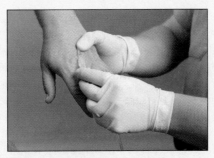

10-8e   Connect the IV tubing.

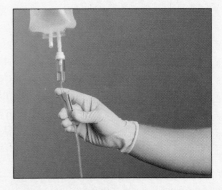

10-8f   Turn on the IV and check the flow.

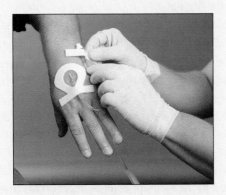

10-8g   Secure the site.

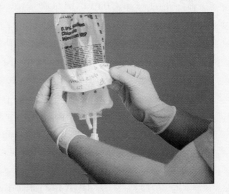

10-8h   Label the intravenous solution bag.

(Photos © Scott Metcalfe)

circulatory system. Carefully remove the metal stylet and promptly dispose of it in the sharps container. Remove the venous constricting band.

8. Obtain venous blood samples as discussed in the section on venous blood sampling.

9. Attach the administration tubing to the cannula. Remove the protective cap from the needle adapter and tightly secure the needle adapter into the cannula hub. Open the flow regulator and allow the fluid to run freely for several seconds. Adjust the flow rate. Do not let go of the cannula and administration tubing until you have secured them as explained in step 10.

10. Apply antibiotic ointment to the site and cover it with an adhesive bandage or other commercial device. Loop the distal tubing and secure with tape. This makes the medication administration port more accessible and attaches the device to the patient more securely. Continue by taping the administration tubing to the patient, proximal to the venipuncture site.

11. Label the intravenous solution bag with the following information:
    — Date and time initiated
    — Person initiating the intravenous access

12. Continually monitor the patient and flow rate.

INTRAVENOUS ACCESS IN THE EXTERNAL JUGULAR VEIN

The external jugular vein is a large peripheral blood vessel in the neck, between the angle of the jaw and the middle third of the clavicle. It connects into the central circulation's subclavian vein. Since it lies so close to the central circulation, cannulation here offers many of the same benefits afforded by central venous access. Fluids and medications rapidly reach the core of the body from this site.

Consider accessing the external jugular only after you have exhausted other means of peripheral access or when a patient requires immediate fluid administration. This is an extremely painful site to access, so you typically will reserve its use for patients with a decreased or total loss of consciousness.

Cannulating the external jugular vein requires essentially the same equipment as other forms of peripheral IV access, plus a 10-mL syringe. You will not need a constricting band. To access the external jugular, use the following technique (Procedure 10-9):

1. Prepare all equipment as for peripheral IV access in an arm, hand, or leg. In addition, fill the 10-mL syringe with 3 to 5 mL of sterile saline. Attach the distal part of the syringe to the flashback chamber of a large bore, over-the-needle catheter. Apply the proper BSI.

2. Place the patient supine and/or in the Trendelenburg position. This position will increase blood flow to the chest and neck, thus distending the vein and making it easier to see. In addition, the supine-Trendelenburg position decreases the chance of air entering the circulatory system during cannulation.

3. Turn the patient's head to the side opposite of access. This maneuver makes the site easier to see and reach; do not perform it if the patient has traumatic head and/or neck injuries.

4. Cleanse the site with antiseptics. Start at the site of intended puncture and work outward 1 to 2 inches in ever increasing circles.

5. Occlude venous return by placing a finger on the external jugular just above the clavicle. This should distend the vein, again allowing greater visualization and ease of puncture. Never apply a venous constricting band around the patient's neck.

Consider accessing the external jugular only after you have exhausted other means of peripheral access or when a patient requires immediate fluid administration.

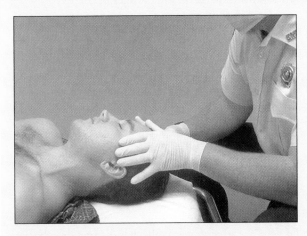

10-9a   Place the patient supine or in the Trendelenburg position.

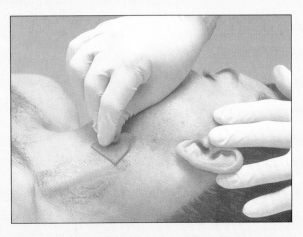

10-9b   Turn the patient's head to the side opposite of access and cleanse the site.

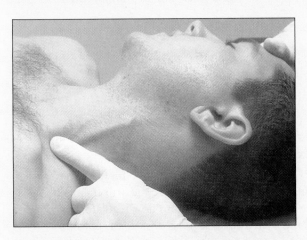

10-9c   Occlude venous return by placing a finger on the external jugular just above the clavicle.

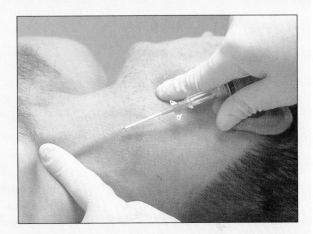

10-9d   Point the catheter at the medial third of the clavicle and insert it, bevel up, at a 10° to 30° angle.

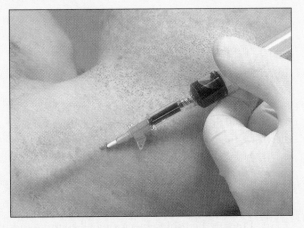

10-9e   Enter the external jugular while withdrawing on the plunger of the attached syringe.

6. Position the intravenous cannula parallel with the vein, midway between the angle of the jaw clavicle. Point the catheter at the medial third of the clavicle and insert it, bevel up, at a 10° to 30° angle.

7. Enter the external jugular while withdrawing on the plunger of the attached syringe. You will see blood in the syringe or feel a pop as the cannula enters the vein. Once inside the vein, advance the entire angiocatheter another 0.5 cm so the tip of the Teflon catheter lies within the lumen of the vein. Then slide the Teflon catheter into the vein and remove the metal stylet as previously described. Immediately dispose of the metal stylet.

8. Obtain venous blood samples as discussed in the section on venous blood sampling.

9. Attach the administration tubing to the IV catheter. Allow the intravenous solution to run freely for several seconds. Set the flow rate and secure as appropriate.

10. Monitor the patient for complications.

While using the external jugular vein has advantages, it also has distinct drawbacks. You may inadvertently puncture the airway or damage the nearby arterial vessels. Additionally, this is a painful entry site for the conscious patient. To minimize risks, perform the procedure very carefully.

INTRAVENOUS ACCESS WITH A MEASURED VOLUME ADMINISTRATION SET

When using a measured volume administration set, follow this procedure (Procedure 10-10):

1. Prepare the tubing by closing all clamps, and insert the flanged spike into the IV solution bag's spike port.

2. Open the airway handle. Open the uppermost clamp and fill the burette chamber with approximately 20 mL of fluid. Squeeze the drip chamber until the fluid reaches the fill line. Open the bottom flow regulator to purge air through the tubing. When all air is purged, close the bottom flow regulator.

3. Continue to fill the burette chamber with the designated amount of solution.

4. Close the uppermost clamp and open the flow regulator until you reach the desired drip rate. Leave the airway handle open, so that air replaces the displaced fluid.

To refill the burette chamber, open the uppermost clamp until you have delivered the desired volume; then repeat step 4.

You can also use measured volume administration sets for continuous fluid administration. Fill the burette chamber with at least 30 mL of solution and close the airway handle. Leave the uppermost clamp open and adjust the rate with the lower flow regulator.

INTRAVENOUS ACCESS WITH BLOOD TUBING

To establish an IV with blood tubing, use the following procedure (Procedure 10-11):

1. Prepare the tubing by closing all clamps, and insert the flanged spike into the spike port of the blood and/or normal saline solution (Y-configured tubing).

Intravenous Access with a Measured Volume Administration Set

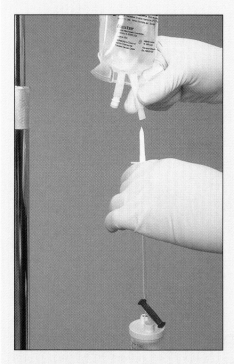

10-10a   Spike the solution bag.

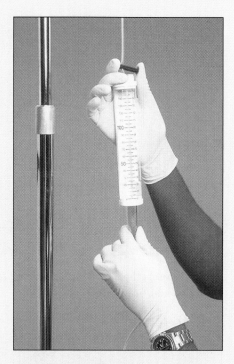

10-10b   Open the uppermost clamp and fill the burette chamber with the desired volume of fluid.

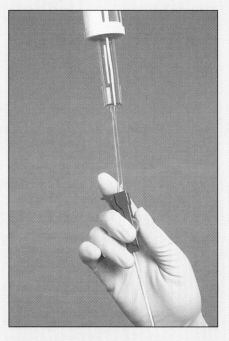

10-10c   Close the uppermost clamp and open the flow regulator.

Intravenous Access with Blood Tubing

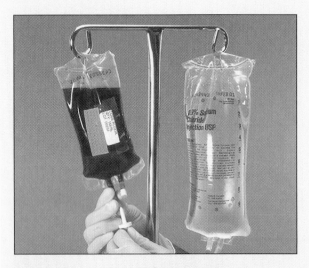

10-11a   Insert the flanged spike into the spike port of the blood and/or normal saline solution.

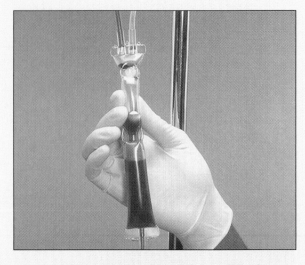

10-11b   Squeeze the drip chamber until it is one-third full and blood covers the filter.

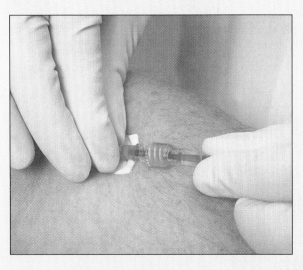

10-11c   Attach blood tubing to the intravenous cannula or into a previously established IV line.

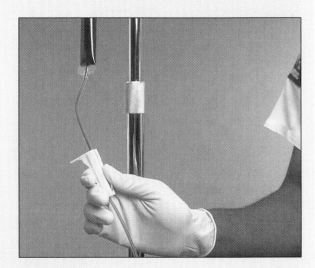

10-11d   Open the clamp(s) and/or flow regulator(s) and adjust the flow rate.

2. Squeeze the drip chamber until it is one-third full and blood covers the filter. Repeat for the normal saline if you are using Y tubing.

3. If you are using straight tubing, piggyback a secondary line of normal saline into the blood tubing, unless you plan to piggyback the straight blood tubing into a large bore primary line.

4. Flush all tubing with normal saline and blood as appropriate.

5. Attach blood tubing to the intravenous cannula or into a previously established IV line.

6. Ensure patency by infusing a small amount of normal saline. Shut down when you have confirmed patency.

7. Open the clamp(s) and/or flow regulator(s) that allows blood to move from the bag to the patient. Adjust the flow rate accordingly.

8. When blood therapy is complete or must be discontinued, shut down the flow regulator from the blood supply and open the regulator(s) for the normal saline solution.

FACTORS AFFECTING INTRAVENOUS FLOW RATES

If an IV does not flow properly, check for the following problems and correct them as appropriate.

★ *Constricting band.* Has the venous constricting band been removed? This is probably the most common mistake both in and out of the hospital. Additionally, ensure that the patient is not wearing restrictive clothing that interferes with venous blood flow.

★ *Edema at the puncture site.* Swelling at the IV site indicates fluid collection caused by infiltration. This **extravasation** occurs if you accidentally puncture the vein more than once, thus allowing IV solution and blood to escape from the second puncture and accumulate in the surrounding tissue. An infiltrated IV site is not usable.

★ *Cannula abutting the vein wall or valve.* If the distal tip of the cannula butts against a wall or valve, carefully reposition it. You may have to untape and retape the cannula once you have achieved an adequate flow rate. Additionally, you may need to use an arm board to keep the patient's extremity straight, as flexion may kink the vein at the site and impede the solution's flow.

★ *Administration set control valves.* Ensure that the flow regulator is open. Be sure to check the flow regulator and clamps of both the primary and any secondary or extension tubing.

★ *IV bag height.* When you move the patient, you may raise the cannulation site above the IV solution bag. This interrupts the solution's gravitational flow from the bag into the patient.

★ *Completely filled drip chamber.* Is the drip chamber completely filled? You can easily correct this by inverting the bag and squeezing the fluid from the drip chamber back into the bag.

★ *Catheter patency.* A blood clot at the end of the Teflon catheter or needle may obstruct the flow of solution from the IV solution bag into the body. If the flow slows, increase the IV drip rate to keep the catheter or needle clear. If the flow stops completely, cleanse the medication administration port closest to the IV entry site with alcohol preparations and insert a syringe and hypodermic needle. Gently aspirate back on the syringe until

 Review

Content

IV Troubleshooting

Constricting band still in place?
Edema at puncture site?
Cannula abutting vein wall or valve?
Administration set control valves closed?
IV bag too low?
Completely filled drip chamber?
Catheter patency

extravasation *leakage of fluid or medication from the blood vessel that is commonly found with infiltration.*

the blood clot is pulled into the syringe. Never flush an IV that has stopped running because of a clot. Flushing will force the clot into the circulatory system and can cause occlusions in the heart or lungs.

If flow remains inadequate after you have eliminated all of these possible causes, lower the IV bag below the insertion site. If blood flows into the IV administration tubing, the site is patent and the problem lies elsewhere. If the problem persists, remove the IV and reestablish it on another extremity, using all new equipment. If you do not observe blood return, the site is inoperable.

pyrogen *foreign protein capable of producing fever.*

embolus *foreign particle in the blood.*

COMPLICATIONS OF PERIPHERAL INTRAVENOUS ACCESS

Even though it is a routine procedure, intravenous access is not trouble free. It can cause a number of complications.

Pain   Pain at the puncture site occurs during needle penetration or with extravasation. To minimize pain, use a smaller gauge catheter or use a 1 percent lidocaine solution (without epinephrine) to anesthetize the overlying skin before insertion.

Local Infection   Local infection occurs if you do not properly cleanse the site and thus introduce pathogens through the puncture. This complication does not become apparent until after the IV has been established for several hours.

Pyrogenic Reaction   **Pyrogens** (foreign proteins capable of producing fever) in the administration tubing or IV solution can cause a pyrogenic reaction. The abrupt onset of fever (100° F to 106° F), chills, backache, headache, nausea, and vomiting characterize these reactions. Cardiovascular collapse may also result.

Typically, a pyrogenic reaction will occur within one-half to one hour after you initiate an IV. If you suspect a pyrogenic reaction, immediately terminate the IV and reestablish access in the opposite side with new equipment and fluid.

Typically, pyrogenic reactions occur secondary to the use of intravenous solutions that have been contaminated with a microorganism or other foreign matter. Pyrogenic reactions underscore the need to discard any fluid that is cloudy or any equipment that has been opened.

Allergic Reaction   A patient receiving IV therapy may develop an allergic reaction. Most often allergic reactions accompany the administration of blood or colloidal (protein-containing) solutions. In addition, some patients may react to the latex in some types of IV administration tubing.

The sudden onset of hives (urticaria), itching (pruritis), localized or systemic edema, or shortness of breath may signify an allergic reaction. If you suspect an allergic reaction, stop the IV infusion and remove the IV catheter. Treat the patient as discussed in Volume 3, Chapter 5.

Catheter Shear   A catheter shear can occur if you pull the Teflon catheter through or over the needle after you have advanced it into the vein. The soft plastic catheter will easily snag on the metal stylet's sharp point and shear off, thus forming a plastic **embolus.** Therefore, never draw the Teflon catheter over the metal stylet after you have advanced it.

Inadvertent Arterial Puncture   Because arteries may lie close to veins, accidental arterial puncture may occur. Arterial blood is bright red and characteristically spurts with each contraction of the heart. When an arterial puncture occurs, immediately remove the catheter and apply direct pressure to the site for at least 5 minutes. Do not release the pressure until the hemorrhage has stopped.

Circulatory Overload   **Circulatory overload** occurs if you administer too much fluid for the patient's condition. You must monitor flow rates carefully, especially for patients with medical conditions such as kidney failure or heart failure who are intolerant of excessive fluid. Continually examine the patient for signs of circulatory overload (crackles, tachypnea, dyspnea, and jugular venous distention, as discussed in Volume 2, Chapter 2). If you encounter circulatory overload, adjust the flow rate.

circulatory overload   an excess in intravascular fluid volume.

Thrombophlebitis   **Thrombophlebitis,** or inflammation of the vein, is particularly common in long-term intravenous therapy. Redness and edema at the puncture site are typical signs of thrombophlebitis. This complication may also present as pain along the course of the vein, sometimes accompanied by inflammation and tenderness. Typically, thrombophlebitis does not occur until several hours after IV initiation. When you suspect thrombophlebitis, terminate the IV and apply a warm compress to the site.

thrombophlebitis inflammation of the vein.

Thrombus Formation   A **thrombus,** or blood clot, can form if IV access injures the vessel wall. A thrombus may form around the catheter and occlude the movement of fluid between the IV and the blood vessel. If you suspect a thrombus, restart the IV using new equipment. Do not attempt to dislodge the clot with a fluid bolus, as this may create an embolus that causes neurological or pulmonary complications.

thrombus   blood clot.

Air Embolism   **Air embolism** occurs when air enters the vein. Air embolus is most likely to occur during central venous access or when administration tubing has not been properly flushed. Failure to tamponade larger veins during cannulation may allow air into the vein.

air embolism   air in the vein.

Necrosis   **Necrosis,** or the sloughing off of dead tissue, occurs later in IV therapy as medication has extravasated into the interstitial space.

necrosis   the sloughing off of dead tissue.

Anticoagulants   **Anticoagulant** drugs such as aspirin, Coumadin, or heparin increase the chance of bleeding and impede hemorrhage control during IV establishment. They drastically increase the complications of hematoma or infiltration.

anticoagulant   drug that inhibits blood clotting.

CHANGING AN IV BAG OR BOTTLE

You may sometimes have to change an IV bag or bottle. This generally occurs when only 50 mL of solution remain and you must continue therapy after those 50 mL are depleted. Changing the solution bag or bottle is a sterile process. If the equipment becomes contaminated you should dispose of it.

To change the IV solution bag or bottle, use the following technique:

1. Prepare the new IV solution bag or bottle by removing the protective cover from the IV tubing port.

2. Occlude the flow of solution from the depleted bag or bottle by moving the roller clamp on the IV administration tubing.

3. Remove the spike from the depleted IV bag or bottle. Be careful not to drop or contaminate the spike in any way.

4. Insert the spike into the new IV bag or bottle. Ensure that the drip chamber is filled appropriately.

5. Open the roller clamp to the appropriate flow rate.

If air becomes entrained within the administration tubing during this process, cleanse the medication administration port below the trapped air and insert a hypodermic needle and syringe. Pull the plunger back to aspirate the trapped air into the syringe. After you have removed the air, adjust the IV flow rate as needed.

INTRAVENOUS DRUG ADMINISTRATION

Medications can be delivered through an existing IV line. As the IV line is seated directly into a vein, the blood rapidly absorbs these medications and distributes them throughout the body. Intravenous administration avoids many of the barriers to drug absorption in other routes. For example, drugs given via the gastrointestinal tract face enzymes and other chemicals that may deactivate, exacerbate, or in some other way alter the medication being administered. Likewise, local tissues can absorb drugs administered via the subcutaneous or intramuscular routes, thus preventing the total dosage from reaching the bloodstream for delivery. The two methods for administering drugs through an IV line are intravenous bolus and intravenous infusion.

Intravenous Bolus

An intravenous bolus involves injecting the circulatory system with a concentrated dose of drug through the medication administration port of an established IV. This procedure requires the following equipment:

★ BSI protection
★ Alcohol antiseptic preparation
★ Packaged medication
★ Syringe (size depends upon the volume of drug you will administer)
★ 18- to 20-gauge hypodermic needle, 1 to $1\frac{1}{2}$ inch long
★ Existing intravenous line with medication port

To administer an intravenous medication bolus, use the following technique (Procedure 10-12):

1. Assure that the primary IV line is patent.
2. Confirm the drug, indication, dosage, and need for an IV bolus.
3. Draw up the medication or prepare a prefilled syringe as appropriate.
4. Cleanse the medication port nearest the IV site with an alcohol antiseptic preparation.
5. Insert a hypodermic needle through the port membrane.
6. Pinch the IV line above the medication port. This prevents the medication from traveling toward the fluids bag, forcing it instead toward the patient.
7. Inject the medication as appropriate.
8. Remove the hypodermic needle and syringe and release the tubing.
9. Open the flow regulator to allow a 20-cc fluid flush. The fluid will push the medication into the patient's circulatory system.
10. Dispose of the hypodermic needle and syringe as appropriate. Monitor the patient for desired or undesired effects.

Intravenous Drug Infusion

Many cardiac drugs and antibiotics are given as intravenous infusions (IV piggybacks). Intravenous drug infusions deliver a steady, continual dose of medication through an existing IV line. You may give them either as an initial dosage or to maintain drug levels after delivering an initial bolus.

Never administer intravenous infusions as a primary IV line.

Intravenous Bolus Administration

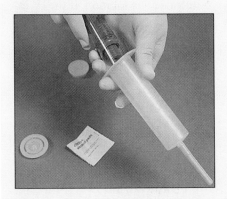

10-12a   Prepare the equipment.

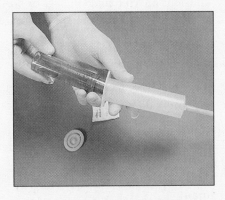

10-12b   Prepare the medication.

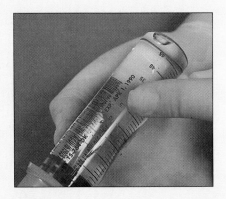

10-12c   Check the label.

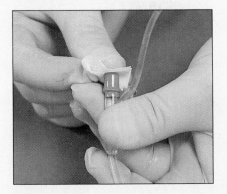

10-12d   Select and clean an administration port.

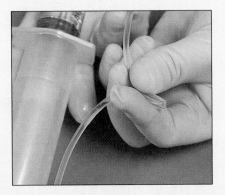

10-12e   Pinch the line.

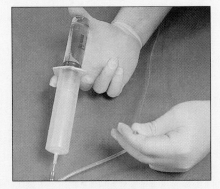

10-12f   Administer the medication.

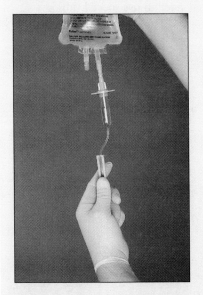

10-12g   Adjust the IV flow rate.

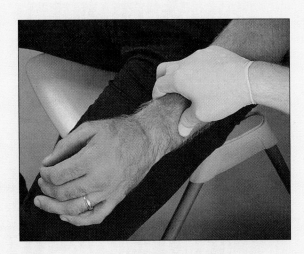

10-12h   Monitor the patient.

Piggybacking IV infusions through an existing intravenous line gives you greater control over medication delivery and allows you to easily discontinue the infusion when therapy is complete or must be stopped. Never administer intravenous infusions as a primary IV line.

IV infusions are contained in bags or bottles of intravenous solution. If the IV infusion is premixed, read the label on the bag for the following information:

★ Name of medication

★ Total dosage in weight mixed in bag

★ Concentration (weight per single cc)

★ Expiration date

If the infusion is not premixed, make a label listing this information and attach it to the bag (Figure 10-34 ■). Additionally, note the date and time you mixed the infusion, and initial it.

Use the following technique to administer a medication as an IV infusion (Procedure 10-13):

1. Establish a primary IV line and assure patency.

2. Confirm administration indications and patient allergies.

3. Prepare the infusion bag or bottle. (If the infusion is premixed, continue to step 4.)

   a. Draw up the appropriate quantity of medication from its source with a syringe.

   b. Cleanse the IV bag or bottle's medication port with an alcohol antiseptic wipe.

   c. Insert the hypodermic needle into the medication port and inject the medication.

   d. Gently agitate the bag or bottle to mix its contents.

   e. Label the bag or bottle.

4. Connect administration tubing to the medication bag or bottle and fill the drip chamber to the fluid line. Most infusions require microdrip tubing. If you use a mechanical infusion pump, you may need to use special tubing.

■ Figure 10-34   If an IV solution is not premixed, you will have to mix and label it yourself.

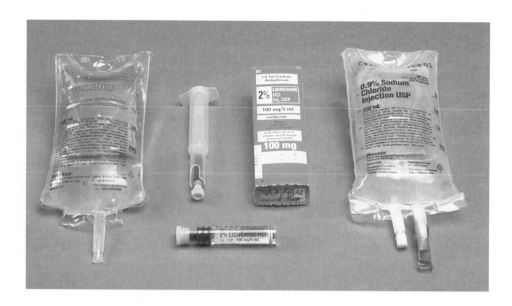

Intravenous Infusion Administration

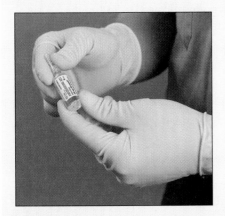

10-13a   Select the drug.

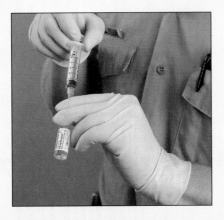

10-13b   Draw up the drug.

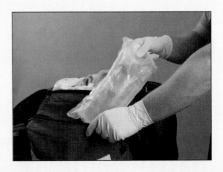

10-13c   Select IV fluid for dilution.

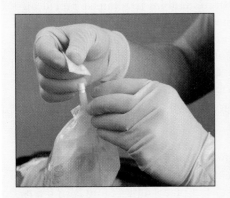

10-13d   Clean the medication addition port.

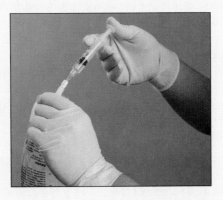

10-13e   Inject the drug into the fluid.

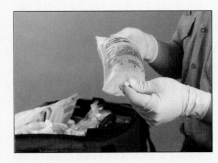

10-13f   Mix the solution.

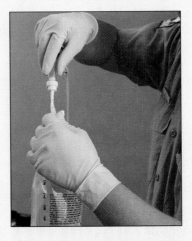

10-13g   Insert an administration set and connect it to the main IV line with a needle.

(Photos © Scott Metcalfe)

5. Place the hypodermic needle on the administration tubing's needle adapter and flush the tubing with solution. (The needle adapter typically accepts a 20-gauge needle.)

6. Cleanse the medication administration port on the primary line with alcohol and insert the secondary line's hypodermic needle. Secure the hypodermic needle and the secondary administration line with tape or another securing device.

7. Reconfirm the indication, drug, dose, and route of administration.

8. Shut down the primary line so that no fluid will flow from the primary solution bag.

9. Adjust the secondary line to the desired drip rate. If you are using a mechanical infusion pump set it accordingly.

10. Properly dispose of the needle and syringe.

When the infusion is complete, shut down the secondary line with the flow regulator or a clamp. Open the primary line and adjust it to the indicated drip rate. Remove the hypodermic needle from the medication administration port and properly dispose of all contents. If required by your local protocols, retain the medication bag to verify administration and for quality assurance.

You can also use measured volume administration tubing to administer medicated infusions. First, fill the burette chamber of a measured volume administration device with a specific volume of fluid. Then you can inject the drug through the medication injection site on top of the burette chamber. You must adjust the flow rate to deliver the precise amount of medication required. In addition, you can mix the medication within the IV bag or bottle as previously described and use the measured volume administration tubing solely for administering the infusion rather than for mixing it.

Heparin Lock and Saline Lock

heparin lock *peripheral IV cannula with a distal medication port used for intermittent fluid or medication infusions. Flushes of heparin solution, which inhibit blood coagulation, are used to maintain patency of the device.*

saline lock *peripheral IV cannula with a distal medication port used for intermittent fluid or medication infusions. Saline is injected into the device to maintain its patency.*

When a patient requires occasional IV medication drips or boluses but does not need continuous fluid, heparin locks are used. A **heparin lock** is a peripheral IV port that does not use a bag of fluid. Like a typical IV start, it places an IV cannula into a peripheral vein; however, instead of IV administration tubing, it has attached short tubing with a clamp and a distal medication port (Figure 10-35 ■). A heparin lock decreases the risk of accidental fluid overload and electrolyte derangement. You also may withdraw blood samples from the lock if it is in a suitable vein. For short-term use, **saline locks** may be used. Sterile saline is injected following the drug. Saline remains in the lock to keep it open. For long-term use, a heparin lock is preferred. Although it functions the same as a saline lock, a heparin lock is filled with a low-concentration solution of heparin, which aids in keeping any blood that gets into the device from clotting. Typically, a drug will be administered through the heparin lock. This is followed by a saline flush to assure that no drug remains in the lock or hub. Then, the lock and hub are filled with a heparin solution. This aids in keeping the IV site open for a long period of time.

Initiating a heparin lock requires the following equipment:

★ IV cannula

★ Heparin lock

★ Syringe with 3 to 5 cc sterile saline or commercial saline injection device

★ Tape or commercial securing device

★ Venous blood drawing equipment

★ Venous constricting band

★ Antiseptic swab (betadine/alcohol)

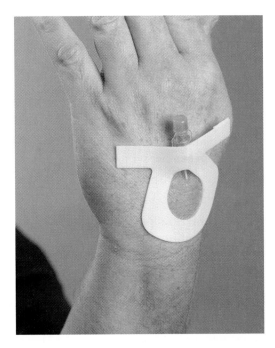

To place a heparin lock, follow these steps:

1. Select the venipuncture site.
2. Place the constricting band proximal to the puncture site.
3. Cleanse the venipuncture site with alcohol or betadine antiseptics.
4. Insert the intravenous cannula into the vein.
5. Slide the Teflon catheter into the vein.
6. Carefully remove the metal stylet and promptly dispose of it into the sharps container. Remove the venous constricting band.
7. Obtain venous blood samples, as explained under Venous Blood Sampling.
8. Attach the heparin lock tubing to the angiocatheter hub.
9. Cleanse the medication port and inject 3 to 5 mL of sterile saline into the lock. Easy flow of the saline without edema at the puncture site indicates patency. If you encounter resistance or if edema forms, restart the procedure with new equipment.
10. Apply antibiotic ointment to the site and cover with an adhesive bandage or other commercial device. Secure the tubing to the patient.

To administer an IV medication bolus through a heparin lock, assemble the following equipment and supplies:

★ BSI protection
★ Alcohol antiseptic preparation
★ Packaged medication
★ Syringe (the size depends on the volume being administered)
★ 18- to 20-gauge hypodermic needle 1 to $1\frac{1}{2}$ inch long

After you have gathered all equipment and supplies, use the following technique to administer an IV medication bolus with a heparin lock:

1. Confirm the drug, indication, dosage, and need for an IV bolus.
2. Draw up the medication or prepare a prefilled syringe as appropriate.

3. Cleanse the medication port nearest the IV site with alcohol antiseptic preparation.

4. Ensure that the plastic clamp is open.

5. Insert the hypodermic needle through the port membrane.

6. Inject the medication as appropriate.

7. Remove the hypodermic needle and dispose of it in the sharps container.

8. Follow the medication administration with a 10- to 20-mL saline flush from another syringe.

9. Properly dispose of the hypodermic needle and syringe. Monitor the patient for desired or undesired effects.

If fluid administration becomes necessary, you can unscrew the medication port and insert IV administration tubing. Periodically flush with sterile saline or heparin to prevent clot formation and occlusion at the Teflon catheter's distal end.

Venous Access Device

venous access device
surgically implanted port that permits repeated access to central venous circulation.

A **venous access device** is a surgically implanted port that permits repeated access to the central venous circulation. Implanted just under the skin, venous access devices are constructed of a plastic or stainless steel injection port and flexible catheter. The injection port, which lies just beneath the skin, contains a self-sealing septum that allows repeated penetration and access into the venous circulation. The self-sealing septum is connected to a flexible catheter that is placed within the lumen of a central vein, most often the superior vena cava.

Typically, patients with venous access devices have chronic illnesses that require repeated intravenous access for medication administration, long-term intravenous therapy, or blood sampling. Generally, venous access devices are placed on the anterior chest near the third or fourth rib lateral to the sternum. A venous access device is apparent as a raised circle just beneath the skin.

Huber needle   *needle that has an opening on the side of the shaft instead of the tip.*

Use of an indwelling central venous access device requires special training. Delivering a medication through the venous access device requires a special needle specific for the venous access device in question. A common needle, the **Huber needle,** has an opening on the side of its shaft instead of at the tip. When placed into the injection port, this configuration allows easy administration of medication into the venous access device. Never access a venous access device unless you have the specific needle unique for the particular device. Always ask the patient, family, or nursing staff about the type of venous access device. Often, they will have a supply of needles for the device.

To administer fluids, medication, or blood through a venous access device, you must first prepare the site using the following technique:

1. Take BSI measures.

2. Fill a 10-mL syringe with approximately 7 mL of normal saline.

3. Place a 21- or 22-gauge Huber needle (or other specialized needle) on the end of the syringe.

4. Cleanse the skin over the injection port with povidone-iodine or alcohol preparations.

5. Stabilize the site with one hand while inserting the Huber needle at a 90° angle. Gently advance it until it meets resistance. This signals that the needle has contacted the floor of the injection port.

6. Pull back on the plunger and observe for blood return. The presence of blood confirms placement.

7. Slowly inject the normal saline to assure patency.

To administer the medication by intravenous bolus, use the following technique:

1. Prepare the medication, fluid, or blood for administration.
2. Attach a 21- or 22-gauge Huber needle (or other specialized needle) to the end of the syringe.
3. Cleanse the skin over the injection port with povidone-iodine or alcohol preparations.
4. Insert the needle into the injection port at a 90° angle until the needle cannot be further advanced. Pull back on the plunger of the syringe and observe for the return of blood. The presence of blood confirms proper placement.
5. Inject the medication as appropriate.
6. Remove and dispose of the syringe appropriately.
7. With another syringe and attached specialized needle, administer a bolus of heparinized saline to clear the catheter of any blood clots or other obstruction.

If the venous access device is not patent or access proves difficult, contact medical direction for further directives.

To administer IV fluids, use the following technique:

1. Prepare a primary IV line. Be sure to prime or flush the air from the administration tubing.
2. Attach a 21- or 22-gauge Huber needle (or other specialized needle) to the primary IV administration tubing. Insert a 10-mL syringe and hypodermic needle filled with 7 mL of normal saline solution into the tubing medication delivery port nearest the venous access device.
3. Cleanse the skin over the injection port with povidone-iodine or alcohol preparations.
4. Insert the needle into the injection port at a 90° angle until it encounters resistance.
5. Pinch the administration tubing above the medication administration port and pull back on the syringe plunger. Observe for the return of blood. The presence of blood confirms proper placement.
6. Gently inject the 7 mL of normal saline solution.
7. Set the primary line to the appropriate flow rate.

If administering a secondary medicated infusion, continue as follows:

1. Prepare a secondary line containing the fluid, blood, or medicated solution for infusion.
2. Attach a hypodermic needle to the needle adapter of the secondary line. Insert the secondary line into a medication administration port on the primary tubing.
3. Shut down the primary line and infuse the medicated solution as appropriate. Look for ease of administration as a sign of patency.
4. When infusion is complete, administer a bolus of heparinized saline to clear the catheter of any blood clots or other obstruction.

Using a venous access device is a very sterile procedure. You must take care to clean the site before delivering medications. Other complications of using a venous access device include infection, thrombus formation, and dislodgment of the catheter tip from the vein.

Figure 10-36 Infusion
pump.

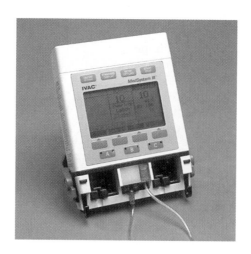

Electromechanical Infusion Devices

Electromechanical infusion devices permit the precise delivery of fluid and/or medications through electronic regulation. Anytime that intravenous infusion occurs, electromechanical infusion pumps provide optimal delivery. Infusion devices are classified as either infusion controllers or infusion pumps.

infusion controller *gravity-flow device that regulates fluid's passage through an electromechanical pump.*

extravascular *outside the vein.*

infusion pump *device that delivers fluids and medications under positive pressure.*

Infusion Controllers Infusion **controllers** are gravity-flow devices that regulate the fluid's passage through the pump. Because infusion controllers do not use positive pressure, they will not force fluids into the **extravascular** space if you infiltrate the vein.

Infusion Pumps Infusion **pumps** deliver fluids and medications under positive pressure (Figure 10-36 ▪). This pressure can cause complications such as hematoma or extravasation if you infiltrate the vein. Some infusion pumps contain a pressure monitor and will warn you if they encounter the increased resistance that occurs with infiltration.

Syringe-type infusion pumps are gaining popularity for medical transport. Syringe pumps deliver their medications from a medical syringe without a hypodermic needle instead of from IV solution bags, fluids, or liquid medications (Figure 10-37 ▪). You place the syringe containing the medications in the pump, which uses computerized mechanics to gradually depress the plunger at the correct rate. These compact pumps prove advantageous during transport.

Figure 10-37 Syringe-type infusion pump.

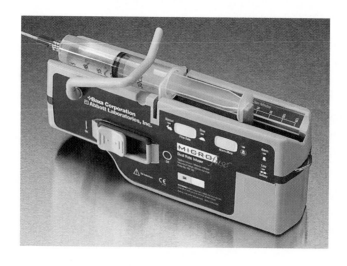

Manufacturers make many different electromechanical infusion pumps. Depending on the maker, pump compatibility may require specialized administration tubing. With some computerized pumps, you can enter the basic information and then the pump will perform all medical calculations internally and automatically set the drip rate. Most infusion pumps contain internal monitoring devices that sound an alarm for problems such as infiltration, occlusion, or fluid source depletion. Electronic devices are prone to malfunction, so you must be prepared to perform all calculations and set the drip rate manually.

VENOUS BLOOD SAMPLING

The laboratory analysis of blood can provide valuable information about the sick and/or injured patient. The concentrations of electrolytes, gases, hormones, or other chemicals in blood can often shed light on the underlying causes of vague complaints such as dizziness or generalized weakness. Additionally, blood evaluation can confirm suspected conditions. For example, elevated cardiac enzymes in a patient's blood can confirm a suspected myocardial infarction.

In the field, you often will be the first to assess and treat an ill or injured patient. Many of your interventions can alter the blood's composition and erase important information. If you obtain venous blood samples before performing those interventions, they will enable the physician to evaluate the patient's original status.

Venous blood is commonly obtained via venipuncture. Thus, paramedics, who routinely initiate intravenous access, can simultaneously obtain blood samples. Doing so saves considerable hospital time and avoids multiple needle sticks.

You should obtain venous blood in the following situations:

★ During peripheral access

★ Before drug administration

★ When drug administration may be needed

Never stop to draw blood if it will delay critical measures such as drug administration in cardiac arrest or transport in a multisystems trauma.

> Never stop to draw blood if it will delay critical measures.

Equipment for Drawing Blood

You will need the following equipment to obtain venous blood.

Blood tubes Blood tubes are made of glass and have color-coded, self-sealing rubber tops. Blood tube sizes for adults generally range from 5 to 7 mL; for pediatrics, from 2 to 3 mL (Figure 10-38 ■). They are vacuum packed, and some contain a chemical anticoagulant. The different-colored tops correspond to specific anticoagulants. A label on every blood tube identifies the type of additive and its expiration date. Do not use a blood tube after its expiration date, as both the anticoagulant and the vacuum lose their effectiveness.

blood tube *glass container with color-coded, self-sealing rubber top.*

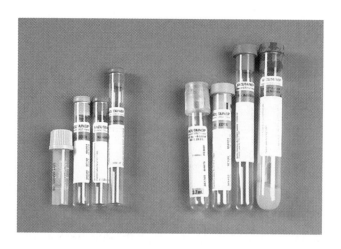

Table 10–1	Blood Tube Sequence	
	Anticoagulant	Color of Top
1.	none	red
2.	citrate	blue
3.	heparin	green
4.	EDTA	purple
5.	fluoride	gray

Using blood tubes in their correct order is essential. If you do not follow the proper sequence, the various anticoagulants will cause cross-contamination, skewing the results and rendering the blood useless. Table 10–1 lists anticoagulants, the order in which you should use them, and the colors of their tops.

Miscellaneous Equipment   Depending upon the technique you use to obtain venous blood, you will also need syringes, hypodermic needles, and commercially manufactured plastic sleeves called vacutainers.

Obtaining Venous Blood

Obtaining venous blood is a simple process; however, if the blood is to remain usable, you must pay strict attention to detail. You can obtain blood either from an angiocath or directly from the vein. Which technique you use will depend on the situation. In either case, venous blood samples are best obtained from sturdy veins such as the cephalic, basilic, or median. Smaller veins such as those on the back of the hand are more likely to collapse during retrieval, making the procedure difficult to complete.

Obtaining Venous Blood from an IV Angiocath   The most convenient way to obtain venous blood is through an angiocath at the time of peripheral vascular access. In addition to blood tubes, you will need a tube holder (Figure 10-39 ■). The tube

■ Figure 10-39   Vacutainer with Luer sampling needle.

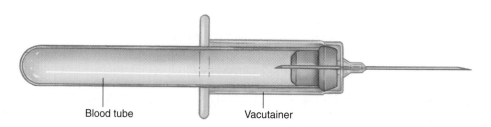

Blood tube   Vacutainer

holder is commonly referred to as a **vacutainer.** A special needle called a multi-draw needle fits into the tube holder. The **multi-draw needle** has a rubber-covered needle used to puncture the self-sealing top of the blood tube. The remaining portion of the multi-draw needle protrudes from the tube holder and fits snugly into the hub of the angiocath.

vacutainer *device that holds blood tubes.*

To obtain blood directly from the angiocath, use the following procedure:

1. Assemble and prepare all equipment. Inspect the blood tubes for expiration or damage and insert the multi-draw needle into the vacutainer.

   Note: Never place blood tubes into the assembled vacutainer and multi-draw needle until you are ready to draw blood. This will destroy the vacuum and render the blood tube useless.

2. Establish IV access with the angiocatheter. Do not connect IV administration tubing.

3. Attach the end of the multi-draw needle adapter to the hub of the cannula.

4. In correct order, insert the blood tubes so that the rubber-covered needle punctures the self-sealing rubber top. Blood should be pulled into the blood tube.

5. Fill all blood tubes completely, as the amount of anticoagulant is proportional to the tube's volume. Gently agitate the tubes to mix the anticoagulant evenly with the blood.

6. Tamponade the vein and remove the vacutainer and multi-draw needle. Attach the IV and assure patency.

7. Properly dispose of all sharps.

8. Label all blood tubes with the following information:

   — Patient's first and last name

   — Patient's age and gender

   — Date and time drawn

   — Name of the person drawing the blood

If commercial equipment is not available, use a 20-mL syringe (Figure 10-40 ■). Attach the syringe's needle adapter to the angiocath hub and gently pull back the plunger. Blood will fill the syringe. When the syringe is full, remove it from the angiocath and place the IV line into the angiocath. Carefully attach a hypodermic needle to the syringe to puncture the tops of the blood tubes. In the appropriate order, place the collected blood into the blood tubes and gently agitate. When finished, properly dispose of all sharps and label the blood tubes.

Obtaining Blood Directly from a Vein When IV access is difficult or unobtainable, you may draw blood directly from the vein with a hypodermic needle. This technique is useful for routine sampling that will not require further IV access. To draw blood directly from a vein, you will need the same equipment as for obtaining blood from an angiocath, but you will use a **Luer sampling needle** (Figure 10-41 ■). A Luer sampling needle is similar to a multi-draw needle, but instead of an angiocath adapter it has a long, exposed needle. The Luer sampling needle screws into the vacutainer, and you insert the exposed needle directly into the vein. You will also need a constricting band and antiseptic wipes.

Luer sampling needle *long, exposed needle that screws into the vacutainer and is inserted directly into the vein.*

To obtain blood directly from a vein, use the following procedure:

1. Assemble and prepare all equipment. Inspect the blood tubes for expiration or damage, and insert the multi-draw needle into the vacutainer.

2. Apply the constricting band and select an appropriate puncture site.

3. Cleanse the site with alcohol or betadine.

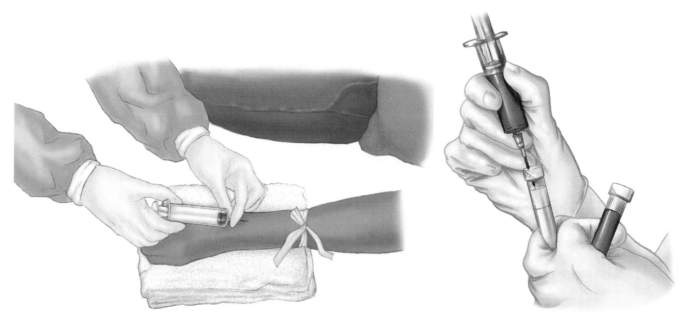

Figure 10-40   Obtaining a blood sample with a 20-mL syringe.

Figure 10-41   Luer sampling needle.

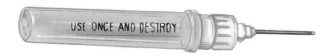

USE ONCE AND DESTROY

4. Insert the end of the Luer sampling needle into the vein and remove the constricting band.

5. In the correct order, insert each blood tube so that the rubber-covered needle punctures the self-sealing rubber top. Blood should be pulled into the tube.

6. Gently agitate the tube to evenly mix the anticoagulant with the blood. Completely fill all blood tubes, as the anticoagulant is proportional to the volume of the tube.

7. Place sterile gauze over the site and remove the sampling needle. Properly dispose of all sharps.

8. Cover the puncture site with gauze and tape or an adhesive bandage.

9. Label all blood tubes with the following information:

   — Patient's first and last name

   — Patient's age and gender

   — Date and time drawn

   — Person drawing the blood

Again, if commercial equipment is not available, you may use a 20-mL syringe. When using a syringe, attach an 18-gauge hypodermic needle to the end of the syringe and insert it into the vein. Gently pull back the plunger to fill the syringe with blood. When the syringe is full, remove the syringe and dress the puncture site. In the appropriate order, inject the collected blood into the blood tubes and gently agitate. When you have finished, properly dispose of all sharps and label the blood tubes.

Complications from drawing blood include damage to the vein wall, inadvertent removal of the IV angiocath, and hemoconcentration and hemolysis of the blood sample. **Hemoconcentration** occurs when the constricting band is left in place too long, elevating the numbers of red and white blood cells in the sample. **Hemolysis** is the destruction of red blood cells. When red blood cells are destroyed, they release hemoglobin and potassium, thus rendering the blood unusable. Causes of hemolysis include vigorously shaking the blood tubes after they are filled, using too small a needle for retrieval, or too forcefully aspirating blood into or out of a syringe.

hemoconcentration *elevated numbers of red and white blood cells.*

hemolysis *the destruction of red blood cells.*

REMOVING A PERIPHERAL IV

You should remove any IV that will not flow or has fulfilled its need. To do so, completely occlude the tubing with the flow regulator and/or clamp. Remove all tape or other securing devices from the tubing and patient. Place a sterile gauze pad over the puncture site. Apply pressure to the gauze with the fingers or thumb of your nondominant hand. With your dominant hand, grasp the cannula at its hub and swiftly remove it, pulling straight back. The site may bleed, so apply direct pressure with the gauze for 5 minutes. Immediately dispose of all materials in the appropriate biohazard container. Apply an adhesive bandage or tape clean gauze over the site to protect against infection.

Remove any IV that will not flow or has fulfilled its need.

INTRAOSSEOUS INFUSION

Intraosseous (IO) infusions involve inserting a rigid needle into the cavity of a long bone or into the sternum (*intra-*, within; *os,* bone). The bone marrow contains a network of venous sinusoids that drain into the nutrient and emissary veins. These sinusoids accept fluids and drugs during intraosseous infusion and transport them to the venous system. Any solution or drug that can be administered intravenously, either bolus or infusion, can be administered by the intraosseous route.

intraosseous *within the bone.*

Generally, you will use IO infusions for the critical patient less than 5 years old when you cannot establish peripheral IV access. Less commonly, you may use intraosseous infusions in adult patients. These patients have different access sites than pediatric patients, and rapid volume administration may not be as effective. Situations that might require an intraosseous insertion include shock, status epilepticus, trauma, cardiac arrest, and critical pediatric patients where rapid IV access cannot be obtained. Initiate intraosseous lines only after 90 seconds or three unsuccessful attempts to establish peripheral IV access.

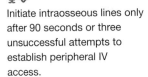

Initiate intraosseous lines only after 90 seconds or three unsuccessful attempts to establish peripheral IV access.

ACCESS SITE

The bone most commonly used for intraosseous access is the tibia. For pediatric access, the proximal tibia is most commonly used. The tibia (both proximal and distal) and sternum can also be used for IO access in the adult patient. To properly locate appropriate sites and avoid complications, you must understand the anatomy and physiology of the tibia (Figure 10-42 ■) and sternum. The three main sections of the tibia are the diaphysis, which comprises the middle, and the two epiphyses, one at either end. Epiphyseal disks, or growth plates, between the diaphysis and the epiphyses allow the tibia to grow and develop and are present in children. Damage to these disks during intraosseous access can cause long-term growth complications or abnormalities in children.

On either side of the proximal tibia are the medial and lateral condyles. You can identify the proximal epiphysis by palpating the condyles. Within the diaphysis, the medullary canal contains the bone marrow. When placed correctly, the distal part of the intraosseous needle will lie in the medullary canal.

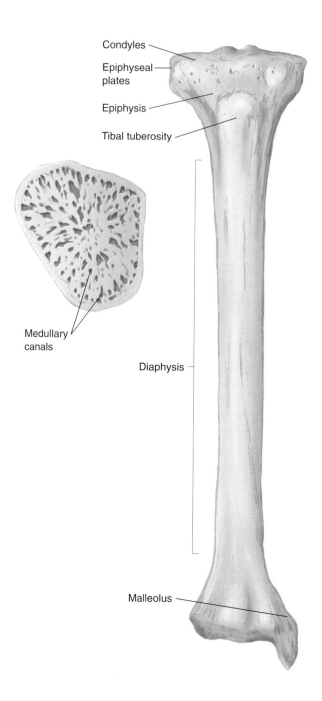

■ Figure 10-42   Tibia.

Condyles

Epiphyseal plates

Epiphysis

Tibal tuberosity

Medullary canals

Diaphysis

Malleolus

Between the condyles, on the top of the anterior tibial crest, is a palpable bump called the tibial tuberosity. The tibial tuberosity lies at the level of the epiphyseal growth plate. Consequently, the tibial tuberosity is extremely important in locating the appropriate pediatric intraosseous access site.

At the distal end of the leg lie the lateral malleolus and the medial malleolus. These aid in location of the distal epiphyseal portion of the tibia and are important landmarks for intraosseous placement in the adult patient.

For the pediatric patient (under 5 years old), you will establish intraosseous access on the medial aspect of the proximal tibia (Figure 10-43a ■). This site is from two to three finger-breadths below the tibial tuberosity. At this level, place the needle on the flat area medial to the anterior tibial crest. For adult or geriatric patients, place the nee-

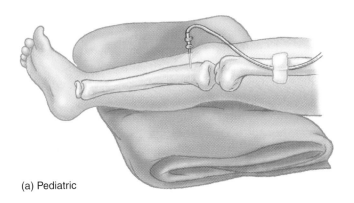

(a) Pediatric

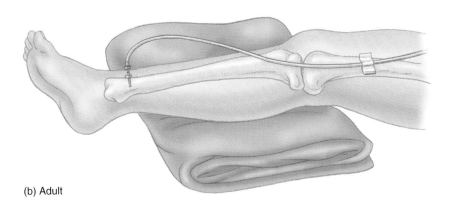

(b) Adult

dle at the distal part of the tibia, one to two finger-breadths above the medial malleolus (Figure 10-43b).

EQUIPMENT FOR INTRAOSSEOUS ACCESS

Intraosseous placement requires a specially designed needle and a 10-mL syringe. Manufactured specifically for IO access, an intraosseous needle is a 14- to 18-gauge hollow cannula with a sharp metal **trocar** inside (Figure 10-44 ■). The trocar gives strength for puncture and prevents occlusion during insertion. Upon placement, the trocar is removed. The intraosseous needle has a plastic handle for insertion and an adjustable plastic disk to stabilize the needle once it is in place. You will attach a 10-mL syringe containing 3 to 5 cc of sterile saline to the intraosseous needle. The syringe and saline are used similarly to IV access of the external jugular vein. A large-bore spinal needle with a trocar in place is an acceptable substitute for an intraosseous needle.

trocar   *a sharp, pointed instrument.*

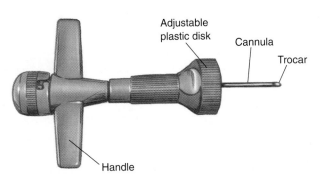

Adjustable
plastic disk

Cannula

Trocar

Handle

■ Figure 10-44   Intraosseous needle.

Other equipment for intraosseous placement is similar to that for a peripheral intravenous access line (fluid, administration tubing, tape, antiseptics, and gauze). A pressure infuser is often needed for IO fluid administration. Some IO devices require a specialized adapter for flushing or using a pressure infuser. Depending upon the specific intraosseous needle, you may need an adapter to connect the administration tubing and the needle.

Several commercial devices are available for both pediatric and adult intraosseous access. While these devices differ in their mechanism and location, they still must be placed through the cortex of a bone and into the marrow cavity where fluids and medications can be administered. Examples of commercial IO access devices include:

★ *Bone Injection Gun (B.I.G.).* The Bone Injection Gun (B.I.G.) was developed in Israel and is available in an adult and a pediatric model. (Figures 10-45 a and b ■).

★ *F.A.S.T.1.* The F.A.S.T.1 allows adult IO placement into the sternum. This site is easy to access and the device is easy to insert. A special needle introducer guides insertion, and a dome protects the site after placement. A special remover is required to extract the needle from the sternum (Figure 10-46 ■).

★ *EZ-IO.* The EZ-IO uses a small drill to place the needle into the bone. The drill is reusable. The manufacturer recommends placement in the proximal tibia for adults. The device is presently approved only for adults (Figure 10-47 ■).

PLACING AN INTRAOSSEOUS INFUSION

To place an intraosseous line use the following technique (Procedure 10-14):

1. Determine the indication for intraosseous access.

2. Assemble and check all equipment.

3. Position the patient. Rotate the leg toward the outside to expose the medial, proximal aspect of the tibia.

4. Locate the access site. Palpate the tibia and use all landmarks.

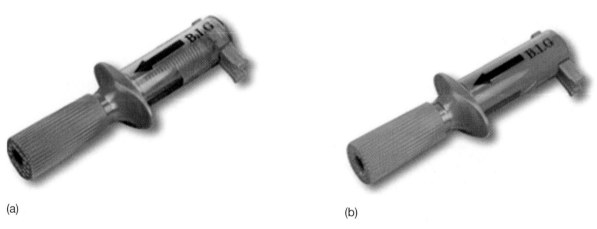

(a)

(b)

■ Figure 10-45   The Bone Injection Gun (B.I.G.): (a) adult model (b) pediatric model. *(Both: WaisMed, Ltd.)*

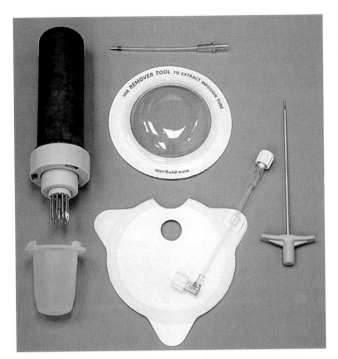

■ Figure 10-46 The F.A.S.T.1 allows IO placement in the sternum of an adult. *(Pyng Technologies Corp.)*

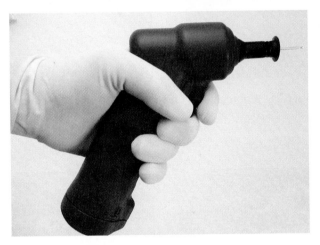

■ Figure 10-47 The EZ-IO, which uses a small drill to place the needle into the bone, is presently approved only for adults. *(Vida-Care Corporation)*

— *Pediatric.* Locate the tibial tuberosity. Move from one to two finger-breadths below the tibial tuberosity and find the flat expanse medial to the anterior tibial crest.

— *Adult or geriatric.* Find the medial malleolus. Move from one to two finger-breadths above the medial malleolus and locate the flat expanse medial to the anterior tibial crest.

5. Cleanse the site with alcohol or betadine. Start at the puncture site and work outward in an expanding circular motion.

6. Perform the puncture. Holding the needle perpendicular to the puncture site, insert it with a twisting motion until you feel a decrease in resistance or a "pop." When this occurs, the needle is in the medullary canal. Do not advance it any further. Generally, you will need to insert the needle only 2 to 4 mm for entry.

7. Remove the trocar and attach the syringe. Slowly pull back the plunger to attempt aspiration into the syringe. Easy aspiration of bone marrow and blood confirms correct medullary placement.

Intraosseous Medication Administration

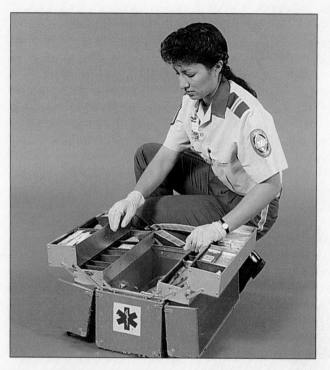

10-14a   Select the medication and prepare equipment.

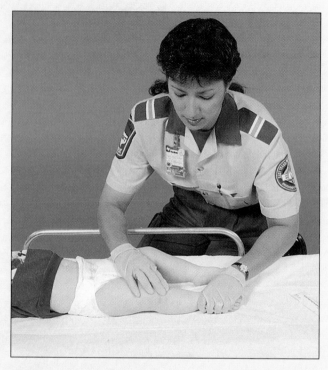

10-14b   Palpate the puncture site and prep with an antiseptic solution.

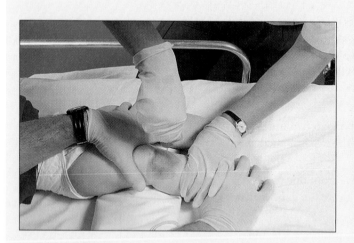

10-14c   Make the puncture.

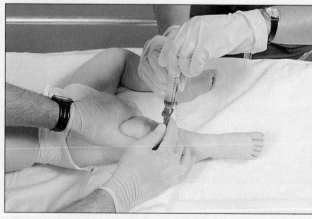

10-14d   Aspirate to confirm proper placement.

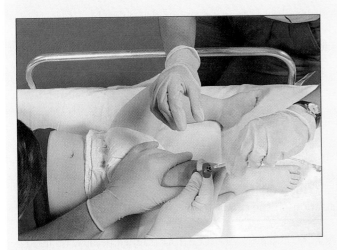

10-14e   Connect the IV fluid tubing.

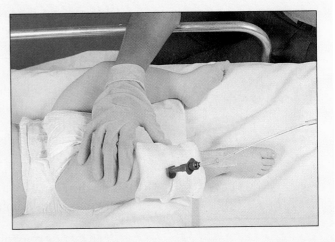

10-14f   Secure the needle appropriately.

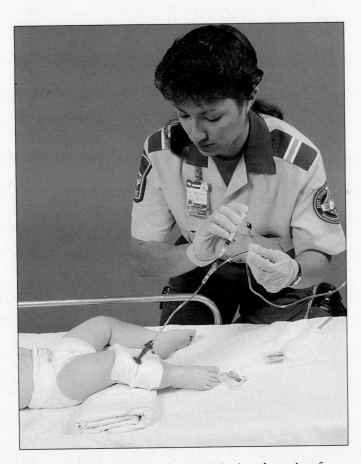

10-14g   Administer the medication. Monitor the patient for effects.

8. Once you have confirmed placement, rotate the plastic disk toward the skin to secure the needle.

9. Remove the syringe and attach the prepared administration tubing and solution. Set the appropriate flow rate.

10. Secure the intraosseous needle as if securing an impaled object by surrounding it with bulky dressings and taping them securely in place. Commercial devices for securing an intraosseous needle are available.

After establishing intraosseous access, you must periodically flush the intraosseous needle to keep it patent. Failure to do so may allow the needle to become occluded, hindering medication administration.

Because the intraosseous needle is connected to the primary IV administration set and fluid, any solution or drug that can be administered by IV bolus or continuous infusion can also be delivered by the intraosseous route. To administer medications or solutions through the intraosseous route, use the medicinal administration port on the primary administration tubing with the techniques as described under Intravenous Drug Administration (Intravenous Drug Bolus and Intravenous Drug Infusion).

If an intraosseous infusion is complete or must be discontinued because of an adverse reaction, shut down the secondary line with the flow regulator or a clamp. Open the primary line and adjust it to the indicated drip rate. Remove the hypodermic needle from the medication administration port and properly dispose of all contents if the infusion has been exhausted.

Review

Content

Intraosseous Access Complications

Fracture
Infiltration
Growth plate damage
Complete insertion
Pulmonary embolism
Infection

INTRAOSSEOUS ACCESS COMPLICATIONS AND PRECAUTIONS

Intraosseous access poses serious potential complications:

★ *Fracture.* Too large a needle or too forceful an insertion can fracture the tibia, particularly in very young children.

★ *Infiltration.* Infiltration occurs when IV solution collects in the local tissues instead of in the intramedullary canal. Infiltration may occur if you run fluids through an incorrectly placed needle or if a fracture has occurred. An infusion that does not run freely or the formation of an edema at the puncture site indicates infiltration. If infiltration occurs, immediately discontinue infusion and restart on the other leg.

★ *Growth plate damage.* An improperly located puncture may damage the growth plate and result in long-term growth complications. Locating the site with proper technique is the most effective way to avoid this complication.

★ *Complete insertion.* Complete insertion occurs when the needle passes through both sides of the tibia, rendering the site useless. To avoid complete puncture, stop advancing the needle once you feel the pop. If complete puncture occurs, remove the intraosseous needle with a reverse twisting motion and start again on the other leg. Apply direct pressure and a sterile dressing over the site(s) for at least 5 minutes.

★ *Pulmonary embolism.* If bone, fat, or marrow particles make their way into the circulatory system, pulmonary embolism may result. Proper technique and vigilance for signs associated with pulmonary embolism (sudden onset of chest pain or shortness of breath) are important to establishing and maintaining intraosseous access.

Other complications of intraosseous access are similar to those of peripheral intravenous access. They include local infection, thrombophlebitis, air embolism, circulatory overload, and allergic reaction.

CONTRAINDICATIONS TO INTRAOSSEOUS PLACEMENT

Do not attempt intraosseous placement in the following situations:

* ★ Fracture to the tibia or femur on the side of access
* ★ Osteogenesis imperfecta—a congenital bone disease that results in fragile bones
* ★ Osteoporosis
* ★ Establishment of a peripheral IV line

Intraosseous placement is a relatively safe intervention that can be used for the critically ill patient (most commonly the pediatric patient under the age of 5 years). Its location allows access while you perform other interventions such as CPR or endotracheal intubation. Because you probably will use intraosseous access only infrequently, you must continually refresh this skill so that you can perform it properly when needed.

You must continually refresh your intraosseous access skills so that you can perform this technique properly when needed.

Part 3: Medical Mathematics

Proper drug administration requires basic mathematical proficiency. Because drug dosages are not always standardized, you may have to calculate amounts according to your patient's age, weight, or other medically related criteria. To properly prepare and administer medications, you must understand roman numerals and be proficient in the following mathematical skills:

* ★ Multiplication
* ★ Division
* ★ Fractions
* ★ Decimal fractions
* ★ Proportions
* ★ Percentages

If you are deficient in one or more of these areas, refer to any text on basic and intermediate math.

METRIC SYSTEM

Medication doses are most often expressed and measured in metric units. Accepted worldwide, the metric system is pharmacology's principal system of measurement. Once you become familiar with it, the metric system is easy to use.

Cultural Considerations

The Metric System Although the United States has been slow to adopt the metric system, it is widely used in science and medicine. As a paramedic, you must be familiar with the metric system and be able to make calculations using it.

Table 10-2	Metric Prefixes	
Prefix	Multiplier	Abbreviation
kilo	1,000	(k)
hecto	100	(h)
deka	10	(D)
deci	1/10 or 0.1	(d)
centi	1/100 or 0.01	(c)
milli	1/1,000 or 0.001	(m)
micro	1/1,000,000 or 0.000001	(mcg or μg)

✓ **Review**

Fundamental Metric Units

Grams—mass
Meters—distance
Liters—volume

The metric system's three fundamental units are grams (mass), meters (distance), and liters (volume). In pharmacology, you will frequently encounter dosages greater or less than these fundamental units. To avoid long numbers with repetitive zeros when measurements are substantially less than or greater than the fundamental unit, the metric system adds prefixes to the fundamental units. Table 10–2 lists metric prefixes.

The most commonly used prefixes in pharmacology are *kilo-, centi-, milli-,* and *micro-.* Prefixes above the fundamental units denote quantities larger than the standard gram, liter, or meter, while those below are smaller. The prefix *milli-* is smaller than the fundamental unit and *m* refers to 1/1,000. Thus, a *milliliter* equals 1/1,000 of a liter. If you divided a liter into one thousand equal parts, a milliliter would equal one of those parts. Similarly, a milligram is 1/1,000 of a gram. If you divided a gram into one thousand equal parts, a milligram would equal one of those parts. The prefix *micro-* expresses 1/1,000,000. A *microgram* is 1/1,000,000 of a gram.

CONVERSION BETWEEN PREFIXES

If you know the prefixes and their numeric equivalents, you can easily convert measurements to smaller or larger units. To convert a measurement to a smaller unit, multiply the original measurement by the numerical equivalent of the smaller measurement's prefix.

Example 1. Convert 3 grams to milligrams.

Milligrams (1/1,000) are smaller than grams; therefore, multiply 3 by 1,000:

$$3 \text{ (grams)} \times 1,000 \text{ (milli)} = 3,000$$
$$3 \text{ grams} = 3,000 \text{ milligrams}$$

Example 2. Convert 2.67 liters to milliliters.

Milliliters (1/1,000) are smaller than a liter; therefore multiply 2.67 by 1,000:

$$2.67 \text{ liters} \times 1,000 \text{ (milli)} = 2,670$$
$$2.67 \text{ liters} = 2,670 \text{ milliliters}$$

To convert a measurement to a larger unit, divide the original measurement by the numerical equivalent of the smaller measurement's prefix.

Example 3. Convert 1,600 micrograms to grams.

A microgram is 1/1,000,000 the size of a gram; therefore, divide 1,600 by 1,000,000:

$$1,600/1,000,000 = 0.0016 \text{ grams}$$
$$1,600 \text{ micrograms} = 0.0016 \text{ grams}$$

When converting a measurement to or from a prefix that is not the fundamental unit, first convert the *existing* measurement to the *fundamental* measurement. Then convert the fundamental measurement to the desired unit.

Example 4. Convert 5.6 milligrams to micrograms.

First, convert the 5.6 milligrams to grams:

$$5.6 \text{ milligrams}/1{,}000 = 0.0056 \text{ grams (g)}$$
$$5.6 \text{ milligrams} = 0.0056 \text{ grams}$$

Now, convert 0.0056 grams to micrograms as previously described:

$$0.0056 \text{ (grams)} \times 1{,}000{,}000 = 5{,}600 \text{ micrograms}$$
$$5.6 \text{ milligrams} = 5{,}600 \text{ micrograms}$$

For the beginner, this technique avoids confusion. The more experienced provider will be able to make a direct conversion from milligrams to micrograms.

HOUSEHOLD AND APOTHECARY SYSTEMS OF MEASURE

In the past, pharmacology traditionally used the household and apothecary systems to measure drug dosages. Gradually, the metric system has replaced those systems, but you may occasionally encounter their remnants. Table 10–3 gives the metric equivalents of the household and apothecary units you will most likely confront.

WEIGHT CONVERSION

Some medications' dosages are calculated according to kilograms of body weight. To convert pounds to kilograms use the following formula:

$$\text{kilograms} = \text{pounds}/2.2$$

Example 5.   How many kilograms does a 182-lb. person weigh?

$$\text{kilograms} = 182 \text{ lbs.}/2.2$$
$$\text{kilograms} = 82.7$$

TEMPERATURE

The international thermometric scale measures temperature in degrees Celsius. While degrees Celsius is often cited interchangeably with degrees centigrade, the two scales are slightly different. For practical purposes, however, you can think of them both as dividing the interval between the freezing and boiling points of water into 100 equal

Table 10–3	Metric Equivalents	
Household	**Apothecary**	**Metric**
1 gallon	4 quarts	3.785 liters
1 quart	1 quart	0.946 liters
16 ounces	approximately 1 pint	473 milliliters
1 cup	approximately ½ pint	approximately 250 milliliters
1 tablespoon		approximately 16 milliliters
1 teaspoon		approximately 4 to 5 milliliters

parts, with 0° being the freezing point and 100° being the boiling point. The household measurement system, in contrast, divides the interval between the freezing and boiling points of water into 180 equal parts, with 32° being the freezing point and 212° being the boiling point. When taking a body temperature, use the following formulas to convert between degrees Fahrenheit and degrees Celsius:

$$°F = 9/5 \, °C + 32$$
$$°C = 5/9 \, (°F − 32)$$

Example 6. Convert 98.2° F to °C

$$°C = 5/9 \, (98.2 − 32)$$
$$°C = 5/9 \, (66.2)$$
$$°C = 36.8$$
$$36.8° \, C = 98.2° \, F$$

Example 7. Convert 28.4° C to °F

$$°F = 9/5 \, (28.4) + 32$$
$$°F = 51.12 + 32$$
$$°F = 83.1$$
$$83.1° \, F = 28.4° \, C$$

Converting between the different prefixes and between different systems of measurement is crucial in calculating drug dosages. You should continually practice all conversions, not only during your formal education but throughout your career in the emergency medical services.

Continually practice all mathematical conversions throughout your career in the emergency medical services.

UNITS

unit *predetermined amount of medication or fluid.*

Some medications are measured in **units.** Penicillin, heparin, and insulin are administered in units. Units do not convert between the metric, household, and apothecary systems.

MEDICAL CALCULATIONS

Always check drug dosage calculations twice.

Frequently you will have to apply basic mathematical principles to calculate specific quantities before administering medications and fluids. In prehospital care, the following forms of medications often require calculation:

★ Oral medications

★ Liquid parenteral medications

★ Intravenous fluid administration

★ Intravenous medication infusions

stock solution *standard concentration of routinely used medications.*

Most medications are provided in **stock solution.** Therefore, you must calculate the exact amount of medication to remove from the stock for administration. To calculate basic drug dosage, you will need three facts:

★ Desired dose

★ Dosage on hand

★ Volume on hand

Desired Dose The **desired dose** is the specific quantity of medication needed. Most dosages are expressed as a weight (grams, milligrams, or micrograms). Dosages may be standard or calculated according to body weight or age.

desired dose *specific quantity of medication needed.*

Dosage and Volume on Hand All liquid medications are packaged as concentrations. *Concentration* refers to weight per volume. A liquid medication's concentration is the drug's weight (grams, milligrams, or micrograms) per volume of liquid (mL) in which it is dissolved. For example, 50 percent Dextrose (D_{50}) is packaged as a concentration of 25 grams (weight) dextrose in 50 mL (volume) of water. From the concentration, you can determine the **dosage on hand** (weight) and the **volume on hand.** For 50 percent Dextrose, the dosage on hand is 25 grams and the volume on hand is 50 mL. Concentrations are identified on all drug packaging and labels.

Because you cannot see the desired dose dissolved in liquid, you must convert its weight to volume, a readily visible measurement, using the following formula:

concentration *weight per volume.*

dosage on hand *the amount of drug available in a solution.*

volume on hand *the available amount of solution containing a medication.*

$$\text{Volume to be administered} = \frac{\text{Volume on hand (desired dose)}}{\text{Dosage on hand}}$$

To use this formula, you must express all weight and volume measurements with the same metric prefix. For example, if the desired dose is expressed in *milli*grams, the dosage on hand must also be expressed in *milli*grams, volume on hand in *milli*liters.

CALCULATING DOSAGES FOR ORAL MEDICATIONS

The following example illustrates how to calculate the volume of a specific drug dosage:

> **Example 1.** A physician orders you to administer 90 mg of acetaminophen to a pediatric patient. The liquid acetaminophen is packaged as a concentration of 500 mg in 8 mL of solution. How much of the medication will you administer?

Because you cannot see the 90 mg of acetaminophen, you must convert this weight to a volume. To do so you need these facts:

$$\text{Desired dose} = 90 \text{ mg}$$
$$\text{Dosage on hand} = 500 \text{ mg}$$
$$\text{Volume on hand} = 8 \text{ mL}$$

Use the formula to calculate the dosage's volume:

$$\text{Volume on hand (8 mL)} \times \text{Desired dose (90 mg)}$$

$$\text{Volume to be administered} = \frac{\text{Volume on hand (8 mL)} \times \text{Desired dose (90 mg)}}{\text{Dosage on hand (500 mg)}}$$

$$\text{Volume to be administered} = (8 \times 90)/500$$
$$\text{Volume to be administered} = 720/500$$
$$\text{Volume to be administered} = 1.44$$

Administer 1.44 mL of solution to deliver 90 mg of acetaminophen.

Another way to calculate drug dosages is the ratio (fraction) and proportion method. A ratio (fraction) illustrates a relationship between two numbers. A proportion

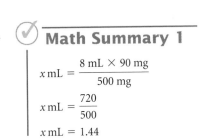

Math Summary 1

$$x \text{ mL} = \frac{8 \text{ mL} \times 90 \text{ mg}}{500 \text{ mg}}$$
$$x \text{ mL} = \frac{720}{500}$$
$$x \text{ mL} = 1.44$$

is the comparison of two numerically equivalent ratios. Using the variable x, the previous problem can be stated:

$$8 \text{ mL}/500 \text{ mg} = x \text{ mL}/90 \text{ mg}$$

To solve the problem, cross-multiply the numerals:

$$8/500 = x/90$$
$$720/500 = x$$
$$1.44 = x$$
$$x = 1.44 \text{ mL}$$

Math Summary 2

$$\frac{8 \text{ mL}}{500 \text{ mg}} = \frac{x \text{ mL}}{90 \text{ mg}}$$
$$x \text{ mL} = \frac{720}{500}$$
$$x = 1.44 \text{ mL}$$

CONVERTING PREFIXES

The following example shows how to calculate the volume to be administered when the desired dose, the dosage on hand, and the volume on hand are not all expressed in metric units with the same prefix.

Example 2. A physician orders you to give 250 mg of a drug via IV bolus. The multidose vial contains 2 grams of the drug in 10 mL of solution. How much of the medication should you administer?

Because the desired dose is expressed as *milli*grams, the dosage on hand must be converted from grams to milligrams. In the metric system, 2 grams equal 2,000 milligrams. You now know:

$$\text{Desired dose} = 250 \text{ mg}$$
$$\text{Dosage on hand} = 2,000 \text{ mg}$$
$$\text{Volume on hand} = 10 \text{ mL}$$

Now you can use the formula to calculate the volume to be administered:

Math Summary 3

$$x \text{ mL} = \frac{10 \text{ mL} \times 250 \text{ mg}}{2,000 \text{ mg}}$$
$$x \text{ mL} = \frac{2,500}{2,000}$$
$$x \text{ mL} = 1.25$$

$$\text{Volume to be administered} = \frac{\text{Volume on hand (10 mL)} \times \text{Desired dose (250 mg)}}{\text{Dosage on hand (2,000 mg)}}$$
$$\text{Volume to be administered} = (10 \times 250)/2,000$$
$$\text{Volume to be administered} = 2,500/2,000$$
$$\text{Volume to be administered} = 1.25$$

Administer 1.25 mL of solution to deliver 250 mg of medication.
You can also solve this problem using the ratio proportion as follows:

$$10 \text{ mL}/2,000 \text{ mg} = x \text{ mL}/250 \text{ mg}$$
$$2,500 = 2,000 \, x$$
$$2,500/2,000 = x$$
$$1.25 = x$$
$$x = 1.25 \text{ mL}$$

Math Summary 4

$$\frac{10 \text{ mL}}{2,000 \text{ mg}} = \frac{x \text{ mL}}{250 \text{ mg}}$$
$$x \text{ mL} = \frac{2,500}{2,000}$$
$$x = 1.25 \text{ mL}$$

Tablets also come in stock doses. If the dosage of one tablet or pill is more than needed, divide the tablet or pill to make the correct dose. Do not divide enteric or time-release capsules.

CALCULATING DOSAGES FOR PARENTERAL MEDICATIONS

You can use the same formula to calculate specific doses and volume for parenteral medication delivery.

Example 3. A physician wants you to administer 5 milligrams of medication subcutaneously. The ampule contains 10 mg of the drug in 2 mL of solvent. How much medication should you use?

$$\text{Desired dose} = 5 \text{ mg}$$
$$\text{Dosage on hand} = 10 \text{ mg}$$
$$\text{Volume on hand} = 2 \text{ mL}$$

$$\text{Volume to be administered} = \frac{\text{Volume on hand (2 mL)} \times \text{Desired dose (5 mg)}}{\text{Dosage on hand (10 mg)}}$$

$$\text{Volume to be administered} = (2 \times 5)/10$$
$$\text{Volume to be administered} = 10/10$$
$$\text{Volume to be administered} = 1 \text{ mL}$$

Administer 1 mL of solution to deliver 5 mg of the medication.
Using the ratio and proportion method, the problem is solved as follows:

$$2 \text{ mL}/10 \text{ mg} = x \text{ mL}/5 \text{ mg}$$
$$10/10 = x$$
$$1 = x$$
$$x = 1.0 \text{ mL}$$

Math Summary 5

$$\frac{2 \text{ mL}}{10 \text{ mg}} = \frac{x \text{ mL}}{5 \text{ mg}}$$
$$x \text{ mL} = \frac{10}{10}$$
$$x = 1.0 \text{ mL}$$

CALCULATING WEIGHT-DEPENDENT DOSAGES

Occasionally, you will have to calculate the desired dose according to the patient's weight.

Example 4. You must administer 1.5 mg/kg of lidocaine via IV bolus to a patient in stable ventricular tachycardia. The concentration of lidocaine is 100 mg in a prefilled syringe containing 10 mL of solution. The patient weighs 158 lbs.

Start by converting the patient's weight to kilograms:

$$\text{Kilograms} = \text{pounds}/2.2$$
$$\text{Kilograms} = 158 \text{ lbs}/2.2$$
$$\text{Kilograms} = 71.82$$

The patient weighs approximately 72 kg.

Calculate the desired dose:

$$1.5 \text{ mg} \times 72 \text{ kg} = 108 \text{ mg}$$

You now know these three facts:

$$\text{Desired dose} = 108 \text{ mg}$$
$$\text{Dosage on hand} = 100 \text{ mg}$$
$$\text{Volume on hand} = 10 \text{ mL}$$

Math Summary 6

$$x \text{ mL} = \frac{10 \text{ mL} \times 108 \text{ mg}}{100 \text{ mg}}$$

$$x \text{ mL} = \frac{1,080}{100}$$

$$x = 10.8 \text{ mL}$$

Math Summary 7

$$\frac{10 \text{ mL}}{100 \text{ mg}} = \frac{x \text{ mL}}{108 \text{ mg}}$$

$$x \text{ mL} = \frac{1,080}{100}$$

$$x = 10.8 \text{ mL}$$

Math Summary 8

$$x \text{ drops/min} = \frac{500 \text{ mL} \times 60 \text{ gtts/mL} \times 2 \text{ mg}}{2,000 \text{ mg}}$$

$$x \text{ drops/min} = \frac{60,000}{2,000}$$

$$x \text{ drops/min} = 30$$

Use the same formula as before to calculate the volume to be administered:

$$\text{Volume to be administered} = \frac{\text{Volume on hand (10 mL)} \times \text{Desired dose (108 mg)}}{\text{Dosage on hand (100 mg)}}$$

Volume to be administered = $(10 \times 108)/100$

Volume to be administered = $1,080/100$

Volume to be administered = 10.8

Administer 10.8 mL of solution to deliver 108 mg of lidocaine.

After you have calculated the desired dose, you can solve this problem using the ratio and proportion method as previously illustrated.

CALCULATING INFUSION RATES

To deliver fluid or medication through an IV infusion, you must calculate the correct infusion rate in drops per minute. To do so you must know the administration tubing's drip factor, as well as the volume on hand, desired dose, and dosage on hand.

Medicated Infusions

To calculate the correct IV infusion rate, use the following formula:

$$\text{Drops/minute} = \frac{\text{Volume on hand (ml)} \times \text{Drip factor (gtts/mL)} \times \text{Desired dose (mg/min)}}{\text{Dosage on hand (mg)}}$$

Example 5. A physician wants you to administer 2 mg per minute of lidocaine to a patient. To prepare the infusion, you mix 2 grams of lidocaine in an IV bag containing 500 milliliters of 5 percent dextrose in water (D_5W). You will use a microdrip administration set (60 gtts/mL). Calculate the infusion rate.

Desired dose = 2 mg

Dosage on hand = 2,000 mg (2 grams)

Volume on hand = 500 mL

Drip factor = 60 gtts/mL

$$\text{Drops/minute} = \frac{\text{Volume on hand (500 mL)} \times \text{Drip factor (60 gtts/mL)} \times \text{Desired dose (2 mg)}}{\text{Dosage on hand (2,000 mg)}}$$

Drops/minute = $(500 \times 60 \times 2)/2,000$

Drops/minute = $(60,000)/2,000$

Drops/minute = 30

Run the infusion at 30 drops/minute to infuse 2 mg of lidocaine per minute.

Fluid Volume Over Time

Fluids with or without medications may require administration over a specific period of time. To deliver the fluid correctly you must calculate volume/time. This calculation requires the following information:

★ Volume to be administered

★ Drip factor of the administration set (gtts/mL)

★ Total time of infusion (minutes)

To calculate the **infusion rate,** use this formula:

$$\text{Drops/minute} = \frac{\text{Volume to be administered (drip factor)}}{\text{Time in minutes}}$$

infusion rate *speed at which a medication is delivered intravenously.*

Example 6. A physician tells you to administer 500 milliliters of normal saline solution to a patient over 1 hour (60 minutes). The administration tubing is a macrodrip set with a drip factor of 10 gtts/mL. At what drip rate would you run this infusion?

$$\text{Volume to be administered} = 500 \text{ mL}$$
$$\text{Administration set drip factor (gtts/mL)} = 10 \text{ gtts/mL}$$
$$\text{Total time of infusion (minutes)} = 60 \text{ minutes}$$

Calculate the infusion rate:

$$\text{Drops/minute} = \frac{(500 \text{ mL})\,(10 \text{ gtts/mL})}{60 \text{ minutes}}$$
$$\text{Drops/minute} = (500 \times 10)/60$$
$$\text{Drops/minute} = 5,000/60$$
$$\text{Drops/minute} = 83.3$$

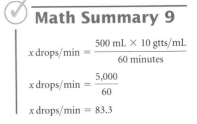

Math Summary 9

$$x \text{ drops/min} = \frac{500 \text{ mL} \times 10 \text{ gtts/mL}}{60 \text{ minutes}}$$
$$x \text{ drops/min} = \frac{5,000}{60}$$
$$x \text{ drops/min} = 83.3$$

Set the flow rate at approximately 83 drops per minute to infuse 500 milliliters of normal saline in almost exactly 60 minutes.

You can use the same formula to determine how long it will take to use all the fluid in a container.

Example 7. You are transporting a patient with an IV antibiotic. The infusion rate is 45 gtts/minute and the administration tubing is a microdrip set (60 gtts/mL). 150 milliliters remain in the 500 milliliter bag of D_5W. How long until the antibiotic will complete infusion?

Use the same formula as in example 6; however, in this instance you will find time in minutes.

$$45 \text{ drops/minute} = \frac{(150 \text{ mL})\,(60 \text{ gtts/mL})}{\text{Time}}$$
$$45 = (150 \times 60)/\text{time}$$
$$45 = 9,000/\text{time}$$
$$\text{Time} = 9,000/45$$
$$\text{Time} = 200$$
$$45 \text{ drops/minute} = 200 \text{ minutes}$$

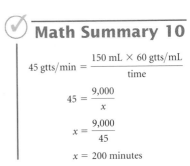

Math Summary 10

$$45 \text{ gtts/min} = \frac{150 \text{ mL} \times 60 \text{ gtts/mL}}{\text{time}}$$
$$45 = \frac{9,000}{x}$$
$$x = \frac{9,000}{45}$$
$$x = 200 \text{ minutes}$$

The antibiotic will complete infusion in 200 minutes, or 3 hours and 20 minutes.

Calculating Dosages and Infusion Rates for Infants and Children

Infants and children cannot tolerate under- or overdoses of medication and fluids. When you administer infusions to pediatric patients, you must calculate exact flow rates. Because infants and children differ drastically from adults in size and internal development, their dosages often depend on weight. Most weight-dependent dosages express the patient's weight in kilograms, so you must make the appropriate conversion from pounds as discussed earlier. Occasionally, you may encounter a medication that is based on body surface area (BSA). Chemotherapeutic agents for children are often based on body surface area. While you will not initiate such drugs, you may encounter them on critical care transports either by ground or air. Many aids for calculating pediatric drug doses and infusion rates are available, including charts, forms, and length-based resuscitation tapes. While these devices are helpful, you should not rely on them exclusively. They are no substitute for knowledge.

Summary

Drug administration is a fundamental skill used in the treatment of the sick and injured. For medications to be effective, they must be *safely* delivered into the body by the *appropriate* route. Many different routes for drug delivery are available to the paramedic; however, specific drugs require specific routes for administration.

It is your responsibility to be familiar with all routes of drug delivery and the techniques for establishing and utilizing them. You will use some routes of medication administration infrequently, and they will quickly fade from memory. Nonetheless, someone's well-being may depend on your ability to utilize such a route in an emergency. Therefore, periodic review of all routes used in medication administration is highly recommended. In addition, you must accurately calculate many drug dosages. Dosage errors and inappropriate medication administration harm patient care and cast serious doubt on your ability.

You Make the Call

You have been called for a 53-year-old male patient experiencing chest pain and shortness of breath. After assessing the patient, you find him to be alert and oriented, with a clear airway, and breathing adequately at a rate of 16 breaths per minute. His distal pulses are strong, and his skin is cool and slightly diaphoretic. Your partner obtains the following vital signs: blood pressure 142/88 mmHg, pulse 92 beats per minute, and respirations 16 and easy. The patient exhibits no jugular venous distention or peripheral edema, and breath sounds are clear bilaterally. The 12-lead cardiac monitor shows a sinus rhythm with ST segment elevation in leads V_1 through V_3. The patient has no medical allergies and is on no medications. He denies any previous medical history.

In addition to high-flow, high-concentration oxygen, you elect to administer nitroglycerin, morphine sulfate, and aspirin, based on your suspicion of an acute myocardial infarction. Accordingly, you quickly establish an IV line.

1. Before administering aspirin or any other medication orally (p.o.), what major consideration must you be sure of?
2. Of the following medications and routes of delivery, which will provide the fastest and most predictable rate of absorption?
   - aspirin—enteral tract
   - nitroglycerin—sublingual
   - morphine sulfate—IV bolus

3. When administered sublingually, how is the nitroglycerin absorbed into the body?
4. You elect to administer 3 mg of morphine sulfate to the patient. The medication is packaged as 10 mg in 5 mL of solution in a multidose vial. How many milliliters must you administer to give the 3 mg of morphine?

See Suggested Responses at the back of this book.

Review Questions

1. The simplest and often the most neglected form of BSI is:
   a. hand washing.
   b. donning a gown.
   c. wearing gloves.
   d. wearing eye goggles.

2. A cleansing agent that is toxic to living tissue is:
   a. sterile.
   b. antiseptic.
   c. disinfectant.
   d. medically clean.

3. A drug administered through the mucous membranes of the ear and ear canal is a(n):
   a. buccal medication.
   b. nasal medication.
   c. aural medication.
   d. ocular medication.

4. "Within the dermal layer of the skin" defines:
   a. buccal.
   b. intradermal.
   c. subcutaneous.
   d. intramuscular.

5. The state in which solutions on opposite sides of a semipermeable membrane are in equal concentration describes a(n) _____ state.
   a. colloid
   b. isotonic
   c. hypertonic
   d. hypotonic

6. To minimize the chances of a catheter shear reaching the patient's central circulation, always leave the venous constricting band in place until you have completely removed the needle from the catheter. However, never leave the constricting band in place more than _____ minutes.
   a. 1.5
   b. 2
   c. 3
   d. 4

7. Medically clean techniques include:
   a. hand washing.
   b. glove changing.
   c. discarding equipment in opened packages.
   d. all of the above.

8. To minimize or eliminate the risk of an accidental needle stick, the paramedic must:
   a. recap needles only as a last resort.
   b. minimize the tasks performed in a moving ambulance.
   c. immediately dispose of used sharps in a sharps container.
   d. all of the above.

9. The abbreviation _____ designates the right eye.
   a. o.u.
   b. o.p.
   c. o.d.
   d. o.s.

10. In an acute respiratory emergency involving a patient with a metered dose inhaler, always use a(n) _____ instead of the MDI.
    a. LMA
    b. ET tube
    c. nebulizer
    d. nasal airway

11. When using an endotracheal tube, you must increase conventional IV dosages from _____ – _____ times.
    a. 1–2
    b. $2–2\frac{1}{2}$
    c. 2–3
    d. $3\frac{1}{2}$–4

12. A _____ is a liquid that contains small particles of solid medication.
    a. syrup
    b. elixir
    c. emulsion
    d. suspension

13. _____ denotes any drug administration outside of the gastrointestinal tract.
    a. enema
    b. enteral
    c. parenteral
    d. suppository

14. Which of the following is not a parenteral drug delivery route?
    a. sublingual route
    b. intravenous access
    c. intraosseous infusion
    d. intramuscular injection

15. All of the following are examples of colloidal solutions except:
    a. Dextran.
    b. Hespan.
    c. lactated Ringer's.
    d. salt poor albumin.

16. _____, or inflammation of the vein, is particularly common in long-term intravenous therapy.
    a. necrosis
    b. air embolism
    c. thrombus formation
    d. thrombophlebitis

17. _____ is an HBOC derived from expired donated human blood.
    a. Oxygent
    b. Hemopure
    c. PolyHeme
    d. LiquiVent

18. Advantages of heparin locks include all of the following except:
    a. provides a peripheral IV port.
    b. does not need continuous fluid infusion.
    c. blood samples cannot be withdrawn from the lock.
    d. decreases the risk of accidental electrolyte derangement.

19. Causes of hemolysis include:
    a. using too small a needle for retrieval.
    b. vigorously shaking the blood tubes after they are filled.
    c. too forcefully aspirating blood into or out of a syringe.
    d. all of the above.

20. Which of the following is not considered a complication of intraosseous access?
    a. local infection
    b. air embolism
    c. fat embolism
    d. thrombophlebitis

21. The bone most commonly used for intraosseous access is the:
    a. tibia.
    b. femur.
    c. fibula.
    d. humerus.

22. The three fundamental units of the metric system are:
    a. meters, liters, grains.
    b. grams, meters, liters.
    c. inches, pints, pounds.
    d. grams, liters, ounces.

23. 1,000 milligrams equal:
    a. 1 kilogram.
    b. 1 gram.
    c. 0.001 gram.
    d. 10 grams.

24. A patient weighs 90 kg. What is his weight in pounds?
    a. 180
    b. 41
    c. 75
    d. 198

25. The metric prefix *hecto-* means:
    a. 1.
    b. 10.
    c. 100.
    d. 1,000.

26. The metric system is based upon what number system?
    a. ratios
    b. decimals
    c. fractions
    d. percentages

27. Medical control orders you to administer Valium, 2.0 mg. The medication is in a prefilled syringe labeled 10 mg. in 2 cc. You draw up the correct dose which is:
    a. 0.20 mL.
    b. 2.0 mL.
    c. 0.4 cc.
    d. 4.0 cc.

28. To administer 35 mg of Benadryl from a syringe labeled 50 mg/cc you would give:
    a. 1.5 cc.
    b. 0.8 cc.
    c. 0.7 mL.
    d. 0.7 mg.

29. 0.75 liters converted to milliliters is:
    a. 1,075 mL.
    b. 1.075 mL.
    c. 75 mL.
    d. 750 mL.

30. Two grams is equal to:
    a. 1,000 mg.
    b. 2,000 mg.
    c. 3,000 mg.
    d. 2,000 mL.

31. 2.5 grams is equal to:
    a. 150 mg.
    b. 1,500 mg.
    c. 2,500 mg.
    d. 2,000 mg.

32. 1 kilogram is equal to:
    a. 2.0 pounds.
    b. 2.2 pounds.
    c. 0.2 pounds.
    d. 2.2 kilograms.

See Answers to Review Questions at the back of this book.

Further Reading

Bledsoe, Bryan E. and Dwayne Clayden. *Prehospital Emergency Pharmacology.* 6th ed. Upper Saddle River, N.J.: Pearson Education/Prentice Hall, 2005.

Campbell, John Emory, and the Alabama Chapter of the American College of Emergency Physicians. *Basic Trauma Life Support for Paramedics and Other Advanced Care Providers.* 5th ed. Upper Saddle River, N.J.: Pearson/Prentice Hall, 2004.

Chung, Michele B. *Math Principles and Practice: Preparing for Health Career Success.* Upper Saddle River, N.J.: Prentice Hall, 1999.

Dalton, Alice L., et al. *Advanced Medical Life Support.* 2nd ed. Upper Saddle River, N.J.: Pearson/Prentice Hall, 2003.

Kee, Joyce L., and Evelyn R. Hayes. *Pharmacology: A Nursing Process Approach.* 4th ed. Philadelphia, Pa.: W. B. Saunders Company, 2003.

Martini, Frederick. *Fundamentals of Anatomy and Physiology.* 6th ed. San Francisco: Benjamin Cummings, 2004.

McKenny, Leda M., and Evelyn Salerno. *Pharmacology in Nursing.* 21st ed. St. Louis: Mosby, 2003.

McSwain, Norman E., and Scott Frame. *Prehospital Trauma Life Support.* 5th ed. St. Louis: Mosby, 2003.

Mikolaj, Alan A. *Drug Dosage Calculations for the Emergency Care Provider.* 2nd ed. Upper Saddle River, N.J.: Pearson/Prentice Hall, 2003.

On the Web

Visit Brady's Paramedic Website at **www.bradybooks.com/paramedic.**

Therapeutic Communications

Objectives

After reading this chapter, you should be able to:

1. Define communication. (p. 466)
2. Identify internal and external factors that affect a patient/bystander interview. (pp. 466–467)
3. Identify strategies for developing rapport with the patient. (pp. 467–468, 473–474)
4. Provide examples of open-ended and closed, or direct, questions. (pp. 471–472)
5. Discuss common errors made when interviewing patients. (p. 474)
6. Identify the nonverbal skills used in patient interviewing. (pp. 469–471)
7. Summarize methods used to assess mental status based on interview techniques. (pp. 472–473)
8. Discuss strategies for interviewing a patient who is not motivated to talk. (pp. 473, 474–475)
9. Differentiate strategies used when interviewing a patient who is hostile compared to one who is cooperative. (pp. 473, 479)
10. Summarize the developmental considerations of various age groups that influence patient interviewing. (pp. 469, 472, 475–477)
11. Define the unique interviewing techniques for patients with special needs. (pp. 474–479)
12. Discuss interviewing considerations used in cross-cultural communications. (pp. 477–479)
13. Given several preprogrammed simulated patients, provide a patient interview using therapeutic communication. (pp. 466–479)

Key Terms

Case Study

I've been teaching EMS for 20 years, and I couldn't describe the impact of good interpersonal communication better than this student does. Here is his report. Read it and see what you think.

"What a study in contrasts the last two nights have been. As a paramedic student observer, I went from riding with one crew, whose members demonstrated what must be the worst possible insensitivity and callousness, to another crew, whose members showed compassion and kindness.

"Two nights ago, there was a call to an emergency for a possible heart attack. Without going into a lot of detail, I can only say that the experience was dismal. The closest EMS First Responders were sent, in case CPR was needed, but when they saw the patient was awake, they quickly realized that there was little they could do while they waited for us. In the meantime, all the way there, the paramedics continued an ongoing discussion about the problems with the ambulance company's management.

"When we arrived, I noticed that the two First Responders were leaning disdainfully against their vehicle. I overheard one of them say to the medics, 'You got a middle-of-the-night turkey here.' I have to admit, I found their attitude shocking, and I was interested to see how the label they placed on this woman affected the paramedics. Well, they approached the patient with an obvious negative attitude, and things went from bad to worse. Concerned family and friends—about four people—were rudely pushed aside and ignored. No one seemed to think it was important to interact with them at all. You can imagine the snide remarks that were made later when the crew found out the 'heart attack' had been abdominal gas. I'm sure the whole experience left that family feeling very unhappy with EMS.

"Then, last night, I had an entirely different experience. This paramedic crew couldn't have been more different, even though the call was very similar to the one the night before: another possible heart attack. As we arrived on scene, we saw the First Responders working to put the patient and the family at ease. The one in charge introduced the patient by name to the paramedics, and then told the paramedics what he had already learned. The paramedics introduced themselves to the patient, and then talked her through everything they were going to do. Their questions were polite and their manner exceptionally soothing. Everyone was efficient, kind, and calm. Someone was even assigned to help the husband get ready and into the ambulance for the ride to the hospital.

"What an amazing difference! So much about the two emergencies was the same, yet I observed absolutely opposite behaviors in the responders. The second crew's collective professionalism and excellent communication skills left me with an absolute trust that they could handle virtually anything. They restored my faith in the positive nature of EMS. They are a credit to our community, and my goal is to be like them."

INTRODUCTION

communication *the exchange of common symbols—written, spoken, or other kinds such as signing and body language.*

Communication should be easy. After all, **communication** is only a matter of exchanging common symbols—written, spoken, or other kinds such as signing and body language. However, as you know, even in the best circumstances, communication can be a challenge. EMS providers have a particularly difficult job of it, because they must communicate with strangers who are in crisis.

As a paramedic, you must learn how to use every available strategy to make sure that you understand your patients and that they, in turn, understand you. You also must be able to communicate well with the patient's relatives, bystanders, and other EMS providers. Strategies you will use include persistently paying attention to word choices, tones of voice, facial expressions, and body language. You will learn to minimize external and internal distractions and to adjust your personal communication style to fit each new situation, especially when dealing with children, elderly people, people of different cultures, and hostile people.

empathy *identification with and understanding of another's situation, feelings, and motives.*

Helpful core traits for effective communication in EMS include a genuine liking for people, a sincere desire to be part of a helping profession, and an understanding of human strengths and weaknesses.

Helpful core traits for effective communication in EMS include a genuine liking for people, a sincere desire to be part of a helping profession, an understanding of human strengths and weaknesses, and **empathy,** or the ability to view the world through another's eyes while remaining true to yourself.

BASIC ELEMENTS OF COMMUNICATION

encode *to create a message.*

Communication consists of a sender, a message, a receiver, and feedback (Figure 11-1 ■). First, the sender has to **encode,** or create a message; that is, he must write, speak, or otherwise place symbols common to both parties in an understandable format. This may

■ Figure 11-1 Communication consists of a sender, a message, a receiver, and feedback.

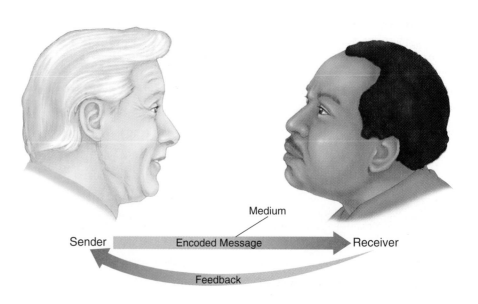

mean translating the message into another language, using words a child can understand, or writing the words on paper. The receiver then must **decode,** or interpret, the message, ideally with the same meaning the sender intended to convey. Finally, the receiver gives the sender **feedback** (a response to the message). If by way of this response, the sender believes the message was received accurately, both parties can congratulate themselves on communicating successfully.

Unfortunately, partial or complete failure to communicate occurs often. There are abundant reasons for this. In EMS those reasons include:

★ Prejudice, or lack of empathy, particularly by the paramedic toward the patient or situation

★ Lack of privacy, which inhibits a patient's responses to questions

★ External distractions, such as traffic, crowds, loud music, EMS radios, or TVs

★ Internal distractions, or thinking about things other than the situation at hand

One way to minimize failure is to keep in mind that patience and flexibility are hallmarks of a good communicator.

TRUST AND RAPPORT

As a representative of EMS, you are granted a certain amount of the public's trust at each new emergency scene. You have to earn the rest by putting the patient and others at ease and by letting them know you are on their side, you respect their comments, and you want to help. Little courtesies such as asking the patient his name and thereafter pronouncing it correctly can help to accomplish this goal. So can recognizing and responding with compassion to signs of discomfort or suffering. Once trust is established, rapport follows.

With good rapport, the people you are serving will follow your lead, even if that means some pain (such as with a needle stick) and inconvenience (such as canceling a trip to have a medical evaluation at the hospital). The people with whom you work also will be more motivated to do difficult and sometimes dangerous tasks. Remember that effective communication begins and ends with trust and rapport. Without them, your safety could be at risk.

PROFESSIONAL BEHAVIORS

First impressions are crucial. What others see in you during the first few seconds of an encounter can lay the foundation for success or failure. The patient relies almost exclusively on visual input, so your physical presentation—from facial expression to the appearance of your clothing—matters. Even though encounters with patients are typically brief, patients usually remember them for a very long time. Make sure your first impression is a positive one. The elements of a good first impression involve all conventional professional standards, including:

★ Clean, neat uniform that allows you to be easily identifiable as a paramedic

★ Good personal hygiene, including clean, cut fingernails and inoffensive breath; also avoiding use of colognes and perfumes

★ Physical fitness

★ Overall professional demeanor that is calm, capable, and trustworthy

★ Facial expression that is open, interested, caring; avoiding expressions of disdain or disgust

★ Confident (not arrogant) stance

decode *to interpret a message.*

feedback *a response to a message.*

✓ Review

Content

Reasons for Failing to Communicate

• Prejudice
• Lack of privacy
• External distractions
• Internal distractions

Patience and flexibility are hallmarks of a good communicator.

Effective communication begins and ends with trust and rapport.

Make sure your first impression is a positive one.

Maintain professional behavior not only on a call with a patient, but when you stop at the mini-mart for a coffee as well!

★ Appropriate gait; avoiding running or strolling

★ Consideration for the patient, such as wiping your feet on the doormat before entering the residence

The next period of interaction with your patient is the time for obtaining in-depth information about the emergency and the patient's medical history. This may be called the **patient interview.** A good starting point is always to assure the patient's privacy, which also minimizes inhibitions and distractions. It helps to be sure that lighting is adequate and noise is minimized. Equipment that might be alarming (such as needles) should be placed out of the patient's sight.

Other ways to help build the trust and rapport you need to conduct a patient interview include the following:

★ *Use your patient's name.* It is a powerful tool for forming a quick bond. A technique for remembering a name involves three steps: First, say the patient's name out loud three times in the first minute. Then "see" the patient's name in your mind in bold capital letters. Finally, "feel" yourself writing the name in your imagination. Some people actually write the name on their paperwork, but this does not work as well as the mental imagery.

★ *Address your patient properly.* Use formal forms of address, such as "Mr." and "Mrs." or "Ms.," as appropriate. Never call patients "honey," "dude," or any name other than their own. Also, be careful about shortening children's names. If a child is introduced to you as "Matthew," use that name, or ask the child if he goes by a nickname such as "Matt."

★ *Modulate your voice.* Pay attention to your volume. Speak quietly and in low tones. If the patient is hard of hearing or difficult to control, speak up. Check your pitch; some people find it hard to hear high voices. Also, check your rate of speaking. Be especially aware that people in crisis may have difficulty taking in information at a normal rate, so slow down.

★ *Use a professional but compassionate tone of voice.* Avoid tones that portray sarcasm, irritation, anger, or other emotions that fail to serve the patient.

★ *Explain what you are doing and why.* This helps to ease your patient's anxiety, especially if he is in pain. For example, if you must immobilize a broken bone, explain that a splint will help to prevent movement and more pain. Also tell the patient that applying a splint may be painful but, once applied, the broken limb should be more comfortable.

Note: Never make false promises or false assurances. They violate your patient's trust.

★ *Keep a kind, calm facial expression.* Remember that facial expressions can reflect a wide variety of emotions and conditions, including relaxation, relief, pain, fear, anger, sorrow, and so on. No matter what the emergency, maintain a kind-looking poker face. It will convince others that you can handle things.

★ *Use the appropriate style of communication.* There is a wide range to choose from. In general, patients will respond well to a calm, reassuring demeanor, but be prepared to use a tough, authoritative approach when needed. Also, if a situation requires you to be firm, be completely firm. Do not let your facial expression, for example, kill the effect (such as one that says, "Gosh, I hope they believe me!").

At the end of a call, a final word or two can be very helpful, particularly after emotional calls. A "goodbye and good luck" can help bring the event to a close for the patient and family.

---

patient interview *interaction with a patient for the purpose of obtaining in-depth information about the emergency and the patient's pertinent medical history.*

Review

Ways to Build Trust and Rapport

- Use the patient's name
- Address the patient properly
- Modulate your voice
- Use a professional but compassionate tone
- Explain what you are doing and why
- Keep a kind, calm expression
- Use an appropriate style of communication

Review

How to Remember a Name

- Say the name out loud three times
- "See" the name in bold capital letters
- "Feel" yourself write the name

COMMUNICATION TECHNIQUES

GENERAL GUIDELINES

Patients generally respond to questioning in one of three ways: They may pour out information easily, they may reveal some things and conceal others that might be embarrassing or shameful, or they may resist, hiding information from themselves and, therefore, from you. The patient who conceals information or resists giving it may be trying to maintain a certain image or may be fearful about how others will respond (perhaps with ridicule or rejection). To get the information you need, you must be consistently professional, nonjudgmental, and willing to talk about any concern the patient may have.

Nonverbal Communication

Nonverbal communication, or body language, consists of gestures, mannerisms, and postures by which a person communicates with others. Your position within the environment and in relation to your patient is part of that language. Examples include the following:

★ *Distance* (Table 11–1). In the United States, the socially acceptable distance between strangers is 4 to 12 feet. A "comfortable" distance may be described as twice the length of a patient's arm. In most cases, paramedics are able to break social convention and quickly enter a patient's "intimate space" (1.5 feet or less) because people intuitively understand the need for medical personnel to get "hands on" with them. However, if the patient stiffens or backs away from you, the best strategy may be to linger at a less-threatening distance until you have built more trust and rapport.

★ *Relative level* (Figure 11-2). A different message is sent to the patient each time you stand at his eye level, above it, or below it. Remaining at eye level indicates equality. Standing above or over the patient imparts an air of authority, but it also can be intimidating. Dropping below eye level indicates a willingness to let the patient have some control of the situation, a strategy that can be especially helpful when your patient is an elderly adult or a child.

 Review

Responses to Questioning

Patients may:
- Pour out information easily
- Reveal some things and conceal others
- Resist responding

To get the information you need, you must be consistently professional, nonjudgmental, and willing to talk about any concern the patient may have.

nonverbal communication *gestures, mannerisms, and postures by which a person communicates with others; also called body language.*

Review

Elements of Nonverbal Communication

- Distance
- Relative level
- Stance

Table 11–1	Interpersonal Zones	
Zone	**Distance**	**Characteristics**
Intimate zone	0 to 1.5 feet	Visual distortion occurs.
		Best for assessing breath and other body odors.
Personal distance, or "personal space"	1.5 to 4 feet	Perceived as extension of self.
		No visual distortion.
		Body odors are not apparent.
		Voice is moderate.
		Much of patient assessment, and sometimes patient interviewing, may occur at this distance.
Social distance	4 to 12 feet	Used for impersonal business transactions.
		Perceptual information is much less detailed than at personal distance.
		Patient interview may occur at this distance.
Public distance	12 feet or more	Allows impersonal interaction with others.
		Voices must be projected.

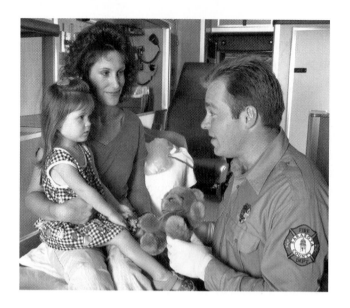

■ Figure 11-2   Getting down to a patient's level can help improve communications on a pediatric call.

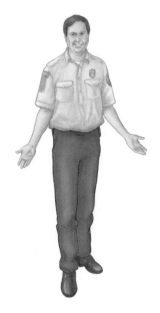

■ Figure 11-3a   An open stance.

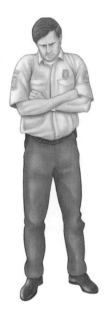

■ Figure 11-3b   A closed stance.

open stance   *a posture or body position that is relaxed and suggests confidence, ease, warmth, and attentiveness.*

closed stance   *a posture or body position that is tense and suggests negativity, discomfort, fear, disgust, or anger.*

★ *Stance* (Figure 11-3 ■). Arms extended, open hands, relaxed large muscles, and a nodding head characterize an **open stance.** A paramedic who has an open stance sends the message that he is confident and at ease. When it is safe to do so, use this stance to communicate warmth and attentiveness.

A **closed stance** is just the opposite. In this position, arms are flexed, or arms are crossed tightly over the chest. The fists are clenched or a finger may be pointing. The head may be shaking negatively. The body is square to the patient or, in some cases, may turn slightly away. This posture suggests disinterest, discomfort, disgust, fear, or anger and sends negative signals to the patient.

Watch your patient's body language, too. It can tell you how well communication with him is going. If the patient has a closed stance, you may need to change your approach.

Eye Contact

A powerful source of effective communication comes with eye contact. While you are interviewing the patient, use it as much as possible. (Always remove sunglasses while working with patients.) Even when you are taking notes, look at the patient frequently. Eye contact is one way to send a message to your patient, whether it is a compassionate "I care about you" or a stern "settle down now." You name it. With eye contact, you can hold the attention of a patient so powerfully that your patient can feel you are helping him hang on in desperate circumstances.

Of course, using eye contact means that the other person is looking at you, too, which can be unnerving, especially if you are unfamiliar with this technique. If you feel uncomfortable, look at the bridge of the other person's nose for a bit of relief. Then try direct eye contact again. Build this skill over time, and it will serve you well.

Compassionate Touch

Another communication skill is touching (Figure 11-4 ■). The ability to hold a hand, or even hug, in the right circumstances can yield information that would otherwise not be given. Some paramedics need to learn this skill the way they learn how to use an IV. That is, it can be awkward at first, but it is worth the effort. Nothing builds trust and rapport, or calms patients, faster than the power of touch. How effective it is depends on the patient's age, gender, cultural background, past experience, and current setting. Be careful to touch appropriately. There is a line between compassion and improper intimacy. Remember that as a paramedic, you must always carefully guard the integrity of the public's trust in you.

> Nothing builds trust and rapport, or calms patients, faster than the power of touch.

INTERVIEW TECHNIQUES

From the moment of your first contact with the patient, your job is to find out all information relevant to the present emergency. You need to identify the patient's chief complaint (the reason why 911 was called), find out the circumstances that caused the emergency, and determine the patient's condition. Much of this is accomplished by asking questions, observing the patient, and listening effectively.

Questioning Techniques

An important part of patient assessment is gathering information that is accurate, complete, and relevant to the present emergency. To begin, you must identify the patient's chief complaint. Although dispatch probably will have given you an idea of what the emergency is about, it is important for you to let the patient state the chief complaint in his own

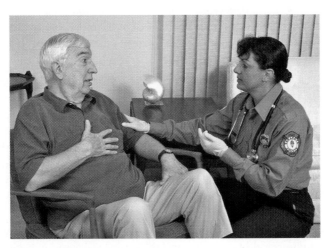

■ Figure 11-4   Use an appropriate compassionate touch to show your concern and support.

leading questions *questions framed to guide the direction of a patient's answers.*

open-ended questions *questions that permit unguided, spontaneous answers.*

words. If you were to ask **leading questions** (ones that guide the patient's replies), such as: "Are you having chest pain?" or "I see you've injured your arm. How does it feel?", you could easily miss a serious problem. So, instead, ask **open-ended questions,** such as: "What happened that led you to call 911?" or "What seems to be the problem?" They will allow your patient to respond in an unguided, spontaneous way. They also encourage patients who are reluctant to speak to describe their complaint in a way that might not be possible otherwise.

The patient's chief complaint should then drive the evolution of all other questions to be asked. For example, if your patient's chief complaint is chest pain, you are required to obtain answers to a specific set of questions. But instead of asking them as if you were reading a shopping list, individualize the process. For example, you would have to find out if a patient with chest pain takes any medications. If your patient tells you that his chief complaint is "chest pain so bad even the nitroglycerin tablets aren't helping," your question about medications might be worded: "What medications do you take in addition to nitroglycerin?" This tells the patient you have been listening, which can yield a greater rapport. Other questioning techniques include the following:

★ *Continue to ask open-ended questions.* They do not limit the patient's responses, which can help to reveal unexpected but important facts. For example, instead of asking a patient with abdominal pain "Did you have breakfast today?" which can be answered with either a "yes" or a "no," ask: "What have you eaten today?"

★ *Use direct questions, when necessary.* Direct questions, or **closed questions,** ask for specific information. ("Did you eat lunch?" or "Does the abdominal pain come and go like a cramp, or is it constant?") These questions are good for three reasons: They fill in information generated by open-ended questions. They help to answer crucial questions when time is limited. And they can help to control overly talkative patients, who might want to tell you about their gallbladder surgery in 1949 when the chief complaint is a sprained ankle.

closed questions *questions that ask for specific information and require only very short or yes-or-no answers; also called direct questions.*

★ *Do not ask leading questions.* Avoiding them means avoiding being taken down a path unrelated to the current emergency.

★ *Ask only one question at a time, and allow complete answers.* If you ask more than one question, the patient may not know which one to answer and may leave out portions of information or become confused.

★ *Listen to the patient's complete response before asking the next question.* By doing so, you might find that you need to ask a question that is different from the one you were expecting to ask.

★ *Use language the patient can understand.* In general, people do not understand medical terms. For example, you may need to use "pee" instead of "urine," or "breaths" instead of "respirations." However, be careful to avoid jargon and slang. Also keep in mind that children are very literal and concrete minded. Never tell a child, for example, that you are going to "take" her blood pressure. Say instead that you are going to "measure" it.

★ *Do not allow interruptions, if possible.* Unless your partner or other EMS personnel need to give you patient care information of a critical nature, interruptions will interfere with your patient's and your trains of thought. Interruptions also can cause you to miss information important to the patient's medical care.

Observing the Patient

Observe the patient during the interview. External signs such as overall appearance, including clothing, jewelry, and other physical signs, may give you some indication of the patient's condition. Other clues you pick up may offer you a way to explore the patient's internal experiences, or mental status.

So, while you are interacting with the patient, observe his level of consciousness and body movements. Assess his rate and clarity of speech, his thinking, and his ability to pay attention, concentrate, and comprehend. You may be able to check the patient's orientation to person, place, and time, and his remote, recent, and immediate memory. Explore his mood and energy level, too. Watch for evidence of autonomic responses (sweating, trembling, and so on) and for unusual facial movements such as a tic around the mouth, nose, or eyes. Note that lack of eye contact can suggest that the patient is shy, withdrawn, confused, bored, intimidated, apathetic, or depressed.

Many people do not cope well with being the center of attention. Be aware of various defense mechanisms people may use, so you can be prepared to deal with them, if necessary. For example, if your patient is self-grooming (fixing hair or straightening clothes), it may be that he needs some reassurance. If the patient keeps shifting focus away from your questions, back off for a bit and then return to the topic from a different angle.

If the patient is acting out and hostile, point out the behavior in a professional manner, ask if the behavior is intentional, let him know that such behavior defeats the purpose of calling for help, and then name behaviors you would rather see. If there is any indication that the patient's hostility may threaten your safety or that of your crew, maintain distance and an exit path. (Additional information about hostile patients appears later in this chapter.)

Effective Listening and Feedback

Few people practice the art of listening well. Usually, they think about what they are going to say next while others are still talking to them. There may be less than a one-half second gap between speakers, and many people cannot even wait that long and instead finish others' sentences for them.

Listening is an active skill, not a passive one. It requires your complete attention, and it requires constant practice. In order to listen well, you must focus on the messenger. Stop doing other things. Discipline yourself to cease any internal dialogue that can distract or interrupt you mentally. Never finish the other person's sentences, and do not consider your response until the speaker has finished speaking. Allow some silence when the speaker has stopped.

Once the speaker has stopped talking, provide feedback to confirm that you have understood his message correctly. Feedback techniques include:

★ *Silence.* Give the patient time to gather his thoughts and add to what has been said.

★ *Reflection.* To check your understanding and to reassure the speaker, echo his message back to him using your own words.

★ *Facilitation.* Encourage the speaker to provide more information.

★ *Empathy.* Let your body language show that you understand, so that the patient feels accepted and more open to talking.

★ *Clarification.* Ask the speaker to help you understand, when you need to eliminate confusion about what has been said.

★ *Confrontation.* Focus the patient on one particular factor of the interview.

★ *Interpretation.* State your interpretation of the information; that is, link events, make associations, identify an implied cause, or draw conclusions.

★ *Explanation.* Share factual or objective information related to the message.

★ *Summarization.* Briefly review the interview and your interpretation of the situation. Ask open-ended questions, if needed, to allow the patient to clarify details.

 Review

Content

Feedback Techniques

- Silence
- Reflection
- Facilitation
- Empathy
- Clarification
- Confrontation
- Interpretation
- Explanation
- Summarization

Traps of interviewing, or common errors made when listening and providing feedback to patients, include the following:

★ *Providing false assurances.* Never make any promises you cannot keep. For example, saying "everything will be all right" is a terrible false reassurance.

★ *Giving advice.* People call 911 because they are seeking advice, but the paramedic must be careful how it is conveyed. Saying "my opinion is that your chest pain should be evaluated at the hospital" is acceptable advice. Saying "I think you would be crazy not to get seen by a doctor" is not.

★ *Authority.* Remember that EMS is not a power trip. Although paramedics are imbued with the power to do a difficult job, that power must never be used inappropriately. A paramedic provides a vital public service. Doing so correctly requires constant attention to protecting the public's trust and avoiding behaviors that might be interpreted as abuse of power.

★ *Using avoidance language.* Avoidance language is "an unproductive conflict strategy in which a person takes mental or physical flight from the actual conflict," according to communication expert Joseph DeVito. For example, a person who chooses to change the conversation rather than get into a discussion about something difficult may use avoidance language. If a paramedic does this, the patient's whole story may not be revealed.

★ *Distancing.* When the paramedic is insensitive to distancing, he may stand too close or too far from the patient to attain optimal rapport. Noticing the effects of distancing and adjusting accordingly is a hallmark of a good communicator.

★ *Professional jargon.* Although it is necessary to make sure the patient knows what you are doing and why, it is unnerving for him to hear that you are going to "slip a line and jam a tube." So, watch your language and make sure you are speaking at your patient's comprehension level.

★ *Talking too much.* Remember that listening is also a part of communication.

★ *Interrupting.* As already discussed, good listening skills require you to wait until your patient answers you fully.

★ *Using "why" questions.* The question "why" often steers a conversation toward blame, such as: "Why did you put your hand in the lawnmower while it was running?" or "Why didn't you call for help 3 hours ago?" This type of question is counterproductive.

Demonstrating good listening and feedback skills on an emergency call is challenging. So many things are happening, it can seem like a whirlwind. It may be necessary to apply monitoring equipment to the patient while you ask questions, for example. If this happens, reassure the patient by saying something like: "I know it seems overwhelming to you, but please understand that I am listening to your answers while I work."

PATIENTS WITH SPECIAL NEEDS

Patients generally are more than willing to answer your questions, though some will require more time and a variety of techniques. Note that difficult interviews stem from several sources. The patient's condition, including a developing cognitive impairment, may impact his ability to talk. The patient may be afraid to talk to you because of a psychological disorder, language or cultural difference, or even the difference between your ages. Or the patient intentionally may want to deceive you (to hide illegal drug abuse, for example).

Use the same techniques on a patient who is reluctant to talk to you as you would on any other patient, but use them in a slightly different way. For example, start your in-

✓ **Review**

Sources of Difficult Interviews

• Patient's physical condition
• Patient's fear of talking
• Patient's intentions to deceive

terview in the usual manner. If the patient does not respond to your questions, take time to develop rapport by reviewing the reason dispatch gave for the call. Attempt to ask open-ended questions. If unsuccessful, try direct questions including ones that require only a yes-or-no response. Accept that you may not be able to obtain any elaboration or details about the facts. Provide positive feedback to any response the patient provides.

If the patient continues to be reluctant, be sure the patient understands your questions. Rule out language barriers and hearing difficulties. Once you know the patient can understand you, continue to ask questions about the critical information you need to know to progress with treatment. If you cannot get even this much, attempt to rule out pathology (disease) by asking family members or others at the scene how long the patient has been uncommunicative.

If you determine that pathology is not the cause, you may need to continue to build trust and rapport with the patient. One way to do this is to encourage him to ask you questions about your equipment, profession, medical care, or any topic that might start conversation. Model how you would like the patient to respond to your questions by fully answering his questions.

Further information on communicating with patients who require a special effort on your part follows. These patients include children and their parents, elderly people, people who are blind or deaf, people of other cultures, and people who are hostile or uncooperative.

Children

Effective communication with pediatric patients (infants, children, and adolescents) depends on their age. Have a good idea of what to expect at each stage of development so that your efforts to communicate can be directed appropriately (Table 11–2).

Table 11–2	Childhood Development by Age	
Common Term	**Age**	**Characteristics and Behaviors**
Infant	Birth to 1 year	Knows the voice and face of parents.
		Will want to be held by a parent or caregiver.
		Responds best to firm, gentle handling and a quiet calm voice.
Toddler	1 to 3 years old	Very curious at this age, and into everything, so be alert to the possibility of poison ingestion.
		May be distrustful and uncooperative. Usually does not understand what is happening, which raises level of fear.
		May be very concerned about being separated from parents or caregivers.
Preschooler	3 to 5 years old	Can see the world from own perspective only.
		Able to talk, but may not understand what is being said.
		Uses simple words, short sentences, and concrete explanations.
		May be scared and believe what is happening is own fault.
School Age	6 to 12 years old	Is more objective and realistic.
		Should cooperate and be willing to follow the lead of parents and EMS provider.
		Has active imagination and thoughts about death.
		May need continual reassurance.
Adolescent	13 to 18 years old	Acts like adult.
		Resents being spoken to as if still a child.
		Considers modesty to be very important.
		Fears permanent scarring or deformity.
		May become involved in "mass hysteria."

In general, you can start by talking to the caregivers, then gradually approach the patient. Remember your body language. When dealing with younger children especially, it will help to get down to their eye level. Children pick up on anxiety easily and often take cues from what they observe, so it is very important to stay calm. Then introduce yourself, and use the child's name often. Be careful not to clam up and work silently.

Even if your own anxieties and the pressure of the medical requirements of the call are taxing your limits, talk! Tell the child everything: what you are looking at ("Now let's look at this arm . . . ") and why it is important (". . . so we can be sure it's okay, too."). Explain your equipment, and if there is time, let the child see how the equipment works. Above all, explain what you intend to do, even to very young children. (For example, you might say, "Alexander, I am going to make your leg hurt less by putting on this splint. I will need to make the leg move first, which might hurt some. But after that, it should be a lot better. Okay?") Never tell a child that something will not hurt when, in actuality, it will. Once you have lost the trust of a child, it is very difficult to regain it.

Most important, you must build trust. Once you have that, a child will put up with a lot. Giving a child a stuffed toy may be helpful (Figure 11-5 ■). Also, be sure to move slowly, talk gently, explain everything, and be honest. To engage children, ask questions, and when you answer their questions, be sure not to talk down. Use straightforward language. Never try to hide the fact that something is wrong. When something will hurt or will be at all uncomfortable, tell them. The more matter-of-fact and informative you can be, the better. If you are fair about the difficult parts and avoid springing nasty surprises, you will find greater overall cooperation. The need to be gentle whenever possible should be obvious.

If a child is especially fearful, let him play with a toy or other object and then gradually increase contact. Do not be in a hurry to touch a child unless the situation is critical. Use lots of eye contact and compassionate touch, too. Keep in mind that even if the child cannot understand you, your tone of voice is reassuring and your words and actions will be meaningful to the family and bystanders. Ask the child for feedback frequently, wait for an answer, and acknowledge that answer. Involve the child in decision making whenever possible. If he is crying, do not take it personally and do not tell him to stop. Instead, try saying, "Go ahead and cry until you don't want to cry any more." Lending control in this way can work wonders.

Never tell a child that something will not hurt when it will. Once you have lost the trust of a child, it is very difficult to regain it.

■ Figure 11-5 Use a small toy to help calm a child.

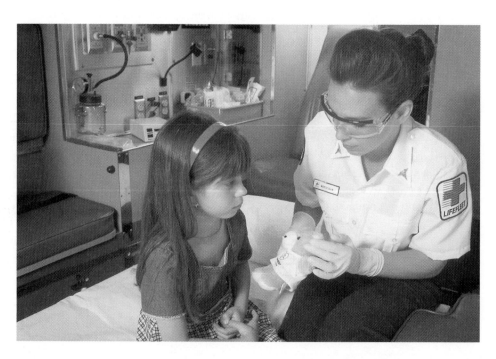

Be aware that young children are very literal. Word choice is important. As noted earlier, do not "take" a pulse, "measure" it. A blood-pressure cuff does not "squeeze," it "hugs." When one child was told that she would fly to the hospital, she started to cry. "I don't know how to fly," she wailed. Think about what you say.

With pediatric patients, it is important to understand that caregivers, especially parents, may be very concerned and upset. Remember that you must manage them as well as your patient. Common responses include crying, emotional outbursts, anger, guilt, and confusion, which may be directed at you. Do not take it personally. You must build trust and rapport with the parents as well as with the child.

Sometimes parents interfere with emergency care and must be separated from the child. Usually, however, it is most effective to let the parents stay and, if appropriate, even hold the child. No matter how parents behave, always treat them with courtesy, respect, and understanding. Avoid raising your voice. Tell them that you know they want help for their child. They need your support and understanding, too.

When possible, allow parents to remain with the pediatric patient.

Note that for younger children (ages 1 to 6), most of your conversation will be with caregivers. Be aware that you are collecting information about the child's history from an adult's point of view, but do not put the caregiver on the defensive. Be careful to be nonjudgmental, especially if it appears that the child has not been provided with proper care or safety before your arrival. Be observant but not confrontational.

Elderly Patients

Be careful of your own prejudices with all special populations, but particularly with the elderly. Be respectful of them. Always use a formal means of address, such as "Mr." and "Mrs." or "Ms." Speak slowly and clearly. Interviews might take longer, because many elders cannot process a lot of information quickly due to interfering physical disabilities and the fact that they can fatigue easily. Remember that the use of compassionate touch can be a welcome and important means of nonverbal support.

Always treat the elderly with the respect that our elders deserve.

Give the elderly patient choices whenever possible. Take along their "living assists," such as walkers, hearing aids, and eyeglasses, and their book of phone numbers to facilitate reaching family or friends. Many elderly people are set in their ways and can be stubborn, but if you respect their dignity and do not rush them, you usually can build enough rapport to work with them effectively.

Patients with Sensory Impairment

Blind people, including the sighted patients whose injuries may require covering the eyes, benefit from verbal communication. Tell them everything you are going to do before doing it. If you need to have them walk, lead them by letting them hold onto your bended arm. Use touch as a form of contact for reassurance.

Ask hearing-impaired and deaf patients their preferred method of communication: lip reading, signing, or writing. Writing often is necessary—and the best method of communication—in the prehospital environment. Always be sure your face is illuminated when you speak to them. At night, also be sure that the deaf person who is trying to lip-read is not blinded by a flashlight. If the patient has some hearing, speak normally and do not exaggerate your enunciation of words or use too much volume, which can distort sound. Be aware that many hearing-impaired patients will nod "yes," even if they do not understand what was said or asked, possibly in a misguided effort to be agreeable.

Language and Cultural Considerations

An emergency situation in which people of different cultures and languages must interact requires you to be especially compassionate. To accomplish this, you must understand that cultures vary and **ethnocentrism,** or viewing your own life as the most desirable, acceptable, or best, and acting in a superior manner, will only hinder communication. Then, you must imagine the additional fear and frustration a patient in crisis

ethnocentrism *viewing one's own life as the most desirable, acceptable, or best, and acting in a superior manner to another culture's way of life.*

Cultural Considerations

Communicating with Hispanic Families Hispanics have become the fastest growing minority in the United States today. Of this community, Mexican Americans comprise over 65 percent. In many first- and second-generation Hispanic families, Spanish remains the language of choice. In many instances, Spanish must be used to adequately convey health care information—particularly in an emergency situation. In this culture, it is important that nonverbal communications be consistent with verbal communications. Furthermore, such communications must have an underlying tone of respect (*respeto*). Spanish language has both informal and formal verb forms. The use of informal verb forms can be seen as a sign of disrespect and should be avoided.

In Mexican American and many Latin American cultures, the grandmother (*abuela*) is often looked to in terms of medical advice and health care decisions. Because of this, the grandmother should often be included in discussions pertaining to the patient. This is particularly true in situations where you have a relatively young mother forced to make health care decisions about her infant. In many cases, despite what medical personnel might say, the grandmother will be sought for advice. Including the grandmother in certain situations will save time and also indicate respect.

---

feels when he tries to explain the emergency to a paramedic who cannot speak his language or understand his attitudes. To really empathize with him, you must be able to avoid **cultural imposition;** that is, avoid imposing on him your own beliefs, values, and patterns of behavior.

cultural imposition *the imposition of one's beliefs, values, and patterns of behavior on people of another culture.*

In a transcultural situation in which your patient also does not speak your language, you have the opportunity to make the experience less stressful by being caring and calm—and finding an interpreter. Some important principles when using an interpreter are:

★ Children of immigrants may act as interpreters. If this occurs, remember to keep what you have to say at the appropriate age level.

★ Recognize that the emergency may cause distressing emotions in the interpreter, especially if the interpreter is a child.

★ Speak slowly.

★ Phrase questions carefully and clearly.

★ Address both the patient and the interpreter.

★ Ask only one question at a time, and wait for a complete response.

★ Understand that the information you receive may not be reliable.

★ Have patience.

Cultural differences include more than just language differences. People of some cultures are more comfortable at a variety of distances when communicating; some expect health care workers to have all the answers to their illnesses; some treat ill or injured family members in different ways. Asian, Native American, Indochinese, and Arab people may consider direct eye contact impolite or aggressive and may thus demonstrate respect to you by averting their eyes. The welts on a feverish Southeast Asian child may not be from abuse, but rather from a folk practice known as "coin rubbing" or "coining," which many believe will draw out fever.

Understand that both you and the patient may bring cultural stereotypes to the situation. If either of you acts as if one culture is superior to the other, the situation could be ripe for problems. As with any call, create an appropriate professional relationship, but keep in mind that the rules about interpersonal space, eye contact, and touching may all be very different from those you know. As you can see, it is a good idea to study the various cultures typical to your area. Be open to the different ways of people, and do not act as if your way is the only correct way to manage things. There is no reason to impose your beliefs, values, and patterns of behavior on others.

Many cultures have established and accepted folk-medicine beliefs. While these may seem strange, they are very important to those who believe and practice them. If you work in an area with a concentration of a particular ethnic group, try to learn about the folk-medicine beliefs and practices of that group.

Hostile or Uncooperative Patients

There are times when you will need to build rapport with someone who cannot or does not want you to. If this is the case, be sure you are not threatening. Avoid confrontation, but keep trying until you are successful. Use the same questioning techniques you usually use. Sometimes patients open up if you clearly explain the benefits and advantages of cooperation. You also may be able to obtain the information you need from observing the scene and from questioning the patient's family, bystanders, or even law enforcement officers.

Set limits and establish boundaries with an uncooperative patient, if necessary. If the patient is sexually aggressive, for example, clarify your professional role for the patient. Tell him in a way that you are certain he understands that you are there to provide emergency medical care. Be sure to document unusual situations, and ask witnesses to document their observations as well. In extreme cases, consider having a same-sex witness ride in the back of your ambulance or tape record all interactions.

If a patient is blatantly hostile, or there is any hint that your safety is jeopardized, be sure to stay far enough away from the patient. Monitor him closely, and never leave the patient alone without adequate assistance. Also, to prevent a hostile situation from getting worse, be sure to have an appropriate show of force (enough personnel to overpower the patient), if necessary. Remember, your personal safety is paramount. Always be sure you have a clear path to the nearest exit, and always position yourself so you can observe others entering or exiting the area. Know local protocols regarding the use of restraints and psychological medications. Don't hesitate to call for law enforcement back-up, if necessary.

TRANSFERRING PATIENT CARE

When you arrive at the scene of an emergency, EMS-trained First Responders may already be there. Before they transfer patient care to you, be sure to listen to their report carefully. Use eye contact, and say the name of the First Responder, if you know it. Integrate the information they give you into the questions you ask your patient; he will trust you more if he sees you have listened to your colleagues. Say something like: "The First Responder said you felt dizzy before you fell today. Were there any other sensations you can remember?"

Transfer of care at the receiving medical facility can be a challenge. Remember to always interact with other emergency colleagues with respect and dignity. If the emergency department is busy, the receiving nurse or doctor may appear to be distracted. If this is true, important medical information could get lost. In noncritical circumstances, therefore, respectfully stand your ground until the nurse or doctor looks at you. Then say, "Are you the person who will be listening to my hand-off report?" If so, follow-up with, "Are you ready to listen, or would you rather wait a moment?" Also, be sure to introduce the patient by name and to say goodbye to the patient before you leave.

Always interact with other emergency colleagues with respect and dignity.

Summary

In a career, a paramedic might handle a thousand patients with chest pain and perform similar medical procedures for each one. But the communication challenges that a paramedic will face will be totally different every time. Indeed, the skills required to manage medical situations are obviously an important part of emergency care. The person who does not study ways to communicate effectively with patients, relatives, bystanders—as well as co-workers—will have missed out on an important part of what it takes to be an excellent practitioner of the art of paramedicine.

Remember, much of the information you will gather from all your patients is extremely personal. (In what other line of work can a perfect stranger approach a person on the street and inquire about bowel or sexual habits?) You will need an enormous degree of sensitivity to recognize and respond to the signs of suffering in order to create an ideal, individualized process of communication. Showing compassion and demonstrating the expertise necessary to assist appropriately will allow you to become an ally to your patients and others.

You Make the Call

You have been sent to a dirty alley near the "red-light district." It is the middle of the night. Upon arrival, you find that a fire crew is on scene. Most of them are leaning disgustedly against the pumper. Thus, you know the situation is not critical before you even get out of the ambulance.

When you do get out, one of the fire crew points down the alley at a small crowd of people standing back from a person who is lying on the street. As you approach, you notice that the lighting is dim but the people all seem calm and under control. Everyone is standing about 12 feet away from the patient. Just as you near the patient, he raises himself up on an elbow and yells drunkenly at you, "I am not letting you or anyone except a real doctor work on me!"

1. Which interaction among the emergency personnel is nonverbal?
2. When the patient expresses his prejudice against you, what techniques can you use to begin the process of building trust and rapport?

See Suggested Responses at the back of this book.

Review Questions

1. When addressing your patient, which of the following forms of address is inappropriate?
   a. Mr.
   b. Mrs.
   c. Dude
   d. Ms.

2. In the United States, the socially acceptable distance between strangers is _____ to _____ feet.
   a. 2–6
   b. 4–5
   c. 4–12
   d. 10–15

3. Arms extended, open hands, relaxed large muscles, and a nodding head characterize a(n):
   a. intimate zone.
   b. open stance.
   c. closed stance.
   d. social distance.

4. Nothing builds trust and rapport, or calms patients, faster than the power of:
   a. touch.
   b. eye contact.
   c. kind voice.
   d. closed stance.

5. A question that guides the patient's replies is a(n):
   a. direct question.
   b. leading question.
   c. closed question.
   d. open-ended question.

6. The feedback technique that gives the patient time to gather his thoughts and add to what has been said is:
   a. empathy.
   b. silence.
   c. facilitation.
   d. clarification.

7. Effective communication with pediatric patients depends on their:
   a. age.
   b. size.
   c. gender.
   d. weight.

8. Viewing your own life as the most desirable, acceptable, or best, and acting in a superior manner to another culture's way of life, is:
   a. idealism.
   b. professionalism.
   c. ethnocentrism.
   d. cultural imposition.

See Answers to Review Questions at the back of this book.

Further Reading

Dernocoeur, K. B. *Streetsense: Communication, Safety, and Control.* 3rd ed. Redmond, WA: Laing Research Services, 1996.

DeVito, J. *Essentials of Human Communication.* 4th ed. New York City: Longman, 2002.

Federal Emergency Management Agency. "EMS Safety: Techniques and Applications." FA-144. Washington, D.C., 1994.

Keeland, B., and L. Jordan. *CommuniMed: Multilingual Patient Assessment Manual.* 3rd ed. St. Louis: Mosby, 1994.

Limmer, D., M. F. O'Keefe, E. T. Dickinson, et al. *Emergency Care.* 9th ed. Fire Service Edition. Upper Saddle River, N.J.: Pearson/Prentice Hall, 2003.

Perez-Sabido, J. *Spanish-English Handbook for Medical Professionals.* 4th ed. Los Angeles: Practice Management Information Corp., 1994.

On the Web

Visit Brady's Paramedic Website at **www.bradybooks.com/paramedic.**

Life-Span Development

Objectives

After reading this chapter, you should be able to:

1. Compare and contrast the physiological and psychosocial characteristics of the following life-span development stages:
   ★ Infant (pp. 484–489)
   ★ Toddler (pp. 489–492)
   ★ Preschooler (pp. 489–492)
   ★ School-age (p. 493)
   ★ Adolescent (pp. 494–495)
   ★ Early adult (p. 495)
   ★ Middle-age adult (pp. 495–496)
   ★ Late-age adult (pp. 496–501)

Key Terms

anxious avoidant
  attachment, p. 488
anxious resistant
  attachment, p. 488
authoritarian, p. 492
authoritative, p. 492
bonding, p. 488
conventional reasoning,
  p. 493
difficult child, p. 489
easy child, p. 489

life expectancy, p. 496
maximum life span, p. 496
modeling, p. 492
Moro reflex, p. 487
palmar grasp, p. 487
permissive, p. 492
postconventional
  reasoning, p. 493
preconventional
  reasoning, p. 493

rooting reflex, p. 487
scaffolding, p. 489
secure attachment, p. 488
slow-to-warm-up child,
  p. 489
sucking reflex, p. 487
terminal-drop hypothesis,
  p. 499
trust vs. mistrust, p. 489

Case Study

You and your partner respond to an early morning call and find several people upset and milling around. As you announce yourselves as paramedics, a woman sticks her head out of a doorway down the hallway and beckons you into a room. There you find a woman in her early 20s. She's lying in bed and seems very uncomfortable. A young man, visibly pale, is sitting on the edge of the bed holding her hand.

The first woman tells you that the patient is in her final month of pregnancy and that she has been experiencing mild contractions for about 12 hours. She spoke with her doctor several hours ago and was told to go to the hospital when her contractions were approximately 5 minutes apart. "Unfortunately, her water broke, and since that time the contractions have been really close together; about 3 minutes apart," the woman tells you. They were afraid to attempt the drive to the hospital, so they decided to call the paramedics.

After asking some pertinent questions, you prepare to examine the patient for crowning. Having done so, you realize it will be necessary to allow the child to be delivered at home. Preparations are made, and within a short time, a beautiful little girl is wrapped in warm blankets and snuggled in her mother's arms. You explain that you will now prepare the mother and baby to be transported to the hospital where they can be examined to be sure there are no problems.

As you leave the room to get your stretcher, the first woman, who is the grandmother of the new baby, is spreading the happy news to the rest of the family. By the time you return to the room, several family members are gathered around a rocking chair where an elderly woman sits, holding her new great-grandchild in her arms. You think to yourself: "Four generations. Wow." Truly a beautiful family event, which you have been privileged to attend.

INTRODUCTION

Though human anatomy and physiology basically stay the same, people do change over the span of a lifetime (Figure 12-1 ■). Besides the obvious changes in size and appearance, there are also changes in vital signs, body systems, and psychosocial development. Some of those changes make it necessary for you to adjust your treatment of patients. For example, the amount of medication a patient receives is based on body size, weight, and the ability of the patient to process it. A child, therefore, usually requires a smaller dosage than a full-grown adult does. Many of the changes experienced over a lifetime can be identified in developmental stages. Those discussed in this chapter are:

- ★ *Infancy*—birth to 12 months
- ★ *Toddler*—12 to 36 months
- ★ *Preschool age*—3 to 5 years
- ★ *School age*—6 to 12 years
- ★ *Adolescence*—13 to 18 years
- ★ *Early adulthood*—19 to 40 years
- ★ *Middle adulthood*—41 to 60 years
- ★ *Late adulthood*—61 years and older

INFANCY

PHYSIOLOGICAL DEVELOPMENT

Vital Signs

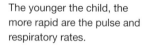

The younger the child, the more rapid are the pulse and respiratory rates.

The greatest changes in the range of vital signs are in the pediatric patient (Table 12–1). The younger the child, the more rapid are the pulse and respiratory rates. At birth, the heart rate ranges from 100 to 180 beats per minute during the first 30 minutes of life

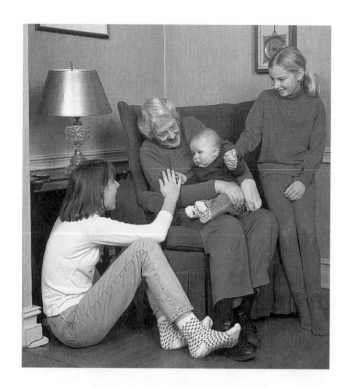

■ Figure 12-1 People change over the span of a lifetime.

Table 12-1	Normal Vital Signs					
	Pulse (beats per minute)	Respiration (breaths per minute)	Blood Pressure (average mmHg)	Temperature		
Infancy:						
At birth:	100–180	30–60	60–90 systolic	98°–100° F	36.7°–37.8° C	
At 1 year:	100–160	30–60	87–105 systolic	98°–100° F	36.7°–37.8° C	
Toddler (12 to 36 months)	80–110	24–40	95–105 systolic	96.8°–99.6° F	36.0°–37.5° C	
Preschool age (3 to 5 years)	70–110	22–34	95–110 systolic	96.8°–99.6° F	36.0°–37.5° C	
School-age (6 to 12 years)	65–110	18–30	97–112 systolic	98.6° F	37° C	
Adolescence (13 to 18 years)	60–90	12–26	112–128 systolic	98.6° F	37° C	
Early adulthood (19 to 40 years)	60–100	12–20	120/80	98.6° F	37° C	
Middle adulthood (41 to 60 years)	60–100	12–20	120/80	98.6° F	37° C	
Late adulthood (61 years and older)	+	+	+	98.6° F	37° C	

+ Depends on the individual physical health status.

and usually settles to around 120 beats per minute after that. The initial respiratory rate is from 30 to 60 breaths per minute but tends to drop to 30 to 40 breaths per minute after the first few minutes of life. Tidal volume is 6 to 8 mL/kg initially and increases to 10 to 15 mL/kg by 12 months of age.

As with the other vital signs, the normal range for blood pressure is related to the age and weight of the infant, tending to increase with age. The average systolic blood pressure increases from a range of 60 to 90 at birth to a range of 87 to 105 at 12 months.

Weight

Normal birth weight of an infant usually is between 3.0 and 3.5 kg. Because of the excretion of extracellular fluid in the first week of life, the infant's weight usually drops by 5 percent to 10 percent; however, infants usually exceed their birth weight by the second week. During the first month, infants grow at approximately 30 grams per day, and they should double their birth weight by 4 to 6 months and triple it at 9 to 12 months (Figure 12-2 ■). The infant's head is equal to 25 percent of total body weight.

Growth charts are good for comparing physical development to the norm, but parents should keep in mind that every child develops at his own rate.

Cardiovascular System

As newborns make the transition from fetal to pulmonary circulation in the first few days of life, several important changes occur. Shortly after birth, the *ductus venosus,* a blood vessel that connects the umbilical vein and the inferior vena cava in the fetus, constricts. As a result, blood pressure changes and the *foramen ovale,* an opening in the interatrial septum of the fetal heart, closes. The *ductus arteriosus,* a blood vessel that connects the pulmonary artery and the aorta in the fetus, also constricts after birth. Once it is closed, blood can no longer bypass the lungs by moving from the pulmonary trunk directly into the aorta.

The infant's head is equal to 25 percent of total body weight.

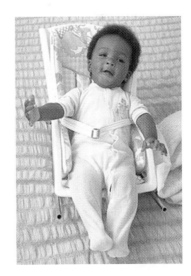

■ Figure 12-2   Infants double their weight by 4 to 6 months old and triple it by 9 to 12 months. *(© Michal Heron)*

These changes lead to an immediate increase in systemic vascular resistance and a decrease in pulmonary vascular resistance. Although the constriction of the ductus arteriosus may be functionally complete within 15 minutes, the permanent closure of the foramen ovale may take from 30 days to 1 year. The left ventricle of the heart will strengthen throughout the first year.

(You may wish to note that in an adult, the ductus venosus becomes a fibrous cord called the *ligamentum venosum,* which is superficially embedded in the wall of the liver. Also, in an adult, the site of the foramen ovale is marked by a depression called the *fossa ovalis,* and the ductus arteriosus is represented by a cord called the *ligamentum arteriosum.*)

Pulmonary System

The first breath an infant takes must be forceful, because until that moment the lungs have been collapsed. Fortunately, the lungs of a full-term fetus continuously secrete surfactant. Surfactant is a chemical that reduces the surface tension that tends to hold the moist membranes of the lungs together. After the first powerful breath begins to expand the lungs, breathing becomes easier.

In general, an infant's airway is shorter, narrower, less stable, and more easily obstructed than at any other stage in life. The infant is primarily a "nose breather" until at least 4 weeks of age; therefore, it is important for the nasal passages to stay clear. A common complaint in infants less than 6 months of age is nasal congestion. This occurs because, as mentioned, young infants are obligate nasal breathers. Even a mild nasal obstruction, as occurs with a viral upper respiratory infection, can cause difficulty breathing, especially during feeding.

An infant's lung tissue is fragile and prone to *barotrauma* (an injury caused by a change in atmospheric pressure). Because of this, prehospital personnel must be careful when applying mechanical ventilation with a bag-valve-mask unit. There are fewer alveoli with decreased collateral ventilation. In addition, the accessory muscles for breathing are immature and susceptible to early fatigue, so they cannot sustain a rapid respiratory rate over a long period of time. Breathing becomes ineffective at rates higher than 60 breaths per minute because air moves only in the upper airway, never reaching the lungs. Rapid respiratory rates also lead to rapid heat and fluid loss.

The chest wall of the infant is less rigid than an adult's, and the ribs are positioned horizontally, causing diaphragmatic breathing. So when you assess respiratory rate and effort in an infant, it is important to observe the abdomen rise and fall. An infant needs less pressure and a lower volume of air for ventilation than an adult does, but the infant has a higher metabolic rate and a higher oxygen-consumption rate than an adult.

Renal System

Usually, the newborn's kidneys are not able to produce concentrated urine, so the baby excretes a relatively dilute fluid with a specific gravity that rarely exceeds 1.0. (Specific gravity is the weight of a substance compared to an equal amount of water. For comparisons, water is considered to have a specific gravity of 1.0.) For this reason, the newborn can easily become dehydrated and develop a water and electrolyte imbalance.

Immune System

During pregnancy, certain antibodies pass from the maternal blood into the fetal bloodstream. As a result, the fetus acquires some of the mother's active immunities against pathogens. Thus, the fetus is said to have naturally acquired passive immunities, which may remain effective for 6 months to a year after birth. A breast-fed baby also receives antibodies through the breast milk to many of the diseases the mother has had.

An infant's airway is shorter, narrower, less stable, and more easily obstructed than at any other stage in life.

Nervous System

Sensation is present in all portions of the body at birth, so a young infant feels pain but lacks the ability to localize it and isolate a response to it. As nerve connections develop, the response to pain becomes much more localized. In addition, motor and sensory development are most advanced in the cranial nerves at birth, because of their life-sustaining function and protective reflexes. Since the cranial nerves control such things as blinking, sucking, and swallowing, the infant has strong, coordinated sucking and gag reflexes. The infant also will have well-flexed extremities, which move equally when the infant is stimulated.

Reflexes The infant has several reflexes that disappear over time. These include the Moro, palmar, rooting, and sucking reflexes. The **Moro reflex,** which is sometimes referred to as the "startle reflex," is the characteristic reflex of newborns. When the baby is startled, he throws his arms wide, spreading his fingers and then grabbing instinctively with the arms and fingers. The reflex should be brisk and symmetrical. An asymmetric Moro reflex (in which one arm does not respond exactly like the other) may imply a paralysis or weakness on one side of the body.

The **palmar grasp** is a strong reflex in the full-term newborn. It is elicited by placing a finger firmly in the infant's palm. The palmar grasp weakens as the hand becomes less continuously fisted. Sometime after 2 months, it merges into the voluntary ability to release an object held in the hand.

The **rooting reflex** causes the hungry infant to turn his head to the right or left when a hand or cloth touches his cheek. If the mother's nipple touches either side of the infant's face, above or below the mouth, the infant's lips and tongue tend to follow in that direction. Stroking the infant's lips causes a sucking movement, or the **sucking reflex,** in the infant. Both the rooting and sucking reflexes should be present in all full-term babies and are most easily elicited before a feeding. They usually last until the infant is 3 or 4 months old; however, the rooting reflex may persist during sleep for 7 or 8 months.

Fontanelles Fontanelles allow for compression of the head during childbirth and for rapid growth of the brain during early life. They are diamond-shaped soft spots of fibrous tissue at the top of the infant's skull where three or four bones will eventually fuse together. The fibrous tissue is strong and, generally, can protect the brain adequately from injury. The posterior fontanelle usually closes in 2 or 3 months, and the anterior one closes between 9 and 18 months. You may wish to note that the fontanelles, especially the anterior one, may be used to provide an indirect estimate of hydration. Normally, the anterior fontanelle is level with the surface of the skull, or slightly sunken. With dehydration, the anterior fontanelle may fall below the level of the skull and appear sunken.

Sleep A newborn usually sleeps for 16 to 18 hours daily, with periods of sleep and wakefulness evenly distributed over a 24-hour period. Sleep time will gradually decrease to 14 to 16 hours per day, with a 9- to 10-hour period at night. Infants usually begin to sleep through the night within 2 to 4 months. The normal infant is easily aroused.

Musculoskeletal System

The developing infant's extremities grow in length from growth plates, which are located on each end of the long bones. The infant also has *epiphyseal plates,* or secondary bone-forming centers that are separated by cartilage from larger (or parent) bones. As each epiphysis grows, it becomes part of the larger bone. Bones grow in thickness by way

Moro reflex occurs when a newborn is startled; arms are thrown wide, fingers spread, and a grabbing motion follows; also called startle reflex.

palmar grasp a reflex in the newborn, which is elicited by placing a finger firmly in the infant's palm.

rooting reflex occurs when an infant's cheek is touched by a hand or cloth; the hungry infant turns his head to the right or left.

sucking reflex occurs when an infant's lips are stroked.

of deposition of new bone on existing bone. Factors affecting bone development and growth include nutrition, exposure to sunlight, growth hormone, thyroid hormone, genetic factors, and general health. Muscle weight in infants is about 25 percent of the entire musculoskeletal system.

Other Developmental Characteristics

Expect rapid changes during an infant's first year of life. At about 2 months of age, he is able to track objects with his eyes and recognize familiar faces. At about 3 months of age, he can move objects to his mouth with his hands and display primary emotions with distinct facial expressions (such as a smile or a frown). At 4 months of age, he drools without swallowing and begins to reach out to people. By 5 months, he should be sleeping through the night without waking for a feeding, and he should be able to discriminate between family and strangers. Teeth begin to appear between 5 and 7 months of age.

At 6 months, the baby can sit upright in a high chair and begin to make one-syllable sounds, such as "ma," "mu," "da," and "di." At 7 months, he has a fear of strangers and his moods can quickly shift from crying to laughing. At 8 months, the infant begins to respond to the word "no," he can sit alone, and he can play "peek-a-boo." At 9 months, he responds to adult anger.

At about 9 months old, the baby begins to pull himself up to a standing position, and explores objects by mouthing, sucking, chewing, and biting them. At 10 months, he pays attention to his name and crawls well. At 11 months, he attempts to walk without assistance and begins to show frustration about restrictions. By 12 months, he can walk with help, and he knows his own name.

PSYCHOSOCIAL DEVELOPMENT

Family Processes and Reciprocal Socialization

The psychosocial development of an individual begins at birth and develops as a result of instincts, drives, capacities, and interactions with the environment. A key component of that environment is the family. The interactions babies have with their families help them to grow and change and help their families do the same. This is called "reciprocal socialization," a model that recognizes the child's active role in its own development.

Raising a baby requires a lot of hard work, but studies show that healthy, happy, and self-reliant children are the products of stable homes in which parents give a great deal of time and attention to their children.

Crying A newborn's only means of communication is through crying. While every cry may seem the same to a stranger, most mothers quickly learn to notice the differences in a basic cry, an anger cry, and a pain cry.

Attachment Infants have their own unique timetables and paths to becoming attached to their parents. **Bonding** is initially based on **secure attachment,** or an infant's sense that his needs will be met by his caregivers. Secure attachment is consistent with healthy development, and leads to a child who is bold in his explorations of the world and competent in dealing with it. It is important for this sense of security to develop within the first 6 months of an infant's life.

When an infant is uncertain about whether or not his caregivers will be responsive or helpful when needed, another type of attachment develops. It is called **anxious resistant attachment.** It leads to a child who is always prone to separation anxiety, causing him to be clinging and anxious about exploring the world.

A third type of attachment is called **anxious avoidant attachment.** It occurs when the infant has no confidence that he will be responded to helpfully when he seeks care. In fact, the infant expects to be rebuffed. This causes him to attempt to live without the love and support of others. The most extreme cases result from repeated rejection or

bonding *the formation of a close personal relationship (as between mother and child), especially through frequent or constant association.*

secure attachment *a type of bonding that occurs when an infant learns that his caregivers will be responsive and helpful when needed.*

anxious resistant attachment *a type of bonding that occurs when an infant is uncertain about whether or not his caregivers will be responsive or helpful when needed.*

anxious avoidant attachment *a type of bonding that occurs when an infant learns that his caregivers will not be responsive or helpful when needed.*

prolonged institutionalization and can lead to a variety of personality disorders from compulsive self-sufficiency to persistent delinquency.

Trust vs. Mistrust　Some psychologists believe that human life progresses through a series of stages, each marked by a crisis that needs to be resolved. Each of the crises involves a conflict between two opposing characteristics. From birth to approximately $1\frac{1}{2}$ years of age, the infant goes through the stage called **trust vs. mistrust.** According to psychologists, the infant wants the world to be an orderly, predictable place where causes and effects can be anticipated. When this is true, the infant develops trust based on consistent parental care. When an infant begins life with irregular and inadequate care, he develops anxiety and insecurity, which have a negative effect on family and other relationships important to the development of trust. This may lead to feelings of mistrust and hostility, which may in turn develop into antisocial or even criminal behavior.

trust vs. mistrust   refers to a stage of psychosocial development that lasts from birth to about $1\frac{1}{2}$ years of age.

Scaffolding

Infants learn in many ways from their parents and others around them. One way they learn—from infancy and throughout their school years—is through **scaffolding,** or building on what they already know. For example, parents or caregivers usually talk to infants as a natural part of caring for them. With scaffolding, the dialogue is maintained just above the level where the child can perform activities independently. As the baby learns, the parent or caregiver changes the nature of the dialogues so that they continue to support the baby but also give him responsibility for the task. In this way, infants continue to build on what they know.

scaffolding   a teaching/learning technique in which one builds on what has already been learned.

Temperament

An infant may be classified as an easy child, a difficult child, or a slow-to-warm-up child. An **easy child** is characterized by regularity of bodily functions, low or moderate intensity of reactions, and acceptance of new situations. A **difficult child** is characterized by irregularity of bodily functions, intense reactions, and withdrawal from new situations. A **slow-to-warm-up child** is characterized by a low intensity of reactions and a somewhat negative mood.

easy child   an infant who can be characterized by regularity of bodily functions, low or moderate intensity of reactions, and acceptance of new situations.

difficult child   an infant, who can be characterized by irregularity of bodily functions, intense reactions, and withdrawal from new situations.

Situational Crisis and Parental-Separation Reactions

Infants who have good relationships with their parents usually follow a predictable sequence of behaviors when they experience a situational crisis (a crisis caused by a particular set of circumstances), such as being separated from parents. The first stage of parental-separation reaction is protest, the second stage is despair, and the last is detachment or withdrawal.

　Protest may begin immediately upon separation and continue for about 1 week. Loud crying, restlessness, and rejection of all adults show how distressed the infant is. In the second stage, despair, the infant's behavior suggests growing hopelessness marked by monotonous crying, inactivity, and steady withdrawal. In the final stage, detachment or withdrawal, the infant displays renewed interest in its surroundings, even though it is usually a remote, distant kind of interest. This phase is apathetic and may persist even if the parent reappears.

slow-to-warm-up child   an infant, who can be characterized by a low intensity of reactions and a somewhat negative mood.

Parental-separation reactions in an infant include protest, despair, and withdrawal.

TODDLER AND PRESCHOOL AGE

PHYSIOLOGICAL DEVELOPMENT

Vital signs for toddlers (12 to 36 months, Figure 12-3 ■) and preschool-age children (3 to 5 years old, Figure 12-4 ■) are not the same as an infant's. The heart rate for toddlers ranges from 80 to 110 beats per minute. Respiratory rate ranges from 24 to 40 breaths

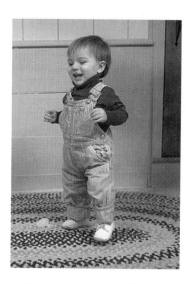

■ Figure 12-3   A toddler beginning to stand and walk on his own. (© Michal Heron)

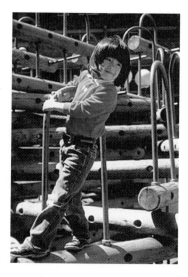

■ Figure 12-4   In the preschool-age child, exploratory behavior accelerates. (© Michal Heron)

per minute. Systolic blood pressure ranges from 95 to 105 mmHg. For preschoolers, heart rate ranges from 70 to 110 beats per minute, respiratory rate from 22 to 34 breaths per minute, and systolic blood pressure from 75 to 110 mmHg. Normal temperature for both ranges from 96.8 to 99.6° F (36.3° C to 37.9° C). In addition, the rate of weight gain is slowing dramatically. The average toddler or preschooler gains approximately 2.0 kg per year.

Changes in body systems include the following:

Remember that toddlers and preschool-age children have immature chest muscles and cannot sustain an excessively rapid respiratory rate for long.

★ *Cardiovascular system.* The capillary beds are now better developed and assist in thermoregulation of the body more efficiently. Hemoglobin levels approach normal adult levels at this point.

★ *Pulmonary system.* The terminal airways continue to branch off from the bronchioles and alveoli increase in number, providing more surfaces for gas exchange to take place in the lungs. It is still important to remember that children have immature chest muscles and cannot sustain an excessively rapid respiratory rate for long. They will tire quickly and their respiratory rate will decrease, indicating the onset of ventilatory failure.

★ *Renal system.* The kidneys are well-developed by the toddler years. Specific gravity and other characteristics of urine are similar to what would be found in an adult.

★ *Immune system.* By this point in life, the passive immunity born with the infant is lost, and the child becomes more susceptible to minor respiratory and gastrointestinal infections. This occurs at the same time the child is being exposed to the infections of other children in child care and preschool. Fortunately, the toddler and preschooler will develop their own immunities to common pathogens as they are exposed to them.

★ *Nervous system.* The brain is now at 90 percent of adult weight. Myelination (the development of the covering of nerves) has increased, which allows for effortless walking as well as other basic skills. Fine motor skills, including the use of hands and fingers in grasping and manipulating objects, begin developing at this stage.

- ★ *Musculoskeletal system.* Both muscle mass and bone density increase during this period.
- ★ *Dental system.* All of the primary teeth have erupted by the age of 36 months.
- ★ *Senses.* Visual acuity is at 20/30 during the toddler years. Hearing reaches maturity at 3 to 4 years old.

In addition, though children are physiologically capable of being toilet trained by the age of 12 to 15 months, they are not psychologically ready until 18 to 30 months of age. So, it is important not to rush toilet training. Children will let their parents know when they are ready. The average age for completion of toilet training is 28 months.

The average age for completion of toilet training is 28 months.

PSYCHOSOCIAL DEVELOPMENT

Cognition

Children begin to use actual words at about 10 months, but they do not begin to grasp that words "mean" something until they are about 1 year of age. Usually, by the time they are 3 or 4 years old, they have mastered the basics of language, which they will continue to refine throughout their childhood. Between 18 and 24 months, they begin to understand cause and effect. Between the ages of 18 and 24 months, they develop separation anxiety, becoming clinging and crying when a parent leaves. Between 24 and 36 months, they begin to develop "magical thinking" and engage in play-acting, such as playing house and similar activities.

By the age of 3 or 4, children have mastered the basics of language.

Between the ages of 18 and 24 months, children develop separation anxiety.

Play

Exploratory behavior accelerates at this stage. The child is able to play simple games and follow basic rules, and he begins to display signs of competitiveness. Play provides an emotional release for youngsters, because it lacks the right-or-wrong, life-and-death feelings that may accompany interactions with adults. Therefore, observations of children at play may uncover frustrations otherwise unexpressed.

Sibling Relationships

While there are many positive aspects to growing up with siblings, there also may be negative ones, which can lead to sibling rivalry. The first-born child often finds it very difficult to share the attention of his parents with a younger sibling. If the older child must also help care for the younger ones, he may become even more frustrated. While first-born children usually maintain a special relationship with parents, they also are expected to exercise more self-control and show more responsibility when interacting with younger siblings. Younger children often see only the apparent privileges extended to the older children, such as later bedtimes and more freedom to come and go. Still, when asked if they would be happier if their siblings did not exist, most prefer to keep them around.

Peer-Group Functions

Peers, or youngsters who are similar in age (within 12 months of each other), are very important to the development of toddler and school-age children. In fact, peer groups actually become more important as childhood progresses. Peers provide a source of information about other families and the outside world. Interaction with peers offers opportunities for learning skills, comparing oneself to others, and feeling part of a group.

Parenting Styles and Their Effects

authoritarian *a parenting style that demands absolute obedience without regard to a child's individual freedom.*

There are three basic styles of parenting: **authoritarian, authoritative,** and **permissive:**

★ *Authoritarian* parents are demanding and desire instant obedience from a child. No consideration is given to the child's view, and no attempt is made to explain why. Frequently, the child is punished for even asking the reason for some decision or directive. This parenting style often leads to children with low self-esteem and low competence. Boys are often hostile and girls are often shy.

authoritative *a parenting style that emphasizes a balance between a respect for authority and individual freedom.*

★ *Authoritative* parents respond to the needs and wishes of their children. While they believe in parental control, they attempt to explain their reasons to the child. They expect mature behavior and will enforce rules, but they still encourage independence and actualization of potential. These parents believe that both they and children have rights and try to maintain a happy balance between the two. This parenting style usually leads to children who are self-assertive, independent, friendly, and cooperative.

permissive *a parenting style that takes a tolerant, accepting view of a child's behavior.*

★ *Permissive* parents take a tolerant, accepting view of their children's behavior, including aggressive behavior and sexual behavior. They rarely punish or make demands of their children, allowing them to make almost all of their own decisions. They may be either "permissive-indifferent" or "permissive-indulgent" parents, but it is very difficult to make the distinction. This parenting style may lead to impulsive, aggressive children who have low self-reliance, low self-control, low maturity, and lack responsible behavior.

Divorce and Child Development

Nearly half of today's marriages end in divorce. As a result of divorce, a child's physical way of life often changes (a new home, for example, or a reduced standard of living). The child's psychological life is also touched. The effects on the child's development, however, depend greatly on the child's age, his cognitive and social competencies, the amount of dependency on his parents, how the parents interact with each other and the child, and even the type of child care. Toddlers and preschoolers commonly express feelings of shock, depression, and a fear that their parents no longer love them. They may feel they are being abandoned. They are unable to see the divorce from their parents' perspective, and therefore believe the divorce centers on them. The parent's ability to respond to a child's needs greatly influences the ultimate effects of divorce on the child.

Television

Virtually every family has at least one television in the home. Most children watch television for several hours each day, many with few, if any, parental restrictions. Television violence increases levels of aggression in toddlers and preschoolers, and it increases passive acceptance of the use of aggression by others. Parental screening of the television programs children watch may be effective in avoiding these outcomes.

modeling *a procedure whereby a subject observes a model perform some behavior and then attempts to imitate that behavior. Many believe it is the fundamental learning process involved in socialization.*

Modeling

Toddlers and preschool-age children begin to recognize sexual differences, and, through **modeling,** they begin to incorporate gender-specific behaviors they observe in parents, siblings, and peers.

SCHOOL AGE

PHYSIOLOGICAL DEVELOPMENT

Between the ages of 6 and 12 years, a child's heart rate is between 65 and 110 beats per minute, respiratory rate is between 18 and 30 breaths per minute, and systolic blood pressure ranges from 97 to 112 mmHg. Body temperature is approximately 98.6° F (37° C). The average child of this age gains 3 kg per year and grows 6 cm per year. In most children, vital signs reach adult levels during this period of time, but their lymph tissues are proportionately larger than those of an adult. In addition, brain function increases in both hemispheres, and primary teeth are being replaced by permanent ones.

Vital signs in most children reach adult levels during the school-age years.

PSYCHOSOCIAL DEVELOPMENT

School-age children (Figure 12-5 ■) have developed decision-making skills, and usually are allowed more self-regulation, with parents providing general supervision. Parents spend less time with school-age children than they did with toddlers and preschoolers.

The development of a self-concept occurs at this age. School-age children have more interaction with both adults and other children, and they tend to compare themselves to others. They are beginning to develop self-esteem, which tends to be higher during the early years of school than in the later years. Often self-esteem is based on external characteristics and may be affected by popularity with peers, rejection, emotional support, and neglect. Negative self-esteem can be very damaging to further development.

As children mature, moral development begins when they are rewarded for what their parents believe to be right and punished for what their parents believe to be wrong. With cognitive growth, moral reasoning appears and the control of the child's behavior gradually shifts from external sources to internal self-control. According to one theory, there are three levels of moral development: **preconventional reasoning, conventional reasoning,** and **postconventional reasoning,** with each level having two stages.

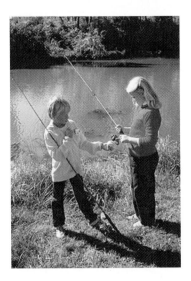

■ Figure 12-5   School-age children are allowed more self-regulation and independence as they grow older. (© Michal Heron)

preconventional reasoning
the stage of moral development during which children respond mainly to cultural control to avoid punishment and attain satisfaction.

conventional reasoning   *the stage of moral development during which children desire approval from individuals and society.*

postconventional reasoning
the stage of moral development during which individuals make moral decisions according to an enlightened conscience.

- ★ *Preconventional reasoning.* Stage one is punishment and obedience; that is, children obey rules in order to avoid punishment. There is no concern about morals. Stage two is individualism and purpose; that is, children obey the rules but only for pure self-interest. They are aware of fairness to others but only as it pertains to their own satisfaction.

- ★ *Conventional reasoning.* In stage three, children are concerned with interpersonal norms, seeking the approval of others and developing the "good boy" or "good girl" mentality. They begin to judge behavior by intention. In stage four, they develop the social system's morality, becoming concerned with authority and maintaining the social order. They realize that correct behavior is "doing one's duty."

- ★ *Postconventional reasoning.* Stage five is concerned with community rights as opposed to individual rights. Children at this level believe that the best values are those supported by law because they have been accepted by the whole society. They believe that if there is a conflict between human need and the law, individuals should work to change the law. Stage six is concerned with universal ethical principles, such as that an informed conscience defines what is right, or people act not because of fear, approval, or law, but from their own standards of what is right or wrong.

According to this theory, individuals will move through the levels and stages of moral development throughout school age and young adulthood at their own rates.

ADOLESCENCE

PHYSIOLOGICAL DEVELOPMENT

Vital signs in adolescents (13 to 18 years old) are as follows: heart rate is between 60 and 90 beats per minute, respiratory rate is between 12 and 26 breaths per minute, and systolic blood pressure is between 112 and 128 mmHg. Body temperature is approximately 98.6° F (37° C). In addition, the adolescent usually experiences a rapid 2- to 3-year growth spurt, beginning distally with enlargement of the feet and hands followed by enlargement of the arms and legs. The chest and trunk enlarge in the final stage of growth. Girls are usually finished growing by the age of 16 and boys by the age of 18. In late adolescence, the average male is taller and stronger than the average female.

At this age, both males and females reach reproductive maturity (Figure 12-6 ■). Secondary sexual development occurs, with noticeable development of the external sexual organs. Pubic and axillary hairs appear and, mostly in males, vocal quality changes. In females, menstruation has begun, breasts and the ductile system of the mammary glands develops, and there is increased deposition of adipose tissue in the subcutaneous layer of the breasts, thighs, and buttocks. In addition, in the female, endocrine system changes include the release of *follicle-stimulating hormone (FSH)*, *luteinizing hormone (LH)*, and *gonadrotropin*, which promotes estrogen and progesterone production. In the male, gonadrotropin promotes testosterone production.

Muscle mass and bone growth are nearly complete at this stage. Body fat decreases in early adolescence and increases later. Females require 18 to 20 percent body fat in order for menarche, or the first menstruation, to occur. Blood chemistry is nearly equal to that of an adult, and skin toughens through sebaceous gland activity. (You may wish to note that a disorder of the sebaceous glands is responsible for acne, which is common in adolescence. In acne, the glands become overactive and inflamed, ducts become plugged, and small red elevations containing blackheads or pimples appear.)

PSYCHOSOCIAL DEVELOPMENT
Family

Adolescence can be a time of serious family conflicts as the adolescent strives for autonomy and parents strive for continued control. The many biological changes that occur at this stage cause inner conflict in both the adolescent and parents. Privacy becomes extremely important at this stage of life and, because of modesty, the adolescent prefers that parents not be present during physical examinations. It also is likely that when a patient history is being taken, questions asked in the presence of parents or guardians may not be answered honestly.

Children experience an increase in idealism during adolescence. They believe that adults should be able to live up to their expectations, which of course they cannot always do, which leads to disappointment.

Development of Identity

At this age, adolescents are trying to achieve more independence. They take "time out" to experiment with a variety of identities, knowing that they do not have to assume responsibility for the consequences of those identities. As they attempt to develop their own identity, self-consciousness and peer pressure increase. They become interested in the opposite sex, and they find this somewhat embarrassing. They really do not know how to handle this increased interest. They want to be treated like adults and do not know how to achieve this.

Both males and females reach reproductive maturity during adolescence.

The many biological changes that occur in adolescence cause inner conflict in both the adolescent and parents.

Adolescents want to be treated like adults.

How well and how fast adolescents progress through the various stages of identity development depends on how well they are able to handle crises. Minority adolescents tend to have more identity crises than others. In general, antisocial behavior usually peaks at around the eighth or ninth grade.

Body image is a great concern at this point in life. Peers continually make comparisons, and certainly the media lead to unrealistic ideas of what the "perfect" body should look like. This is a time when eating disorders are common. It also is a time when self-destructive behaviors begin, such as use of tobacco, alcohol, and illicit drugs. Depression and suicide are more common at this age group than in any other.

Ethical Development

As adolescents develop their capacity for logical, analytical, and abstract thinking, they begin to develop a personal code of ethics. Just as they get disappointed when adults do not live up to their expectations, they tend to get disappointed in anyone who does not meet their personal code of ethics.

EARLY ADULTHOOD

Between the ages of 19 and 40 years, heart rate averages 70 beats per minute, respiratory rate averages between 12 and 20 breaths per minute, blood pressure averages 120/80 mmHg, and body temperature averages 98.6° F (37° C). This is the period of life during which adults develop lifelong habits and routines.

Peak physical condition occurs between the ages of 19 and 26 years of age, when all body systems are at optimal performance levels. At the end of this period, the body begins its slowing process. Spinal disks settle, leading to a decrease in height. Fatty tissue increases, leading to weight gain. Muscle strength decreases, and reaction times level off and stabilize. Accidents are a leading cause of death in this age group.

The highest levels of job stress occur at this point in life, the time in which the young adult strives to find his place in the world. Love develops, both romantic and affectionate. Childbirth is most common in this age group, with new families providing new challenges and stress (Figure 12-7 ■). In spite of all this, this period is not associated with psychological problems related to well-being.

MIDDLE ADULTHOOD

Between the ages of 41 and 60 years, average vital signs are as follows: heart rate, 70 beats per minute; respiratory rate between 12 and 20 breaths per minute; blood pressure at 120/80 mmHg; and body temperature averages 98.6° F (37° C).

The body still functions at a high level with varying degrees of degradation based on the individual (Figure 12-8 ■). There are usually some vision and hearing changes during this period. Cardiovascular health becomes a concern, with cardiac output decreasing and cholesterol levels increasing. Cancer often strikes this age group, weight control becomes more difficult, and for women in the late 40s to early 50s, menopause commences.

Adults in this age group are more concerned with the "social clock" and become more task oriented as they see the time for accomplishing their lifetime goals recede. Still, they tend to approach problems more as challenges than as threats. This is also the time of life for "empty-nest syndrome," or the time after the last offspring has left home. Some women feel depression or a sense of loss and purposelessness at this time, feelings that are made worse by aging and menopause. Sometimes a father also becomes depressed, but the syndrome seems to affect mothers to a greater extent. Many parents,

Depression and suicide are more common during adolescence than in any other age group.

Peak physical condition occurs between the ages of 19 and 26 years of age, when all body systems are at optimal performance levels.

Accidents are a leading cause of death in early adulthood.

Cardiovascular health becomes a concern during middle adulthood.

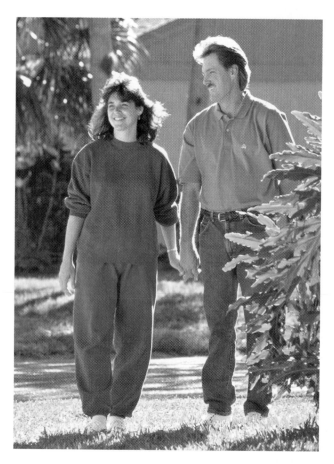

■ Figure 12-7   Peak physical conditions occur in early adulthood.

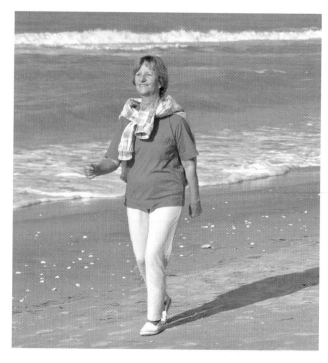

■ Figure 12-8   People in middle adulthood still function at a high level.

however, view the period after children have left home as a time of increased freedom and opportunity for self-fulfillment. Unfortunately, adults in this age group often find themselves burdened by financial commitments for elderly parents, as well as for young adult children.

LATE ADULTHOOD

maximum life span *the theoretical, species-specific, longest duration of life, excluding premature or "unnatural" death.*

life expectancy *based on the year of birth, the average number of additional years of life expected for a member of a population.*

Maximum life span is the theoretical, species-specific, longest duration of life, excluding premature or "unnatural" death. For human beings, maximum life span is approximately 120 years. **Life expectancy,** which is based on the year of birth, is defined as the average number of additional years of life expected for a member of a population. Human beings almost always die of disease or accident before they reach their biological limit.

PHYSIOLOGICAL DEVELOPMENT
Vital Signs

At 61 years of age and older, vital signs—heart rate, respiratory rate, and blood pressure—depend on the individual's physical health status. Body temperature still averages 98.6° F (37° C).

⚷ ───────────────
At 61 years of age and older, vital signs—heart rate, respiratory rate, and blood pressure—depend on the individual's physical health status.

Life Span and Disease The life span of individuals in most countries in the industrialized world continues to increase. This is due to many factors that include better health care, widespread availability of vaccinations, safer agricultural and manufacturing equipment, safer automobiles, the absence of major wars, and many others. With an extended life span, we are starting to commonly see diseases that were once uncommon. For example, only in the last 20 to 30 years have we started to see an increase in cases of Alzheimer's disease. But, is the incidence of Alzheimer's disease now more common or is it just that people are now living long enough for the disease to manifest itself? Although it will take structured research to determine this for sure, the latter part of the statement is surely true. Typically, approximately 10 percent of people age 65 show signs of the disease, while 50 percent of persons age 85 have symptoms of Alzheimer's. The proportion of persons with Alzheimer's begins to decrease after age 85 because of the increased mortality caused by the disease, and relatively few people over the age of 100 have the disease. Thus, the increased incidence of Alzheimer's disease may simply be due to the fact that people are living longer.

Cardiovascular System

During late adulthood, the cardiovascular system changes in ways that affect its overall function. The walls of the blood vessels thicken, causing increased peripheral vascular resistance and reduced blood flow to organs. There is decreased baroreceptor sensitivity and, by 80 years of age, there is approximately a 50 percent decrease in vessel elasticity.

During late adulthood, the cardiovascular system changes in ways that affect its overall function.

In addition, the heart tends to show disease in the heart muscle, heart valves, and coronary arteries. Increased workload causes cardiomegaly (enlargement), mitral and aortic valve changes, and decreased myocardial elasticity. The myocardium is less able to respond to exercise, and the SA node and other cells responsible for producing heartbeats become infiltrated with fibrous connective tissue and fat. Pacemaker cells diminish, resulting in dysrhythmia. Because of prolonged contraction time, decreased response to various medications that would ordinarily stimulate the heart, and increased resistance to electrical stimulation, the heart also becomes less able to contract. Tachycardia (abnormally rapid heart action) is not well tolerated.

Functional blood volume decreases in late adulthood. Decreases also can be expected in platelet count and the number of red blood cells (RBCs), which can lead to poor iron levels.

Respiratory System

The trachea and large airways increase in diameter in late adulthood, and enlargement of the end units of the airway results in a decreased surface area of the lungs. Decreased elasticity of the lungs leads to an increase in lung volume and to a reduction in surface area. The decreased elasticity also causes the chest to expand and the diaphragm to descend. The ends of the ribs calcify to the breastbone, producing stiffening of the chest wall, which increases the workload of the respiratory muscles.

Changes in the respiratory system lead to an increased likelihood for older adults to develop lung disease and progressive declines in lung function.

These changes lead to an increased likelihood for older adults to develop lung disease and progressive declines in lung function. Metabolic changes also may lead to decreased lung function, and because of lifelong exposure to pollutants, diffusion through alveoli is diminished. Coughing also becomes ineffective because of a weakened chest wall and bone structure. Of all the factors that influence lung function, smoking continues to produce the greatest amount of disability.

Endocrine System

During this stage of life, there is a decrease in glucose metabolism and insulin production. The thyroid shows some diminished triiodothyronine (T3) production, cortisol (from the adrenal cortex) is diminished by 25 percent, the pituitary gland is 20 percent less effective, and reproductive organs atrophy in women.

Gastrointestinal System

One way the gastrointestinal system is affected at this stage of life is by way of tooth loss. Age-related dental changes do not necessarily lead to loss of teeth. Usually tooth loss is caused by cavities or periodontal disease, both of which may be prevented by good dental hygiene. With age, the location of cavities in teeth changes and an increasing amount of root cavities and cavities around existing sites of previous dental work are seen. Tooth loss can lead to changes in diet, an increased chance of malnutrition, and serious vitamin and mineral deficiencies.

This is also true when the individual has false teeth, which do not completely restore normal chewing ability and can reduce taste sensation. In addition, alterations in swallowing are more common in older people without teeth because they tend to swallow larger pieces of food. Swallowing takes 50 to 100 percent longer, probably because of subtle changes in the swallowing mechanism. Peristalsis is decreased and the esophageal sphincter is less effective.

In general, the gastrointestinal system shows less age-associated change in function than other body systems. Stomach contractions appear to be normal, but it does take longer to empty liquids from the stomach. The amount of stomach acid secretions decreases, probably because of the loss of the cells that produce gastric acid. There is usually a small amount of atrophy to the lining of the small intestine. In the large intestine, expect to see atrophy of the lining, changes in the muscle layer, and blood vessel abnormalities. Approximately one of every three people over 60 has diverticula, or outpouchings, in the lining of the large intestine resulting from increased pressure inside the intestine. Weakness in the bowel wall also may be a contributing factor.

The number of some opiate receptors increases with aging, which may lead to significant constipation when narcotics are ingested. Changes may occur in the metabolism and in absorption of some sugars, calcium, and iron. Highly fat-soluble compounds such as vitamin A appear to be absorbed faster with age. The activity of some enzymes such as lactase—which aids in the digestion of some sugars, particularly those found in dairy products—appears to decrease. The absorption of fat also may change, and the metabolism of specific compounds, including drugs, can be significantly prolonged in elderly people.

Renal System

With aging, there is a 25 to 30 percent decrease in kidney mass. About 50 percent of nephrons are lost and abnormal glomeruli are more common. Reduced kidney function leads to a decreased clearance of some drugs and decreased elimination. The kidney's hormonal response to dehydration is reduced as is the ability to retain salt under conditions when it should be conserved. The ability of the kidneys to modify vitamin D to a more active form may also lessen.

The Senses

Taste buds diminish during this stage of life, which leads to a loss of taste sensation. Smell declines rapidly after the age of 50 and the parts of the brain involved in smell degenerate significantly so that by age 80, the detection of smell is almost 50 percent poorer than it was at its peak. Since taste and smell work together to make enjoyment of food possible, appetite often declines. Response to painful stimuli is diminished as is kinesthetic sense, or the ability to sense movement.

Visual acuity and reaction time is diminished, and there are actual changes in the organs of hearing. The ear canal atrophies, the eardrum thickens, and there may be degenerative and even arthritic changes in the small joints connecting the bones in the middle ear. Significant changes take place in the inner ear. These changes in structure significantly affect hearing. Hearing loss for pure tones, which increases with age in men and women, is called "presbycusis." With presbycusis, higher frequencies become less audible than lower frequencies. Pitch discrimination plays an important role in speech perception so, with age, speech discrimination declines. When exposed to loud background noise or indistinct speech, older people hear less, but at the same time, they may be very sensitive to loud sounds.

Nervous System

With aging, there is a decrease of neurotransmitters and a loss of neurons in the cerebellum, which controls coordination, and the hippocampus, which is involved in some aspects of memory function. The sleep-wake cycle also is disrupted, causing older adults to have sleep problems.

PSYCHOSOCIAL DEVELOPMENT

While disease may reduce physical and mental capabilities, the ability to learn and adjust continues throughout life, and is greatly influenced by interests, activity, motivation, health, and income (Figure 12-9 ■). However, there is a **terminal-drop hypothesis** that there is a decrease in cognitive functioning over a 5-year period prior to death. The individual may or may not be aware of diffuse changes in mood, mental functioning, or the way his body responds.

terminal-drop hypothesis *a theory that death is preceded by a 5-year period of decreasing cognitive functioning.*

Housing

While most older adults would rather stay in their own homes, it is not always possible because home-care services are not affordably available in all communities as a viable alternative to nursing homes. Home-care services usually provide assistance with household chores such as preparing meals, cleaning and laundry, and performing personal care tasks such as feeding and bathing. Health care services in the home are provided by nurses and physical or speech therapists. In order to be eligible for these services under Medicare, the patient must be home-bound, need an intensive level of services, and be expected to benefit from such services over a reasonable amount of time. Home-care services are usually time-limited.

An alternative to home-care services is "assisted living," or living in a facility that offers a combination of home care and nursing home facilities. There is a greater sense of control, independence, and privacy because the older adult has more choices while still being in an institutional setting. Bedrooms and bathrooms can be locked by residents, but dining and recreational facilities are usually shared.

About 95 percent of older adults live in communities, from simple groupings of homes where mostly older adults live to a relatively new type of living arrangement called the "continuing-care retirement community." The appeal of these communities is that future health care needs are covered in a setting that is an attractive residential campus where cultural and recreational activities are available. Entrance fees to this type of community may be as much as $250,000, plus monthly fees which average $1,000.

Challenges

One of the major challenges for the older adult is maintaining a sense of self-worth. Senior citizens are commonly seen as "over the hill," less intelligent than younger

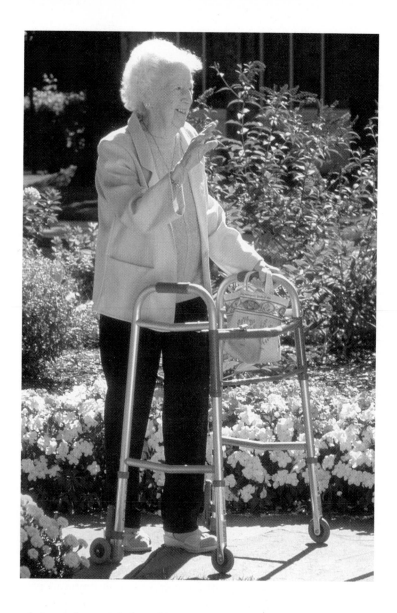

■ Figure 12-9   The ability to learn and adjust continues throughout life.

It is not until adults reach the age of 40 that ill health—as opposed to accidents, homicide, and suicide—becomes the major cause of death.

adults, and certainly less able to care for themselves. Many older adults are forced into retirement because they are seen as less productive. In reality, although older workers may have slowed down a bit, they are often more concerned with producing quality work than younger workers. Another problem older adults face at this stage of life is a feeling of declining well-being. It is not until adults reach the age of 40 that ill health—as opposed to accidents, homicide, and suicide—becomes the major cause of death. Arteriosclerotic heart disease is the major killer after the age of 40 in all age, sex, and racial groups.

Financial Burdens

The duration of each state in the life cycle, and the ages of family members for each stage, will vary from family to family. Obviously, this will have an effect on the financial status of families. For example, a couple who completes their family while in their early adult years will have a different lifestyle when their last child leaves home than a couple with a "change-of-life" child. Late children can cause serious economic problems for retirees on fixed incomes who are trying to meet the staggering costs of education.

Retirement brings about changes for both spouses, but it seems to be particularly stressful for those wives who are not prepared emotionally or financially. Retirement usually means a decrease in income and in the standard of living, which can be very difficult to handle.

A decreasing level of interest in work is natural as one grows older, but it has a severe impact on the income of older people. Almost 22 percent of all older people live in households below the poverty level. More than 50 percent of all single women above the age of 60 live at or below the poverty level. Older women in the United States make up the single poorest group in our society.

Dying Companions or Death

Whether it is the death of a companion or one's own impending death, fear and grief seem to have a great deal in common. Grief not only follows death, but when there is advance warning, grief may well precede death. Frequently, the death or impending death of a companion leads us to fear for our own lives. Psychiatrist Elisabeth Kübler-Ross believes that regardless of whether it is one's own death or the death of a companion, everyone must go through certain emotions. While the five stages in her theory may sometimes overlap, everyone must deal with each of the stages of death before the grieving process ends. (Review Chapter 2 for Kübler-Ross's five stages.)

Note: Human physiological and psychosocial development will be discussed in more detail in Volume 2, *Patient Assessment;* Volume 3, *Medical Emergencies;* Volume 4, *Trauma Emergencies;* and in Volume 5, *Special Considerations/Operations,* the chapters on neonatology, pediatrics, geriatrics, and the challenged patient.

Summary

The changes that take place during the span of a lifetime are innumerable. At some stages, the changes seem to occur almost daily. It is only through experience with patients at all of the various stages of life that you will come to feel comfortable dealing with each of them. Remember that no matter what the stage of development, patience and a sincere desire to help a patient will help you to make the right decisions about emergency care.

You Make the Call

You are dispatched to respond to a patient who is complaining of abdominal pain. When you arrive at the scene, you are met at the door by a middle-aged man who tells you the patient is his daughter. She is upstairs in her bedroom, and her mother is with her. You climb the stairs, followed closely by the father. When you enter the bedroom, you find a 16-year-old female lying on the bed. Her mother is sitting beside her, holding a damp cloth to her forehead. A younger sister is hovering around, trying to help.

The mother tells you that the patient woke about an hour ago, crying that her stomach hurt. The pain has gotten progressively worse over the last hour, and the patient has been complaining of nausea as well.

You begin your assessment of the patient, but she will not allow you to examine her abdomen. When you attempt to ask questions about what led up to this pain, the date of her last menstrual period, whether or not she could possibly be pregnant, she refuses to answer you, shifting her eyes toward her parents and sister who are still in the room. Her mother tells her to please answer your questions, but the patient just begins to cry.

1. Do you believe that this is normal behavior for a patient of this age and in this particular situation?
2. What is a likely reason for this behavior?
3. What might you do to make this patient more cooperative?

See Suggested Responses at the back of this book.

Review Questions

1. At birth, the heart rate ranges from _____ to _____ beats per minute during the first 30 minutes of life.
   a. 90–120
   b. 100–120
   c. 100–180
   d. 160–240

2. The infant's head is equal to _____ percent of total body weight.
   a. 10
   b. 15
   c. 20
   d. 25

3. The _____ _____, a blood vessel that connects the pulmonary artery and the aorta in the fetus, constricts after birth.
   a. ductus venosus
   b. foramen ovale
   c. ductus arteriosus
   d. ligamentum venosum

4. The _____ _____, which is sometimes referred to as the "startle reflex," is the characteristic reflex of newborns.
   a. Moro reflex
   b. rooting reflex
   c. sucking grasp
   d. palmar grasp

5. _____ parents encourage independence but will enforce rules.
   a. mutual
   b. permissive
   c. authoritative
   d. authoritarian

6. In this stage of moral development, children are concerned with interpersonal norms, seeking the approval of others, and developing the "good boy" or "good girl" mentality.
   a. permissive reasoning
   b. conventional reasoning
   c. preconventional reasoning
   d. postconventional reasoning

7. The theoretical, species-specific, longest duration of life, excluding premature or "unnatural" death, is:
   a. life expectancy.
   b. early adulthood.
   c. maximum life span.
   d. middle adulthood.

8. As adults reach the age of _____, ill health—as opposed to accidents, homicide, and suicide—becomes the major cause of death.
   a. 25
   b. 30
   c. 40
   d. 60

See Answers to Review Questions at the back of this book.

Further Reading

Bowlby, J. *A Secure Base: Parent-Child Attachment and Healthy Human Development.* Philadelphia: Basic Books, Inc., 1990.

Dacey, J., J. Travers, and D. Neuki. *Human Development Across the Lifespan.* 5th ed. Dubuque, IA: McGraw Hill, 2004.

Dickenson, E. T., et al. "Geriatric Utilization of Emergency Medical Services." *Annals of Emergency Medicine* 27(2) (1996): 199–203.

Hole, J. W., Jr. *Hole's Human Anatomy and Physiology.* 9th ed. Dubuque, IA: McGraw Hill, 2002.

Williams, M. E., M. D. *The American Geriatrics Society's Complete Guide to Aging and Health.* New York: Harmony Books, 1995.

On the Web

Visit Brady's Paramedic Website at **www.bradybooks.com/paramedic.**

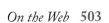

Airway Management and Ventilation

Objectives

After reading this chapter, you should be able to:

1. Explain the primary objective of airway maintenance. (p. 508)
2. Identify commonly neglected prehospital skills related to the airway. (p. 538)
3. Describe the anatomy and function of the upper and lower airway structures in detail, including landmarks for direct laryngoscopy. (pp. 509–515)
4. Explain the differences between adult and pediatric airway anatomy. (pp. 514–515)
5. Discuss the following functions of the respiratory system:
   ★Mechanics of ventilation (pp. 516–517)
   ★Pulmonary circulation (p. 517)
   ★Gas exchange in the lungs (pp. 517–520)
   ★Diffusion of the respiratory gases (p. 519)
6. Describe oxygen transport in the blood and factors that affect it. (pp. 519–520)
7. Describe carbon dioxide transport in the blood and factors that affect it. (p. 520)
8. Describe the voluntary and involuntary regulation of respiration. (pp. 521–522)
9. List the concentration of gases that comprise atmospheric air. (pp. 517–518)

10. Describe the various measures of respiratory function, and give the average normal values for each, including the normal respiratory rates for the adult, child, and infant. (pp. 522–523)

11. Describe assessment of the airway and the respiratory system. (pp. 525–537)

12. Describe the modified forms of respiration and list the factors that affect respiratory rate and depth. (pp. 528–529)

13. Discuss the methods for measuring oxygen and carbon dioxide in the blood and their prehospital use. (pp. 531–537)

14. Define and explain the implications of partial airway obstruction with good and poor air exchange and complete airway obstruction. (p. 523)

15. Describe the common causes of upper airway obstruction, including:
    ★ The tongue (pp. 523–524)
    ★ Foreign body aspiration (p. 524)
    ★ Laryngeal spasm (p. 524)
    ★ Laryngeal edema (p. 524)
    ★ Trauma (p. 524)

16. Describe complete airway obstruction maneuvers, including:
    ★ Heimlich maneuver (p. 587)
    ★ Removal with Magill forceps (p. 587)

17. Describe causes of respiratory distress, including:
    ★ Upper and lower airway obstruction (pp. 523–525)
    ★ Inadequate ventilation (p. 525)
    ★ Impairment of respiratory muscles (pp. 516–517)
    ★ Impairment of nervous system (pp. 516–517)

18. Explain the risk of infection to EMS providers associated with airway management and ventilation. (p. 603)

19. Describe manual airway maneuvers, including:
    ★ Head-tilt/chin-lift maneuver (pp. 538–539)
    ★ Jaw-thrust maneuver (pp. 539–540)
    ★ Modified jaw-thrust maneuver (p. 540)

20. Discuss the indications, contraindications, advantages, disadvantages, complications, special considerations, equipment, and techniques of the following:
    ★ Upper airway and tracheobronchial suctioning (pp. 597–600)
    ★ Nasogastric and orogastric tube insertion (p. 600)
    ★ Oropharyngeal and nasopharyngeal airway (pp. 542–546)
    ★ Ventilating a patient by mouth-to-mouth, mouth-to-nose, mouth-to-mask, one-, two-, or three-person bag-valve mask, flow-restricted oxygen-powered ventilation device, and automatic transport ventilator (pp. 602–607)

21. Compare the ventilation techniques used for an adult patient to those used for pediatric patients, and describe special considerations in airway management and ventilation for the pediatric patient. (pp. 572–576, 605)

22. Identify types of oxygen cylinders and pressure regulators, and explain safety considerations of oxygen storage and delivery, including steps for delivering oxygen from a cylinder and regulator. (p. 601)

23. Describe the indications, contraindications, advantages, disadvantages, complications, liter flow range, and concentration of delivered oxygen for the following supplemental oxygen delivery devices (pp. 601–602)
    ★ Nasal cannula
    ★ Simple face mask
    ★ Partial rebreather mask
    ★ Nonrebreather mask
    ★ Venturi mask

24. Describe the use, advantages, and disadvantages of an oxygen humidifier. (p. 602)

25. Describe the indications, contraindications, advantages, disadvantages, complications, equipment, and technique for the following:
    ★ Endotracheal intubation by direct laryngoscopy (pp. 546–563, 572–576)
    ★ Digital endotracheal intubation (pp. 563–566)
    ★ Dual lumen airway (pp. 580–584)
    ★ Nasotracheal intubation (pp. 576–579)
    ★ Rapid sequence intubation (pp. 568–572)
    ★ Endotracheal intubation using sedation (pp. 568–572)
    ★ Open cricothyrotomy (pp. 592–596)
    ★ Needle cricothyrotomy (translaryngeal catheter ventilation) (pp. 588–592)
    ★ Extubation (pp. 579–580)

26. Describe the use of cricoid pressure during intubation. (pp. 541–542)

27. Discuss the precautions that should be taken when intubating the trauma patient. (pp. 566–568)

28. Discuss agents used for sedation and rapid sequence intubation. (pp. 569–571)

29. Discuss methods to confirm correct placement of the endotracheal tube. (pp. 559–563)

30. Define the following: gag reflex, atelectasis, FiO_2, hypoxia, hypoxemia, pulsus paradoxus, gastric distention, Sellick maneuver, and laryngectomy. (pp. 511, 512, 514, 520, 521, 528, 529, 596, 600)

Key Terms

Case Study

Ellis County Unit 947 is dispatched to a motor vehicle collision on rural County Road 664, approximately 8 miles from town. This particular stretch of road is well known to paramedics because of a number of serious crashes over the last several months. The road contains numerous sharp curves and is under construction in several locations. Today, Unit 947 is staffed by paramedics Crystal Jernigan and Charles Allen. In addition, paramedic student Sharon Rodriquez is assigned to the unit for her paramedic field internship.

On arrival at the scene, they find one vehicle that has apparently run off the road and struck a telephone pole. Witnesses to the crash estimate the vehicle was traveling at approximately 45 miles per hour before striking the pole. The lone 24-year-old male occupant was ejected from the vehicle and lies face down in a ditch approximately 50 feet from the car. After assuring scene safety and donning the appropriate body substance isolation (BSI) measures, Crystal assesses the patient. She finds him to be unresponsive. Charles and Sharon help her to log-roll the patient to a supine position with cervical-spine precautions applied. Sharon holds in-line cervical spine stabilization while Crystal opens the airway with the modified jaw-thrust technique.

The patient exhibits agonal respirations. In addition, gurgling noises are heard with each breath. After suctioning bloody secretions from his mouth, Crystal attempts to insert an oropharyngeal airway. However, the patient's teeth are tightly clenched and the airway will not pass. Crystal provides ventilatory support with a bag-valve-mask unit and 100 percent oxygen. The Glasgow Coma Score is 5. In anticipation of endotracheal intubation, the cardiac monitor and pulse oximeter are applied. An IV of lactated Ringer's is established. Because the patient's jaws remain tightly clenched, satisfactory control of the airway cannot be obtained. Crystal decides to perform rapid-sequence intubation to obtain a definitive airway. The equipment and supplies are readied. As they prepare for the procedure, Charles applies the Sellick maneuver while Sharon continues to hold cervical spine stabilization.

One-hundred milligrams of lidocaine and five milligrams of midazolam (Versed) are administered intravenously as directed in the system's prehospital standing orders. Following this, 100 milligrams of succinylcholine (Anectine) are administered through the IV. After approximately 90 seconds, adequate neuromuscular blockade is obtained. Crystal quickly suctions the airway and inserts an 8.0-mm endotracheal tube under direct visualization. The tube easily passes through the vocal cords. The cuff is inflated and an end-tidal CO_2 detector is connected to the endotracheal tube. The patient is ventilated with a bag-valve device and 100 percent oxygen. Auscultation of the chest reveals bilateral, symmetrical breath sounds and the absence of breath sounds over the epigastrium (the area over the patient's stomach). In addition, there is a color change on the end-tidal CO_2 detector and a continuously improving pulse oximetry reading, all of which help confirm endotracheal placement of the tube.

While Crystal secures the tube, the initial assessment is completed and a rapid trauma exam is conducted. The patient is placed into a cervical collar and secured to a backboard, while assessment and treatment continue. The patient has no obvious injuries. His blood pressure is 150/90 and his pulse rate is 64. Respirations are being assisted at a rate of 20 breaths per minute. With mechanical ventilation, pulse oximetry reveals an oxygen saturation reading of 98 percent. The finger stick glucose is 88 mg/dL. ALS unit 947 transports the patient to the emergency department without further incident.

Following the initial emergency department assessment, a nonenhanced computed tomography (CT) scan of the brain is obtained. The patient is found to have a large subdural hematoma that requires emergent surgical drainage. Following surgery, the patient regains consciousness. He spends 24 hours in the ICU and is then moved to a regular hospital room. The paramedics stop by the hospital and visit on their next duty shift. The patient has no recall of the crash whatsoever. The last thing he remembers is looking on the floor of the car for a CD that he dropped. One week after the crash, he is discharged with no neurologic deficits.

Airway management and ventilation are the first and most critical steps in the initial assessment of every patient you will encounter.

Your deliberate and precise use of simple, basic airway skills is the key to successful airway management and good patient outcome.

INTRODUCTION

Airway management and ventilation are the first and most critical steps in the initial assessment of every patient you will encounter. You must immediately establish and maintain an open airway while providing adequate oxygen delivery and carbon dioxide elimination for all patients. Without adequate airway maintenance and ventilation, the patient will succumb to brain injury or even death in as little as 6 to 10 minutes. Early detection and intervention of airway and breathing problems, including bystander action, are vital to patient survival.

Your deliberate and precise use of simple, basic airway skills is the key to successful airway management and good patient outcome. Once you have applied the basic airway techniques to properly provide oxygenation and ventilation for your patient, you can use more sophisticated airway maneuvers and skills to further stabilize his airway. You must continually monitor and reassess the airway, being careful to watch for displacement of the endotracheal tube, mucous plugging, equipment failure, or the development of a pneumothorax.

This chapter will provide the information and skills you will need to manage even the most difficult airway. It begins with a review of the respiratory system's anatomy and physiology and then explores the initial assessment and management of the airway and ventilation. Finally it details enhanced airway management options for the more experienced paramedic.

ANATOMY OF THE RESPIRATORY SYSTEM

The respiratory system provides a passage for **oxygen,** a gas necessary for energy production, to enter the body and for **carbon dioxide,** a waste product of the body's metabolism, to exit. This gas exchange, called **respiration,** requires a patent, open airway as well as adequate respiratory function. Many pathological processes can inhibit respiration. To understand the interventions that you will use to maintain adequate airway and ventilatory function, you must thoroughly understand the anatomy of the upper and lower airway.

UPPER AIRWAY ANATOMY

The *upper airway* extends from the mouth and nose to the larynx (Figure 13-1 ■). It includes the nasal cavity, oral cavity, and pharynx. The larynx joins the upper and lower airways.

oxygen   *gas necessary for energy production.*

carbon dioxide   *waste product of the body's metabolism.*

respiration   *the exchange of gases between a living organism and its environment.*

✓ **Review**

Content

Upper Airway Components

- Nasal cavity
- Oral cavity
- Pharynx

■ Figure 13-1   Anatomy of the upper airway.

NASAL CAVITY

— Superior, middle and inferior turbinates

— Hard and soft palates

NASOPHARYNX

— Tonsils/adenoids

— Uvula

OROPHARYNX

— Tongue

LARYNGOPHARYNX (HYPOPHARYNX)

— Vallecula

— Epiglottis

LARYNX

— Esophagus

— Trachea

Glottic opening

Vocal cords

Thyroid cartilage

Cricothyroid membrane

Cricoid cartilage

Thyroid gland

The Nasal Cavity

The nasal cavity is the most superior part of the airway. The maxillary, frontal, nasal, ethmoid, and sphenoid bones comprise the lateral and superior walls of the nasal cavity. The hard palate forms the floor of the nasal cavity. The cartilaginous and highly vascular nasal **septum** separates the right and left nasal cavities.

Several different structures connect with the nasal cavity. These include the sinuses, the eustachian tubes, and the lacrimal ducts. The **sinuses** are air-filled cavities that are lined with a mucous membrane. There are four pairs of sinuses: the ethmoid sinuses, the frontal sinuses, the maxillary sinuses, and the sphenoid sinuses. The sinuses, named for the bone where they are contained, help reduce the overall weight of the head and are thought to assist in heating, purifying, and moistening the inhaled air. The sinuses help trap bacteria entering the nasal cavity. Because of this, they can become infected. Fractures of the upper sinuses (sphenoids) can occasionally cause cerebrospinal fluid (CSF) to leak from the cranial cavity into the nasal cavity. Clinically this presents with clear fluid draining from the nose (rhinorrhea) and can provide a direct route for the transmission of pathogens to the brain and associated structures. The **eustachian tubes,** or auditory tubes, connect the ear with the nasal cavity and allow for equalization of pressure on each side of the tympanic membrane. Swallowing can assist in equalizing this pressure. The **nasolacrimal ducts** drain tears and debris from the eyes into the nasal cavity. This can cause the nose to run when someone cries.

Air enters the nasal cavity through the external **nares** (nostrils). Nasal hairs just inside the external nares initially filter the incoming air. The air then proceeds into the nasal cavity, where it strikes three bony projections, the superior, middle, and inferior turbinates, or conchae. These shelflike structures, which are parallel to the nasal floor, serve as conduits into the sinuses, increase the surface area of the nasal cavity, and cause turbulent airflow. This turbulence helps to filter the air by depositing airborne particles on the **mucous membrane** lining the nasal cavity. Hairlike fibers called cilia propel those trapped particles to the back of the pharynx, where they are swallowed. Because the mucous membrane is covered with **mucus** and has a rich blood supply, it also immediately warms and humidifies the air entering the nose. By the time the air reaches the lower airway, it is at body temperature (37° C), 100 percent humidified, and virtually free of airborne particles. Air proceeds from the nasal cavity through internal nares into the nasopharynx.

The tissue of the nasal cavity is extremely delicate and vascular. Because of this, it is susceptible to trauma. Always remember that improper or overly aggressive placement of tubes or mechanical airways can cause significant bleeding that direct pressure might not control.

The Oral Cavity

The cheeks, the hard and soft palates, and the tongue form the mouth, or oral cavity. The lips that surround the mouth's opening are fleshy folds of skin. Behind the lips lie the gums and teeth, normally numbering 32 in the adult. Significant force is required to avulse (dislodge) or fracture the teeth. Broken or dislodged teeth can potentially obstruct the airway. The hard palate anteriorly and the soft palate posteriorly form the top of the oral cavity and separate it from the nasal cavity. The tongue, a large muscle on the bottom of the oral cavity, is the most common airway obstruction. It attaches to the mandible and the hyoid bone through a series of muscles and ligaments. The U-shaped hyoid bone is located just beneath the chin. The hyoid bone is unique. It is the only bone in the axial skeleton that does not articulate with any other bone. Instead, it is suspended by ligaments from the styloid process of the temporal bone and serves to anchor the tongue and larynx, as well as to support the trachea.

septum *cartilage that separates the right and left nasal cavities.*

sinus *air cavity that conducts fluids from the eustachian tubes and tear ducts to and from the nasopharynx.*

eustachian tube *a tube that connects the ear with the nasal cavity.*

nasolacrimal ducts *tubular vessels that drain tears and debris from the eyes into the nasal cavity.*

nare *nostril.*

mucous membrane *lining in body cavities that handle air transport; usually contains small, mucous-secreting cells.*

mucus *slippery secretion that lubricates and protects airway surfaces.*

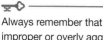

Always remember that improper or overly aggressive placement of tubes or mechanical airways can cause significant bleeding that direct pressure might not control.

The Pharynx

The **pharynx** is a muscular tube that extends vertically from the back of the soft palate to the superior aspect of the esophagus. It allows the air to flow into and out of the respiratory tract and food and liquids to pass into the digestive system. It contains several openings, including the internal nares, the mouth, the larynx, and the esophagus.

The pharynx is divided into three regions: the nasopharynx, the oropharynx, and the laryngopharynx (hypopharynx). The nasopharynx is the uppermost region, extending from the back of the nasal opening to the plane of the soft palate. The oropharynx extends from the plane of the soft palate to the hyoid bone. The adenoids, lymphatic tissue in the mouth and nose, filter bacteria. Either hypertrophy or swelling of the adenoids from infection may make them large enough to obscure your view. The laryngopharynx extends posteriorly from the hyoid bone to the esophagus and anteriorly to the larynx. The laryngopharynx is especially important in airway management.

Because the mouth and pharynx serve dual purposes for respiration and digestion, a number of mechanisms help prevent accidental blockage. To prevent foreign material from entering the trachea and lungs, sensitive nerves activate the body's cough and swallowing mechanisms as well as the **gag reflex.**

Located anteriorly in the hypopharynx is the epiglottis, a leaf-shaped cartilage that prevents food from entering the respiratory tract during swallowing. Just anterior and superior to the epiglottis is the **vallecula,** a fold formed by the base of the tongue and the epiglottis. It is an important landmark for endotracheal **intubation.** A series of ligaments and muscles connect the epiglottis to the hyoid bone and mandible. Immediately behind the hypopharynx are the fourth and fifth cervical vertebral bodies.

The Larynx

The **larynx** is the complex structure that joins the pharynx with the trachea (Figure 13-2 ▦). Lying midline in the neck, it is attached to and lies just inferior to the hyoid bone and anterior to the esophagus. It consists of the thyroid and cricoid cartilage (both considered tracheal cartilage), glottic opening, vocal cords, arytenoid cartilage, pyriform fossae, and cricothyroid membrane.

The main laryngeal cartilage is the shield-shaped thyroid cartilage. Larger in males than in females, the thyroid cartilage forms the anterior prominence called the Adam's apple. The arytenoid cartilage, which forms a pyramid-shaped attachment for the vocal cords posteriorly, is an important landmark for endotracheal intubation. Posteriorly,

pharynx *a muscular tube that extends vertically from the back of the soft palate to the superior aspect of the esophagus.*

 Review

Regions of Pharynx

- Nasopharynx
- Oropharynx
- Laryngopharynx

gag reflex *mechanism that stimulates retching, or striving to vomit, when the soft palate is touched.*

vallecula *depression between the epiglottis and the base of the tongue.*

intubation *passing a tube into a body opening.*

larynx *the complex structure that joins the pharynx with the trachea.*

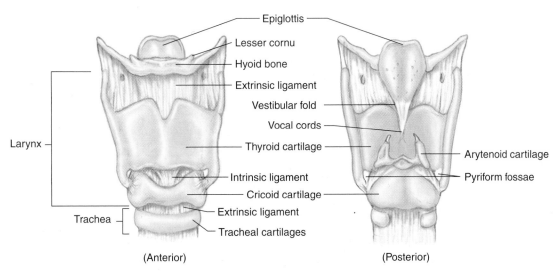

Epiglottis
Lesser cornu
Hyoid bone
Extrinsic ligament
Vestibular fold
Vocal cords
Thyroid cartilage
Intrinsic ligament
Cricoid cartilage
Extrinsic ligament
Tracheal cartilages
Larynx
Trachea
Arytenoid cartilage
Pyriform fossae
(Anterior)
(Posterior)

▦ Figure 13-2   Internal anatomy of the upper airway.

glottis *liplike opening between the vocal cords.*

Sellick maneuver *pressure applied in a posterior direction to the anterior cricoid cartilage; occludes the esophagus.*

aspiration *inhaling foreign material such as vomitus into the lungs.*

cricothyroid membrane *membrane between the cricoid and thyroid cartilages of the larynx.*

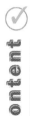

Review

Lower Airway Components

- Trachea
- Bronchi
- Alveoli
- Lung parenchyma
- Pleura

trachea *10- to 12-cm long tube that connects the larynx to the mainstem bronchi.*

smooth muscle closes a gap in the thyroid cartilage. Directly behind the Adam's apple, the thyroid cartilage houses the glottic opening, the narrowest part of the adult trachea, which is bordered by the vocal cords. The patency of the glottic opening, or **glottis,** depends heavily on muscle tone. On either side of the glottic opening are the pyriform fossae, recesses that form the lateral borders of the larynx. The thyrohyoid membrane attaches the upper end of the thyroid cartilage to the hyoid bone.

Within the laryngeal cavity lie the true vocal cords, white bands of cartilage that regulate the passage of air through the larynx and produce voice by contraction of the laryngeal muscles. The vocal cords can also close together to prevent foreign bodies from entering the airway. The passage of an endotracheal tube between the vocal cords interferes not only with the creation of sound, but also with the protective function of coughing.

Beneath the thyroid cartilage is the cricoid cartilage, which forms the inferior border of the larynx. Often it is considered the first tracheal ring. Unlike the thyroid and other tracheal cartilages, whose posterior surfaces are open and not fused, the cricoid cartilage forms a complete ring. The esophagus lies behind the cricoid cartilage, so pressure applied in a posterior direction to the anterior cricoid cartilage occludes the esophagus (**Sellick maneuver**), thus inhibiting vomiting and subsequent **aspiration** during airway management. In children, the cricoid cartilage is the narrowest part of the laryngeal airway. The fibrous **cricothyroid membrane** connects the inferior border of the thyroid cartilage with the superior aspect of the cricoid cartilage. It is the site for surgical airway techniques.

A mucous membrane lines most of the larynx. Rich with nerve endings from the vagus nerve, it is so sensitive that any irritation sparks a cough, or forceful exhalation of a large volume of air. First, air is drawn into the respiratory passageways. Next, the glottic opening shuts tightly, trapping the air within the lungs. Then the abdominal and thoracic muscles contract, pushing against the diaphragm and increasing intrathoracic pressure. The vocal cords suddenly open, and a burst of air forces foreign particles out of the lungs. The laryngeal mucous membrane is so sensitive that its stimulation by a laryngoscope or endotracheal tube can cause bradycardia (slow pulse rate), hypotension (low blood pressure), and decreased respiratory rate.

Other structures proximate to the larynx and of particular interest when you perform surgical airways are the thyroid gland, carotid arteries, and jugular veins. The thyroid gland is a "bow-tie" shaped endocrine gland located in the neck. It is highly vascular and lies inferior to the cricoid cartilage. It contains two lobes, one on each side of the trachea. These lobes are joined in the middle by the isthmus that extends across the trachea. The carotid arteries run closely along the trachea. Several branches of the carotid arteries cross the trachea. Likewise, the jugular veins lie very close to the trachea. Several branches of the jugular veins, such as the superior thyroid vein, cross the trachea.

LOWER AIRWAY ANATOMY

The lower airway extends from below the larynx to the alveoli (Figure 13-3 ■). This is where the respiratory exchange of oxygen and carbon dioxide occurs. Helpful landmarks are the fourth cervical vertebra at the posterior superior border, and the xiphoid process anterior inferiorly, though the posterior lung extends beyond this inferiorly.

The Trachea

As air enters the lower airway from the upper airway, it first enters and then passes through the **trachea.** The trachea is a 10- to 12-centimeter-long tube that connects the larynx to the two mainstem bronchi. It contains cartilaginous, C-shaped, open rings that form a frame to keep it open. The trachea is lined with respiratory epithelium containing cilia and mucous-producing cells. The mucus traps particles that the upper airway did not filter. The cilia then move the trapped particulate matter up into the mouth where it is swallowed or expelled.

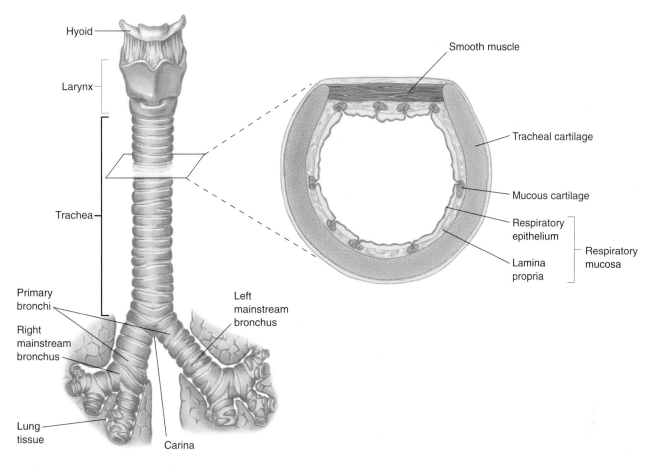

Labels on figure:
Hyoid
Larynx
Trachea
Primary bronchi
Right mainstream bronchus
Lung tissue
Carina
Left mainstream bronchus
Smooth muscle
Tracheal cartilage
Mucous cartilage
Respiratory epithelium
Lamina propria
Respiratory mucosa

■ Figure 13-3   Anatomy of the lower airway.

The Bronchi

At the carina, the trachea divides, or bifurcates, into the right and left mainstem **bronchi.** The right mainstem bronchus is almost straight, while the left mainstem bronchus angles more acutely to the left. Because of this, the right mainstem is often the site of aspirated foreign bodies. In addition, when an endotracheal tube is inserted too far, it tends to enter the right mainstem bronchus, thus ventilating only the right lung. Mainstem bronchi enter the lung tissue at the hilum, and then divide into the secondary and tertiary bronchi. The secondary and tertiary bronchi ultimately branch into the bronchioles, or small airways. The bronchioles are encircled with smooth muscle that contains beta-2 (β_2) adrenergic receptors. When stimulated, these beta-2 receptors relax the bronchial smooth muscle, thus increasing the airway's diameter. This bronchodilation can increase the amount of air transported through the bronchiole. Conversely, parasympathetic receptors, when stimulated, cause the bronchial smooth muscles to contract, thus reducing the diameter of the bronchiole. This bronchoconstriction can inhibit the movement of air through the bronchiole.

After approximately 22 divisions, the bronchioles turn into the respiratory bronchioles. These structures contain only muscular connective tissue and have a limited capacity for gas exchange. The respiratory bronchioles terminate at the alveoli.

The Alveoli

The respiratory bronchioles divide into the alveolar ducts, which terminate in balloon-like clusters of **alveoli** called alveolar sacs (Figure 13-4 ■). The alveoli contain an alveolar membrane that is only one or two cell layers thick. Because of this, the alveoli comprise the key functional unit of the respiratory system. Most oxygen and carbon

bronchi *tubes from the trachea into the lungs.*

alveoli *microscopic air sacs where most oxygen and carbon dioxide gas exchanges take place.*

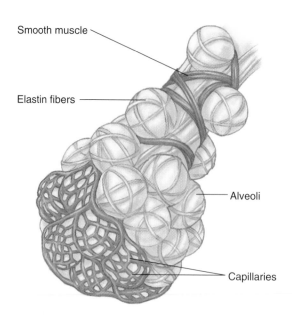

■ Figure 13-4 Anatomy of the alveoli.

Smooth muscle

Elastin fibers

Alveoli

Capillaries

dioxide gas exchanges take place here, although limited gas exchange may occur in the alveolar ducts and respiratory bronchioles. The alveoli become thinner as they expand. This facilitates diffusion of oxygen and carbon dioxide. The alveoli's surface area is massive, totaling more than 40 square meters—enough to cover half of a tennis court. These hollow structures resist collapse largely because of the presence of surfactant, a chemical that decreases their surface tension and makes it easier for them to expand. Alveolar collapse (**atelectasis**) can occur if surfactant is insufficient or if the alveoli are not inflated. No gas exchange takes place in atelectatic alveoli.

atelectasis   alveolar collapse.

The Lung Parenchyma

The alveoli are the terminal ends of the respiratory tree and the functional units of the lungs. As such, they are the core of the lung **parenchyma.** The lung parenchyma is arranged in two pulmonary lobules that form the anatomic division of the lungs. These lobules are further organized into lobes. The right lung has three lobes, the upper lobe, the middle lobe, and the lower lobe. The left lung, which shares thoracic space with the heart, has only two lobes, the upper lobe and the lower lobe.

parenchyma   principal or essential parts of an organ.

The Pleura

Membranous connective tissue called **pleura** covers the lungs. The pleura consists of two layers, visceral and parietal. The visceral pleura envelopes the lungs and does not contain nerve fibers. In contrast, the parietal pleura lines the thoracic cavity and does contain nerve fibers. The potential space between these two layers, called the pleural space, usually holds a small amount of fluid that reduces friction between the pleural layers during respiration. Occasionally, the pleura can become inflamed, causing significant pain with respiration. This condition, called pleurisy, is a common cause of chest pain, particularly in cigarette smokers.

pleura   membranous connective tissue covering the lungs.

THE PEDIATRIC AIRWAY

The pediatric airway is fundamentally the same as an adult's, but you will need to know the differences in relative size and position of some components. The airway is smaller in all aspects, particularly the diameters of the openings and passageways.

In the pharynx, the jaw is smaller and the tongue relatively larger, resulting in greater potential airway encroachment (Figure 13-5 ■). The epiglottis is much floppier

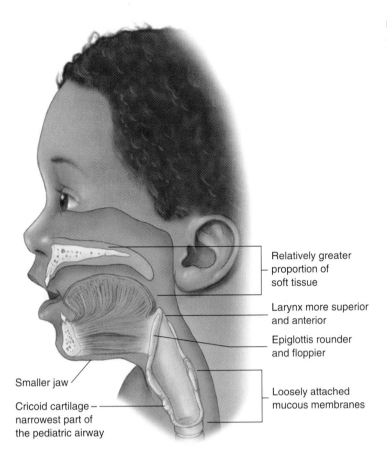

Relatively greater
proportion of
soft tissue

Larynx more superior
and anterior

Epiglottis rounder
and floppier

Smaller jaw

Loosely attached
mucous membranes

Cricoid cartilage –
narrowest part of
the pediatric airway

and rounder ("omega" shaped). The dental (alveolar) ridge and teeth are softer and more fragile than an adult's and potentially more subject to damage from airway maneuvers.

The larynx lies more superior and anterior in children and is funnel-shaped because the cricoid cartilage is undeveloped. Before the age of 10, the cricoid cartilage is the narrowest part of the airway. Most significantly, even a small foreign body or a limited degree of swelling in the pediatric airway can be life threatening. Because of this, young children tend to suffer more problems related to the trachea than do older children. A common example is croup (laryngotracheobronchitis), a viral infection that causes the soft tissues below the glottis to swell. This can reduce the diameter of the airway, potentially causing serious problems.

The ribs and the cartilage of the pediatric thoracic cage are softer and more pliable. This lack of rigidity lessens the thoracic wall's and accessory muscles' ability to assist lung expansion during inspiration. As a result, infants and children tend to rely more on their diaphragms for breathing. Always pay close attention to these differences when treating pediatric patients, especially those with respiratory complaints.

PHYSIOLOGY OF THE RESPIRATORY SYSTEM

Just as successful airway management requires a firm understanding of airway anatomy, a good outcome for these patients requires a working knowledge of the mechanics of oxygenation and ventilation. Your knowledge of normal respiratory physiology will lay the groundwork for your comprehension of important pathophysiology and will help you to determine which actions will assure optimal patient care.

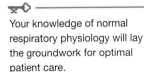

Your knowledge of normal respiratory physiology will lay the groundwork for optimal patient care.

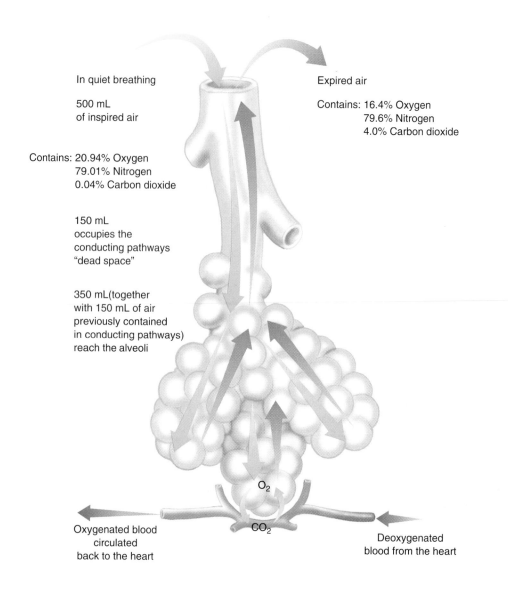

■ Figure 13-6   Diffusion of gases across an alveolar membrane.

In quiet breathing

500 mL
of inspired air

Contains: 20.94% Oxygen
79.01% Nitrogen
0.04% Carbon dioxide

150 mL
occupies the
conducting pathways
"dead space"

350 mL(together
with 150 mL of air
previously contained
in conducting pathways)
reach the alveoli

Expired air

Contains: 16.4% Oxygen
79.6% Nitrogen
4.0% Carbon dioxide

O_2

CO_2

Oxygenated blood
circulated
back to the heart

Deoxygenated
blood from the heart

RESPIRATION AND VENTILATION

Respiration is the exchange of gases between a living organism and its environment. Pulmonary, or external, respiration occurs in the lungs when the respiratory gases are exchanged between the alveoli and the red blood cells in the pulmonary capillaries through the capillary membranes (Figure 13-6 ■). Cellular, or internal, respiration, however, occurs in the peripheral capillaries. It is the exchange of the respiratory gases between the red blood cells and the various body tissues. Cellular respiration in the peripheral tissue produces carbon dioxide (CO_2). The blood picks up this waste product in the capillaries and transports it as bicarbonate ions through the venous system to the lungs. While respiration describes the process of gas exchange in the lungs and peripheral tissues, **ventilation** is the mechanical process that moves air into and out of the lungs. Ventilation is necessary for respiration to occur.

ventilation *the mechanical process that moves air into and out of the lungs.*

The Respiratory Cycle

Nothing within the lung parenchyma makes it contract or expand. Pulmonary ventilation, therefore, depends upon changes in pressure within the thoracic cavity. These changes occur in a respiratory cycle involving coordinated interaction among the respiratory system, the central nervous system, and the musculoskeletal system.

The thoracic cavity is a closed space, opening to the external environment only through the trachea. The diaphragm separates the thoracic cavity from the abdomen. When the diaphragm contracts, it draws downward, away from the thoracic cavity, thus enlarging it. Likewise, when the muscles between the ribs, or intercostal muscles, contract, they draw the rib cage upward and outward, away from the thoracic cavity, further increasing its volume.

The respiratory cycle begins when the lungs have achieved a normal expiration and the pressure inside the thoracic cavity equals the atmospheric pressure. At this point, respiratory centers in the brain communicate with the diaphragm by way of the phrenic nerve, signaling it to contract and thus initiate the respiratory cycle. As the size of the thorax increases in relation to the volume of air it holds, pressure within the thorax decreases, becoming lower than atmospheric pressure. This negative intrathoracic pressure invites air into the thorax through the airway. Because the visceral and parietal pleura remain in contact with each other under normal circumstances, the highly elastic lungs immediately assume the thoracic cavity's internal contour. These combined factors move air into the lungs (inspiration). At the same time, the alveoli inflate with the lungs. They become thinner as they expand, allowing oxygen and carbon dioxide to diffuse across their membranes.

When the pressure in the thoracic cavity again reaches that of the atmosphere, the alveoli are maximally inflated. Pulmonary expansion stimulates microscopic stretch receptors in the bronchi and bronchioles. These receptors signal the respiratory center by way of the vagus nerve to inhibit inspiration, and the air influx stops. This process is primarily protective, as it prevents overinflation of the lungs.

At the end of inspiration, the respiratory muscles now relax, thus decreasing the size of the chest cavity, and in turn increasing the intrathoracic pressure. The naturally elastic lungs recoil, forcing air out through the airway (expiration) until intrathoracic and atmospheric pressure are equal once again. Normal expiration is a passive process, while inspiration is an active process, using energy. In respiratory inadequacy, when this process fails to provide satisfactory gas exchange, the patient may use accessory respiratory muscles such as the strap muscles of his neck and his abdominal muscles to augment his efforts to expand the thoracic cavity.

Pulmonary Circulation

Respiration also requires an intact circulatory system. In fact, during each cardiac cycle, the heart pumps as much blood to the lungs as it pumps to the peripheral tissues. In the capillaries, these cells take oxygen from red blood cells coming from the arterial system and give up carbon dioxide to blood returning to the venous system. The venous system carries this deoxygenated blood to the right side of the heart, and the right ventricle pumps it into the pulmonary artery (Figure 13-7 ■). The pulmonary artery immediately branches into the right and the left pulmonary arteries, each supplying its respective lung. In turn, both branches quickly fan into smaller arteries that end in the pulmonary capillaries. These capillaries are spread over the surfaces of the alveoli, where the red blood cells exchange carbon dioxide for oxygen. The pulmonary capillaries recombine into larger veins, eventually terminating in the pulmonary vein. The pulmonary vein empties the oxygenated blood into the left atrium of the heart. Finally, the heart transports the oxygenated blood through the left ventricle and into the systemic arterial system via the aorta and its tributaries.

The lungs themselves receive little of their blood supply from the pulmonary arteries or veins. Instead, bronchial arteries that branch from the aorta supply most of their blood. Bronchial veins return this blood from the lungs to the superior vena cava.

MEASURING OXYGEN AND CARBON DIOXIDE LEVELS

You can determine the amount of oxygen and carbon dioxide in the blood by measuring their partial pressures. **Partial pressure** is the pressure exerted by each component

partial pressure *the pressure exerted by each component of a gas mixture.*

■ Figure 13-7   Pulmonary circulation.

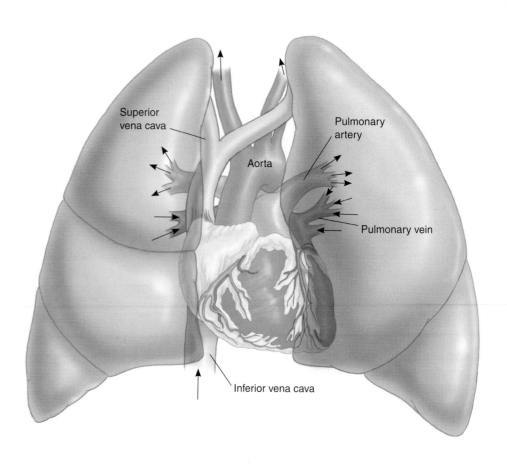

Superior
vena cava

Pulmonary
artery

Aorta

Pulmonary vein

Inferior vena cava

Table 13-1	Partial Pressures and Concentrations of Gases			
	Partial Pressure		*Concentration*	
	Atmospheric	**Alveolar**	**Atmospheric**	**Alveolar**
Nitrogen	597.0 torr	569.0 torr	78.62%	74.9%
Oxygen	159.0 torr	104.0 torr	20.84%	13.7%
Carbon dioxide	0.3 torr	40.0 torr	0.04%	5.2%
Water	3.7 torr	47.0 torr	0.50%	6.2%
TOTAL	760.0 torr	760.0 torr	100.00%	100.0%

of a gas mixture. In other words, the partial pressure of a gas is its percentage of the mixture's total pressure. The partial pressure of oxygen at normal atmospheric pressure, for example, is the percentage of oxygen in atmospheric air (21 percent) multiplied by the atmospheric pressure at sea level (760 torr, or 14.7 pounds per square inch):

$$0.21 \times 760 \text{ torr} = 159.6 \text{ torr}$$

(Note that torr and mmHg are the same measures of pressure.) Earth's atmosphere consists of four major respiratory gases: nitrogen (N_2), oxygen (O_2), carbon dioxide (CO_2), and water (H_2O). Although nitrogen is metabolically inert, it is needed to inflate gas-filled body cavities such as the chest. Table 13–1 lists these four respiratory gases' partial pressures and concentrations in the environment and in the alveoli.

Since alveolar partial pressure and arterial partial pressure are essentially the same in the normal lung, normal arterial partial pressures for oxygen and carbon dioxide may be expressed:

$$\text{Oxygen } (PaO_2) = 100 \text{ torr (average} = 80\text{–}100)$$
$$\text{Carbon dioxide } (PaCO_2) = 40 \text{ torr (average} = 35\text{–}45)$$

Alveolar partial pressures are abbreviated **PA** (PAO_2 and $PACO_2$), whereas arterial partial pressures are abbreviated **Pa** (PaO_2 and $PaCO_2$). Because these values are usually the same, however, they typically appear as the shortened notations PO_2 and PCO_2.

PA *alveolar partial pressure.*

Pa *arterial partial pressure.*

Diffusion

Diffusion is the movement of a gas from an area of higher concentration (partial pressure) to an area of lower concentration, attempting to reach equilibrium. Diffusion transfers gases between the lungs and the blood and between the blood and the peripheral tissues. The rate of diffusion of a gas across the pulmonary membranes depends on the gas's solubility in water. For example, carbon dioxide is 21 times more soluble in water than oxygen and readily crosses the pulmonary capillary membranes. In the peripheral tissues, the gradient (direction of diffusion) for CO_2 is from the tissue, where its concentration is high, to the capillary blood, where its concentration is low.

diffusion *movement of a gas from an area of higher concentration to an area of lower concentration.*

In the lungs, oxygen dissolves in water at the alveolar membrane and leaves the area of higher PO_2, the alveoli, and enters the area of lower PO_2, the venous blood in the pulmonary capillaries. Concurrently, carbon dioxide leaves the area of higher PCO_2, the arterial blood, and enters the area of lower PCO_2, the alveoli. The blood returns from the pulmonary vein to the heart and then moves into the systemic circulation.

Oxygen Concentration in the Blood

Oxygen diffuses into the blood plasma, where most of it combines with hemoglobin and is measured as oxygen saturation (SpO_2). The remainder is dissolved in the blood and is measured as the PaO_2. Hemoglobin approaches 100 percent saturation when the PaO_2 of dissolved oxygen reaches 90 to 100 torr. Each gram of saturated hemoglobin carries 1.34 milliliters of oxygen. Oxygen saturation is the ratio of the blood's actual oxygen content to its total oxygen-carrying capacity:

$$\text{Oxygen saturation} = O_2 \text{ content}/O_2 \text{ capacity} \times 100(\%)$$

The hemoglobin molecule carries the vast majority of oxygen in the blood (approximately 97 percent). Very little oxygen dissolves in the plasma. Since partial pressure measurements detect only the amount of oxygen dissolved in the plasma and do not always reflect the total oxygen saturation, they can be misleading. For example, a patient who has suffered carbon monoxide poisoning cannot transport enough oxygen to the peripheral tissues since carbon monoxide displaces oxygen from the hemoglobin molecule. But an arterial blood gas sample might reveal a normal or high PaO_2. This would indicate that adequate oxygen was reaching the blood. In fact, however, an inadequate amount of hemoglobin would be available to transport the oxygen to the peripheral tissues, thus resulting in peripheral hypoxia.

Several factors can affect oxygen concentrations in the blood:

★ Decreased hemoglobin concentration (anemia, hemorrhage)

★ Inadequate alveolar ventilation due to low inspired-oxygen concentration, respiratory muscle paralysis, and pulmonary conditions such as emphysema, asthma, or pneumothorax

hypoventilation *reduction in breathing rate and depth.*

pneumothorax *accumulation of air or gas in the pleural cavity.*

hemothorax *accumulation in the pleural cavity of blood or fluid containing blood.*

pulmonary embolism *blood clot that travels to the pulmonary circulation and hinders oxygenation of the blood.*

FiO_2 *concentration of oxygen in inspired air.*

Never withhold oxygen from any patient whose clinical condition indicates its need.

★ Decreased diffusion across the pulmonary membrane when diffusion distance increases or the pulmonary membrane changes; for example, when fluid enters the space between the alveolar membrane and the pulmonary capillary membrane, as in pneumonia, chronic obstructive pulmonary disease (COPD), or pulmonary edema (swelling)

★ Ventilation/perfusion mismatch occurs when a portion of the alveoli collapses, as in atelectasis. Blood travels past these collapsed alveoli without oxygenation (shunting), without carbon dioxide, and without oxygen uptake. This can result from **hypoventilation,** which can occur secondary to pain or inability to inspire (traumatic asphyxia). When the lung collapses, as in **pneumothorax, hemothorax,** or a combination of the two, less surface area is available for gas exchange. Alternately, a ventilation/perfusion mismatch can occur when blood is prevented from reaching the alveolar capillary membranes but alveolar ventilation remains adequate. This occurs when a blood clot travels to or is formed in the pulmonary arterial system, a condition known as pulmonary thromboembolism

You can correct oxygen derangements by increasing ventilation, administering supplemental oxygen, using intermittent positive-pressure ventilation (IPPV), or administering drugs to correct underlying problems such as pulmonary edema, asthma, or **pulmonary embolism.** The emergency being treated determines the desired fractional concentration of oxygen (**FiO_2**) to be delivered. It is crucial to remember not to withhold oxygen from any patient whose clinical condition indicates its need.

Carbon Dioxide Concentrations in the Blood

The blood transports carbon dioxide mainly in the form of bicarbonate ion (HCO_3^-). It carries approximately 70 percent as bicarbonate and approximately 20 percent combined with hemoglobin. Less than 7 percent is dissolved in the plasma. Several factors influence carbon dioxide's concentration in the blood, including increased CO_2 production and/or decreased CO_2 elimination:

★ Hyperventilation lowers CO_2 levels and can be the result of an increased respiratory rate or deeper respiration, both of which increase the minute volume. (We discuss minute volume more completely later in this chapter.)

★ Causes of increased CO_2 production include:

–Fever

–Muscle exertion

–Shivering

–Metabolic processes resulting in the formation of metabolic acids.

★ Decreased CO_2 elimination (increased CO_2 levels in the blood) results from decreased alveolar ventilation. Common causes include hypoventilation due to:

–Respiratory depression by drugs

–Airway obstruction

–Impairment of the respiratory muscles

–Obstructive diseases such as asthma and emphysema.

hypercarbia *excessive pressure of carbon dioxide in the blood.*

Increased CO_2 levels (**hypercarbia**) are usually treated by increasing the rate and/or volume of ventilation and by correcting the underlying cause.

REGULATION OF RESPIRATION
Voluntary and Involuntary Respiratory Controls

The number of times a person breathes in 1 minute, the **respiratory rate,** is unique in that both voluntary and involuntary nervous system mechanisms control it. We do not ordinarily need to make a conscious effort to breathe; our brains automatically regulate this function. However, we can voluntarily override our involuntary respirations until physical and chemical mechanisms signal the nervous system's respiratory centers to provide involuntarily impulses and correct any breathing irregularities.

Nervous Impulses from the Respiratory Center   The main respiratory center lies in the *medulla,* located in the brainstem. Various neurons within the medulla initiate impulses that result in respiration. A rise in the frequency of these impulses increases the respiratory rate. Conversely, a decrease in their frequency decreases the respiratory rate. The medulla is connected to the respiratory muscles primarily via the vagus nerve. This is an involuntary pathway. If the medulla fails to initiate respiration, an additional control center in the pons, called the *apneustic center,* assumes respiratory control to ensure the continuation of respirations. A third center, the *pneumotaxic center,* also in the pons, controls expiration.

Stretch Receptors   During inspiration, the lungs become distended, activating stretch receptors. As the degree of stretch increases, these receptors fire more frequently. The impulses they send to the brainstem inhibit the medullary cells, decreasing the inspiratory stimulus. Thus, the respiratory muscles relax, allowing the elastic lungs to recoil and expel air from the body. As the stretch decreases, the stretch receptors stop firing. This process, called the *Hering-Breuer reflex,* prevents overexpansion of the lungs.

Chemoreceptors   Other involuntary respiration controls include central chemical receptors in the medulla and peripheral chemoreceptors in the carotid bodies and in the arch of the aorta. These chemoreceptors are stimulated by decreased PaO_2, increased $PaCO_2$, and decreased pH. (The pH scale expresses the degree of acidity or alkalinity. A lower pH indicates greater acidity; a higher pH indicates greater alkalinity; Chapter 8 discusses pH in greater detail.) Cerebrospinal fluid (CSF) pH is the primary control of respiratory center stimulation. The CSF pH responds very quickly to changes in arterial PCO_2. Any increase in PCO_2 will decrease CSF pH, which will in turn stimulate the central chemoreceptors to increase respiration. Conversely, low $PaCO_2$ levels will raise CSF pH, in turn decreasing chemoreceptor stimulation and slowing respiratory activity. Because $PaCO_2$ is inversely related to CSF pH, $PaCO_2$ is seen as the normal neuroregulatory control of respirations. Additionally, any increase in the arterial PCO_2 stimulates the peripheral chemoreceptors to signal the brainstem to increase respiration, thus speeding CO_2 elimination from the body.

Hypoxic Drive   The body also constantly monitors the PaO_2 and the pH. In fact, **hypoxemia** (decreased partial pressure of oxygen in the blood) is a profound stimulus of respiration in a normal individual. People with chronic respiratory disease such as emphysema and chronic bronchitis tend to retain CO_2 and, therefore, have a chronically elevated $PaCO_2$. Chemoreceptors in the periphery eventually become accustomed to this chronic condition, and the central nervous system stops using $PaCO_2$ to regulate respiration. This activates a default mechanism called **hypoxic drive,** which increases respiratory stimulation when PaO_2 falls and inhibits respiratory stimulation when PaO_2 climbs. High-volume oxygen administration to people with

respiratory rate   *number of times a person breathes in 1 minute.*

hypoxemia   *decreased partial pressure of oxygen in the blood.*

hypoxic drive   *mechanism that increases respiratory stimulation when PaO_2 falls and inhibits respiratory stimulation when PaO_2 climbs.*

this condition can cause respiratory arrest. Because high-flow, high-concentration oxygen can quickly double or even triple the PaO_2, peripheral chemoreceptors stop stimulating the respiratory centers, causing apnea (cessation of breathing). Although this is a potential threat, it is never appropriate to withhold oxygen from a patient for whom oxygen therapy is indicated. However, you must be prepared to assist with ventilations if the patient's respiratory effort becomes inadequate.

Measures of Respiratory Function

The respiratory rate is the number of respiratory cycles per minute, normally 12 to 20 breaths per minute in adults, 18 to 24 in children, and 40 to 60 in infants. Several factors affect respiratory rate:

* *Fever*—increases rate
* *Emotion*—increases rate
* *Pain*—increases rate
* *Hypoxia* (inadequate tissue oxygenation)—increases rate
* *Acidosis*—increases rate
* *Stimulant drugs*—increase rate
* *Depressant drugs*—decrease rate
* *Sleep*—decreases rate

Paramedics must fully understand ventilatory mechanics and capacities for the average adult's respiratory system. This knowledge will enable you to adapt your mechanical ventilation techniques to your patient's size, lung compliance, need for hyperventilation, or other individual requirements. It is especially crucial in situations that call for advanced mechanical ventilator skills. Respiratory capacities and measurements with which you must be familiar include:

total lung capacity *maximum lung capacity.*

* ***Total lung capacity*** (TLC). This is the maximum lung capacity—the total amount of air contained in the lung at the end of maximal inspiration. In the average adult male, this volume is approximately 6 liters.

tidal volume *average volume of gas inhaled or exhaled in one respiratory cycle.*

* ***Tidal volume*** (V_T). The tidal volume is the average volume of gas inhaled or exhaled in one respiratory cycle. In the adult male this is approximately 500 mL (5 to 7 cc/kg).

* *Dead space volume* (V_D). The dead space volume is the amount of gas in the tidal volume that remains in air passageways unavailable for gas exchange. It is approximately 150 mL in the adult male. Anatomic dead space includes the trachea and bronchi. Obstructions or diseases such as chronic obstructive pulmonary disease or atelectasis can cause physiologic dead space.

* *Alveolar volume* (V_A). The alveolar volume is the amount of gas in the tidal volume that reaches the alveoli for gas exchange. It is the difference between tidal volume and dead-space volume (approximately 350 mL in the adult male):

$$V_A = V_T - V_D$$

minute volume *amount of gas inhaled and exhaled in 1 minute.*

* ***Minute volume*** (V_{min}). The minute volume is the amount of gas moved in and out of the respiratory tract in 1 minute:

$$V_{min} = V_T \times \text{respiratory rate}$$

* *Alveolar minute volume* ($V_{A\text{-}min}$). The alveolar minute volume is the amount of gas that reaches the alveoli for gas exchange in 1 minute:

$$V_{A\text{-}min} = (V_T - V_D) \times \text{respiratory rate}$$

or

$$V_{A\text{-}min} = V_A \times \text{respiratory rate}$$

★ *Inspiratory reserve volume (IRV)*. The inspiratory reserve volume is the amount of air that can be maximally inhaled after a normal inspiration.

★ *Expiratory reserve volume (ERV)*. The expiratory reserve volume is the amount of air that can be maximally exhaled after a normal expiration.

★ *Residual volume (RV)*. The residual volume is the amount of air remaining in the lungs at the end of maximal expiration.

★ *Functional residual capacity (FRC)*. The functional residual capacity is the volume of gas that remains in the lungs at the end of normal expiration:

$$\text{FRC} = \text{ERV} + \text{RV}$$

★ *Forced expiratory volume (FEV)*. The forced expiratory volume is the amount of air that can be maximally expired after maximum inspiration.

RESPIRATORY PROBLEMS

Respiratory emergencies can pose an immediate life threat to the patient. You must calmly and quickly assess the severity of his illness or injury while considering the potential causes of and treatment for his respiratory distress. Often, he will give you little help, either because of anxiety or difficulty speaking. His respiratory difficulty may be due to airway obstruction, injury to upper or lower airway structures, inadequate ventilation caused by worsening of an underlying lung disease and fatigue, or central nervous system problems that threaten the airway or respiratory effort.

AIRWAY OBSTRUCTION

Blockage of the airway is an immediate threat to the patient's life and a true emergency. **Upper airway obstruction** may be defined as an interference with air movement through the upper airway.

Airway obstruction may be either partial or complete. Partial obstruction allows either adequate or poor air exchange. Patients with adequate air exchange can cough effectively; those with poor air exchange cannot. They often emit a high-pitched noise while inhaling (stridor), and their skin may have a bluish appearance (cyanosis). They also may have increased breathing difficulty, which can manifest as choking, gagging dyspnea, or dysphonia (difficulty speaking). When you cannot feel or hear airflow from the nose and mouth, or when the patient cannot speak (aphonia), breathe, or cough, his airway is completely obstructed. He will quickly become unconscious and die if you do not relieve the obstruction. In the absence of breathing, difficulty ventilating the patient will indicate complete airway obstruction.

Causes of Airway Obstruction

The tongue, foreign bodies, teeth, spasm or edema, vomitus, and blood can all obstruct the upper airway.

The Tongue The tongue is the most common cause of airway obstruction (Figure 13-8 ■). Normally, the submandibular muscles directly support the tongue and indirectly support the epiglottis. Without sufficient muscle tone, though, the relaxed tongue falls back against the posterior pharynx, thus occluding the airway. This may produce

upper airway obstruction *an interference with air movement through the upper airway.*

Blockage of the airway is an immediate threat to the patient's life and a true emergency.

 Review

Causes of Airway Obstruction

- Tongue
- Foreign bodies
- Trauma
- Laryngeal spasm and edema
- Aspiration

The tongue is the most common airway obstruction.

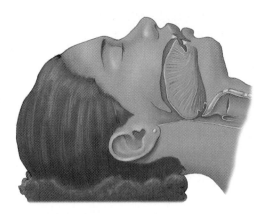

snoring respiratory noises. At the same time, the epiglottis also may block the airway at the larynx. This at least diminishes airflow into the respiratory system, and the patient's breathing efforts may inadvertently suck the base of his tongue into an obstructing position. The patient's tongue can block his airway whether he is lateral, supine, or prone; however, the blockage depends on the position of the patient's head and jaw, so simple airway maneuvers such as the jaw-thrust can usually open his airway.

Foreign Bodies   Large, poorly chewed pieces of food can obstruct the upper airway by becoming lodged in the hypopharynx. These cases often involve alcohol consumption and denture dislodgement. Because they frequently occur in restaurants and are mistaken for heart attacks, they are commonly called "café coronaries." The patient may clutch his neck between the thumb and fingers, a universal distress signal. Children, especially toddlers, often aspirate foreign objects, as they have the tendency to put objects into their mouths.

Trauma   In trauma, particularly when the patient is unresponsive, loose teeth, facial bone fractures, and avulsed or swollen tissue may obstruct the airway. Secretions such as blood, saliva, and vomitus may compromise the airway and risk aspiration. Additionally, penetrating or blunt trauma may obstruct the airway by fracturing or displacing the larynx, allowing the vocal cords to collapse into the tracheal lumen.

Since the glottis is the narrowest part of an adult's airway, edema or spasm of the vocal cords is potentially lethal.

Laryngeal Spasm and Edema   Since the glottis is the narrowest part of an adult's airway, edema (swelling) or spasm (spasmotic closure) of the vocal cords is potentially lethal. Even moderate edema can severely obstruct airflow and cause asphyxia (the inability to move air into and out of the respiratory system). Just beneath the mucous membrane that covers the vocal cords is a layer of loose tissue where blood or other fluids can accumulate. This tissue may swell following injury, and the swelling will be slow to subside. Causes of laryngeal spasm and edema include trauma, anaphylaxis, epiglottitis, and inhalation of superheated air, smoke, or toxic substances. The most common cause of spasm is overly aggressive intubation. It often occurs, too, immediately upon **extubation,** especially when the patient is semiconscious. Some authors propose that laryngeal spasm can sometimes be partially overcome by strengthening ventilatory effort, forceful upward pull of the jaw, or the use of muscle relaxants, although the success of these maneuvers is quite variable.

extubation *removing a tube from a body opening.*

Aspiration   Vomitus is the most commonly aspirated material. Patients most at risk for this are those who are so obtunded (drowsy) that they cannot adequately protect their airways. This can occur with hypoxia, central nervous system toxins, or brain injury, among other causes. In addition to obstructing the airway, aspiration's other effects also significantly increase patient mortality. Vomitus consists of food particles, protein-dissolving enzymes, hydrochloric acid, and gastrointestinal bacteria that have been regurgitated from the stomach into the hypopharynx and oropharynx. If this mixture enters the lungs, it can result in increased interstitial fluid and pulmonary edema. The consequent marked increase in alveolar/capillary distance seriously impairs gas exchange, thus causing hypoxemia and hypercarbia. Aspirated materials can also severely damage the delicate bronchiolar tissue and alveoli. Gastrointestinal bacteria can produce overwhelming infections. These complications occur in 50 to 80 percent of patients who aspirate foreign matter.

INADEQUATE VENTILATION

Insufficient minute volume respirations can compromise adequate oxygen intake and carbon dioxide removal. Additionally, oxygenation may be insufficient when conditions increase metabolic oxygen demand or decrease available oxygen. A reduction of either the rate or the volume of inhalation leads to a reduction in minute volume. In some cases, the respiratory rate may be rapid but so shallow that little air exchange takes place. Among the causes of such decreased ventilation are depressed respiratory function as from impairment of respiratory muscles or nervous system, bronchospasm from intrinsic disease, fractured ribs, pneumothorax, hemothorax, drug overdose, renal failure, spinal or brainstem injury, or head injury. In some conditions, such as sepsis, the body's metabolic demand for oxygen can exceed the patient's ability to supply it. Additionally, the environment may contain a decreased amount of oxygen, as in high-altitude conditions or a house fire, which also produces toxic gases like cyanide and carbon monoxide. These situations of inadequate ventilation can lead to hypercarbia and hypoxia.

RESPIRATORY SYSTEM ASSESSMENT

Vigilance is the key to airway management in every patient. The trauma patient whose airway and breathing initially looked fine on exam may become symptomatic with the pneumothorax that was not initially evident. The asthma patient who initially responded to nebulizer treatment may have a sudden bronchospasm and worsen acutely. Minute-by-minute reassessment of the adequacy of every patient's airway and breathing is essential. The changes may be subtle increases in rate, worsening or onset of irregularity, or increased difficulty speaking. Assessment of the respiratory system begins with the initial assessment and should continue through the focused history and physical exam and the ongoing assessment. (Volume 2, Chapter 3, discusses the initial assessment and the focused history and physical exam in detail.)

Vigilance is the key to airway management in every patient.

INITIAL ASSESSMENT

The initial assessment's purpose is to identify any immediate threats to the patient's life, specifically *a*irway, *b*reathing, and *c*irculation problems (**ABCs**). First, assess the airway to assure that it is patent. Snoring or gurgling may indicate potential airway problems. Next determine the adequacy of breathing. If the patient is comfortable, with a normal respiratory rate, alert, and speaking without difficulty, you may generally assume that his airway is patent and breathing is adequate.

ABCs *airway, breathing, and circulation.*

Patients with altered mental status warrant further evaluation. Feel for air movement with your hand or cheek (Figure 13-9 ■). Look for the chest to rise and fall normally with each respiratory cycle (Figure 13-10 ■). Listen for air movement and equal bilateral breath sounds (Figure 13-11 ■). The absence of breath sounds on one side may indicate a pneumothorax or hemothorax in the trauma patient. In an adult patient, the respiratory rate generally ranges between 12 and 20 breaths per minute. Breathing

Figure 13-9   Feel. *(© Scott Metcalfe)*

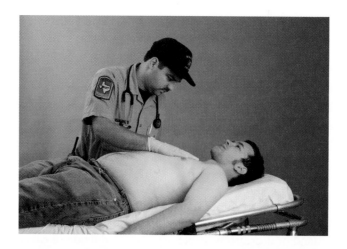

Figure 13-10   Look. *(© Scott Metcalfe)*

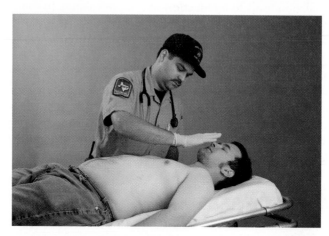

Figure 13-11   Listen. *(© Scott Metcalfe)*

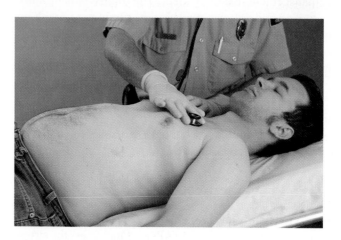

paradoxical breathing
assymetrical chest wall movement that lessens respiratory efficiency.

flail chest   *defect in the chest wall that allows a segment to move freely, causing paradoxical chest wall motion.*

should be spontaneous, effortless, and regular. Irregular breathing suggests a significant problem and usually requires ventilatory support. Observe the chest wall for any asymmetrical movement. This condition, known as **paradoxical breathing,** may suggest a **flail chest.** Patients who show increased respiratory effort; insisting on upright, sniffing, or semi-Fowler's positioning; or those refusing to lie supine should be considered to be in significant respiratory distress.

If the patient is not breathing, or if you suspect airway problems, open the airway using the head-tilt/chin-lift or jaw-thrust maneuver, as described later in this chapter.

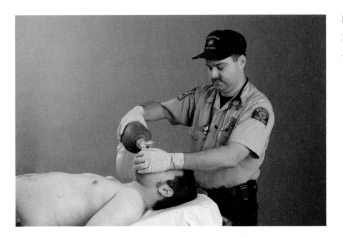

■ Figure 13-12 Bag-valve-mask ventilation. (© Scott Metcalfe)

If trauma is possible, use the jaw-thrust maneuver while stabilizing the cervical spine in the neutral position. Once the airway is open, reevaluate the breathing status. If breathing is adequate, provide supplemental oxygen and assess circulation. Consider the use of airway adjuncts, as discussed later. If breathing is inadequate or absent, begin artificial ventilation (Figure 13-12 ■). When assisting a patient's breathing with a ventilatory device (bag-valve mask or other positive-pressure device), or after placing an airway adjunct (nasopharyngeal airway or oropharyngeal airway), or endotracheally intubating, monitor the chest's rise and fall to determine correct usage and placement. (We will discuss these ventilatory devices and mechanical airways in detail later in this chapter.)

FOCUSED HISTORY AND PHYSICAL EXAMINATION

After you complete the initial assessment and correct any immediate life threats, conduct a focused history and physical exam while continuously monitoring the patient's airway, breathing, and circulation.

Focused History

The time when the patient and his family noted the onset of symptoms is important information, as is whether the acute event occurred suddenly or gradually. Identifying possible triggers such as allergens or heat also can help the patient avoid them in the future. Additionally, the symptoms' course of development since onset will help direct diagnosis and treatment. Have they been progressively worsening, recurrent, or continuous? Associated symptoms will further help to assess the cause of the patient's problem. Has he had fever or chills, productive cough, chest pain, nausea or vomiting, or diaphoresis? Does he think his voice sounds normal?

The patient's past medical history will put his present complaints into perspective and help to identify the risk factors for a variety of likely diagnoses. Determine whether the present episode is similar to any past episodes of shortness of breath, what medical evaluations have been done, and what they have found. Has the patient ever been admitted to the hospital for his complaints? Has he ever been intubated?

The recent history leading to the onset of symptoms is also important. Did the patient run out of medication? Has he been noncompliant with (not taken) his medications? Did he drink too much fluid or alcohol? Did he seize or vomit? Did he eat something that might induce an allergy? Did he receive any trauma? If an injury is involved, evaluate the mechanism of injury. Keep in mind that blunt trauma to the neck may have injured the larynx. Anything that makes the patient's condition better (ameliorates) or worse (exacerbates, aggravates) is also significant.

Physical Examination

Your physical examination of a patient with respiratory problems should continue the evaluation of his airway, breathing, and circulation begun during your initial assessment. Now you will use the physical examination techniques of inspection, auscultation, and palpation to evaluate his injury or illness in more detail and determine your plan of action. (Volume 2, Chapter 2, explains these techniques in detail.)

Inspection   Begin the physical assessment by inspecting the patient. Evaluate the adequacy of his breathing. Note any obvious signs of trauma. Always remember to assess the skin color as an indicator of oxygenation status. Early in respiratory compromise, the sympathetic nervous system will be stimulated to help offset the lack of oxygen. When this happens, the skin will often appear pale and diaphoretic. **Cyanosis** (bluish discoloration) is another sign of respiratory distress. When oxygen binds with the hemoglobin, the blood appears bright red. Deoxygenated hemoglobin, however, is blue and gives the skin a bluish tint. This is not a reliable indicator, however, since severe tissue hypoxia is possible without cyanosis. In fact, cyanosis is considered a late sign of respiratory compromise. When it does appear, it usually affects the lips, fingernails, and skin. A red skin rash, especially if accompanied by hives, may indicate an allergic reaction. A cherry-red skin discoloration may on rare occasions be associated with carbon monoxide poisoning, as can bullae (large blisters).

Observe the patient's position. Tripod positioning (seated, leaning forward, with one arm forward to stabilize the body) may indicate COPD or asthma exacerbation; orthopnea (increased difficulty breathing while lying down) may indicate congestive heart failure, or asthma.

Next, inspecting for **dyspnea**—an abnormality of breathing rate, pattern, or effort—is essential. Dyspnea may cause or be caused by **hypoxia.** Prolonged dyspnea without successful intervention can lead to **anoxia** (the absence or near-absence of oxygen), which without intervention is a premorbid (occurring just before death) event, as the brain can survive only 4 to 6 minutes in this state. Remember that all interventions are useless if you do not establish a patent airway.

Also observe for the following modified forms of respiration:

★ *Coughing*—forceful exhalation of a large volume of air from the lungs. This performs a protective function in expelling foreign material from the lungs.

★ *Sneezing*—sudden, forceful exhalation from the nose. It is usually caused by nasal irritation.

★ *Hiccoughing (hiccups)*—sudden inspiration caused by spasmodic contraction of the diaphragm with spastic closure of the glottis. It serves no known physiologic purpose. It has, occasionally, been associated with acute myocardial infarctions on the inferior (diaphragmatic) surface of the heart.

★ *Sighing*—slow, deep, involuntary inspiration followed by a prolonged expiration. It hyperinflates the lungs and reexpands atelectatic alveoli. This normally occurs about once a minute.

★ *Grunting*—a forceful expiration that occurs against a partially closed epiglottis. It is usually an indication of respiratory distress.

Note any decrease or increase in the respiratory rate, one of the earliest indicators of respiratory distress. Also, look for use of the accessory respiratory muscles—intercostal, suprasternal, supraclavicular, and subcostal retractions—and the abdominal muscles to assist breathing. This indicates increased respiratory effort secondary to respiratory distress. In infants and children, nasal flaring and grunting indicate respiratory distress. COPD patients having difficulty breathing will purse their lips during exhalation. Monitor the patient's blood pressure, including any differences noted during ex-

cyanosis   *bluish discoloration.*

dyspnea   *an abnormality of breathing rate, pattern, or effort.*

hypoxia   *oxygen deficiency.*

anoxia   *the absence or near-absence of oxygen.*

piration versus inspiration. Patients with severe chronic obstructive pulmonary disease may sustain a drop in blood pressure during inspiration. This drop is due to increased pressure within the thoracic cavity that impairs the ability of the ventricles to fill. Thus, decreased ventricular filling leads to decreased blood pressure. A drop in blood pressure of greater than 10 torr is termed **pulsus paradoxus** and may be indicative of severe obstructive lung disease.

Determine if the pattern of respirations is abnormal—deep or shallow in combination with a fast or slow rate. Some common abnormal respiratory patterns include:

pulsus paradoxus *drop in blood pressure of greater than 10 torr during inspiration.*

* ★ *Kussmaul's respirations*—deep, slow or rapid, gasping breathing, commonly found in diabetic ketoacidosis
* ★ *Cheyne-Stokes respirations*—progressively deeper, faster breathing alternating gradually with shallow, slower breathing, indicating brainstem injury
* ★ *Biot's respirations*—irregular pattern of rate and depth with sudden, periodic episodes of apnea, indicating increased intracranial pressure
* ★ *Central neurogenic hyperventilation*—deep, rapid respirations, indicating increased intracranial pressure
* ★ *Agonal respirations*—shallow, slow, or infrequent breathing, indicating brain anoxia

Finally, observing altered mentation may be key in determining if breathing is adequate or if significant hypoxia may be present. If the patient's mental status is not normal, you must determine his usual baseline mental status before you can make this assessment.

Auscultation   Following inspection, listen at the mouth and nose for adequate air movement. Then listen to the chest with a stethoscope (auscultate) (Figure 13-13 ■). In a prehospital setting, you should auscultate the right and left apex (just beneath the clavicle), the right and left base (eighth or ninth intercostal space, midclavicular line), and the right and left lower thoracic back or right and left midaxillary line (fourth or fifth intercostal space, on the lateral aspect of the chest). When the patient's condition permits, you can monitor six locations on the posterior chest, three right and three left. The posterior surface is preferable because heart sounds do not interfere with auscultation at this location. However, since patients are usually supine during airway

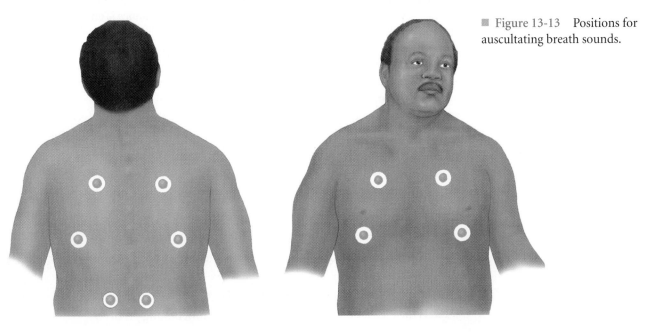

■ Figure 13-13   Positions for auscultating breath sounds.

management, the anterior and lateral positions usually prove more accessible. Breath sounds should be equal bilaterally. Sounds that point to airflow compromise include:

★ *Snoring*—results from partial obstruction of the upper airway by the tongue
★ *Gurgling*—results from the accumulation of blood, vomitus, or other secretions in the upper airway
★ *Stridor*—a harsh, high-pitched sound heard on inhalation, associated with laryngeal edema or constriction
★ *Wheezing*—a musical, squeaking, or whistling sound heard in inspiration and/or expiration, associated with bronchiolar constriction
★ *Quiet*—diminished or absent breath sounds are an ominous finding and indicate a serious problem with the airway, breathing, or both

Beware of the quiet chest!

Sounds that may indicate compromise of gas exchange include:

★ *Crackles (rales)*—a fine, bubbling sound heard on inspiration, associated with fluid in the smaller bronchioles
★ *Rhonchi*—a coarse, rattling noise heard on inspiration, associated with inflammation, mucus, or fluid in the bronchioles

When you assess the effectiveness of ventilatory support or the correct placement of an airway adjunct, remember that air movement into the epigastrium may sometimes mimic breath sounds. Thus, listening to the chest should be only one of several means that you use to assess air movement. Another method of checking correct placement of an airway adjunct is to auscultate over the epigastrium; it should be silent during ventilation. When you provide ventilatory support, watch for signs of gastric distention. They suggest inadequate hyperextension of the neck, undue pressure generated by the ventilatory device, or improper placement of airway adjuncts.

Palpation   Finally, palpate. First, using the back of your hand or your cheek, feel for air movement at the mouth and nose. (If an endotracheal tube is in place, you can check for air movement at the tube's adapter.) Next, palpate the chest for rise and fall. In addition, palpate the chest wall for tenderness, symmetry, abnormal motion, crepitus, and subcutaneous emphysema.

compliance *the stiffness or flexibility of the lung tissue.*

When ventilating with a bag-valve device, gauge airflow into the lungs by noting compliance. **Compliance** refers to the stiffness or flexibility of the lung tissue, and it is indicated by how easily air flows into the lungs. When compliance is good, airflow meets minimal resistance. When compliance is poor, ventilation is harder to achieve. Compliance is often poor in diseased lungs and in patients suffering from chest wall injuries or tension pneumothorax. If a patient shows poor compliance during ventilatory support, look for potential causes. Upper airway obstructions, which cause difficulty with mechanical ventilation, can mimic poor compliance. If ventilating the patient is initially easy but then becomes progressively more difficult, repeat the initial assessment and look for the development of a new problem, possibly related to the mechanical airway maneuvers. The following questions will aid this assessment:

★ Is the airway open?
★ Is the head properly positioned in extension (nontrauma patients)?
★ Is the patient developing tension pneumothorax?
★ Is the endotracheal tube occluded (a mucous plug or aspirated material)?
★ Has the endotracheal tube been inadvertently pushed into the right or left mainstem bronchus?
★ Has the endotracheal tube been displaced into the esophagus?
★ Is the mechanical ventilatory equipment functioning properly?

Pulse rate abnormalities may also suggest respiratory compromise. Tachycardia (an abnormally fast pulse) usually accompanies hypoxemia in an adult, while bradycardia (an abnormally slow pulse) hints at anoxia with imminent cardiac arrest.

A fall in the pulse rate in a patient with airway compromise is an ominous finding.

NONINVASIVE RESPIRATORY MONITORING

Several available devices will help you measure the effectiveness of oxygenation and ventilation. Those measurements used most commonly in prehospital care are pulse oximetry, capnography, and esophageal detection devices. Peak expiratory flow testing can also be useful in the prehospital setting for some respiratory diseases.

Pulse Oximetry

Pulse oximetry is widely used in prehospital emergency care. A pulse oximeter measures hemoglobin oxygen saturation in peripheral tissues (Figure 13-14 ■). It is noninvasive (does not require entering the body), rapidly applied, and easy to operate. Pulse oximetry readings are accurate and continually reflect any changes in peripheral oxygen delivery. In fact, oximetry often detects problems with oxygenation faster than assessments of blood pressure, pulse, and respirations.

To determine peripheral oxygen saturation, you place a sensor probe over a peripheral capillary bed such as a fingertip, toe, or earlobe. In infants, you can wrap the sensor around the heel and secure it with tape. The sensor contains two light-emitting diodes and two sensors. One diode emits near-red light, a wavelength specific for oxygenated hemoglobin; the other emits infrared light, a wavelength specific for deoxygenated hemoglobin. Each hemoglobin state absorbs a certain amount of the emitted light, preventing it from reaching the corresponding sensor. Less light reaching the sensor means more of its type of hemoglobin is in the blood. The oximeter then calculates the ratio of the near-red and infrared light it has received to determine the **oxygen saturation percentage (SpO_2)**.

Pulse oximeters display the SpO_2 and the pulse rate as detected by the sensors. They show the SpO_2 either as a number or as a visual display that also shows the pulse's waveform. The relationship between SpO_2 and the partial pressure of oxygen in the blood (PaO_2) is very complex. However, the SpO_2 does correlate with the PaO_2. The greater

pulse oximetry *a measurement of hemoglobin oxygen saturation in the peripheral tissues.*

oxygen saturation percentage (SpO_2) *the saturation of arterial blood with oxygen as measured by pulse oximetry expressed as a percentage.*

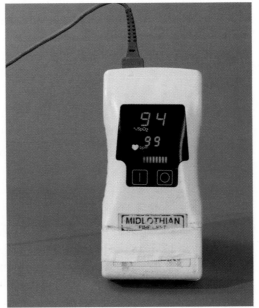

■ Figure 13-14 Pulse oximeter. (© *Scott Metcalfe*)

the PaO_2, the greater will be the oxygen saturation. Since hemoglobin carries 98 percent of oxygen in the blood while plasma carries only 2 percent, pulse oximetry accurately analyzes peripheral oxygen delivery.

Pulse oximetry is often called the "fifth vital sign." When available, you should use it in virtually any situation to determine the patient's baseline value, to guide patient care, and to monitor the patient's responses to your interventions. As a guide, normal SpO_2 varies between 95 and 99 percent. Readings between 91 and 94 percent indicate mild hypoxia and warrant further evaluation and supplemental oxygen administration. Readings between 86 and 91 percent indicate moderate hypoxia. You should generally give these patients 100 percent supplemental oxygen, exercising caution in those with COPD. Readings of 85 percent or lower indicate severe hypoxia and warrant immediate intervention, including the administration of 100 percent oxygen, ventilatory assistance, or both. Your goal is to maintain the SpO_2 in the normal (95 to 99 percent) range.

False readings with pulse oximetry are infrequent. When they do occur, the oximeter often generates an error signal or a blank screen. Causes of false readings include carbon monoxide poisoning, high-intensity lighting, and certain hemoglobin abnormalities. The absence of a pulse in an extremity also will cause a false reading. In hypovolemia and in severely anemic patients, the pulse oximetry reading may be misleading. While the SpO_2 reading may be normal, the total amount of hemoglobin available to carry oxygen may be so markedly decreased that the patient will remain hypoxic at the cellular level.

Pulse oximetry provides key information about the patient and is an important part of emergency care, including prehospital care. However, it is only one more assessment tool and does not replace other physical assessment or monitoring skills. Do not depend solely on pulse oximetry readings to guide care. Always consider and treat the whole patient.

Capnography

End-tidal carbon dioxide ($ETCO_2$) monitoring is a noninvasive method of measuring the levels of carbon dioxide (CO_2) in the exhaled breath. Recordings or displays of exhaled CO_2 measurements are called **capnography.**

Various terms have been applied to capnography, and a review of them may help you to understand the material in this section. These terms include:

capnography *a recording or display of the measurement of exhaled carbon dioxide concentrations.*

* *Capnometry.* Capnometry is the measurement of expired CO_2. It typically provides a numeric display of the partial pressure of CO_2 (in Torr or mmHg) or the percentage of CO_2 present.
* *Capnography.* Capnography is a graphic recording or display of the capnometry reading over time.
* *Capnograph.* A capnograph is a device that measures expired CO_2 levels.
* *Capnogram.* A capnogram is the visual representation of the expired CO_2 waveform.
* *End-tidal CO_2 ($ETCO_2$).* End-tidal CO_2 is the measurement of the CO_2 concentration at the end of expiration (maximum CO_2).
* *$PETCO_2$.* $PETCO_2$ is the partial pressure of end-tidal CO_2 in a mixed gas solution.
* *$PaCO_2$.* The $PaCO_2$ represents the partial pressure of CO_2 in the arterial blood.

CO_2 is a normal end product of metabolism and is transported by the venous system to the right side of the heart. It is then pumped from the right ventricle to the pulmonary artery and eventually enters the pulmonary capillaries. There it diffuses into the alveoli and is removed from the body through exhalation. When circulation is normal, $ETCO_2$ levels change with ventilation and are a reliable estimate of the partial pressure

Table 13–2 | Basic Rules of Capnography

Symptom	Possible Cause
Sudden drop of $ETCO_2$ to zero	• Esophageal intubation • Ventilator disconnection or defect in ventilator • Defect in CO_2 analyzer
Sudden decrease of $ETCO_2$ (not to zero)	• Leak in ventilator system; obstruction • Partial disconnect in ventilator circuit • Partial airway obstruction (secretions)
Exponential decrease of $ETCO_2$	• Pulmonary embolism • Cardiac arrest • Hypotension (sudden) • Severe hyperventilation
Change in CO_2 baseline	• Calibration error • Water droplet in analyzer • Mechanical failure (ventilator)
Sudden increase in $ETCO_2$	• Accessing an area of lung previously obstructed • Release of tourniquet • Sudden increase in blood pressure
Gradual lowering of $ETCO_2$	• Hypovolemia • Decreasing cardiac output • Decreasing body temperature; hypothermia; drop in metabolism
Gradual increase in $ETCO_2$	• Rising body temperature • Hypoventilation • CO_2 absorption • Partial airway obstruction (foreign body); reactive airway disease

of oxygen in the arterial system (PaO_2). Normal $ETCO_2$ is 1 to 2 mm less than the partial pressure of carbon dioxide ($PaCO_2$), or approximately 5 percent. A normal partial pressure of end-tidal CO_2 ($PETCO_2$) is approximately 38 mmHg (0.05×760 mmHg = 38 mmHg). ($ETCO_2$ is normally expressed as a percentage, while $PETCO_2$, a partial pressure, is expressed in mmHg.) When perfusion decreases, as occurs in shock or cardiac arrest, $ETCO_2$ levels reflect pulmonary blood flow and cardiac output, not ventilation.

Decreased $ETCO_2$ levels can be found in shock, cardiac arrest, pulmonary embolism, bronchospasm, and with incomplete airway obstruction (such as mucous plugging). Increased $ETCO_2$ levels are found with hypoventilation, respiratory depression, and hyperthermia (Table 13–2).

Capnometry provides a noninvasive measure of $ETCO_2$ levels, thus providing medical personnel with information about the status of systemic metabolism, circulation, and ventilation. The use of capnography has become commonplace in the operating room, in the emergency department, and in the prehospital setting.

When first introduced into prehospital care, $ETCO_2$ monitoring was used exclusively to verify proper endotracheal tube placement in the trachea. The presence of adequate CO_2 levels following intubation confirms the tube is in the trachea through the presence of exhaled CO_2. CO_2 is detected by using either a colorimetric or an infrared device.

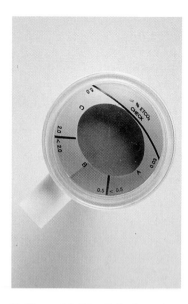

Figure 13-15 Colorimetric end-tidal CO_2 detector.

Colorimetric Devices   The colorimetric device is a disposable $ETCO_2$ detector that contains pH-sensitive, chemically impregnated paper encased within a plastic chamber (Figure 13-15 ■). It is placed in the airway circuit between the patient and the ventilation device. When the paper is exposed to CO_2, hydrogen ions (H^+) are generated, causing a color change in the paper. The color change is reversible and changes breath to breath. A color scale on the device estimates the $ETCO_2$ level. Colorimetric devices cannot detect hyper- or hypocarbia (increased or decreased CO_2 levels). If gastric contents or acidic drugs (e.g., endotracheal epinephrine) contact the paper in the device, subsequent readings may be unreliable.

Electronic Devices   Electronic $ETCO_2$ detectors use an infrared technique to detect CO_2 in the exhaled breath (Figure 13-16 ■). A heated element in the sensor generates infrared radiation. The CO_2 molecules absorb infrared light at a very specific wavelength and can thus be measured. Electronic $ETCO_2$ detectors may be either qualitative (i.e., they simply detect the presence of CO_2) or quantitative (i.e., they determine how much CO_2 is present). Quantitative devices are now routinely used in prehospital care. Most can provide a digital waveform (capnogram) that reflects the entire respiratory cycle (Figure 13-17 ■).

Capnogram   The capnogram reflects CO_2 concentrations over time. It is typically divided into four phases (Figure 13-18 ■).

> ★ *Phase I.* Phase I (AB in Figure 13-18) is the respiratory baseline. It is flat when no CO_2 is present and corresponds to the late phase of inspiration

Figure 13-16   (a) Electronic end-tidal CO_2 detector. (b) Electronic end-tidal CO_2 detector on a patient. *(© Scott Metcalfe)*

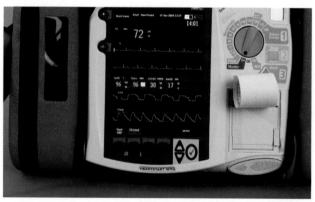

(a)

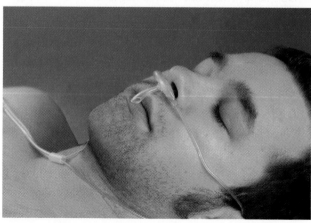

(b)

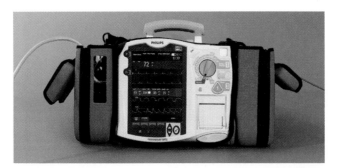

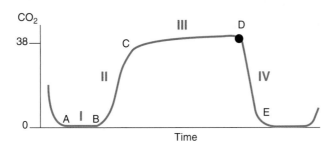

Figure 13-18 Normal capnogram. AB = *Phase I:* late inspiration, early expiration (no CO_2). BC = *Phase II:* appearance of CO_2 in exhaled gas. CD = *Phase III:* plateau (constant CO_2). D = highest point ($ETCO_2$). DE = *Phase IV:* rapid descent during inspiration. EC = respiratory pause.

and the early part of expiration (in which dead-space gases without CO_2 are released).

★ *Phase II.* Phase II (BC in Figure 13-18) is the respiratory upstroke. This reflects the appearance of CO_2 in the alveoli.

★ *Phase III.* Phase III (CD in Figure 13-18) is the respiratory plateau. It reflects the airflow through uniformly ventilated alveoli with a nearly constant CO_2 level. The highest level of the plateau (point D in Figure 13-18) is called the $ETCO_2$ and is recorded as such by the capnometer.

★ *Phase IV.* Phase IV (DE in Figure 13-18) is the inspiratory phase. It is a sudden downstroke and ultimately returns to the baseline during inspiration. The respiratory pause restarts the cycle (EA in Figure 13-18).

Clinical Applications Initially, as noted earlier, $ETCO_2$ detection was used only to determine proper endotracheal tube placement. Typically, a qualitative $ETCO_2$ device was applied to the airway circuit following intubation. If $ETCO_2$ levels were detected, then proper tube placement was verified. However, it is difficult to continuously monitor the airway with a quantitative device. Now, continuous waveform capnography is available and allows continuous monitoring of airway placement and ventilation for intubated patients. Continuous waveform capnography also has utility in monitoring nonintubated patients. By following trends in the capnogram, prehospital personnel can continuously monitor the patient's condition, detect trends, and document the response to medications.

$ETCO_2$ detection is also useful in CPR. During cardiac arrest, CO_2 levels fall abruptly following the onset of cardiac arrest. They begin to rise with the onset of effective CPR and return to near-normal levels with a return of spontaneous circulation. During effective CPR, $ETCO_2$ levels have been found to correlate well with cardiac output, coronary perfusion pressure, and even with the effectiveness of CPR compressions.

Continuous waveform capnography is rapidly becoming a standard of care in EMS (Figure 13-19 ■). Misplaced endotracheal tubes represent a significant area of liability

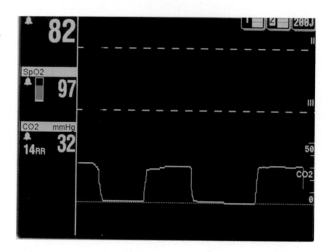

in EMS and the documentation provided by this technology can provide irrefutable evidence of proper endotracheal tube placement.

Esophageal Detector Device

The esophageal detector device (EDD) is a simple and inexpensive tool to help determine whether an endotracheal tube is in the trachea or the esophagus (Figure 13-20 ■). It uses the anatomical principle that the trachea is a rigid tube and will not collapse with negative pressure, while the esophagus is a collapsible tube that flattens with negative pressure and does not allow air to enter the syringe. The EDD may be either a rigid syringe or a bulb syringe (Figure 13-21 ■). Once you have intubated the patient, you attach the EDD to the proximal end of the endotracheal tube (ETT). Then you quickly pull back the syringe, aspirating air from the endotracheal tube. Easily withdrawn air confirms ETT placement in the trachea. If air is difficult or impossible to withdraw, the ETT is in the esophagus.

Peak Expiratory Flow Testing

Peak expiratory flow testing utilizes a disposable plastic chamber into which the patient exhales forcefully after maximal inhalation. It can be used as a crude measure of respiratory efficacy. Improving measurements can indicate good response to treatment of acute respiratory illness.

■ Figure 13-20 Esophageal detector device.

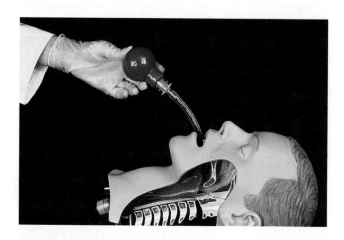

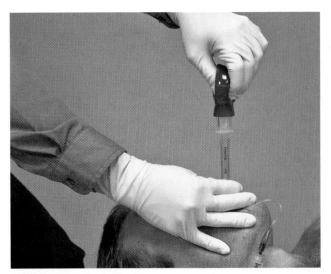

(a)

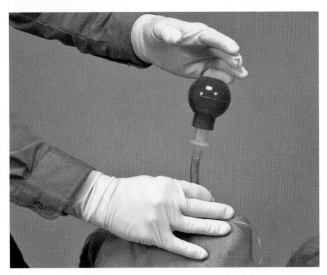

(b)

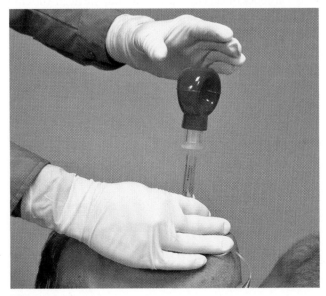

(c)

■ Figure 13-21 An esophageal intubation detector—bulb style. (a) Squeeze the device and then attach it to the endotracheal tube. (b) If the bulb refills easily on release, it indicates correct placement. (c) If the bulb does not refill, the tube is improperly placed.

Back to Basics Always try basic airway maneuvers before resorting to advanced ones.

BASIC AIRWAY MANAGEMENT

Deciding if a patient has a patent airway is the most important step in the initial assessment. Airway management is one of the few prehospital interventions that is known to improve patient survival rates. Once you have determined that intervention is needed, you must use simple manual airway maneuvers and equipment before proceeding with more advanced techniques such as endotracheal intubation or placement of the CombiTube. Always provide supplemental oxygen to all patients for whom it is indicated; never withhold it even from the COPD patient. Be sure to always wear protective eyewear and gloves to avoid contact with the patient's body fluids (Figure 13-22 ■). If you suspect cervical spine injury, perform modified airway techniques in conjunction with appropriate cervical spine stabilization. Once you have secured the airway, frequently reassessing for an adequate airway and ventilation is critical to the patient's survival.

MANUAL AIRWAY MANEUVERS

Manual maneuvers are the simplest airway management techniques. They require no specialized equipment, are safe, and are noninvasive. They are highly effective but often neglected in prehospital care. In the patient who is unconscious or has a decreased level of consciousness, posterior displacement of the tongue is often the cause of airway obstruction. The head-tilt/chin-lift and the jaw-thrust are safe and dependable maneuvers for relieving this obstruction. You should perform one of these techniques on all unconscious patients; do not perform them on responsive patients. If you suspect cervical spine injury, perform the modified jaw-thrust with in-line stabilization of the cervical spine.

Head-Tilt/Chin-Lift

In the absence of cervical spine trauma, the head-tilt/chin-lift is the best technique for opening the airway in an unresponsive patient who is not protecting his own airway

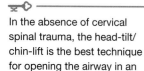

In the absence of cervical spinal trauma, the head-tilt/chin-lift is the best technique for opening the airway in an unresponsive patient who is not protecting his own airway.

■ Figure 13-22   Personal protective equipment.

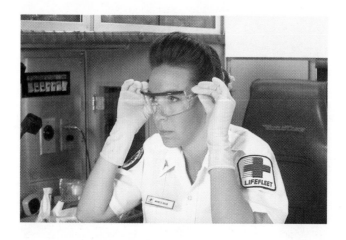

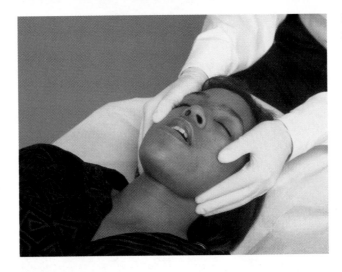

(Figure 13-23 ■). The head-tilt is hazardous to patients with cervical spine injuries; do not use it for those patients. To perform the head-tilt/chin-lift:

1. Place the patient supine and position yourself at the side of the patient's head.
2. Place one hand on the patient's forehead and, using firm downward pressure with your palm, tilt the head back.
3. Put two fingers of the other hand under the bony part of the chin and lift the jaw anteriorly to open the airway.

Caution: Avoid compressing the soft tissues of the neck and chin, which could cause airway obstruction.

Jaw-Thrust Maneuver

A jaw-thrust is also acceptable for an unresponsive patient without the risk of cervical spine injury who cannot protect his airway. Use the following technique (Figure 13-24 ■):

1. Place the patient supine and kneel behind his head.
2. Apply fingers on each side of the jaw at the mandibular angles.
3. Lift the jaw forward (anterior) with a gentle tilting of the patient's head to open the airway.

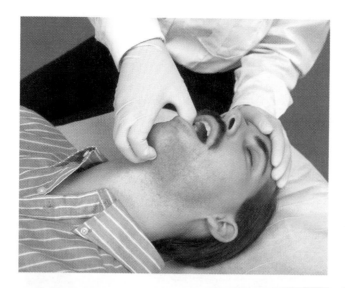

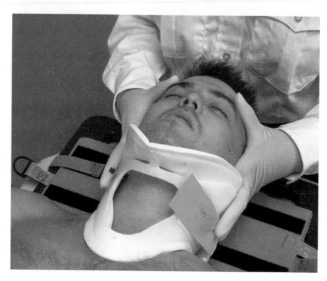

For trauma patients, maintain the cervical spine in neutral position and use either the jaw-thrust without head-tilt or the modified jaw-thrust. You can perform both of these maneuvers with a cervical collar in place:

1. *Jaw-thrust without head-tilt.* Lift the jaw by grasping under the chin and behind the teeth, without tilting the head (Figure 13-25 ■). Use extreme caution with this technique, because even unresponsive patients can clench their teeth shut; do not use this method if the patient's mouth resists opening.

2. *Modified jaw-thrust.* Lift the jaw using fingers behind the mandibular angles; do not tilt the head (Figure 13-26 ■). Use this method if the patient's mouth resists opening.

Although they are simple and effective, none of these manual airway maneuvers protects the airway from aspiration. Additionally, the jaw-thrust and modified jaw-thrust are difficult to maintain for an extended time. The jaw-thrust is impossible to maintain if the patient becomes responsive or combative. Using them in conjunction with a bag-valve mask is often difficult and typically requires a second rescuer. Finally, maintaining the jaw-thrust requires you to keep your thumb in the patient's mouth.

Sellick Maneuver

As a patient becomes unresponsive and requires ventilatory assistance, he loses voluntary control and tone of his upper airway. Combined with air overflowing into the stomach during ventilatory support, this frequently results in gastric distention and regurgitation. Aspiration of vomitus can cause serious complications, including very high death rates. To help prevent regurgitation and reduce gastric distention, the Sellick maneuver applies gentle pressure posteriorly on the anterior cricoid cartilage (Figures 13-27 ■ and 13-28 ■). Since the esophagus lies just behind the cricoid cartilage, this maneuver will effectively close the esophagus to pressures as high as 100 cm/H_2O. It also facilitates intubation by moving the larynx posterior, bringing it into view.

To locate the cricoid cartilage, palpate the thyroid cartilage (Adam's apple) and feel the depression just below it (cricothyroid membrane). The prominence just inferior to this depression is the ring of cricoid cartilage. Using the thumb and index finger of one hand, apply pressure to the anterior and lateral aspects of the cricoid cartilage just next

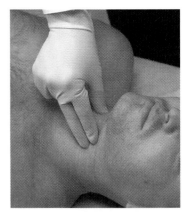

■ Figure 13-27 Sellick maneuver (cricoid pressure).

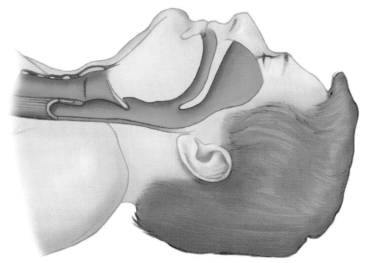

■ Figure 13-28a Airway before applying Sellick.

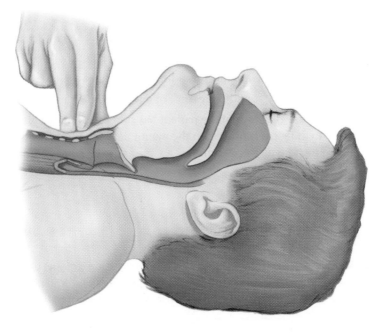

■ Figure 13-28b Airway with Sellick applied (note compression of the esophagus).

to the midline. In infants, use one fingertip and apply gentle downward pressure, taking care to avoid excessive pressure, which may produce tracheal obstruction.

When you use this technique during bag-valve-mask ventilation and endotracheal intubation, a second rescuer is required, and you must remember that the patient will likely regurgitate when you release cricoid pressure. Ideally, therefore, once you have applied the Sellick maneuver, you must maintain it until endotracheal intubation is confirmed and personnel are ready to suction the oropharynx or place a nasogastric tube to decompress the stomach. Additionally, use caution in any patient with a suspected cervical spine injury, as movement of the neck in these patients could cause further spinal cord injury. Complications of the Sellick maneuver include esophageal rupture from unrelieved gastric pressure and obstruction of the trachea or laryngeal trauma from excessive manual pressure.

BASIC MECHANICAL AIRWAYS

In the absence of trauma, secretions, foreign bodies, and edema, basic manual airway maneuvers should clear the tongue from the air passages. However, the tongue often falls back to block the airway again. Two available airway adjuncts, the nasopharyngeal airway and the oropharyngeal airway, correct this. These adjuncts cannot replace good head positioning, but they do help to lift the base of the tongue forward and away from the posterior oropharynx, establishing a patent airway. Always attempt any appropriate manual maneuvers before placing a mechanical airway.

Nasopharyngeal Airway

The **nasopharyngeal airway** is an uncuffed tube made of soft rubber or plastic. The nasopharyngeal airway follows the natural curvature of the nasopharynx, passing through the nose and extending from the nostril to the posterior pharynx just below the base of the tongue. It varies from 17 to 20 cm long, and its diameter ranges from 20 to 36 F (**French**). A funnel-shaped projection at its proximal end helps prevent the tube from slipping inside a patient's nose and becoming lost or aspirated. The distal end is beveled to facilitate passage. You will use the nasopharyngeal airway to relieve soft-tissue upper airway obstruction in cases where an oropharyngeal airway is not advised. Specific indications for the use of the nasopharyngeal airway include obtunded patients (with or without a suppressed gag reflex) and unconscious patients. If the patient does not tolerate the nasopharyngeal airway, you should remove it.

The nasopharyngeal airway's advantages are:

★ It can be rapidly inserted and safely placed blindly.

★ It bypasses the tongue, providing a patent airway.

★ You may use it in the presence of a gag reflex.

★ You may use it when the patient has suffered injury to his oral cavity (anything from trauma to the mandible to significant soft-tissue damage to the tongue or pharynx).

Always attempt any appropriate manual maneuvers before placing a mechanical airway.

nasopharyngeal airway *uncuffed tube that follows the natural curvature of the nasopharynx, passing through the nose and extending from the nostril to the posterior pharynx.*

French *unit of measurement approximately equal to one-third millimeter.*

Legal Notes

Have a Backup Every EMS system should have at least one backup mechanical airway device in the event endotracheal intubation fails. You must be familiar and proficient with any backup airway device used in your system.

★ You may suction through it.

★ You may use it when the patient's teeth are clenched.

Disadvantages of the nasopharyngeal airway are:

★ It is smaller than the oropharyngeal airway.

★ It does not isolate the trachea.

★ It is difficult to suction through.

★ It may cause severe nosebleeds if inserted too forcefully.

★ It may cause pressure necrosis of the nasal mucosa.

★ It may kink and clog, obstructing the airway.

★ Inserting it is difficult if nasal damage (old or new) is present.

★ Use with extreme caution and only as a last resort if basilar skull fracture is suspected.

Do not use the nasopharyngeal airway in patients who are predisposed to nosebleeds or who have a nasal obstruction. Also use with caution when you suspect a basilar skull fracture, because the tube can inadvertently pass into the craninum.

The properly sized nasopharyngeal tube is slightly smaller in diameter than the patient's nostril, and in adults it is equal to or slightly longer than the distance from the patient's nose to his earlobe. Selecting the appropriate size is important. Too small a tube will not extend past the tongue; too long a tube may pass into the esophagus and result in hypoventilation and gastric distention with artificial ventilation (Figures 13-29 ■ and 13-30 ■). To insert the nasopharyngeal airway:

1. If the patient has no history of trauma, hyperextend his head and neck.

2. Assure or maintain effective ventilation. If indicated, ventilate the patient with 100 percent oxygen.

3. Lubricate the exterior of the tube with a water-soluble gel to prevent trauma during insertion. If possible, use a lidocaine gel in the alert or responsive patient; its anesthetic effect on the mucosa will make insertion more comfortable.

4. Push gently up on the tip of the nose and pass the tube into the right nostril. If the septum is deviated and you cannot easily insert the tube into the right nostril, use the left nostril. With the bevel oriented toward the septum, insert the tube gently along the nasal floor, parallel to the mouth.

Never use a nasopharyngeal tube when you suspect a basilar skull fracture, because it can inadvertently pass into the cranial vault.

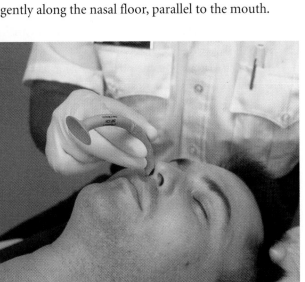

■ Figure 13-29
Nasopharyngeal airway.

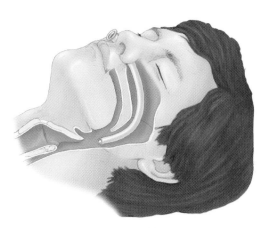

Avoid pushing against any resistance, because this may cause tissue trauma and airway kinking.

5. Verify the appropriate position of the airway. Clear breath sounds and chest rise indicate correct placement. Also, feel at the airway's proximal end for airflow on expiration.

6. Ventilate the patient with 100 percent oxygen, if indicated.

While semiconscious patients tolerate a nasopharyngeal airway better than an oropharyngeal airway, it too may cause vomiting and laryngospasm. Insertion of the nasopharyngeal airway may injure the nasal mucosa, leading to bleeding, aspiration of clots, and the need for suctioning. Forceful insertion of the airway may lacerate the adenoids, causing considerable bleeding.

Oropharyngeal Airway

oropharyngeal airway
semicircular device that follows the palate's curvature.

The **oropharyngeal airway** is a noninvasive semicircular plastic or rubber device designed to follow the palate's curvature. It holds the base of the tongue away from the posterior oropharynx, thus preventing it from obstructing the glottis. Its use is indicated in patients with no gag reflex.

When properly positioned, this device has several advantages:

★ It is easy to place using proper technique.

★ Air can pass around and through the device.

★ It helps prevent obstruction by the teeth and lips.

★ It helps manage unconscious patients who are breathing spontaneously or need mechanical ventilation.

★ It makes suction of the pharynx easier, as a large suction catheter can pass on either side of the device.

★ It serves as an effective bite block in case of seizures or to protect the endotracheal tube.

Disadvantages of the oropharyngeal airway are:

★ It does not isolate the trachea or prevent aspiration.

★ It cannot be inserted when the teeth are clenched. It may obstruct the airway if not inserted properly.

★ It is easily dislodged.

★ Return of the gag reflex may produce vomiting.

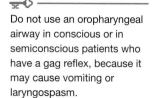

Do not use an oropharyngeal airway in conscious or in semiconscious patients who have a gag reflex, because it may cause vomiting or laryngospasm.

Do not use an oropharyngeal airway in conscious or in semiconscious patients who have a gag reflex, because it may cause vomiting (by stimulating the posterior tongue gag reflexes) or laryngospasm.

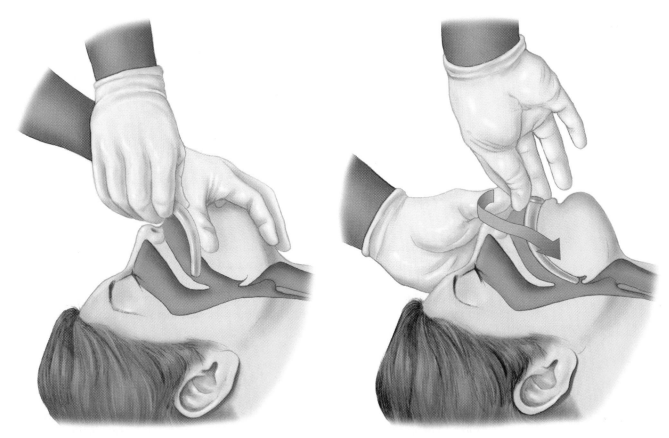

■ Figure 13-31a   Insert the oropharyngeal airway with the tip facing the palate.

■ Figure 13-31b   Rotate the airway 180° into position.

Oropharyngeal airways are available in sizes ranging from #0 (for neonates) to #6 (for large adults). Selecting the proper size is important. If the airway is too long, it can press the epiglottis against the entrance of the larynx, resulting in airway obstruction. If it is too small, it will not adequately hold the tongue forward. To measure for the appropriate oropharyngeal airway, place the flange beside the patient's cheek, parallel to the front of the teeth. A properly sized airway will extend from the patient's mouth to the angle of his jaw (Figure 13-31 ■). To place the oropharyngeal airway:

1. If the patient has no history of trauma, hyperextend his head and neck. Open the mouth and remove any visible obstructions.

2. Assure or maintain effective ventilation; if indicated, ventilate the patient with 100 percent oxygen.

3. Grasp the patient's jaw and lift anteriorly.

4. With your other hand, hold the airway device at its proximal end and insert it into the patient's mouth. Make sure the curve is reversed, with the tip pointing toward the roof of the mouth.

5. Once the tip reaches the level of the soft palate, gently rotate the airway 180° until it comes to rest over the tongue.

6. Verify appropriate position of the airway. Clear breath sounds and chest rise indicate correct placement.

7. Ventilate the patient with 100 percent oxygen, if indicated.

Make sure the airway is correctly positioned. Improper placement can obstruct the airway by pushing the tongue back against the posterior oropharynx (Figure 13-32 ■). The

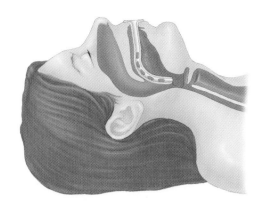

Figure 13-32 Improper placement of oropharyngeal airway.

device's advancing out of the mouth during ventilatory efforts indicates improper placement. Improper technique can also cause dental or pharyngeal trauma. An alternative insertion method useful in both pediatric and adult patients is to press the tongue upward and forward with a tongue blade. Then, the airway can be advanced until the flange is seated at the teeth. This is the preferred method of airway insertion in infants and children.

ADVANCED AIRWAY MANAGEMENT

Inserting advanced mechanical airways requires special training. The preferred method of airway management is endotracheal intubation, because it is the only procedure that effectively isolates the trachea. In some EMS systems, endotracheal intubation is not available. These systems use other airway devices such as the Esophageal Tracheal CombiTube (ETC), laryngeal mask airway (LMA), pharyngotracheal Lumen (PtL), the esophageal gastric tube airway (EGTA), or the esophageal obturator airway (EOA).

Endotracheal intubation is clearly the preferred method of advanced airway management in prehospital emergency care, because it allows the greatest control of the airway.

Review

Endotracheal Intubation Equipment

- Laryngoscope (handle and blade)
- Endotracheal tube
- 10-mL syringe
- Stylet
- Bag-valve mask
- Suction device
- Bite block
- Magill forceps
- Tape or tube-holding device

ENDOTRACHEAL INTUBATION

Endotracheal intubation involves inserting an endotracheal tube into the trachea in order to provide the patient with a definitive, protected airway. It is clearly the preferred method of advanced airway management in prehospital emergency care, because it allows the greatest control of the airway in conjunction with a bag-valve-mask unit or ventilator. Under most circumstances, it requires direct visualization of the larynx with a laryngoscope, though alternative methods are available. Successfully accomplishing endotracheal intubation requires more training than other techniques, and you must maintain ongoing proficiency to ensure patient safety. To assure the quality of your judgment and skill, you must continuously review field intubations and the criteria for performing them. You must also remember that, although endotracheal intubation affords the most effective airway control, you are bypassing important physiological functions of the upper airway—warming, filtering, and humidifying the air before it enters the lower airway.

Equipment

The equipment needed for endotracheal intubation includes: a laryngoscope (handle and blade), an appropriate-size endotracheal tube, a 10-mL syringe, a stylet, a bag-valve mask, a suction device, a bite block, Magill forceps, and tape or a commercial tube-holding device.

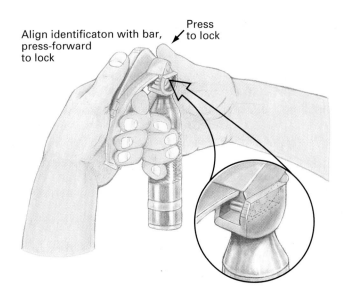

Align identificaton with bar, press-forward to lock

Press to lock

Laryngoscope   The **laryngoscope** is an instrument for lifting the tongue and epiglottis out of the way so that you can see the vocal cords. You will typically use it to place an endotracheal tube, but you may also use it in conjunction with Magill forceps to retrieve a foreign body obstructing the upper airway.

A laryngoscope consists of a handle and a blade. The handle may be either reusable or disposable. It houses batteries that power a light in the blade's distal tip. This light illuminates the airway, making it easier to see upper airway structures. The point attaching the handle and the blade is called the fitting. It locks the blade in place and provides electrical contact between the batteries and the bulb (Figure 13-33 ■).

To prepare for intubation, attach the indentation on the proximal end of the laryngoscope's blade to the bar of the handle. It will click into place when properly seated. To determine if the laryngoscope is functional, raise the blade to a right angle with the handle until it clicks into place (Figure 13-34 ■). The light should turn on and be bright and steady. A yellow, flickering light will not sufficiently illuminate the anatomical structures. If the light fails to go on, the problem may be either dead batteries or a loose bulb. Every airway kit should include spare parts. Infrequently, the contact points or the wire that runs through the blade to the bulb will fail.

laryngoscope   *instrument for lifting the tongue and epiglottis in order to see the vocal cords.*

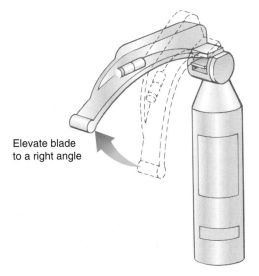

Elevate blade to a right angle

■ Figure 13-34   Activating the laryngoscope light source.

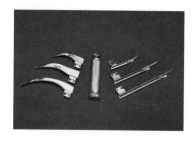

■ Figure 13-35 Laryngoscope blades.

Like the handle, the blade may be reusable or disposable. Two common types of blades are the curved blade (Macintosh blade) and the straight blade (often referred to as the Miller, Miller-Abbott, Wisconsin, or Flagg blade). Laryngoscope blades range in size from 0 for infants to 4 for large adults (Figure 13-35 ■).

The curved blade is designed to fit into the vallecula (Figure 13-36 ■). When you lift its handle anteriorly, the blade elevates the tongue and, indirectly, the epiglottis, allowing you to see the glottic opening. Because the curved blade does not touch the larynx itself, it should not traumatize or stimulate the very sensitive gag receptors on the posterior surface of the epiglottis. The curved blade also permits more room for viewing and ETT insertion. The straight blade, however, is designed to fit under the epiglottis (Figure 13-37 ■). When you lift its handle anteriorly, the blade directly lifts the epiglottis out of the way.

Several new laryngoscope blades have been developed to aid in adequately visualizing the airway. They include the Grandview (Figure 13-38 ■) and the Viewmax (Figure 13-39 ■). These offer magnification of the airway through specialized viewing lenses.

Which blade you use is largely a matter of individual preference, but you should be skilled with both in order to accommodate patients' anatomical differences. A straight blade is better for endotracheal intubation in infants, because it stabilizes their floppier epiglottises and provides greater displacement of their relatively larger tongues. It also is better for the occasional adult patient with a floppy epiglottis or large tongue.

ETT *endotracheal tube.*

Endotracheal Tubes   The endotracheal tube (**ETT**) is a flexible, translucent tube open at both ends and available in lengths ranging from 12 to 32 cm, with centimeter markings along its length (Figure 13-40 ■). The proximal end has a standard 15-mm inside diameter/22-mm outside diameter connector that attaches to the ventilatory device, usually a BVM. The ETT is available with internal tube diameters ranging from 2.5 to 4.5 mm (uncuffed) and from 5.0 to 9.0 mm (cuffed). The distal end has a beveled tip to facilitate smooth movement through airway passages. When present, an inflatable 5- to 10-mL cuff at the distal end of ETT sizes from 5.0 to 9.0 mm provides a seal between the ETT and the trachea. A thin inflation tube runs the length of the main tube from the distal cuff to a syringe. A one-way valve at the proximal end of the inflation

■ Figure 13-36   Placement of Mcintosh blade into vallecula.

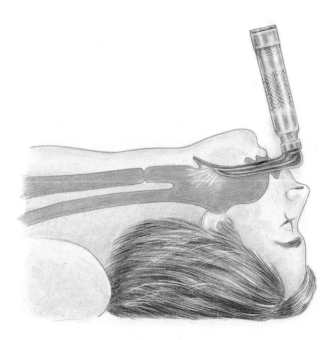

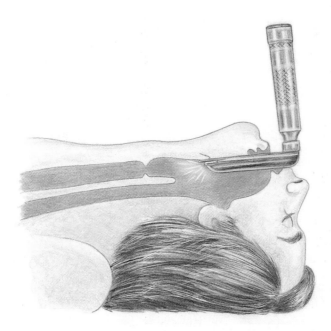

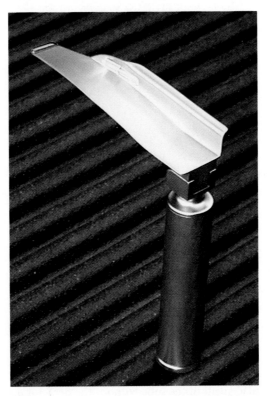

■ Figure 13-38 Grandview laryngoscope blade. *(Photo courtesy of Hartwell Medical)*

tube permits the syringe to push air into the distal cuff or pull it out, but prevents air from escaping the cuff when the syringe is removed. A pilot balloon at the inflation tube's proximal end indicates whether the distal cuff is properly inflated. The pilot balloon should be partially inflated but soft, to avoid overinflating the distal cuff and inadvertently pressuring the tracheal mucosa. This could cause ischemia of the tracheal wall. Always check the distal cuff for leaks before insertion.

Suppliers typically prewrap an ETT in a curved shape. This is because the trachea lies anteriorly in the neck, and the tube must be directed upward to enter the glottic opening. On the Endotrol ETT, an O-shaped ring attaches to a plastic wire that runs the

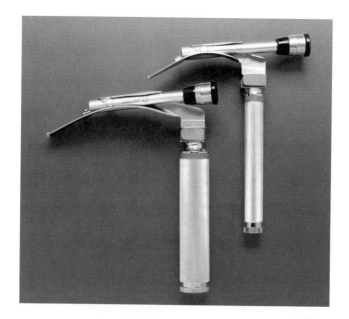

■ Figure 13-39 ViewMax laryngoscope blade. (*Viewmax™, Rüsch Inc. a division of Teleflex Medical*)

■ Figure 13-40 ETT and syringe.

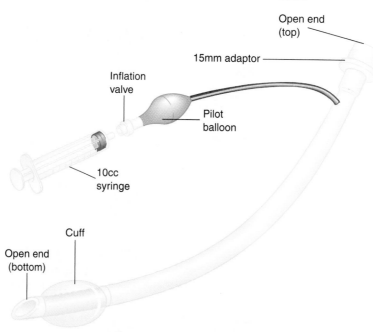

Open end (top)

15mm adaptor

Inflation valve

Pilot balloon

10cc syringe

Cuff

Open end (bottom)

length of the tube and terminates distally (Figure 13-41 ■). Pulling the ring bends the distal end of the tube upward and directs it into the glottic opening. This can facilitate placement of the tube without the need for a stylet.

Endotracheal tubes come in a variety of sizes. Markings on the tubes indicate their internal diameter in millimeters. The typical tube sizes for average-sized adult patients are 7.0 to 9.0 mm (females, 7.0 to 8.0 mm; males, 7.5 to 8.5 mm). A generally acceptable size for both male and female adults is 7.5 mm. (We discuss endotracheal intubation of children in detail later in this chapter.)

Stylet *plastic-covered metal wire used to bend the ETT into a J or hockey-stick shape.*

Stylet The malleable **stylet** is a plastic-covered metal wire used to direct the ETT anteriorly by bending its distal end into a J or hockey-stick shape (Figures 13-42a and 13-42b ■). It is particularly useful in patients with extremely anterior laryngeal anatomy or those with short, fat necks with which head positioning can be difficult. Although

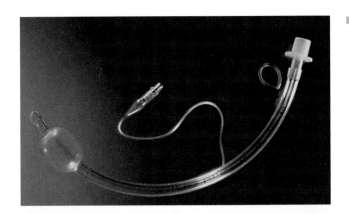

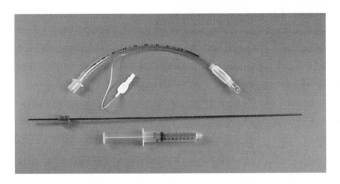

■ Figure 13-42a   ETT, stylet, and syringe, unassembled.

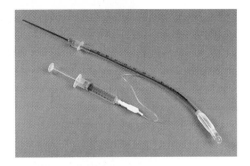

■ Figure 13-42b   ETT, stylet, and syringe, assembled for intubation.

using stylets is not mandatory, many paramedics prefer to use them in the prehospital setting because they afford greater control of the ETT. The wire stylet may damage tissues during intubation if it extends past the distal end of the ETT; therefore, you should keep it recessed at least 2 cm from the tip of the tube.

Gum Elastic Bougie   The gum elastic Bougie (also called the Eschmann tracheal tube introducer) is a straight, semirigid stylet-like device with a bent tip that is covered with a protective resin (Figure 13-43 ■). It is used to facilitate endotracheal intubations when intubation is (or is anticipated to be) difficult. Patients who often present airway difficulties include those who have:

★ Short, thick (bull) neck

★ Other anatomical variation

★ Laryngeal edema (anaphylaxis, burns)

★ Supraglottic tumors

★ Pregnancy

★ Inability to be positioned properly (entrapment, confined space)

The gum elastic Bougie is 60–70 cm long and suitable for use with endotracheal tubes that have an internal diameter of 6.0 mm or greater. During laryngoscopy, the Bougie is carefully advanced into the larynx and through the cords until the tip enters well into the trachea. While maintaining the laryngoscope and Bougie in position, an assistant threads an ETT over the end of the Bougie into the larynx. Once the ETT is in place, the Bougie is removed. The patient can then be ventilated normally.

The gum elastic Bougie should not be used in children less than 14 years of age.

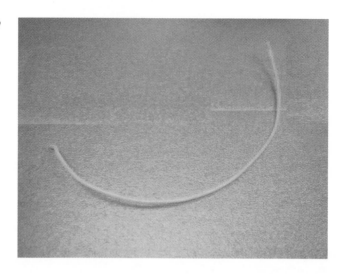

10-mL Syringe   The syringe allows you to inflate the distal cuff just enough to avoid air leaks around the ETT without causing tracheal ischemia.

Tube-Holding Devices   Tie-downs or tape secure the endotracheal tube once it is in the trachea. The reasons for securing the ETT are twofold. First, moving the patient about during resuscitation or transportation can easily dislodge the tube. Even if the ETT is not actually dislodged, its movement can still cause cardiovascular stimulation, an elevation in intracranial pressure, or injury to the tracheal mucosa. Second, the person providing ventilatory support may inadvertently push down on the ETT, forcing it into the right or left mainstem bronchus. Using tape requires extra care, as it can loosen when either the patient's face or the tube is moist. A number of commercial tube-holding devices are available.

Magill forceps scissor-style *clamps with circular tips.*

Magill Forceps   The **Magill forceps** are scissor-style clamps with circular tips. You will use them to remove foreign bodies or to redirect the endotracheal tube during nasotracheal intubation (Figure 13-44 ■).

Lubricant   Water-soluble lubricants facilitate inserting the ETT. Do not use petroleum-based lubricants; they may damage the ETT and cause tracheal inflammation.

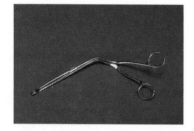

Suction Unit   A suction unit helps to remove secretions and foreign materials from the oropharynx during intubation attempts. It is a vital element that you must never forget. (We discuss suction units in more detail later in this chapter.)

■ Figure 13-44 Magill forceps.

End-Tidal CO_2 Detector or Other Confirmation Device   These adjuncts to intubation are becoming the standard of care in most areas. You must be familiar with the devices, their role in intubation, and your local protocols' requirements for their use.

Additional Airways   You should also have an oropharyngeal airway available during endotracheal intubation. You will occasionally use it as a block to prevent the patient from biting down on and collapsing the ETT.

Protective Equipment   Endotracheal intubation, like many airway procedures, carries the risk of exposure to body substances. Because of this, it is essential to employ body substance isolation procedures. These include, but are not limited to, gloves, mask, protective eyewear, and possibly a gown. Remember, personal safety comes first!

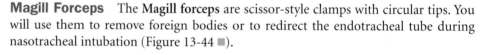

Endotracheal Intubation Indications

Monitoring success rates for particular skills is not hard with an appropriate quality assurance program. Evaluating your ability to judge which patients you should intubate is considerably more difficult. Often the patient's condition may warrant trying nebulizer treatments or supplemental oxygen before deciding to intubate. A patient's continued distress and failure to respond to treatment clearly indicate intubation. In conjunction with the medical director, you are responsible for continually improving your judgment regarding the use of advanced airway management techniques. This includes recognizing subtle indicators that the patient's condition is worsening, before the onset of respiratory arrest.

Endotracheal intubation provides a definitive, secure, open airway for patients who are experiencing, or are likely to experience, upper airway compromise. Some of the indications for endotracheal intubation in these patients include respiratory or cardiac arrest; unresponsiveness without a gag reflex; inability to protect the airway, resulting in an increased risk of aspiration; and obstruction due to foreign bodies, trauma, burns, or anaphylaxis. Endotracheal intubation also improves oxygenation and ventilation in patients with extreme lower airway difficulty. Some lower airway indications include severe respiratory distress due to diseases such as asthma, COPD, CHF, or pneumonia, as well as pneumothorax, hemothorax, or hemopneumothorax with respiratory difficulty. Clearly, then, endotracheal intubation may be indicated in breathing and apneic patients, though caution must be used in any patient with an intact gag reflex.

Do not attempt endotracheal intubation in the prehospital setting if epiglottitis is present, unless airway failure is imminent. Attempts to manipulate the airway in epiglottitis are very likely to result in vigorous laryngospasm. The most prudent management of epiglottitis is oxygenation of the patient without agitation. The preferred treatment for epiglottitis is rapid transport to the operating room for endotracheal intubation under more controlled conditions. This is carried out with the necessary equipment for emergency tracheostomy opened and ready for immediate use. Sometimes, these patients steadily worsen and loss of their airway is imminent and inevitable. In this case, the benefits from endotracheal intubation outweigh the risks. Regardless, the most experienced member of the crew should perform the procedure. Also, it is important to remember that there may be significant laryngeal edema and it may be necessary to insert a smaller-than-normal endotracheal tube. This should be kept in mind before undertaking this procedure. Always follow local protocols and contact medical direction regarding endotracheal intubation in cases where epiglottitis is present or suspected.

Advantages of Endotracheal Intubation

★ It isolates the trachea and permits complete control of the airway.

★ It impedes gastric distention by channeling air directly into the trachea.

★ It eliminates the need to maintain a mask seal.

★ It offers a direct route for suctioning of the respiratory passages.

★ It permits administration of the medications *l*idocaine, *e*pinephrine, *a*tropine, and *n*aloxone via the endotracheal tube. (Use the mnemonic LEAN to remember these medications.)

Disadvantages of Endotracheal Intubation

★ The technique requires considerable training and experience.

★ It requires specialized equipment.

★ It requires direct visualization of the vocal cords.

★ It bypasses the upper airway's function of warming, filtering, and humidifying the inhaled air.

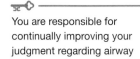

You are responsible for continually improving your judgment regarding airway management.

 Review

Endotracheal Intubation Indicators

- Respiratory or cardiac arrest
- Unconsciousness or obtusion without gag reflex
- Risk of aspiration
- Obstruction due to foreign bodies, trauma, burns, or anaphylaxis
- Respiratory *extremis* due to disease
- Pneumothorax, hemothorax, or hemopneumothorax with respiratory difficulty

Negligence and Malpractice Suits Although negligence and malpractice lawsuits against EMS personnel are still relatively uncommon, many of those that do arise involve issues related to airway management. Improper airway management—such as failure to recognize a displaced endotracheal tube—can result in death or serious disability. Because of this, paramedics must take great care to make certain that airway management procedures are properly performed.

Always remain competent in endotracheal intubation. If you work in a system where there is limited opportunity for its use, then you should increase your in-service education and possibly arrange to spend some time in the hospital performing intubations.

Always make sure that all airway equipment is functioning properly. This includes checking ET tube cuffs, laryngoscope light bulbs, mechanical ventilation devices, and other adjuncts. These must be kept in a readily accessible location and checked on a regular basis.

After performing endotracheal intubation, it is essential to confirm and document proper tube placement by at least three methods. Esophageal detector devices are good, but end-tidal carbon dioxide detectors and capnography are better. Following intubation, periodically and religiously check and confirm continued proper tube placement. For a complete legal record, these findings must be documented. If there is a doubt in regard to tube placement, the tube should be checked or removed and mechanical ventilation continued.

Remember, the greatest chances of tube displacement occur with patient movement. This is especially true when the stretcher with the patient is moved out of the ambulance. When a one-person stretcher is lowered to a level position, care must be taken to ensure that the ET tube has not been dislodged.

The skill of endotracheal intubation does not end after successful placement of the tube. Continuous and vigilant monitoring of tube placement should occur until the patient is turned over to the hospital staff.

Complications of Endotracheal Intubation

Intubation presents a number of potential complications. Properly attending to detail and taking appropriate precautions will help you to avoid these problems.

Equipment Malfunction Equipment malfunctions consume valuable time when you are establishing a definitive airway and effective oxygenation and ventilation. Having a preassembled airway kit that is checked regularly will lessen the chances of this occurring. Ideally someone should check the airway kit daily to be sure that all needed supplies are present and that the bulb, batteries, and blade are in good working condition.

Teeth Breakage and Soft-Tissue Lacerations Endotracheal intubation can injure the lips and teeth, but you can eliminate this hazard by carefully using the laryngoscope as an instrument, not a tool. When inserting the blade into the mouth and pharynx, guide it gently into place, avoiding pressure on the teeth. When manipulating the jaw anteriorly, use gentle traction upward and toward the feet rather than rotating and flexing your wrist, which will make the laryngoscope function as a lever. All levers require a fulcrum—and the only fulcrums available in your patient's mouth will be his upper incisors. A rotating/flexing action may thus break teeth. To avoid this hazard, lift the laryngoscope's handle (exposing the epiglottis) after you have applied the blade to the base of the tongue. After this, keep your wrist straight and do any lifting with your shoulder and arm.

If you use the laryngoscope too roughly, you can lacerate the patient's lips, tongue, or pharyngeal structures, producing profuse bleeding that is hard to control. This can also happen if you direct the tube away from the midline into the pyriform sinuses or allow the stylet to protrude from the distal end of the ETT. In the larynx and lower airway, you might damage the vocal cords, cause laryngeal edema, or tear the trachea if you are not careful. A gentle technique and attention to detail are the keys to avoiding these complications.

Hypoxia   Delays in oxygenation, either from interruption of basic airway techniques and BVM ventilation with 100 percent oxygen or from prolonged intubation attempts, can produce profound, life-threatening hypoxia. Each patient's unique anatomy and unusual clinical situations can challenge even the most experienced paramedic. One basic rule that helps to avoid hypoxia during intubation is to limit each intubation attempt to no more than 30 seconds before reoxygenating the patient. To gauge this interval, some paramedics hold their breath from the time they stop ventilating the patient until they start again.

To avoid hypoxia during intubation, limit each intubation attempt to no more than 30 seconds before reoxygenating the patient.

If you cannot pass the tube through the vocal cords on the first attempt, at least identify your landmarks and note any unique or difficult features that you may need to address. For example, too much edema might indicate a smaller ETT. Or the patient's larynx might be more anterior than you realized from his external anatomy, and you will need to use a different blade or change the ETT angle. You can then pass the tube on a subsequent attempt, after hyperventilating the patient with basic airway techniques and 100 percent oxygen using a BVM device.

Esophageal Intubation   Misplacement of the ETT into the esophagus deprives the patient of oxygenation and ventilation. It is potentially lethal, resulting in severe hypoxia and brain death if you do not recognize it immediately. It also directs air into the stomach, encouraging regurgitation, which can lead to aspiration. Indicators of esophageal intubation include:

Esophageal intubation is potentially lethal if you do not recognize it immediately.

- ★ An absence of chest rise and absence of breath sounds with mechanical ventilation
- ★ Gurgling sounds over the epigastrium with each breath delivered
- ★ Distention of the abdomen
- ★ An absence of breath condensation in the endotracheal tube
- ★ A persistent air leak, despite inflation of the tube's distal cuff
- ★ Cyanosis and progressive worsening of the patient's condition
- ★ Phonation (noise made by the vocal cords)
- ★ No color change with colorimetric $ETCO_2$ detector
- ★ A falling pulse oximetry reading

If you have any suspicion that the tube is in the esophagus, remove it immediately. Hyperventilate the patient with 100 percent oxygen and attempt endotracheal intubation with another tube.

Endobronchial Intubation   If you pass the endotracheal tube successfully through the vocal cords and advance it too far, it likely will enter either the right or left mainstem bronchus. As discussed earlier, the ETT may be misplaced to either side, but it is more likely to pass into the right mainstem, which angles away from the trachea less acutely than does the left. In either case, the ETT ventilates only one lung and the result is hypoventilation and hypoxia from inadequate gas exchange. Also, when the bag-valve device **insufflates** enough air for two lungs into the smaller area of only one lung, it can

insufflate   *to blow into.*

create enough pressure to cause barotrauma such as a pneumothorax, worsening the patient's condition.

You can avoid inserting the ETT too far by following these guidelines:

1. Advance the distal cuff no more than 1 to 2 cm past the vocal cords.
2. Once the tube is positioned, hold it in place with one hand to prevent it from being pushed any farther.
3. Inflate the cuff and firmly secure the tube in place with tape or a commercial tube-holding device.
4. Note the number marking on the side of the ETT where it emerges from the patient's mouth at the teeth, gums, or lips. This will allow you to quickly recognize any changes in tube placement. Approximate ETT depth for the average adult is 21 cm at the teeth for women and 23 cm at the teeth for men, though this will vary.

Findings in endobronchial intubation include:

★ Breath sounds present on one side of the chest but diminished or absent on the other
★ Poor compliance (resistance to ventilations with the bag-valve device)
★ Cyanosis, cardiac dysrhythmias, or other evidence of hypoxia

To resolve the problem, loosen or remove any securing devices and withdraw the ETT until breath sounds are present and equal bilaterally. Be certain to deflate the cuff when pulling back on the ETT.

Tension Pneumothorax Any tear in the lung parenchyma can cause a pneumothorax. If this is allowed to progress untreated, a tension pneumothorax, an accumulation of air or gas in the pleural cavity, may develop. A tension pneumothorax is a large pneumothorax that affects other structures in the chest. The expanding tension pneumothorax will adversely affect the other lung, the heart, and the structures of the mediastinum. It will eventually displace these structures away from the side of the chest with the tension pneumothorax. In addition to mainstem bronchus intubation, tension pneumothorax can result if you use too much of the bag-valve device's volume on a small adult or child or use the full bag-valve-device volume against diseased lungs with poor compliance. Tension pneumothorax is marked by progressively worsening compliance (more difficulty in ventilating), diminished unilateral breath sounds, hypoxia with hypotension, and distended neck veins. Often the trachea will deviate away from the side of the chest with the pneumothorax. Also, the marked increase in intrathoracic pressure resulting from the tension pneumothorax can prevent the ventricles from adequately filling. This can cause a decrease in cardiac output and will worsen the patient's overall condition. If you suspect tension pneumothorax, needle decompression of the chest is indicated, as described in Volume 4, Chapter 10.

Orotracheal Intubation Technique

The most widely preferred and, therefore, the most commonly used path for endotracheal intubation is the orotracheal route. Many medical personnel favor this route because it involves direct visualization of the vocal cords and a clear view of the ETT's passage through them. It is thus the most accurate method of intubation and the least likely to induce trauma to the airway. To perform orotracheal intubation in the absence of suspected trauma (Procedure 13–1):

1. Place the patient supine.
2. After using basic manual and adjunctive airway maneuvers to open the airway, ventilate the patient with 100 percent oxygen.

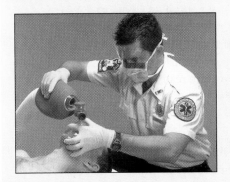

13-1a Ventilate the patient.

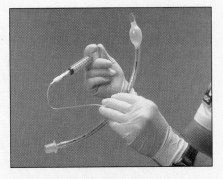

13-1b Prepare the equipment.

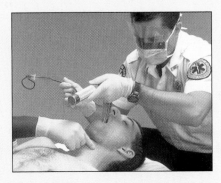

13-1c Apply the Sellick maneuver and insert laryngoscope.

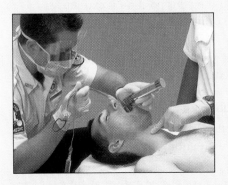

13-1d Visualize the larynx and insert the ETT.

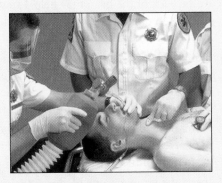

13-1e Inflate the cuff, ventilate, and auscultate.

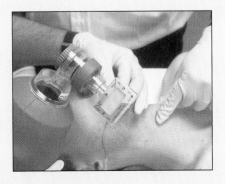

13-1f Confirm placement with an $ETCO_2$ detector.

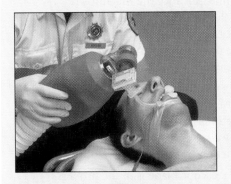

13-1g Secure the tube.

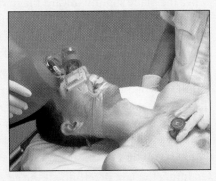

13-1h Reconfirm ETT placement.

(Photos © Scott Metcalfe)

3. While your partner ventilates the patient, prepare your intubation equipment, including suction, and be certain that all needed equipment is present and in good working order. Assemble and check the laryngoscope blade and handle to be certain you have a steady, bright light—then close the handle. Insert the stylet into the ETT, making sure to keep the distal end of the stylet at least 2 cm proximal to the distal tip of the ETT. You may choose to bend the distal end of the ETT into a "hockey stick" shape just proximal to the distal cuff to help direct the ETT anteriorly. Apply water-soluble lubricant to the distal end of the ETT and reinsert. Leaving the ETT partially in its packaging until you are ready to insert it helps to keep it as clean as possible. Fill the 10-mL syringe with 5 to 10 mL of air and attach it to the valve at the proximal end of the ETT, using a twisting motion to lock it in place. Check the cuff for air leaks.

4. Turn on the suction and attach an appropriate tip.

5. Position the patient's head and neck. Remove any dentures or partial dental plates. To visualize the larynx, you must align the three axes of the mouth, the pharynx, and the trachea. To do this, place the patient's head in a "sniffing position" by flexing the neck forward and the head backward. Inserting a rolled towel or sheet under the patient's shoulders or the back of the head may help. Establishing this position is extremely difficult in patients with short, fat necks or whose motion is limited by such conditions as arthritis.

6. Hold the laryngoscope in your left hand whether you are right- or left-handed. Most laryngoscopes are designed for right-handed people; that is, the right-handed person must hold the laryngoscope in his left hand in order to manipulate the endotracheal tube with his right.

7. If you have not already done so, have your partner apply the Sellick maneuver (cricoid pressure) and maintain it until you confirm ETT placement in the trachea.

8. Insert the laryngoscope blade gently into the right side of the patient's mouth. With a gentle sweeping action, displace the tongue to the left. This pushes the tongue out of your line of vision and allows more room to manipulate the endotracheal tube.

9. Move the blade slightly toward the midline. Advance the Macintosh (curved) blade until the distal end is at the base of the tongue in the vallecula; advance the Miller (straight) blade until the distal end is under the epiglottis. As you advance the blade, move the patient's lower lip away from the blade using the index finger of your right hand.

10. Lift the laryngoscope handle slightly upward and toward the feet to displace the jaw. Be careful not to put pressure on the teeth. At this point, you can see any vomitus, blood, or secretions in the posterior pharynx. You likely will have to suction the airway clear. If the secretions are thick or copious, you may need to remove the suction tip and use the suction hose.

11. On lifting the jaw, determine if the laryngoscope blade is in the proper position. You may need to adjust it before you can visualize the vocal cords. If you cannot see landmarks clearly, gently withdraw the blade, slowly and slightly. This may bring the vocal cords into view. If it does not, you might need to gently advance the blade farther into the hypopharynx.

12. Keeping your left wrist straight, use your left shoulder and arm to continue lifting the mandible and tongue to a 45° angle to the ground (up and toward the feet) until the glottis is exposed (Figure 13-45 ■). Often

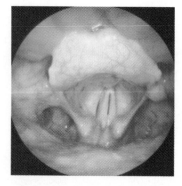

■ Figure 13-45 Glottis visualized through laryngoscopy. (*Phototake, NYC*)

you may not see the entire glottis, but you should see at least its posterior third or half. If the larynx lies anteriorly, a slight increase in your partner's pressure on the Sellick maneuver should improve your view of the vocal cords. Occasionally, your partner will need to lessen the cricoid pressure slightly to allow you to visualize the vocal cords. Be ready to instruct him to apply more or less cricoid pressure.

13. Hold the ETT in your right hand with your fingertips as you would a dart or a pencil; this gives you control to gently maneuver the ETT. Advance the tube through the right corner of the patient's mouth, and direct it toward the midline.

14. Directly visualizing the vocal cords, pass the ETT gently through the glottic opening until its distal cuff disappears beyond the vocal cords; then advance it another 1 to 2 cm.

15. Hold the tube in place with your hand to prevent its displacement; do not let go under any circumstance until it is taped or tied securely in place. Attach a bag-valve device to the 15/22-mm connector on the tube; have the ETCO$_2$ detector attached to the bag-valve device as your local protocols require.

16. Inflate the distal cuff with 5 to 10 mL of air. To avoid tracheal trauma or ischemia from excessive cuff pressure, apply only enough pressure to prevent air leakage around the ETT during ventilation. Listen for any air leak and adjust the cuff's pressure as needed. When cuff pressure is correct, remove the syringe, using a twisting motion to prevent any air leak.

17. Check for proper tube placement. While listening for equal bilateral breath sounds over the chest, watch to see that the chest rises and falls symmetrically. Listen over the epigastrium to be certain you hear no gastric sounds. Look for moisture condensation in the exhaled breath; it should appear in the ETT during each exhalation.

18. Ventilate the patient with 100 percent oxygen. Gently insert an oropharyngeal airway to serve as a bite block.

19. Secure the ETT with umbilical tape, while maintaining ventilatory support. Loop the tape around the tube at the level of the patient's teeth, attaching it tightly to the tube without kinking or pinching it. Then wrap the tape around the patient's head, and tie it at the side of his neck. Alternatively, use a commercial tube-holding device.

20. Repeat step 17 periodically to confirm proper ETT placement. Also repeat step 17 after any major patient movement or movement of his head or neck. (Neck manipulation can displace the tube up to 5 cm.) Continue to support the tube manually while maintaining ventilatory support.

Verification of Proper Endotracheal Tube Placement   Continuously checking and rechecking tube placement is an important responsibility during endotracheal intubation. The hypervigilance with which you must monitor the patient's clinical condition cannot be overemphasized. You can employ a number of methods in the field to confirm correct ETT placement. You should put them to maximum use, but do not become overly reliant on technology. The patient's clinical condition should be the deciding factor in your patient management decisions.

The most reliable method of confirming proper ETT placement is direct visualization of its passage through the vocal cords. This requires the proper use of a laryngoscope and continued visualization of the vocal cords throughout intubation. If you do this, you have little chance of inadvertently intubating the esophagus.

The hypervigilance with which you must monitor the patient's clinical condition cannot be overemphasized.

Following ETT placement, watch to be sure that the patient's chest rises with ventilations. If the ETT is misplaced in the esophagus, the chest will not rise. You also should auscultate for breath sounds. Their equal presence over both sides (apices and bases) of the chest and their absence over the epigastrium helps to confirm proper ETT placement. Conversely, their absence over the chest and their presence over the epigastrium indicates an esophageal intubation. Breath sounds present on one side but absent or diminished on the other indicate that the ETT may be advanced too deeply into one of the mainstem bronchi, that bronchial obstruction may be present, or that a pneumothorax is present. Absent breath sounds bilaterally may indicate esophageal intubation.

End-tidal CO_2 detectors and esophageal detector devices can be helpful. Adequate levels of exhaled carbon dioxide, as detected by an end-tidal CO_2 detector, confirm proper endotracheal tube placement. The ability to withdraw air readily from an esophageal detector device's syringe further confirms placement of the ETT in the trachea. Resistance to air withdrawal, or the creation of a vacuum, denotes esophageal intubation.

Also observe the endotracheal tube's contents. Exhaled air approaches 100 percent humidity. Usually, the ambient relative humidity is less than 100 percent. Thus, condensation inside the ETT suggests its proper placement. Because the gastric sphincter relaxes in critically ill patients and the high pressures of a bag-valve mask create gastric distention, patients frequently vomit and aspirate during resuscitation. If you misplace the ETT into the esophagus, you may observe an efflux of gastric contents through the ETT, particularly with subsequent ventilation attempts. Because aspiration into the trachea also may have occurred, you might see vomitus in the ETT even with proper endotracheal intubation; nonetheless, this finding always should raise suspicion of esophageal intubation and prompt further investigation.

It is important to assure proper endotracheal tube placement. Allegations of improperly placed endotracheal tubes are a major reason for paramedic malpractice suits. Because of this, it is important to verify *and document* proper endotracheal tube placement. In fact, it is ideal to verify and document at least three different indicators of proper placement. These may include:

- ★ Visualization of the tube passing between the cords
- ★ Presence of bilateral breath sounds
- ★ Absence of breath sounds over the epigastrium
- ★ Positive end-tidal CO_2 change on an $ETCO_2$ device
- ★ Verification of endotracheal placement by an esophageal detector device
- ★ Presence of condensation inside the endotracheal tube
- ★ Absence of vomitus inside the endotracheal tube
- ★ Absence of phonation, or vocal sounds, once the tube is placed

In addition, an increase in the oxygen saturation will help support proper placement of the endotracheal tube. Likewise, a rise and fall of the chest indicates endotracheal intubation. Worsening gastric distention may indicate possible esophageal placement. Any gastric distention should be investigated. Remember, though, it is not uncommon for gastric distention to develop prior to endotracheal intubation due to mechanical ventilation. Even in experienced hands, it is very difficult to avoid gastric distention with mechanical ventilation until an endotracheal tube is placed.

Transillumination Intubation Since a bright light in the trachea is visible (transilluminates) through the soft tissue of the anterior neck, an ETT with a lighted stylet can facilitate correct intubation (Figure 13-46 ■). The stylet is a plastic cable with a malleable, retractable wire running through its center and a small, high-intensity bulb at its distal end. An on-off switch and power supply at the stylet's proximal end control

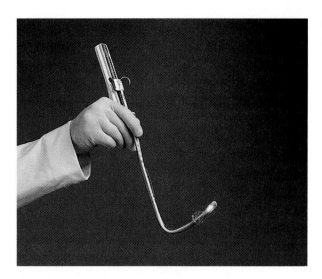

the bulb, which begins to blink about 30 seconds after it is turned on. This blinking makes detecting the light's transilluminations easier.

You can confirm correct ETT placement by observing the stylet's light through the anterior neck's soft tissue; esophageal intubation results in little or no light being visible. Because you can place the ETT safely and correctly without directly visualizing the glottic opening, you can perform endotracheal intubation without manipulating a trauma patient's head and neck. Several studies have shown the transillumination technique to be fast, dependable, and atraumatic.

This technique's biggest limitation is that bright ambient light can make the transillumination difficult to see. Therefore, it works best in a darkened room and with thin patients. When attempting this procedure, reduce ambient light; in direct or bright daylight, shade the patient's neck.

To perform transillumination intubation:

1. While maintaining ventilatory support, ventilate the patient with 100 percent oxygen.

2. Prepare and check your equipment. The endotracheal tube's diameter should be 7.5 to 8.5 mm. You will need to cut the ETT to a length of 25 to 27 cm to accommodate the stylet. Place the stylet in the ETT and lock the ETT in place at its proximal end. Using the sliding mechanism on the handle, adjust the stylet and bend it into a hockey-stick shape just proximal to the distal cuff.

3. With the patient supine and his head in neutral position, kneel along either his right or left side, facing his head.

4. Turn on the stylet light.

5. With your index and middle fingers inserted deeply into the patient's mouth and your thumb under his chin, lift his tongue and jaw forward (Figure 13-47 ■).

6. With the proximal end of the ETT directed toward the patient's feet, insert the tube/stylet into the mouth and advance it gently through the oropharynx into the hypopharynx.

7. Use a "hooking" action with the tube/stylet to lift the epiglottis out of the way (Figure 13-48 ■).

8. When you see a circle of light at the patient's Adam's apple, the stylet is placed correctly (Figure 13-49 ■). A diffuse, dim, hard-to-see, or absent

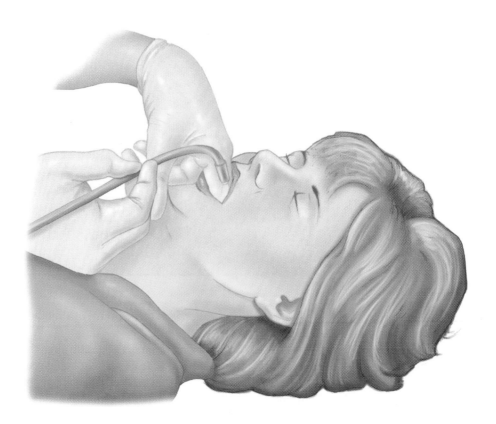

■ Figure 13-47 Insertion of lighted stylet/ETT.

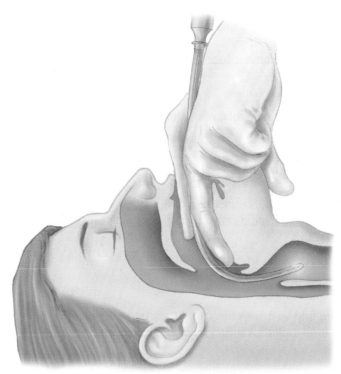

■ Figure 13-48 Lighted stylet/ETT in position.

light indicates that the ETT/stylet combination is in the esophagus. A bright light lateral and superior to the Adam's apple indicates that it has moved into the right or left pyriform fossa. To correct either of these placements, withdraw the tube and reattempt intubation after ventilating the patient with 100 percent oxygen for several minutes, using proper basic manual and adjunct airway maneuvers.

Tube stat

9. After the ETT is properly placed, hold the stylet stationary. Advance the tube off the stylet into the larynx approximately 1 to 2 cm, while simultaneously retracting the internal wire from the stylet using the O-ring at its proximal end.

10. Once the light is in the correct position and you have partially advanced the ETT while partially retracting the stylet wire, hold the tube firmly in place with one hand and remove the stylet.

11. Attach the bag-valve device to the endotracheal tube's 15/22-mm connector and deliver several breaths, inflating the distal ETT cuff and checking for proper placement as usual.

12. Secure the ETT, recheck placement, and maintain ventilatory support. Continue periodic assessment of the airway.

Digital Intubation   Some situations may require you to perform digital intubation. This technique dates to the eighteenth century, when people performed intubations without the benefit of a laryngoscope. Instead, they used digital (finger), or tactile (touch), intubation (Figure 13-50 ■).

Digital intubation is still useful for a number of situations in the prehospital setting. It is suggested when a patient is deeply comatose or in cardiac arrest and when proper positioning is difficult. The classic example is an unresponsive trauma patient with a suspected cervical spine injury. Since the digital technique does not require manipulation of the head and neck, it is of great value here. It may also be useful in extrication situations where the confined space prevents properly positioning the patient. Also, because digital intubation does not require visualization, it may be helpful when

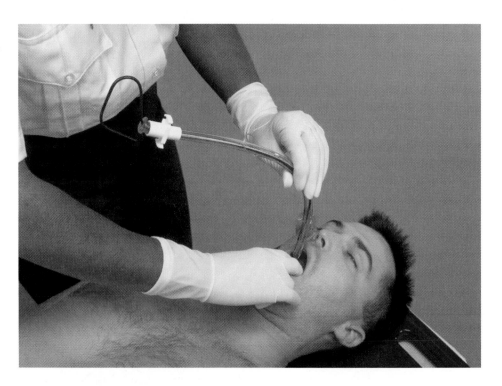

■ Figure 13-50 Blind orotracheal intubation by digital method.

facial injuries distort the patient's anatomy or when you cannot suction copious amounts of blood, vomitus, or other secretions for a proper view of the airway.

Digital intubation is risky for the paramedic; it may stimulate even a deeply comatose patient to clamp down and bite your finger. Do not use it with conscious patients or with unconscious patients who have a gag reflex. To perform digital intubation:

1. Use blood and body fluid precautions.

2. While maintaining ventilatory support with basic manual and adjunctive airway maneuvers, ventilate the patient with 100 percent oxygen.

3. Prepare and check your equipment. You will need the following items: an appropriately sized ETT, a malleable stylet, water-soluble lubricant, a 5- to 10-mL syringe, a bite block, and umbilical tape or a commercial anchoring device. Insert the stylet into the endotracheal tube and bend the ETT/stylet into a J shape.

4. While another team member stabilizes the patient's head and neck in an in-line (neutral) position, kneel at the patient's left shoulder, facing his head. Place a bite block device between the patient's molars to help protect your fingers.

5. Insert your left middle and index fingers into the patient's mouth (Figure 13-51 ■). By alternating fingers, "walk" your hand down the midline while simultaneously tugging gently forward on the tongue. You may also use gauze to hold and extend the tongue more effectively, which may facilitate palpation of the glottis. This lifts the epiglottis up and away from the glottic opening, within reach of your probing fingers.

6. Palpate the arytenoid cartilage posterior to the glottis and the epiglottis anteriorly with your middle finger (Figure 13-52 ■). Press the epiglottis forward, and insert the endotracheal tube into the mouth, anterior to your fingers (Figure 13-53 ■).

7. Advance the tube, pushing it gently with your right hand. Use your left index finger to keep the tip of the ETT against your middle finger. This will direct the tip to the epiglottis.

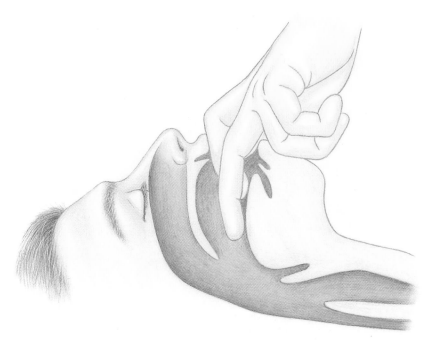

■ Figure 13-51 Digital intubation. Insert your middle and index fingers into the patient's mouth.

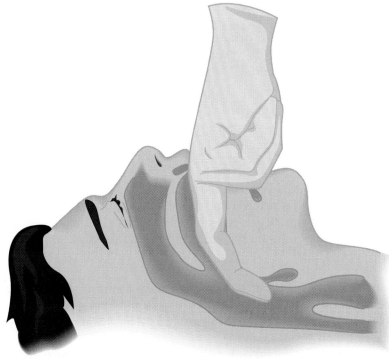

■ Figure 13-52 Digital intubation. Walk your fingers and palpate the patient's epiglottis.

8. Use your middle and index fingers to direct the tip of the ETT between the epiglottis (in front) and your fingers (behind). Then with your right hand advance the ETT through the cords while simultaneously maneuvering it forward with your left index and middle fingers. This will prevent it from slipping posteriorly into the esophagus.

9. Hold the tube in place with your hand to prevent its displacement. Attach a bag-valve device with an $ETCO_2$ detector to the 15/22-mm connector on the ETT; inflate the distal cuff with 5 to 10 mL of air; check for proper tube placement.

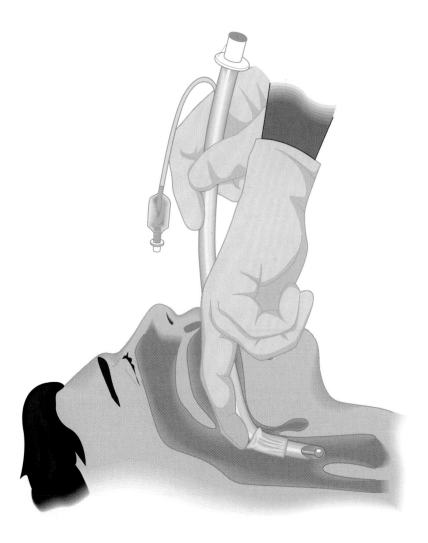

10. Ventilate the patient with 100 percent oxygen. Gently insert an oropharyngeal airway to serve as a bite block. Secure the ETT with umbilical tape. Repeat steps to confirm proper ETT placement and maintain ventilatory support. Continue your airway assessment periodically.

Trauma Patient Intubation   Airway management and ventilatory support in the trauma patient are essential for a successful outcome. Appropriate treatment of all other injuries is meaningless if you do not assure a patent airway and adequate oxygenation and ventilation.

The trauma patient presents a number of obstacles to effective airway management and ventilation. Some of them may be the need for extrication, blood in the oropharynx, distorted anatomy due to injury, and the need to protect the cervical spine. Getting an adequate seal on a mask is very difficult when the patient is being extricated or has significant facial trauma. You must keep the cervical spine in a neutral, in-line position throughout your management of all patients with known or suspected cervical spine trauma. Digital intubation, transillumination intubation, and nasotracheal intubation (described later in this chapter) provide potential solutions for some patients when trauma complicates airway management, but visualizing the vocal cords is still preferable. You can do this effectively using direct laryngoscopy-assisted orotracheal intubation with manual in-line stabilization of the cervical spine (Procedure 13–2).

Appropriate treatment of a trauma patient's other injuries is meaningless if you do not assure a patent airway and adequate oxygenation and ventilation.

Endotracheal Intubation with In-line Stabilization

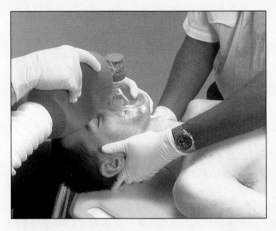

13-2a   Ventilate the patient and apply manual C-spine stabilization.

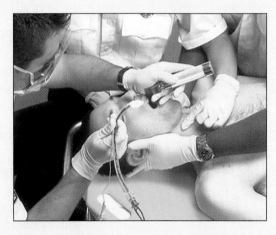

13-2b   Apply Sellick maneuver and intubate.

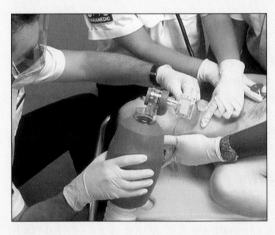

13-2c   Ventilate the patient and confirm placement.

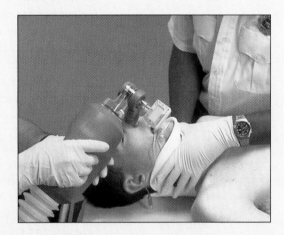

13-2d   Secure the ETT and place a cervical collar.

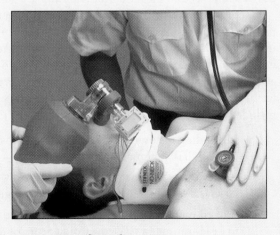

13-2e   Reconfirm placement.

To perform orotracheal intubation with in-line stabilization:

1. After basic manual and adjunctive airway maneuvers, have your partner maintain in-line stabilization while kneeling at the patient's side, facing his head. This is done by placing both hands over the patient's ears with the little, ring, and middle fingers under the occiput, the index fingers anterior to the ears, and the thumbs on the face over the maxillary sinuses.

2. Apply slight pressure in a caudal direction (toward the feet) to support and immobilize the head.

3. Proceed gently with orotracheal intubation, remembering the need to minimize movement of the cervical spine.

Rapid Sequence Intubation

Your most immediate concern with every patient you treat is to maintain a patent airway and adequate oxygenation and ventilation. Clearly, if a patient is in cardiac or respiratory arrest, or is unconscious or obtunded and not protecting his airway, endotracheal intubation is indicated. Quite commonly, however, you may have an awake patient, perhaps with significantly altered mental status, who is hypoxic even on 100 percent oxygen because of respiratory distress or a worsening airway disorder. This patient is working his hardest to breathe but does not have adequate gas exchange to support life. His altered mental status indicates that some level of significant hypoxia is putting essential brain functions at risk.

You cannot perform orotracheal intubation on this patient until he fatigues enough to have respiratory failure, with resultant unconsciousness and decreased muscle tone. By then, however, he will have suffered prolonged hypoxia, possibly accompanied by a myocardial infarction, brain damage, or vomiting with aspiration. If a patient clearly is precipitously failing maximal aggressive medical management, or if the history of his problem clearly indicates that he will not be able to or already cannot protect his airway, then active intervention is appropriate to control the airway and provide adequate ventilation. The safest way to do this is an advanced airway procedure called rapid sequence induction or **rapid sequence intubation (RSI).** Classic rapid sequence induction is an anesthetic procedure whereby patients rapidly receive induction of general anesthesia followed by endotracheal intubation. In emergency medicine, we do not administer general anesthesia, but we have borrowed other elements of this technique in order to rapidly obtain an airway in a patient who has altered mental status. While the term *rapid sequence induction (RSI)* describes the classic procedure, it has been modified in the emergency medicine setting to *rapid sequence intubation (RSI)*. Again, the difference is that the latter does not utilize a general anesthetic agent.

Rapid sequence intubation involves preoxygenating the patient to the best level possible given his condition, carefully monitoring him, and giving medications to induce (sedate) and temporarily paralyze him. You then proceed with orotracheal intubation in a controlled manner. Patients who are candidates for RSI are either awake, responsive, agitated, or combative, or have a significant gag reflex, clenched teeth, or too much airway muscle tone to allow intubation. Indications for RSI include:

★ Impending respiratory failure due to intrinsic pulmonary disease such as COPD, CHF, asthma, or pneumonia

★ Acute airway disorder that threatens airway patency such as facial burns, laryngeal or upper airway trauma, and epiglottitis

★ Altered mental status with significant risk of vomiting and aspiration, as in head trauma (a Glasgow Coma Score of 8 or less), drug or alcohol intoxication, status epilepticus

rapid sequence intubation
giving medications to sedate (induce) and temporarily paralyze a patient and then performing orotracheal intubation.

The basic physiology involved in rapid sequence intubation centers around the neuromuscular junction—the connection between peripheral nerves and skeletal muscle. Nerve impulses travel down the nerve and release a chemical (neurotransmitter) which stimulates (depolarizes) skeletal muscle, resulting in contraction. Acetylcholine is the primary neurotransmitter, and blocking its action results in relaxation of skeletal (voluntary) muscle. There are two ways to block the neuromuscular junction. Depolarizing agents substitute themselves into the neuromuscular junction in place of acetylcholine. They have a stimulating effect as they work, which produces fasciculations (generalized involuntary muscle twitching). Succinylcholine is a depolarizing agent, and is the most commonly used paralytic agent for RSI. Nondepolarizing agents block the uptake of acetylcholine and do not allow stimulation of the muscle. Thus they do not cause fasciculations. Vecuronium, atracurium, and pancuronium are typical examples of nondepolarizing neuromuscular blocking agents.

Paralyzing the patient causes complete muscular relaxation and allows you to take control of his precarious clinical condition. In addition to paralyzing the airway muscles, these agents also immobilize the respiratory muscles, so the patient becomes apneic and requires mechanical ventilation. Esophageal and stomach muscles, and therefore sphincter tone, also relax, posing the risk of vomiting and aspiration. Succinylcholine (Anectine), the agent preferred for neuromuscular blockade in emergency medical care, is a depolarizing drug. As mentioned, it causes fasciculations just before initiating paralysis. These fasciculations may increase the tendency to vomit and may increase intracranial pressure. Conditions that elevate serum potassium preclude the use of succinylcholine, which transiently increases serum potassium, and thus can lead to life-threatening hyperkalemia. Side effects, which are dose related, include bradycardia and other dysrhythmias, as well as hypertension. The guidelines for using succinylcholine include:

* Dose: 1.5 mg/kg, IV bolus in adults; 2.0 mg/kg, IV bolus in children less than 10 years old

* Onset of action: 60 to 90 seconds

* Duration: 3 to 5 minutes

* Contraindications: penetrating eye injuries, patients with burns greater than 8 hours' duration, massive crush injuries, and neurologic injuries greater than 1 week out

Vecuronium (Norcuron) is a nondepolarizing agent; thus, it does not cause fasciculations. It is generally the second-line paralytic when succinylcholine is contraindicated, because it has fewer cardiac and hypotensive side effects than other nondepolarizing agents. In much smaller doses as a premedication, or priming dose, to succinylcholine or to a paralyzing dose of vecuronium it effectively lessens or prevents fasciculations. It also blunts succinylcholine's bradycardic effect. This priming (or premedication) dose is given 2 minutes before the paralytic agent. Guidelines for using vecuronium include:

* Dose: 0.15 mg/kg IV bolus (paralyzing)
     0.01 mg/kg IV bolus (priming)

* Onset: 2 to 3 minutes

* Duration: 45 minutes

Atracurium (Tracrium) is a nondepolarizing paralytic useful for patients with kidney or liver disease because these conditions do not prolong its duration. Some patients experience hypotension from the histamine release that this drug causes. The usual dosage of 0.5 mg/kg IV has a duration of 20 to 30 minutes.

Pancuronium (Pavulon) is a nondepolarizing paralytic that has been used frequently in the past. The advantage of its relatively rapid onset (3 to 5 minutes) is offset

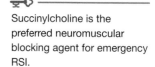

Succinylcholine is the preferred neuromuscular blocking agent for emergency RSI.

 Review

Content

Common Paralytic Agents

* Succinylcholine
* Vecuronium
* Atracurium
* Pancuronium

by its major disadvantage, a long (60-minute) duration. It also produces tachycardia due to its effects on the heart. Better agents are currently available.

If you cannot intubate a paralyzed patient he has no definitive airway. You must ventilate him mechanically for the duration of the paralysis (assuming you can mechanically maintain a patent airway). If the airway is lost during the procedure, you must be prepared to initiate a surgical airway (cricothyrotomy). Nothing works as fast as succinylcholine or is of as short a duration; therefore, it is the preferred neuromuscular blocking agent for emergency RSI.

Neuromuscular blocking agents do not affect mental status or pain sensation; therefore, you must use sedating and amnestic drugs to ease the awake, aware patient's anxiety and discomfort and to decrease his gag reflex, thereby increasing patient compliance and enhancing the ease of intubation. If the patient is already obtunded (from a drug overdose or head injury, for example), sedating him is pointless; omit that step. If the patient's injuries are causing significant pain and his clinical condition does not contraindicate their use, give small doses of pain medications as indicated.

When hypovolemia is present or when significant trauma is present with hypotension or a strong likelihood for hypotension, avoid induction agents that cause hypotension. Agents that blunt ICP response are good choices for the patient with head injury. Table 13–3 details general guidelines for common sedative (induction) agents. If you are able to identify that the patient has an allergy or sensitivity to a particular agent, you should not administer that agent.

Two other agents, atropine and lidocaine, are appropriate for use as premedication agents in RSI, if indicated. Table 13–4 outlines their use.

Most patients with emergent airway conditions have eaten or drunk something within a few hours before the onset of their emergency conditions. Thus, you should consider every emergency patient to have a full stomach and be at risk of vomiting and aspiration. This is another reason why you should expediently intubate the patient after the onset of paralytic effect and **apnea.** Remember to always have a working suction device at the patient's side during airway maneuvers. Likewise, application of Sellick maneuver will help prevent aspiration.

apnea *temporary stop in breathing.*

Table 13–3	Guidelines for Sedative (Induction) Agents				
Induction Agent	Dose	Onset	Duration (min)	Advantages	Disadvantages
Midazolam (Versed)	0.1–0.3 mg/kg	1–3 min	20–30 min	Amnesia effects, good sedative	Hypotension
Diazepam (Valium)	0.2–0.5 mg/kg	2–3 min	30–40 min	Amnesia effects	Hypotension, respiratory depression
Etomidate (Amidate)	0.3 mg/kg	1–2 min	5 min	Little effect on blood pressure, decreases intracranial pressure (ICP)	Suppresses cortisol → not good for head-injured patients
Ketamine (Ketalar)	1–2 mg/kg	≤ 1 min	10–20 min	Decreases bronchospasm, little hypotension, amnesia	Increases ICP
Sodium thiopental	3–5 mg/kg	≤ 1 min	5 min	Blunts ICP changes	Significant hypotension, bronchospasm
Propofol (Diprivan)	1–1.5 mg/kg	≤ 1 min	3–5 min	Rapid onset, good sedative effects	Significant hypotension
Fentanyl	3–5 mcg/kg	1–2 min	30–40 min	Little effect on blood pressure; blunts ICP changes	Can cause muscle rigidity in chest wall

Table 13–4	Adjunctive RSI Agents		
Agent	Dose	Indication	Contraindication Precaution
Atropine	0.01-0.02 mg/kg (min.–max./0.1–0.4)	Pediatric patients, bradycardia	Cannot give less than 0.1 mg
Lidocaine	1 mg/kg	Head injury	Allergy

To perform rapid sequence intubation:

1. Preoxygenate the patient with 100 percent oxygen using basic manual and adjunctive maneuvers, and using a bag-valve mask, if indicated.

2. Prepare your equipment, supplies, and patient. In addition to the usual intubation equipment, be certain you have at least one, and preferably two, secure and working IV lines. Place the patient on a cardiac monitor and pulse oximeter. Draw the appropriate doses of medications into syringes and label them.

3. If the patient is alert, administer a sedative (induction) agent, such as midazolam (Versed), prior to administering any neuromuscular blocking agents.

4. Apply the Sellick maneuver (cricoid pressure) and maintain until you confirm proper ETT placement.

5. Per local protocols, consider premedicating the patient with a priming dose of vecuronium. This is especially important in children, where fasciculations from succinylcholine can cause musculoskeletal trauma. Also, if indicated in local protocols, consider premedicating with lidocaine and atropine.

6. Paralyze the patient, administering succinylcholine 1.5 mg/kg IV bolus and continue oxygenation. Alternatively, vecuronium (Norcuron) can be used as a blocking agent. It has a slower onset of action.

7. Once adequate relaxation is obtained, insert the ETT through the patient's vocal cords at the onset of apnea and jaw relaxation, using the orotracheal intubation procedure previously explained. Because you have preoxygenated the patient, BVM ventilation is generally not indicated before the first intubation attempt, unless prolonged. Not ventilating the patient at this juncture will help prevent gastric distention and regurgitation. If you are unable to pass the tube after 20 to 30 seconds, stop, hyperventilate the patient with 100 percent oxygen for 2 minutes, and then try again. Remember that the patient's lower esophageal sphincter tone is decreased, so ventilating during paralysis makes gastric distention and vomiting more likely, even with cricoid pressure. Your goal is to rapidly place the ETT properly in the trachea to minimize these complications. Use 100% oxygen but avoid hyperventilation.

8. Confirm proper placement of the ETT into the trachea. Inflate the distal cuff, ventilate with a bag-valve device with a CO_2 detector attached, and look for the appropriate color change. Watch for the chest to rise and fall with ventilations. Auscultate with each ventilation for bilateral breath sounds over the chest and no gastric sounds over the stomach.

9. Release the Sellick maneuver.

10. Insert a bite block device, secure the ETT in place, reconfirm placement, and continue ventilating the patient. Continually assess the patient's condition and recheck ETT placement.

11. Check with medical direction or follow your local protocol for indications for continuing paralysis with vecuronium during transport. This will depend largely on your patient's medical condition and combativeness after the paralytic and induction agent wear off, as well as on your anticipated transport time to the hospital.

Pediatric Intubation

Pediatric airway emergencies generally produce more anxiety than adult emergencies among both medical care providers and the family. It is important to take appropriate steps to separate the parent from the pediatric patient with significant respiratory distress or apnea in order to effectively manage the airway. While the indications, procedures, and precautions for airway management in children are fundamentally the same as in adults, you must take additional precautions and remember several significant differences. These concerns revolve around variances in anatomy, as discussed earlier in this chapter. To review the anatomical features of the pediatric airway:

★ The structures are proportionally smaller and more flexible than an adult's.

★ The tongue is larger in relation to the oropharynx.

★ The epiglottis is floppy and round ("omega" shaped).

★ The glottic opening is higher and more anterior in the neck.

★ The vocal cords slant upward, toward the back of the head, and are closer to the base of the tongue.

★ The narrowest part of the airway is the cricoid cartilage, not the glottic opening as in adults.

A straight laryngoscope blade is preferred for most pediatric patients, although straight or curved may be useful for adolescents. Also, selecting the appropriate tube diameter for children is critical. Too large a tube can cause tracheal edema and/or damage to the vocal cords, while too small a tube may not allow exchange of adequate ventilatory volumes. Table 13–5 lists general guidelines for selecting ETT size according to the child's age. Another guide for children's sizes is:

$$\text{ETT size (mm)} = (\text{Age in years} + 16) \div 4$$

Table 13–5	Approximate Size of ETT for Pediatrics			
Patient's Age	ETT Size	Type	Depth of ETT Insertion	Laryngoscope Blade Size
Premature infant	2.5–3.0	Uncuffed	8 cm	0 straight
Full-term infant	3.0–3.5	Uncuffed	8–9.5 cm	1 straight
Infant to 1 year	3.5–4.0	Uncuffed	9.5–11 cm	1 straight
Toddler	4.0–5.0	Uncuffed	11–12.5 cm	1–2 straight
Preschool	5.0–5.5	Uncuffed	12.5–14 cm	2 straight
School age	5.5–6.5	Uncuffed	14–20 cm	2 straight
Adolescent	7.0–8.0	Cuffed	20–23 cm	3 straight or curved

Correct tube size for an 8-year-old, for instance, would be $(8 + 16) \div 4$, or 6 mm. You can also measure tube size by matching it to the diameter of the child's smallest finger. Usually you will use noncuffed endotracheal tubes with infants and children under the age of 8 years, because the round narrowing of these patients' cricoid cartilage forms a suitable cuff.

The depth of insertion of the distal tip for pediatric endotracheal tubes should be 2 to 3 cm below the vocal cords, as deeper insertion may result in mainstem intubation or injury to the carina. The uncuffed ETT has a black glottic marker at its distal end that should be placed at the level of the vocal cords. The cuffed ETT should be placed so that the cuff is just below the vocal cords. For detailed guidelines regarding the depth of insertion for different age groups, refer to Table 13–5. Alternately, you can use the formula $(3 \times \text{ETT inside diameter}) - 1$.

Also remember that infants and small children have greater vagal tone than adults. Therefore, laryngoscopy and passage of an endotracheal tube are more likely to precipitate a vagal response, dramatically slowing the child's heart rate and decreasing cardiac output and blood pressure. To guard against this complication, you must monitor heart rate throughout the procedure, and you may give atropine (0.02 mg/kg, 0.1 mg minimum) IV bolus. If heart rate falls below 60 beats per minute stop the procedure and reinitiate ventilations with 100 percent oxygen.

The indications for endotracheal intubation in a pediatric patient are the same as those for adults:

★ Ventilatory support with a bag-valve mask is inadequate.

★ Cardiac or respiratory arrest.

★ It is necessary to provide a route for drug administration (LEAN) or ready access to the airway for suctioning.

★ Prolonged artificial ventilation is needed.

Additionally, if local protocols allow, you may use endotracheal intubation in a child with epiglottitis if his condition is rapidly deteriorating.

To perform endotracheal intubation on a pediatric patient (Procedure 13–3):

1. After initiating basic manual and adjunctive maneuvers, ventilate the patient with 100 percent oxygen, using the appropriately sized BVM.

2. Prepare and check your equipment. As stated earlier, a straight blade laryngoscope is usually preferred in infants and small children, since it provides greater displacement of the tongue and better visualization of the relatively cephalad and anterior epiglottis. Also, with children younger than 8 years old, you will typically use an uncuffed endotracheal tube. Due to the short distance between the mouth and the trachea, you rarely need a stylet to position the tube properly. Remember to lubricate the ETT with water-soluble gel.

3. Place the patient's head and neck in an appropriate position. You should maintain a pediatric patient's head in a sniffing position (perhaps by placing a towel under his head), unless you know of or suspect trauma. In case of trauma, proceed with manual in-line stabilization of the cervical spine.

4. Have your partner apply gentle cricoid pressure (Sellick maneuver).

5. Hold the laryngoscope in your left hand and insert it gently into the right side of the patient's mouth. With a sweeping action, displace the tongue to the left.

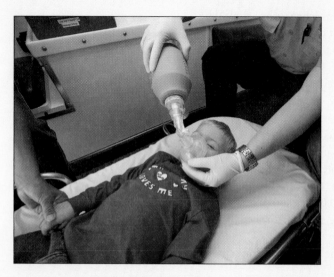

13-3a   Ventilate the child.

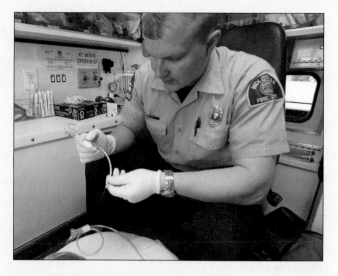

13-3b   Prepare the equipment.

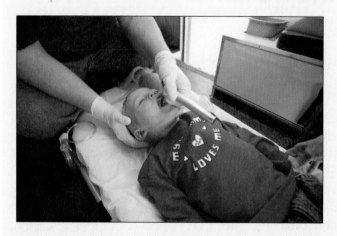

13-3c   Insert the laryngoscope.

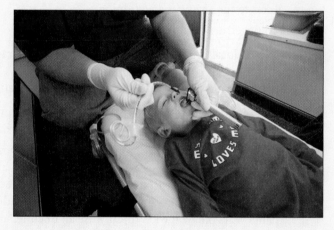

13-3d   Visualize the child's larynx and insert the ETT.

(Photos © Scott Metcalfe)

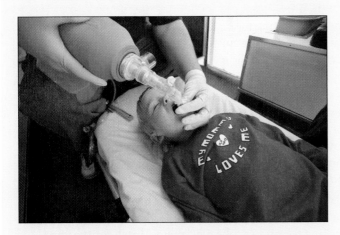

13-3e   Ventilate, inflate the ETT cuff (if it is a cuffed tube), and auscultate.

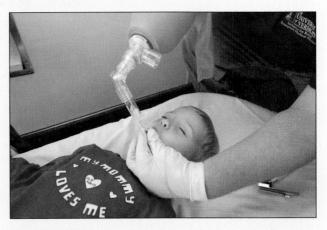

13-3f   Confirm placement with an $ETCO_2$ detector or waveform capnography.

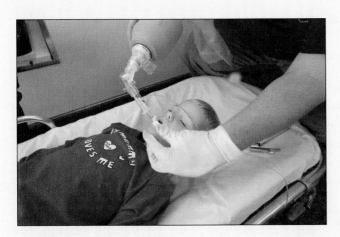

13-3g   Secure the tube.

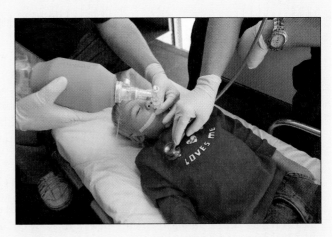

13-3h   Reconfirm proper ETT placement.

6. Move the blade slightly toward the midline, and then advance it until the distal end reaches the base of the tongue.

7. Look for the tip of the epiglottis, and position the laryngoscope properly. Keep in mind that a child—particularly an infant—has a shorter airway and a higher glottis than an adult. Because of this, you may see the cords much sooner than you expect.

8. If you cannot see the glottis, bring the blade gently and slowly out until the vocal cords fall into view. Lift the epiglottis gently with the tip of the laryngoscope. Be certain not to use the teeth or gums as a fulcrum.

9. Grasp the endotracheal tube in your right hand and, under direct visualization of the vocal cords, insert it through the right corner of the patient's mouth into the glottic opening. Pass it through until the distal 10 mm or distal cuff of the ETT disappears 2 to 3 cm beyond the vocal cords. In some cases, advancing an endotracheal tube will be difficult at the level of the cricoid. Do not force the ETT through this region, as it may cause laryngeal edema and bleeding.

10. Hold the tube in place with your left hand, and attach an infant- or child-size bag-valve device to the 15/22-mm connector and deliver several breaths, checking for proper tube placement. Watch for the chest to rise and fall symmetrically with each ventilation. Auscultate for equal, bilateral breath sounds at the lateral chest wall, high in the axilla. Breath sounds over the epigastrium should be absent with ventilations. The patient should improve clinically, with pinker color and increased heart rate. Additionally, use the end-tidal CO_2 detector as previously discussed.

11. If the tube has a distal cuff, inflate it with just enough air to prevent any air leaks.

12. Secure the ETT with tape or a commercial device as with an adult patient, note placement of the distance marker at teeth/gums, recheck for proper placement, and continue ventilatory support. Periodically reassess ETT placement, and watch the patient carefully for any clinical signs of difficulty. As with the adult patient, allow no more than 30 seconds to pass without ventilating your patient.

NASOTRACHEAL INTUBATION

nasotracheal route *through the nose and into the trachea.*

The orotracheal route is usually preferred for intubation as it affords more control over the airway. In a few circumstances, however, the **nasotracheal route** (through the nose and into the trachea) may be useful. As a rule this is a "blind" procedure without direct visualization of the vocal cords. To perform nasotracheal intubations, you can often visualize the vocal cords with a laryngoscope and guide the ETT with Magill forceps. But if this is possible, orotracheal intubation is generally feasible and preferred. Potential indications for blind nasotracheal intubation include:

★ Possible spinal injury
★ Clenched teeth, preventing opening the patient's mouth
★ Fractured jaw, oral injuries, or recent oral surgery
★ Significant angioedema (facial and airway swelling)
★ Obesity
★ Arthritis, preventing placement in the sniffing position

Nasotracheal intubation is not recommended in the following situations:

- ★ Suspected nasal fractures
- ★ Suspected basilar skull fractures
- ★ Significantly deviated nasal septum or other nasal obstruction
- ★ Cardiac or respiratory arrest
- ★ Unresponsive patient

Advantages of Nasotracheal Intubation

When the patient's condition indicates its use, nasotracheal intubation offers the following advantages:

- ★ The head and neck can remain in neutral position.
- ★ It does not produce as much gag response and is better tolerated by the awake patient.
- ★ It can be secured more easily than an orotracheal tube.
- ★ The patient cannot bite the ETT.

Disadvantages of Nasotracheal Intubation

The following disadvantages of nasotracheal intubation discourage its use unless clearly indicated by the patient's condition:

- ★ It is more difficult and time consuming to perform than orotracheal intubation.
- ★ It is potentially more traumatic for patients. Passage of the tube may lacerate the pharyngeal mucosa or larynx during insertion.
- ★ The tube may kink or clog more easily than an orally placed endotracheal tube.
- ★ It poses a greater risk of infection, because the ETT introduces nasal bacteria into the trachea.
- ★ Improper placement is more likely when performing blind nasotracheal intubation, as the tube's passage through the glottic opening cannot be visualized.
- ★ Blind nasotracheal intubation requires that the patient be breathing.

Nasotracheal Intubation Technique

To perform blind nasotracheal intubation (Figure 13-54 ■):

1. Using basic manual and adjunctive maneuvers, open the airway and ventilate the patient with 100 percent oxygen.
2. Prepare your equipment and place the patient supine. If you suspect cervical spine injury, maintain the head and neck in neutral position with manual in-line stabilization.
3. Inspect the nose and select the larger nostril as your passageway.
4. Apply topical anesthesia with Hurricaine spray or topical lidocaine.
5. Insert the ETT into the nostril, with the bevel along the floor of the nostril or facing the nasal septum. This will help avoid damage to the turbinates. Next, gently guide the ETT from anterior to posterior.
6. As you feel the tube drop into the posterior pharynx, listen closely at its proximal end for the patient's respiratory sounds. These sounds are

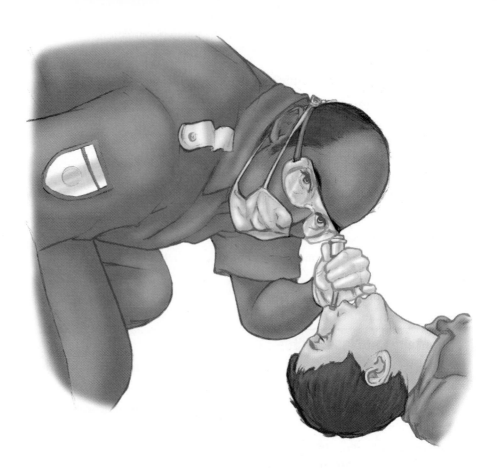

■ Figure 13-54 Blind nasotracheal intubation.

loudest when the ETT is proximal to the epiglottis. When the ETT's tip reaches the posterior pharyngeal wall, you must take care to direct it toward the glottic opening. At this point, the tip of the ETT may catch in the pyriform sinus. If it does, you will feel resistance, and the skin on either side of the Adam's apple will tent. To resolve pyriform sinus placement, slightly withdraw the ETT and rotate it to the midline.

7. With the patient's next inhaled breath, advance the ETT gently but quickly into the glottic opening. Continue passing the ETT until the distal cuff is just past the vocal cords. At this point, the patient may cough, buck, or strain. Gagging or vocal sounds are signs of esophageal placement, while slight bulging and anterior displacement of the larynx usually indicate correct tracheal placement. When you place the ETT correctly in the trachea, you will see the patient's exhaled air as condensation in the ETT and feel it coming from the proximal end of the ETT.

8. Holding the ETT with one hand to prevent displacement, inflate the distal cuff with 5 to 10 mL of air, connect a bag-valve device with an $ETCO_2$ detector attached, ventilate the patient with 100 percent oxygen, and confirm proper placement of the ETT. Observe the chest rise and fall with ventilations, auscultate breath sounds over the chest bilaterally, and verify no gastric sounds with each ventilation.

9. Secure the ETT and reconfirm proper placement. Continue to observe the patient's condition, maintain ventilatory support, and frequently recheck ETT placement.

Nasotracheal Tube Auscultation Device Nasotracheal tube auscultation devices (e.g., the Burden nasoscope) can be used to facilitate blind nasotracheal intubation (Figures 13-55a and b ■). With this device, you can listen closely to the

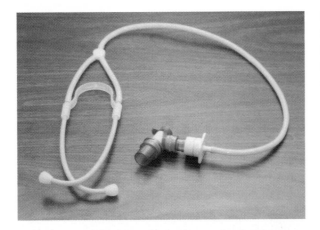

Figure 13-55a The Burden nasoscope, a commercial nasotracheal tube auscultation device. *(Photo courtesy of Brant Burden, EMT-P)*

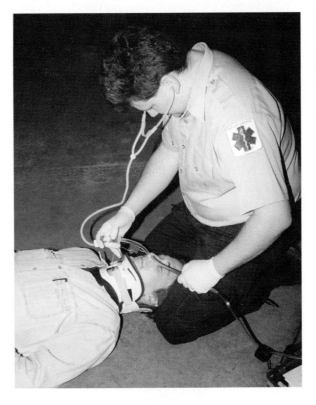

■ Figure 13-55b The nasotracheal tube auscultation device is inserted in order to hear breath sounds better during nasotracheal tube insertion. *(Photo courtesy of Brant Burden, EMT-P)*

patient's breathing when blindly inserting a nasotracheal tube. The device functions like a stethoscope with an in-line diaphragm that connects to the endotracheal tube. Most of these devices are disposable single-use items. They can be used only in patients who are breathing.

FIELD EXTUBATION

Infrequently, an intubated patient will awaken and be intolerant of the ETT. This happens most often with respiratory distress patients who undergo rapid sequence intubation. When the paralytic medications wear off and they awaken from the induction medications, they may struggle against the intubation and ventilation. This usually indicates sedation and, perhaps, repeat paralysis, because extubation will cause continued respiratory distress with loss of a definitive airway. If the patient is clearly able to maintain and protect his airway and accomplish adequate spontaneous respirations and is not under the influence of any sedating agents, and if reassessment indicates the problem that led to endotracheal intubation is resolved, extubation may be indicated. However, you must consider the high risk of laryngospasm, involuntary closure of the glottis upon extubation, especially in the awake patient. Laryngospasm may prohibit successful reintubation attempts. Additionally, in repeat attempts at rapid sequence intubation the medications will produce variable responses and do not ensure relaxation of the laryngospasm. The need for field extubation is extremely rare.

To perform field extubation:

1. Continue blood and body fluid precautions. Ensure patient's oxygenation. A crude method for accomplishing this in the field is to be certain that the patient's mental status, skin color, and pulse oximetry are optimal on room air with the ETT in place.

2. Prepare intubation equipment and suction.

3. Confirm patient responsiveness.

4. Suction the patient's oropharynx.

5. Deflate the ETT cuff.

6. Remove the ETT upon cough or expiration.

7. Provide supplemental oxygen as indicated.

8. Reassess the adequacy of the patient's ventilation and oxygenation.

ESOPHAGEAL TRACHEAL COMBITUBE

The **Esophageal Tracheal CombiTube** (ETC) is a dual-lumen airway with a ventilation port for each **lumen.** The longer, blue port (#1) is the proxial port; the shorter, clear port (#2) is the distal port, which opens at the distal end of the tube. The ETC has two inflatable cuffs—a 100-mL cuff just proximal to the distal port and a 15-mL cuff just distal to the proximal port.

The ETC is inserted blindly through the mouth into the posterior oropharynx and then gently advanced. The tube enters either the trachea or the esophagus (Figures 13-56 ■ and

Esophageal Tracheal CombiTube *dual-lumen airway with a ventilation port for each lumen.*

lumen *the tunnel through a tube.*

✓ Review

Intubation Devices

- Endotracheal tube (ETT)
- Esophageal Tracheal CombiTube (ETC)
- Laryngeal mask airway (LMA)
- Pharyngo-tracheal lumen airway (PtL)
- Esophageal gastric tube (EGTA)
- Esophageal obturator airway (EOA)

■ Figure 13-56 ETC airway. First ventilate through the longer blue tube (#1). Ventilation will be successful if the tube has been placed (as is most common) in the esophagus.

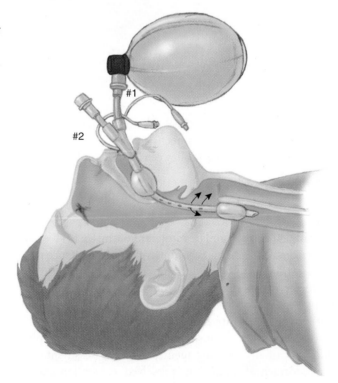

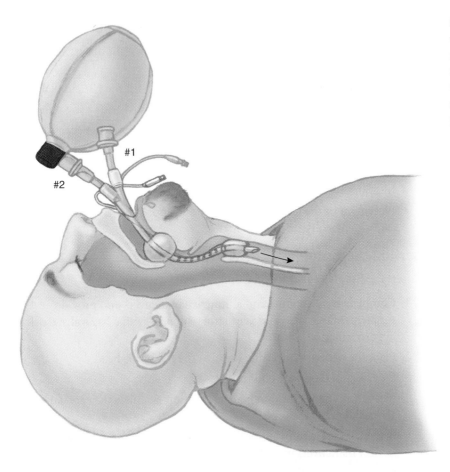

Figure 13-57 ETC airway. If ventilation through tube #1 is not successful, then ventilate through the shorter clear tube (#2). Ventilation will be successful if the tube has been placed in the trachea.

13-57 ■). Esophageal placement is most common. Inflate both cuffs (proximal cuff first and then distal cuff) per the manufacturer's recommendations. Ventilate through the longer blue tube (#1) and auscultate for breath sounds. If breath sounds are present and there is no evidence of gastric insufflation, continue ventilations. This indicates esophageal placement. If breath sounds are absent and auscultation of gastric insufflation is positive, immediately begin ventilating through the shorter clear tube (#2). Confirm ventilation by auscultation of breath sounds and absence of gastric insufflation. This indicates tracheal placement. If auscultation of breath sounds is positive and auscultation of gastric insufflation is negative, continue ventilation. Secure the tube and monitor end-tidal carbon dioxide levels.

Advantages of the Esophageal Tracheal CombiTube

★ It provides alternate airway control when conventional intubation techniques are unsuccessful or unavailable.

★ Insertion is rapid and easy.

★ Insertion does not require visualization of the larynx or special equipment.

★ The pharyngeal balloon anchors the airway behind the hard palate.

★ The patient may be ventilated regardless of tube placement (esophageal or tracheal).

★ It significantly diminishes gastric distention and regurgitation.

★ It can be used on trauma patients, since the neck can remain in neutral position during insertion and use.

★ If the tube is placed in the esophagus, gastric contents can be suctioned for decompression through the distal port.

Disadvantages of the Esophageal Tracheal CombiTube

★ Suctioning tracheal secretions is impossible when the airway is in the esophagus.

★ Placing an endotracheal tube is very difficult with the ETC in place.

★ It cannot be used in conscious patients or in those with a gag reflex.

★ The cuffs can cause esophageal, tracheal, and hypopharyngeal ischemia.

★ It does not isolate and completely protect the trachea.

★ It cannot be used in patients with esophageal disease or caustic ingestions.

★ It cannot be used with pediatric patients.

★ Placement of the CombiTube is not foolproof—errors can be made if assessment skills are not adequate.

Inserting the Esophageal Tracheal CombiTube

To insert the Esophageal Tracheal CombiTube:

1. Complete basic manual and adjunctive maneuvers and provide supplemental oxygen and ventilatory support with a bag-valve mask and hyperventilation.

2. Place the patient supine and kneel at the top of his head.

3. Prepare and check the equipment.

4. Place the patient's head in neutral position. Stabilize the cervical spine if cervical injury is possible.

5. Insert the ETC gently at midline through the oropharynx, using a tongue-jaw-lift maneuver, and advance it past the hypopharynx to the depth indicated by the markings on the tube. The black rings on the tube should be between the patient's teeth.

6. Inflate the pharyngeal cuff with 100 mL of air and the distal cuff with 10 to 15 mL of air.

7. Ventilate through the longer blue proximal port with a bag-valve device connected to 100 percent oxygen, while auscultating over the chest and stomach. If you hear bilateral breath sounds over the chest and none over the stomach, secure the tube and continue ventilating.

8. If you hear gastric sounds over the chest instead of breath sounds, change ports and ventilate through the clear connector. Confirm breath sounds over the chest with no gastric sounds. Use multiple confirmation techniques as previously discussed (visualize, auscultate, use $ETCO_2$ detector, monitor clinical improvement).

9. Secure the tube and continue ventilating with 100 percent oxygen.

10. Frequently reassess the airway and adequacy of ventilation.

PHARYNGO-TRACHEAL LUMEN AIRWAY

pharyngotracheal lumen airway *(PtL) is a two tube system.*

The **pharyngotracheal lumen airway (PtL)** is a two-tube system (Figure 13-58 ■). The first tube is short, with a large diameter; its proximal end is green. A large cuff encircles the tube's lower third. When inflated, the cuff seals the entire oropharynx. Air introduced at this tube's proximal end will enter the hypopharynx. The second tube is long, with a small diameter, and clear. It passes through and extends approximately 10 cm beyond the first tube. This second tube may be inserted blindly into either the trachea or

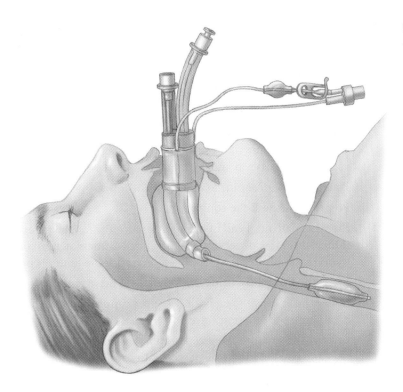

the esophagus. A distal cuff, when inflated, seals off whichever anatomical structure the tube has entered. When the second tube enters the trachea, you will ventilate the patient through it.

Each of the PtL's tubes has a 15/22-mm connector at its proximal end, allowing the attachment of a standard ventilatory device. A semirigid plastic stylet in the clear plastic tube allows redirection of the oropharyngeal cuff while the other cuff remains inflated. An adjustable, cloth neck strap holds the tube in place. When the long, clear tube is in the esophagus, deflating the cuff in the oropharynx allows you to move the device to the left side of the patient's mouth. This may permit endotracheal intubation while continuing esophageal occlusion. However, placement of an endotracheal tube with a PtL already in place is difficult at best.

Advantages of the Pharyngotracheal Lumen Airway

★ It can function in either the tracheal or esophageal position.

★ It has no face mask to seal.

★ It does not require direct visualization of the larynx and, thus, does not require the use of a laryngoscope or additional specialized equipment.

★ It can be used in trauma patients, since the neck can remain in neutral position during insertion and use.

★ It helps protect the trachea from upper airway bleeding and secretions.

Disdvantages of the Pharyngotracheal Lumen Airway

★ It does not isolate and completely protect the trachea from aspiration.

★ The oropharyngeal balloon can migrate out of the mouth anteriorly, partially dislodging the airway.

★ Intubation around the PtL is extremely difficult, even with the oropharyngeal balloon deflated.

★ It cannot be used in conscious patients or those with a gag reflex.

★ It cannot be used in pediatric patients.

★ It can only be passed orally.

Inserting the Pharyngotracheal Lumen Airway

To insert the pharyngotracheal lumen airway:

1. Complete basic manual and adjunctive maneuvers and provide supplemental oxygen and ventilatory support with a BVM ventilation.

2. Place the patient supine and kneel at the top of his head.

3. Prepare and check the equipment.

4. Place the patient's head in the appropriate position. Hyperextend the neck if there is no risk of cervical spine injury. Maintain neutral position with stabilization of the cervical spine if cervical spine injury is possible.

5. Insert the PtL gently, using the tongue-jaw-lift maneuver.

6. Inflate the distal cuffs on both PtL tubes simultaneously with a sustained breath into the inflation valve.

7. Deliver a breath into the green oropharyngeal tube. If the patient's chest rises and you auscultate bilateral breath sounds, the long clear tube is in the esophagus. Inflate the pharyngeal balloon and continue ventilations via the green tube.

8. If the chest does not rise and you auscultate no breath sounds, the long clear tube is in the trachea. Remove the stylet from the clear tube and ventilate the patient through that tube.

9. Attach the bag-valve device to the 15-mm connector, secure the tube, and continue ventilatory support with 100 percent oxygen.

10. Multiple placement confirmation techniques are again essential, as are good assessment skills. Misidentification of placement has been reported. Frequently reassess the airway and adequacy of ventilation.

If the patient regains consciousness or if the protective airway reflexes return, remove the PtL. It is best to remove the PtL before endotracheal intubation.

Complications of PtL placement include:

★ Pharyngeal or esophageal trauma from poor technique

★ Unrecognized displacement of the long tube from the trachea into the esophagus

★ Displacement of the pharyngeal balloon

LARYNGEAL MASK AIRWAY

The laryngeal mask airway (LMA) may assist with ventilations in the unconscious patient without laryngeal reflexes when tracheal intubation is unsuccessful. It has an inflatable distal end (similar to a face mask) which is placed in the hypopharynx and then inflated (Figure 13-59 ■). A bag-valve device at the proximal end assists respirations (similar to an endotracheal tube). The laryngeal mask airway can be disposable and comes in various sizes. Its blind insertion requires less skill and training than endotracheal intubation. The laryngeal mask airway's disadvantage is that it does not isolate the trachea; therefore, it does not protect the airway from regurgitation and aspiration.

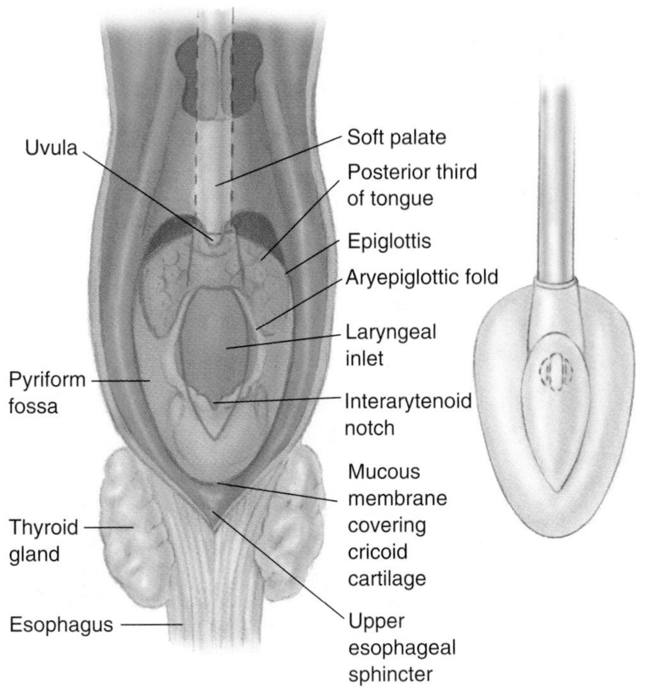

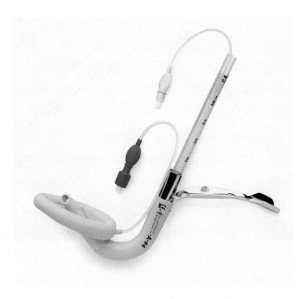

Figure 13-59   Laryngeal mask airway.

Uvula

Soft palate

Posterior third of tongue

Epiglottis

Aryepiglottic fold

Laryngeal inlet

Pyriform fossa

Interarytenoid notch

Mucous membrane covering cricoid cartilage

Thyroid gland

Esophagus

Upper esophageal sphincter

Figure 13-60   Intubating laryngeal mask airway (LMA). *(LMA North America)*

Also, it cannot be used in a patient who has a gag reflex or is semiconscious. You must weigh these disadvantages against the benefits of establishing a patent airway.

Intubating LMA

The intubating LMA (also called the LMA Fastrach) (Figure 13-60 ■) is designed to facilitate endotracheal intubation. It is a rigid, anatomically curved airway tube that is wide enough to accept an 8.0-mm cuffed ETT and is short enough to ensure passage of the ETT cuff beyond the vocal cords. It has a rigid handle to facilitate one-handed insertion, removal, and adjustment of the device's position to enhance oxygenation and alignment with the glottis. There is an epiglottic elevating bar in the mask aperture that elevates the epiglottis as the ETT is passed through and a ramp that directs the tube centrally and anteriorly to reduce the risk of arytenoid trauma or esophageal placement.

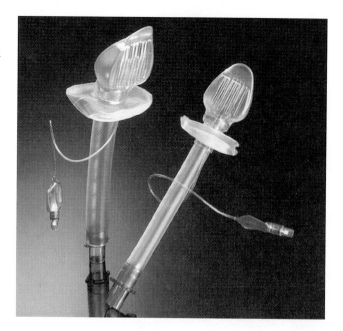

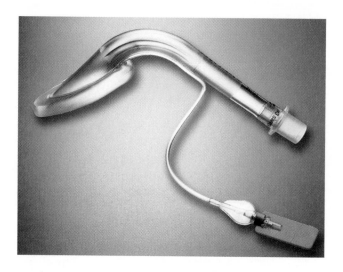

Cobra Perilaryngeal Airway

The Cobra perilaryngeal airway (PLA) is similar to the laryngeal mask in that it is a supraglottic airway (inserted just above the glottis) (Figure 13-61 ■). It is a single-use, disposable airway. The "cobra head" of the airway holds both the soft tissue and the epiglottis out of the way. Ventilations are provided through fenestrated (slotted) openings in the distal airway.

Ambu Laryngeal Mask

The Ambu laryngeal mask is a supraglottic, single-use, disposable airway (Figure 13-62 ■). It features a special curve that replicates the natural human airway anatomy. This curve is molded directly into the tube so that insertion is easy, without abrading the upper airway. The curve ensures that the patient's head remains in a neutral position when the mask is in use.

ESOPHAGEAL GASTRIC TUBE AIRWAY AND ESOPHAGEAL OBTURATOR AIRWAY

Although clearly better devices have made them obsolete, the esophageal gastric tube airway and esophageal obturator airway are still available in some areas. Our discussion is intended solely to familiarize you with these devices. They both stimulate the gag reflex, so you must use them only for patients with no gag reflex. Both can cause esophageal rupture. They can be inserted with the head in neutral position.

The esophageal gastric tube airway (EGTA) is a hollow tube. A cuff just proximal to the distal, open port blocks air to the esophagus. The EGTA is inserted into the esophagus, with ventilation via the attached, inflatable mask through air holes at the level of the hypopharynx. A second port on the face mask allows you to extend a gastric tube through the distal port into the stomach for decompression of contents. If the gastric tube enters the trachea, the airway and gastric suction ports on the mask are not interchangeable.

The esophageal obturator airway (EOA) is a hollow tube with a closed end and a distal cuff intended to block air from the esophagus. It is inserted into the esophagus, with ventilation via an attached face mask through air holes at the level of the hypopharynx. The EOA does not allow gastric suctioning, and improper placement in the trachea introduces a closed tube into the airway.

Contraindications to EOA insertion are:

★ Age less than 16 years

★ Height less than 5 feet or more than 6 feet, 7 inches

★ Possible ingestion of caustic poisons

★ History of esophageal disease or alcoholism

FOREIGN BODY REMOVAL UNDER DIRECT LARYNGOSCOPY

Direct visualization of the larynx with a laryngoscope may enable you to remove an obstructing foreign body using Magill forceps or a suction device (Figure 13-63 ■). Initially, you should carry out basic life support maneuvers for airway obstruction, including the Heimlich maneuver, finger sweep, and chest thrust. As you recall from your basic training, the Heimlich maneuver involves initiating a forceful upward thrust with your fist on the choking patient's abdomen, halfway between the umbilicus and the xiphoid process. Use suction as indicated. If these fail to alleviate the obstruction, direct visualization of the airway for foreign body removal is indicated. The procedure for visualizing the airway is identical to that used for orotracheal intubation.

SURGICAL AIRWAYS

With proper training and frequent practice, including the use of rapid sequence intubation procedures, you will be able to secure most airways in the field by endotracheal intubation. Occasionally, however, extreme circumstances prohibit successful endotracheal intubation. In these situations, performing a surgical airway technique may be the only way to ensure your patient's survival. Two different techniques, **needle cricothyrotomy** (also called translaryngeal cannula ventilation) and **open cricothyrotomy,** both provide access to the airway through the cricothyroid membrane. A needle cricothyrotomy is generally the easier procedure but makes providing adequate ventilation more difficult; an open cricothyrotomy is the more difficult procedure but allows for more effective oxygenation and ventilation.

needle cricothyrotomy *surgical airway technique that inserts a 14-gauge needle into the trachea at the cricothyroid membrane.*

open cricothyrotomy *surgical airway technique that places an endotracheal or tracheostomy tube directly into the trachea through a surgical incision at the cricothyroid membrane.*

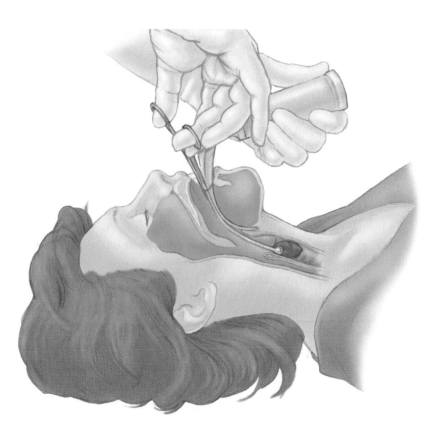

You should use surgical airway procedures only after you have exhausted your other airway skills and have decided that no other means will establish an airway. Even when performed correctly, these procedures are highly invasive and prone to complications which you must recognize and treat immediately. The major long-term complication, tracheal **stenosis,** can cause difficulty if the patient requires intubation at some point in the future. You must master the skills for performing surgical airways and continually practice them under the direct supervision of the physician medical director, who should determine that you can perform the technique and that you understand and can treat its possible complications.

Indications that warrant a surgical cricothyrotomy include problems that prevent intubating or ventilating a patient by the nasal or oral routes. Massive facial or neck trauma is the most common cause. Some cases involve so much facial or airway distortion that you cannot identify normal landmarks. Other indications of a surgical cricothyrotomy include total upper airway obstruction due to epiglottitis, severe anaphylaxis, burns to the face and respiratory tract, posterior laceration of the tongue, or the inability to open the mouth. You can perform surgical airways with the patient's head and neck in neutral position. Contraindications to performing surgical airways in the field include inability to identify anatomical landmarks (including trauma and short, fat necks), crush injury to the larynx, tracheal transection, and underlying anatomical abnormalities such as trauma, tumor, or subglottic stenosis.

Needle Cricothyrotomy

Though it is an invasive surgical procedure that you must master before performing it in the field, a needle cricothyrotomy is technically easier to accomplish than an open cricothyrotomy and has a lower complication rate. It can be rapidly performed, does not manipulate the cervical spine, and provides adequate ventilation when performed properly. It is a temporary airway, used until a larger diameter, definitive airway is provided. It does not interfere with subsequent intubation attempts because it uses a 14-gauge needle, which has a relatively small diameter so that an ETT can pass beside it.

However, because the catheter does not fill the tracheal diameter, needle cricothyrotomy cannot protect the patient against aspiration.

This procedure requires different oxygenation and ventilation techniques than other airway maneuvers. Transtracheal jet insufflation (ventilation) uses a high-pressure jet ventilator to force oxygen through the small-diameter catheter and provide adequate oxygenation and ventilation. Because very high pressures insufflate large volumes of oxygen, **barotrauma,** including pneumothorax, is a potential complication. This procedure is not indicated if exhalation is not possible or if adequate high-pressure ventilation equipment is not available.

barotrauma *injury caused by pressure within an enclosed space.*

Needle Cricothyrotomy Complications   The potential complications of needle cricothyrotomy with jet ventilation include:

★ Barotrauma from overinflation

★ Excessive bleeding due to improper catheter placement

★ Subcutaneous emphysema from improper placement into the subcutaneous tissue, excessive air leak around the catheter, or laryngeal trauma

★ Airway obstruction from compression of the trachea secondary to excessive bleeding or subcutaneous air

★ Hypoventilation from use of improper equipment, incorrect use of the jet ventilator, or misplacement of the catheter

Needle Cricothyrotomy Technique   To perform needle cricothyrotomy with jet ventilation:

1. Place the patient supine and hyperextend the head and neck (maintain neutral position if you suspect cervical spine injury). Position yourself at the patient's side. Manage the patient's airway with basic maneuvers and supplemental oxygen, and prepare your equipment.

2. Gently palpate the inferior portion of the thyroid cartilage and the cricoid cartilage. The indention between the two is the cricothyroid membrane (Figures 13-64 ▓ and 13-65 ▓).

▓ Figure 13-64   Anatomical landmarks for cricothyrotomy.

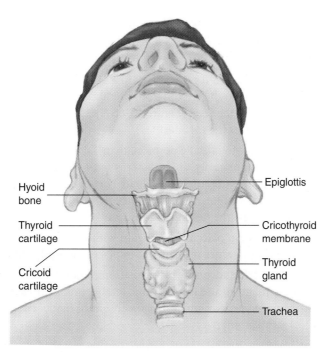

Hyoid bone

Thyroid cartilage

Cricoid cartilage

Epiglottis

Cricothyroid membrane

Thyroid gland

Trachea

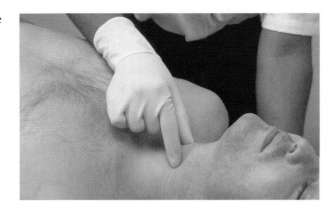

■ Figure 13-65 Locate/palpate the cricothyroid membrane.

■ Figure 13-66 Proper positioning for cricothyroid puncture.

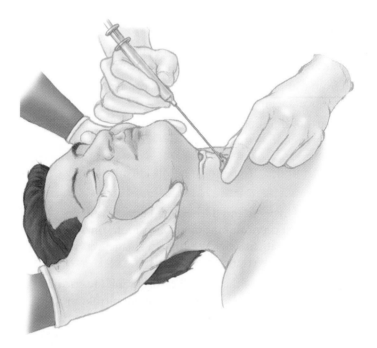

3. Prepare the anterior neck with povidone-iodine swabs. Firmly grasp the laryngeal cartilages and reconfirm the site of the cricothyroid membrane.

4. Attach a large-bore IV needle, with a catheter (adults: 14- or 16-gauge; pediatrics: 18- or 20-gauge) to a 10- or 20-mL syringe. Carefully insert the needle into the cricothyroid membrane at midline, directed 45° caudally (towards the feet) (Figure 13-66 ■). Often you will feel a pop as the needle penetrates the membrane.

5. Advance the needle no more than 1 cm, then aspirate with the syringe. If air returns easily, the catheter is in the trachea. If blood returns or you feel resistance to return, reevaluate needle placement. After you confirm proper placement, hold the needle steady and advance the catheter. Then withdraw the needle (Figure 13-67 ■).

6. Reconfirm placement by again withdrawing air from the catheter with the syringe. Secure the catheter in place (Figure 13-68 ■).

7. Check for adequacy of ventilations. Look for chest rise with each ventilation, and listen for bilateral breath sounds in the chest. If spontaneous ventilations are absent or inadequate, begin transtracheal jet ventilation.

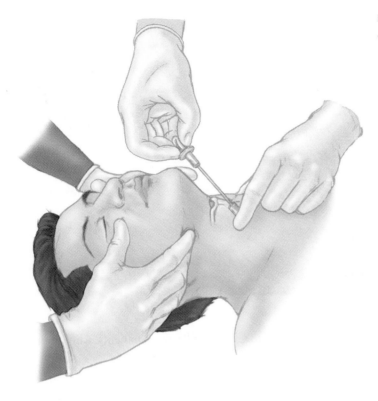

■ Figure 13-67 Advance the catheter with the needle.

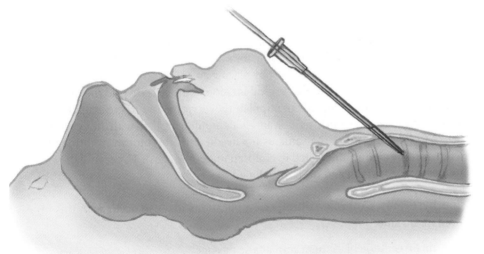

■ Figure 13-68 Cannula properly placed in the trachea.

8. Connect one end of the oxygen tubing to the catheter and the other end to the jet ventilator.

9. Open the release valve to introduce an oxygen jet into the trachea (Figure 13-69 ■). Then adjust the pressure to allow adequate lung expansion (usually about 50 psi, compared with about 1 psi through a regulator).

10. Watch the chest carefully, turning off the release valve as soon as the chest rises. Exhalation then occurs passively through the glottis, due to elastic recoil of the lungs and chest wall. Deliver at least 10-12 breaths per minute to ensure adequate oxygenation and ventilation. The inflation-to-deflation time ratio should be approximately 1:2, as with normal respirations. Keep in mind that you may need to adjust this to the patient's needs,

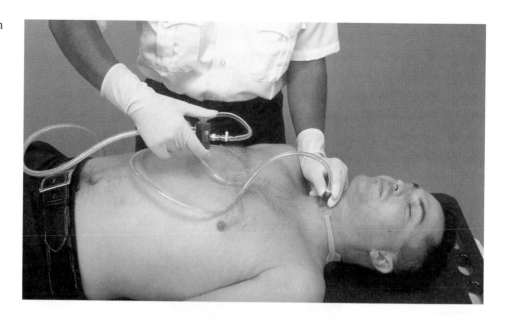

■ Figure 13-69 Jet ventilation with needle cricothryrotomy.

particularly in COPD and asthma patients, who often require a longer expiration time.

11. Continue ventilatory support, assessing for adequacy of ventilations and looking for the development of any potential complications.

Open Cricothyrotomy

An open cricothyrotomy is preferred to needle cricothyrotomy when a complete obstruction prevents a glottic route for expiration. Indications are the same as for needle cricothyrotomy. It involves obtaining an airway by placing an endotracheal or tracheostomy tube directly into the trachea through a surgical incision at the cricothyroid membrane. It can be rapidly performed and does not manipulate the cervical spine. Its greater potential complications mandate even more training and skills monitoring than with the needle method.

Contraindications are the same as for needle cricothyrotomy. Additionally, open cricothyrotomy is contraindicated in children under the age of 12 because the cricothyroid membrane is small and underdeveloped.

Cricothyrotomy Complications   Complications that can occur with this invasive procedure include:

★ Incorrect tube placement into a false passage
★ Cricoid and/or thyroid cartilage damage
★ Thyroid gland damage
★ Severe bleeding
★ Laryngeal nerve damage
★ Subcutaneous emphysema
★ Vocal cord damage
★ Infection

Open Cricothyrotomy Technique   To perform an open cricothyrotomy (Procedure 13–4):

1. Locate the thyroid cartilage and the cricoid cartilage. Find the cricothyroid membrane between the two cartilages.

Open Cricothyrotomy

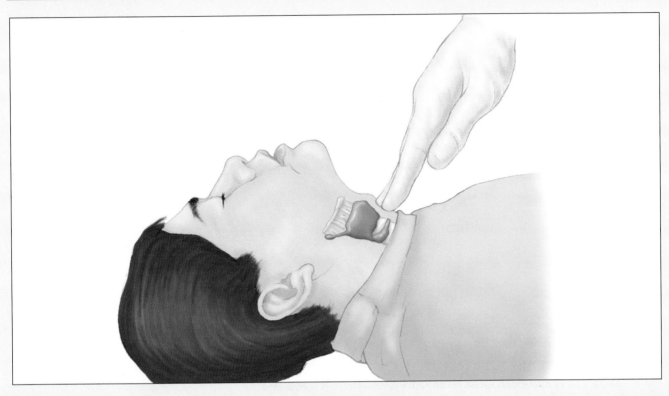

13-4a   Locate the cricothyroid membrane.

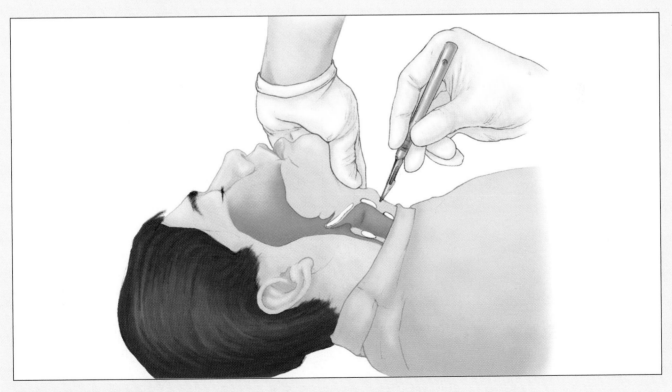

13-4b   Stabilize the larynx and make a 1- to 2-cm skin incision over the cricothyroid membrane.

continued on next page

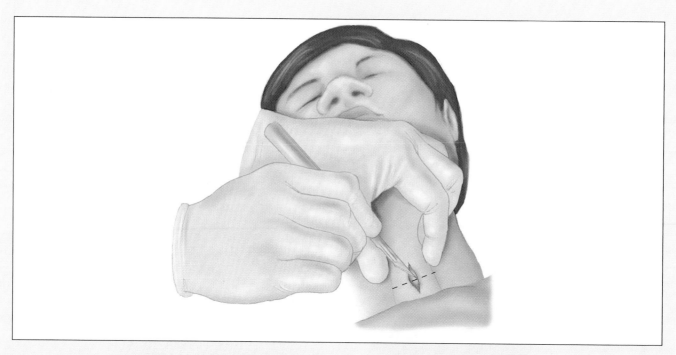

13-4c Make a 1-cm horizontal incision through the cricothyroid membrane.

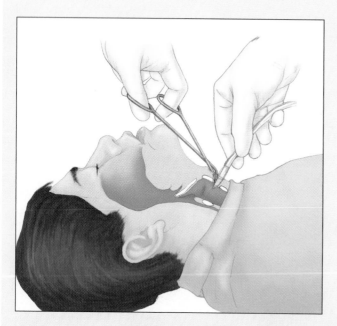

13-4d Using a curved hemostat, spread the membrane incision open.

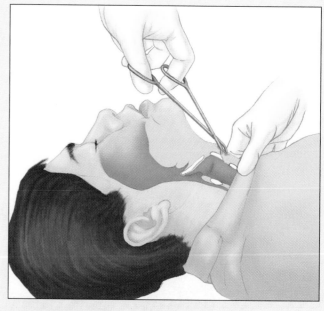

13-4e Insert an ETT (6.0 or 7.0) or Shiley (6.0 or 8.0).

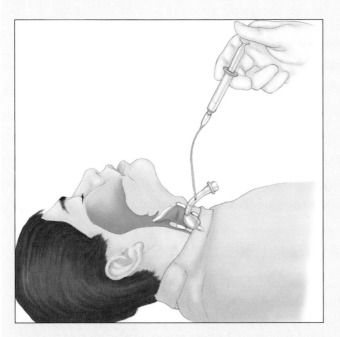

13-4f Inflate the cuff.

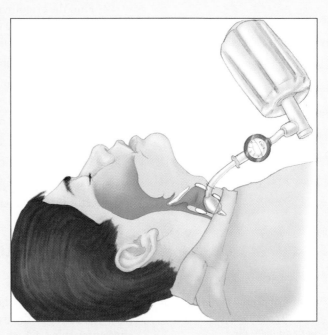

13-4g Confirm placement.

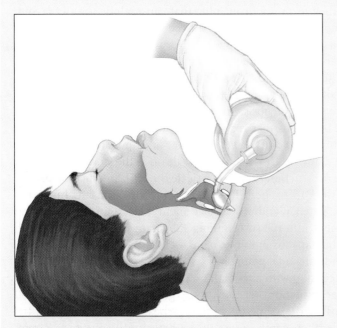

13-4h Ventilate.

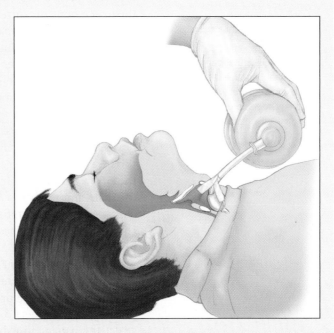

13-4i Secure the tube, reconfirm placement, and evaluate the patient.

2. Clean the area with iodine-containing solution if time permits, while your partner sets up suction, pulse oximetry, and cardiac monitor.

3. Stabilize the cartilages with one hand, while using a scalpel in the other hand to make a 1- to 2-cm vertical skin incision over the membrane.

4. Find the cricothyroid membrane again and make a 1-cm incision in the horizontal plane through the membrane, avoiding nearby veins and arteries, as well as the recurrent laryngeal nerve.

5. Insert curved hemostats into the membrane incision and spread it open.

6. Insert either a cuffed endotracheal tube (6.0 or 7.0 mm) or tracheostomy tube (6 or 8 Shiley), directing the tube into the trachea.

7. Inflate the cuff and ventilate.

8. Confirm placement with auscultation, end-tidal CO_2 detector, and chest rise.

9. Secure the tube in place.

We cannot stress enough that you must continuously practice this skill with the medical director's involvement before you are allowed to perform it.

MANAGING PATIENTS WITH STOMA SITES

stoma *opening in the anterior neck that connects the trachea with ambient air.*

Often patients who have had a laryngectomy (removal of the larynx) or tracheostomy (surgical opening into the trachea) breathe through a **stoma,** an opening in the anterior neck that connects the trachea with the ambient air. These patients frequently have tracheostomy tubes, which consist of an inner and outer cannula, in place to keep the soft-tissue stoma open (Figure 13-70 ■).

A patient with a stoma often has problems with excessive secretions. A laryngectomy produces a less-effective cough, making it more difficult to clear secretions. If these secretions organize, they form a mucous plug that can occlude the stoma and, thus, the airway. A stoma apparatus generally has a fixed outer portion and an inner cannula. The inner cannula can be easily removed and cleaned, then replaced. Timely replacement of the outer cannula is important if it must also be removed, because the stoma can constrict within just a few hours to prohibit its replacement without dilation.

As the external stoma site narrows, so can the inner tracheal diameter; either can produce potentially life-threatening stenosis. Any acute inflammation that leads to soft-tissue swelling can worsen this by further reducing the stoma and tracheal diameter. Further, this stenosis may make the cannula very difficult or impossible to replace. In this case, choose the largest diameter ETT that will pass through the stoma to maintain the airway before complete obstruction occurs. Lubricate the ETT, instruct the patient to exhale, and gently insert the ETT to about 1 to 2 cm beyond the distal cuff. Inflate the cuff, then confirm comfort, patency, and proper placement. Be certain to suspect and check for improper placement into the surrounding subcutaneous tissue, which will produce a false lumen. Subcutaneous emphysema as well as the lack of clinical improvement in the patient indicates a false lumen.

You must use extreme caution with any suctioning, as this process can itself cause soft-tissue swelling. In order to suction, begin by preoxygenating the patient with 100 percent oxygen. Inject 3 mL sterile saline down the trachea through the stoma. Instruct the patient to exhale, then gently insert the catheter until resistance is met. While the patient coughs or exhales, suction the airway during withdrawal of the catheter.

When the patient with a stoma requires ventilatory assistance, the bystander may use the mouth-to-stoma technique, while rescue personnel will generally use a BVM device.

⚷○—
Timely replacement of a stoma device's outer cannula is important because the stoma can constrict within just a few hours to prohibit its replacement without dilation.

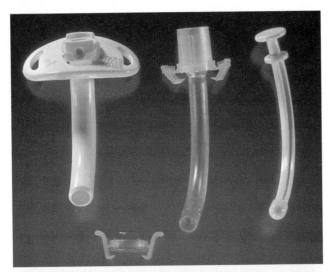

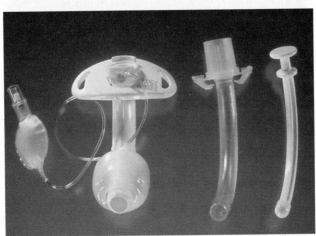

■ Figure 13-70   Tracheostomy cannulae.

If you use the mouth-to-stoma technique, it is preferable to use a pocket mask to cover the stoma for protection from communicable disease. For either technique, locate the stoma site and expose it. Obtain a tight seal around the stoma site, and check for adequate ventilation. Be sure to seal the mouth and nose if you note air leaking from these sites.

SUCTIONING

Anticipating complications when managing airways is the key for successful outcomes. You must be prepared to **suction** all airways in order to remove blood or other secretions and for the patient to vomit. Suctioning equipment must be readily available for all patients, to prevent a simple vomiting episode from becoming a complicated aspiration episode that increases the patient's risk for greater morbidity or mortality.

suction   *to remove with a vacuum-type device.*

SUCTIONING EQUIPMENT

Many different suctioning devices are available. They may be handheld, oxygen-powered, battery-operated, or mounted (nonportable). Table 13–6 details the advantages and disadvantages of each. To suit the prehospital environment, your equipment should be lightweight, portable, durable, generate a vacuum level of at least 300 mmHg

Table 13–6	Advantages and Disadvantages of Various Suction Types	
Type	Advantages	Disadvantages
Hand-powered	Lightweight, portable, inexpensive, simple to operate	Limited volume, manually powered, fluid contact components are not disposable
Oxygen-powered	Small, lightweight	Limited suction power, uses a lot of oxygen
Battery-operated	Lightweight, portable, excellent suction power, simple to operate and troubleshoot in the field	Battery memory decreases with time; mechanically more complicated than hand-powered, some fluid contact components are not disposable
Mounted	Strong suction, adjustable vacuum power, disposable fluid contact components	Not portable, cannot be serviced in the field, no substitute power source

Table 13–7	Types of Suctioning Catheters
Hard/Rigid Catheter	**Soft Catheters**
A large tube with multiple holes at the distal end	Long, flexible tube; smaller diameter than hard-tip catheters
Suctions larger volumes of fluid rapidly	Cannot remove large volumes of fluid rapidly
Standard size	Various sizes
Used in oropharyngeal airway only	Can be placed in the oropharynx, nasopharynx, or down the endotracheal tube
Removes larger particles	Suction tubing without catheter (facilitates suctioning of large debris)

🗝 ——

An adequate and properly functioning suction unit is essential for airway management.

when the distal end is occluded, and allow a flow rate of at least 30 liters per minute when the tube is open. In addition to a portable device, the ambulance should have a mounted, vacuum-powered suction device that can generate stronger suction and can be a backup device in case of equipment failure. The most commonly used suction catheters are either hard/rigid catheters ("Yankauer" or "tonsil tip") or soft catheters ("whistle tip"). Table 13–7 summarizes their differences.

Because suctioning reduces a patient's access to oxygen, you should limit each attempt to 10 seconds. If possible, hyperventilate the patient with 100 percent oxygen before and after each effort. Clear any fluids from the upper airway first, as assisted breathing may cause aspiration. Do not apply suction while inserting the catheter. Apply suction only as you withdraw the catheter after properly positioning it.

Complications of suctioning are related to hypoxia from prolonged suctioning attempts without proper ventilation. The decrease in myocardial oxygen supply can cause cardiac dysrhythmias. Suctioning can also stimulate the vagus nerve, causing bradycardia and hypotension, or the anxiety of being suctioned can cause hypertension and tachycardia. Stimulation of the cough reflex will cause a patient to cough, causing an increase in intracranial pressure and reducing cerebral blood flow.

SUCTIONING TECHNIQUES

You must have suction equipment by any patient who has airway compromise and will need airway management. Do not forget this basic and important skill. To suction a patient:

1. Wear protective eyewear, gloves, and face mask.

2. Preoxygenate the patient; this may require hyperventilating him.

3. Determine the depth of catheter insertion by measuring from the patient's earlobe to his lips.

4. With the suction turned off, insert the catheter into your patient's pharynx to the predetermined depth.

5. Turn on the suction unit and place your thumb over the suction control orifice; limit suction to 10 seconds.

6. Continue to suction while withdrawing the catheter. When using a whistle-tip catheter, rotate it between your fingertips.

7. While maintaining ventilatory support, ventilate the patient with 100 percent oxygen.

In many cases you will suction extremely viscous, or thick, secretions that can obstruct the flow of fluid through the tubing. To reduce this problem, suction water through the tubing between suctioning attempts. This dilutes the secretions and facilitates flow to the suction canister. Most suction units have small water canisters for this purpose.

Tracheobronchial Suctioning

You may have to suction some patients through an endotracheal tube or a tracheostomy tube to remove secretions or mucous plugs that can cause respiratory distress. Suctioning these patients risks hypoxia, so oxygenating them before and after the procedure is essential. If possible, use a sterile technique to avoid contaminating the pulmonary system. Use only the soft-tip catheter to avoid damaging any structures, and be certain to prelubricate it. Once you have preoxygenated the patient with 100 percent oxygen, lubricate the catheter tip with a water-soluble gel and gently insert it until you feel resistance (Figure 13-71 ■). Then apply suction for only 10 to 15 seconds while extracting

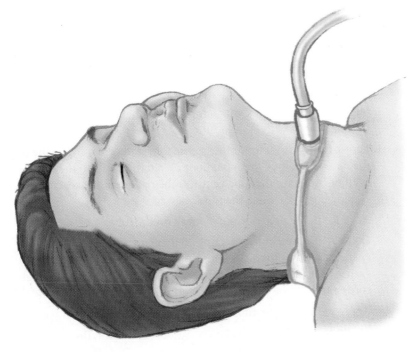

■ Figure 13-71   Tracheostomy suction technique.

the catheter. Ventilation and oxygenation are mandatory immediately after each suctioning attempt. You may have to inject 3 to 5 milliliters of sterile water down the endotracheal tube to help loosen thick secretions.

GASTRIC DISTENTION AND DECOMPRESSION

A common problem with ventilating a nonintubated patient is gastric distention, which occurs when the procedure's high pressures trap air in the stomach. As the stomach expands with this trapped air, the risk of vomiting rises. The enlarged stomach also pushes against the diaphragm, inhibiting the lungs' expansion and increasing their resistance to ventilation. Once the patient has gastric distention, you should place a tube in his stomach for gastric decompression, using either the nasogastric or orogastric approach.

Nasogastric tube placement is generally preferred in awake patients as it allows them to talk, while orogastric tube placement is recommended in patients with facial fractures to avoid placing the tube through a skull fracture into the brain. Indications for gastric tube placement include the need for decompression because of the risk of aspiration or difficulty ventilating. In addition, large-bore gastric tubes are occasionally placed for gastric lavage in hypothermia and some overdose emergencies. The possibility of esophageal bleeding dictates extreme caution in patients with esophageal disease or trauma. Avoid placing gastric tubes in the presence of an esophageal obstruction because of the increased risk of esophageal perforation. Both routes effectively accomplish gastric decompression; the orogastric route adds the advantage of allowing the use of a larger bore tube for lavage. Disadvantages of both routes include discomfort to patients and minor interference with orotracheal intubation. In patients with facial fractures, use orogastric routes to avoid placing the tube through a skull fracture into the brain. When no contraindication exists, nasogastric tube placement for gastric decompression is generally preferred. Both routes put the patient at risk for vomiting, misplacement into the trachea, or trauma and bleeding from poor technique.

As for any other invasive procedure, you should always wear protective eyewear, gloves, and a face shield whenever you place a nasogastric or orogastric tube. To place a nasogastric or orogastric tube:

1. Prepare the patient's head in a neutral position while preoxygenating.

2. Determine the length of tube insertion by measuring from the epigastrium to the angle of jaw, then to the tip of the nares.

3. If the patient is awake, use a topical anesthetic to the nares or oropharynx. Suppress the gag reflex with a topical anesthetic applied into the posterior oropharynx or with IV lidocaine.

4. Lubricate the distal tip of the gastric tube and gently insert the tube into the nares and along the nasal floor or, alternately, into the oral cavity at midline. Advance the tube gently. If the patient is awake, encourage swallowing to facilitate the tube's passage.

5. Advance to the predetermined mark on the tube.

6. Confirm placement by injecting 30 to 50 mL of air while listening to the epigastric region for air sounds. Inability to speak that develops after gastric tube placement indicates malposition of the tube through the vocal cords and into the trachea. If this occurs, you must remove the tube.

7. Apply suction to the tube, and note gastric contents that pass through the tube.

8. Secure the tube in place.

OXYGENATION

Oxygen is an important drug, and you must thoroughly understand its indications and precautions. Providing supplemental oxygen to patients who are frankly hypoxic will diminish the hypoxia's secondary effects on organs such as the brain and the heart. You should provide supplemental oxygen to patients who are in shock or at risk of shock, regardless of their oxygen saturation. Although the patient may be oxygenating his arterial blood well, the oxygen may not be reaching his cells effectively. The increased oxygen levels may help improve perfusion.

Never withhold oxygen from any patient for whom it is indicated. However, use caution with COPD patients. As we discussed earlier in this chapter's section on regulation of respiration, these patients lose the impulse to breathe at normal or supranormal oxygen levels. Their normal respiratory regulatory mechanism (elevated $PaCO_2$) has failed, and their impulse to breathe is triggered by a low PaO_2, or hypoxia. This is termed hypoxic drive. As a general approach, slowly increase these patients' oxygen until their breathing is less labored and they are more comfortable, though not necessarily back to their baseline. Watch your patient closely to be sure his decreased breathing effort does not signal impending respiratory failure due to loss of hypoxic drive. If this occurs, be ready to support the patient's ventilations, using basic maneuvers, adjuncts, and BVM.

> Never withhold oxygen from any patient for whom it is indicated.

OXYGEN SUPPLY AND REGULATIONS

Oxygen is supplied either as a compressed gas or a liquid. Compressed gaseous oxygen is stored in an aluminum or steel tank in 400-liter (D), 660-liter (E), or 3,450-liter (M) volumes. To calculate how long the oxygen will last, use the appropriate formula below—the same formula but with a different constant for each type of cylinder: 0.16 for a D cylinder, 0.28 for an E cylinder, and 1.56 for an M cylinder:

D cylinder tank life in minutes $=$ (tank pressure in psi $\times$ 0.16) $\div$ liters per minute

E cylinder tank life in minutes $=$ (tank pressure in psi $\times$ 0.28) $\div$ liters per minute

M cylinder tank life in minutes $=$ (tank pressure in psi $\times$ 1.56) $\div$ liters per minute

Liquid oxygen is cooled to aqueous form and warmed back to its gaseous state for delivery. Although liquid oxygen requires less storage space than an equal amount of compressed oxygen, you must keep it upright and accommodate other special requirements for its storage and transfer.

Regulators for oxygen tanks are either **high-pressure regulators,** which are used to transfer oxygen at high pressures from tank to tank, or **therapy regulators,** which are used for delivering oxygen to patients. The default pressure for therapy regulators is 50 psi, which is controlled within the regulator to allow for adjustable low-flow oxygen delivery.

> **high-pressure regulator** *regulator used to transfer oxygen at high pressures from tank to tank.*

> **therapy regulator** *pressure regulator used for delivering oxygen to patients.*

OXYGEN DELIVERY DEVICES

Oxygen delivery to patients is measured in liters of flow per minute (L/min). A number of delivery devices are available; the patient's condition will dictate which method you use. You must continually reassess the patient who requires oxygen therapy to be certain that the method of delivery and flow rate are adequate. You should not use these devices for patients with poor respiratory effort, severe hypoxia, or apnea or for patients who exhibit mouth breathing.

> You must continually reassess the patient who requires oxygen therapy to be certain that the method of delivery and flow rate are adequate.

Nasal Cannula The **nasal cannula** is a catheter placed at the nares. It provides an optimal oxygen supplementation of up to 40 percent when set at 6 L/min flow. At flow

> **nasal cannula** *catheter placed at the nares.*

rates above 6 L/min, the nasal mucous membranes become very dry and easily break down. Patients generally tolerate the nasal cannula well. It is indicated for low-to-moderate oxygen requirements and long-term oxygen therapy.

Venturi Mask   The **Venturi mask** is a high-flow face mask that uses a Venturi system to deliver relatively precise oxygen concentrations, regardless of the patient's rate and depth of breathing. As oxygen passes into the mask through a jet orifice in the base of the mask, it entrains room air. The device then delivers the resulting mixture to the patient. Some Venturi masks have dial selectors to control the amount of ambient air taken in; others have interchangeable caps. Either type can deliver concentrations of 24 percent, 28 percent, 35 percent, or 40 percent oxygen. The liter flow depends on the oxygen concentration desired. The Venturi mask is particularly useful for COPD patients, who benefit from careful control of inspired oxygen concentration.

Simple Face Mask   The simple face mask is indicated for patients requiring moderate-to-high oxygen concentrations. Side ports allow room air to enter the mask and dilute the oxygen concentration during inspiration. Flow rates generally range from about 6 to 10 L/min, providing 40 to 60 percent oxygen at the maximum rate, depending on the patient's respiratory rate and depth. Delivery of volumes beyond 10 L/min does not enhance oxygen concentration.

Partial Rebreather Mask   The partial rebreather mask is indicated for patients requiring moderate-to-high oxygen concentrations when satisfactory clinical results are not obtained with the simple face mask. One-way discs that cover the partial rebreather mask's side ports prevent the inspiration of room air. Minimal dilution occurs with inspiration of residual expired air along with the supplemental oxygen. Maximal flow rate is 10 L/min.

Nonrebreather Mask   The nonrebreather mask has one-way side ports as well, but also has an attached reservoir bag to hold oxygen ready to inhale. It provides the highest oxygen concentration of all oxygen delivery devices available, 80 to 95 percent at 15 L/min. It is not indicated as continuing support for poor respiratory effort and severe hypoxia; however, you should place it initially to attempt to preoxygenate these patients while you prepare to intubate them, unless initial ventilatory support with BVM and 100 percent oxygen is indicated.

Small-Volume Nebulizer   Nebulizer chambers containing 3 to 5 cc of fluid are attached to a face mask that allows for delivery of medications in aerosol form (nebulization). Pressurized oxygen or air enters the chamber to create a mist, which the patient then inspires. Oxygen is the usual carrier, but in many COPD cases, supplemental oxygen by nasal cannula with nebulization using air is preferred.

Oxygen Humidifier   You can provide humidified oxygen to the patient by attaching a sterile water reservoir to the oxygen outlet. Humidified oxygen benefits patients with croup, epiglottitis, or bronchiolitis, as well as those patients receiving long-term oxygen therapy.

VENTILATION

Many of your cases in the field will call for ventilatory support. These situations will range from apneic patients to less obvious instances when patients are experiencing depressed respiratory function. Remember that an unconscious patient's respiratory center may not function adequately. A significant decrease in the patient's rate or depth of breathing will lead to decreased respiratory minute volume, hypercarbia, hypoxia, and

Venturi mask *high-flow face mask that uses a Venturi system to deliver relatively precise oxygen concentrations.*

The Venturi mask is particularly useful for COPD patients, who benefit from careful control of inspired oxygen concentration.

✓ Review

Oxygen Delivery Devices

- Nasal cannula
- Venturi mask
- Simple face mask
- Partial rebreather mask
- Nonrebreather mask
- Small-volume nebulizer
- Oxygen humidifier

a lowered pH. If you do not correct this, respiratory or cardiac arrest may occur. Effective ventilatory support requires a tidal volume of at least 800 mL of oxygen at 10-12 breaths per minute.

When providing ventilatory support, you must generate enough force to overcome the elastic resistance of the lungs and chest wall, as well as the frictional resistance in the respiratory passageways, without overinflating the lungs. This is similar to blowing up a balloon; you must overcome the balloon's resistance in order to inflate it. Keep in mind that air will travel the path of least resistance. If you do not maintain a tight seal between the ventilation mask and your patient's face, air will flow out of the gaps rather than through the respiratory passageways.

Effective artificial ventilation requires a patent airway, an effective seal between the mask and the patient's face, and delivery of adequate ventilatory volumes. Exercise care when you attempt to generate enough pressure to ventilate the lungs. Too much pressure may lead to gastric distention and regurgitation. Also, be certain that you allow the patient to exhale between delivered breaths.

MOUTH-TO-MOUTH/MOUTH-TO-NOSE VENTILATION

Mouth-to-mouth and mouth-to-nose ventilation are the most basic methods of rescue ventilation. Both are indicated in the presence of apnea when no other ventilation devices are available. They require no special equipment, yet both allow an adequate seal between the rescuer and the patient and can provide effective ventilatory support, with adequate tidal volumes and oxygenation; however, the capacity of the person delivering the ventilations limits both methods. Also, both methods provide only limited oxygen—the rescuer's expired air will contain only 17 percent oxygen. This procedure's major drawback is its potential for exposing either the rescuer or the patient to communicable diseases through contact with blood and other body fluids. Take care not to hyperinflate the patient's lungs or to hyperventilate yourself.

MOUTH-TO-MASK VENTILATION

The pocket mask is a clear plastic device that you place over an apneic patient's mouth and nose. It prevents direct contact between you and your patient's mouth, thus reducing the risk of contamination and subsequent infection. It may be easier to obtain a good seal on the patient's face using a mask. However, the mask is only useful if it is readily available. Do not use it in awake patients.

A variety of pocket masks are available. Some are reusable, others are disposable. Most are small and compact enough to fit in a pocket or purse, and you should always carry one. Because of the increasing risks of infectious diseases, you should use a disposable mask whenever you ventilate a patient. These devices usually have a one-way valve that prevents you from contacting the patient's expired air. The valve may also provide an inlet for supplemental oxygen; mouth-to-mask ventilation combined with an oxygen flow rate of 10 L/min can deliver an inspired oxygen concentration of approximately 50 percent. To apply the mouth-to-mask technique, position the head to open the airway by one of the previously discussed methods, position the mask to obtain a good seal, and provide adequate ventilatory volumes. As with mouth-to-mouth and mouth-to-nose methods, hyperinflation of the patient's lungs, gastric distention in the patient, and hyperventilation in the rescuer are potential complications.

BAG-VALVE DEVICES

For patients with apnea or an unsatisfactory respiratory effort, prehospital and emergency department personnel most commonly use the bag-valve device. Used correctly

If you do not correct any significant decrease in the patient's rate or depth of breathing, respiratory or cardiac arrest may occur.

Exercise care when you attempt to generate enough pressure to ventilate the lungs.

✓ Review

Content

Ventilation Methods

- Mouth-to-mouth/mouth-to-nose
- Mouth-to-mask
- Bag-valve device
- Demand valve device
- Automatic transport ventilator

Figure 13-72 Bag-valve
mask with built-in colorimetric
$ETCO_2$ detector.

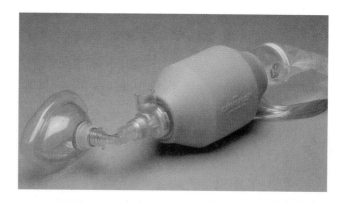

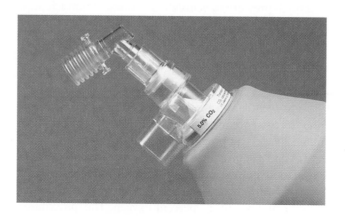

the bag-valve device assists in ventilating patients by expanding the lungs and improving alveolar ventilation, thus preventing hypoxia. When using the bag-valve device with the mask (BVM), the paramedic must still open the airway with either the jaw-thrust or head-tilt/chin-lift maneuver. Nor should you use the BVM in awake patients who do not tolerate the procedure.

The **bag-valve mask** consists of an oblong, self-inflating, silicone or rubber bag with two one-way valves (an air/oxygen-inlet valve and a patient valve) and a transparent plastic face mask, which is available in three sizes: neonatal, child, or adult. Some bag-valve masks have a built-in colorimetric end-tidal CO_2 detector (Figure 13-72 ▪). With the increasing risks of transmitting infectious diseases, bag-valve masks should be disposable. Do not reuse them.

You can use bag-valve masks with or without oxygen. Without oxygen they deliver only room air (21 percent oxygen) to the patient; with oxygen attached, the deliverable amount of oxygen increases to 60 to 70 percent. The bag-valve device also has an adjunct oxygen reservoir or corrugated tubing that can deliver 90 to 95 percent oxygen when coupled with an oxygen source. If possible, connect all patients who require a bag-valve device to an oxygen reservoir with oxygen at 15 L/min.

Bag-valve masks for pediatric cases may have a pop-off valve. Bag-valve masks for adults should not have pop-off valves, because patients with high airway resistance and poor lung compliance will activate the pop-off valve, thus preventing effective ventilation.

One, two, or three rescuers may perform bag-valve-mask ventilation. One-person BVM ventilation is the most difficult method to master because obtaining and maintaining the mask seal can be challenging. You must not only keep the airway open with a jaw-thrust or chin-lift but at the same time keep the mask sealed well and squeeze the BVM to deliver an adequate tidal volume. Two-person BVM ventilation is the most efficient method, providing superior mask seal and tidal volumes when applied correctly. It requires the availability of an adequate number of trained medical personnel. Three-person BVM ventilation also provides excellent mask seal and

bag-valve mask *ventilation device consisting of a self-inflating bag with two one-way valves and a transparent plastic face mask.*

Do not reuse bag-valve masks.

volume delivery, but it requires more personnel, and it crowds access to the patient's airway.

To perform the two-person BVM method, the first rescuer maintains the mask seal while the second squeezes the bag. With the three-person BVM method, the first rescuer applies manual airway maneuvers, the second maintains the mask seal, and the third squeezes the bag. Observe the patient for chest rise, development of gastric distention, and changes in compliance of the bag with ventilation. Complications of BVM ventilation include inadequate volume delivery if there is a poor mask seal or improper technique, barotrauma from overinflation of the lungs, and gastric distention.

Bag-Valve Ventilation of Pediatric Patients

The differences in the pediatric patient's anatomy require some variation in ventilation technique. First, his relatively flat nasal bridge makes achieving mask seal more difficult. Pressing the mask against the child's face to improve the seal can obstruct his airway, which is more compressible than an adult's. You can best achieve the mask seal with the two-person BVM technique, using jaw-thrust to maintain an open airway.

For BVM ventilation, the bag size depends on the child's age. Full-term neonates and infants will require a pediatric BVM with a capacity of at least 450 mL. For children up to 8 years of age, the pediatric BVM is preferred, though for patients in the upper age range you can use an adult BVM with a capacity of 1,500 mL if you do not maximally inflate it. Children older than 8 years require an adult BVM to achieve adequate tidal volumes. Additionally, be certain that the mask fits properly, from the bridge of the nose to the cleft of the chin. If a length-based resuscitation tape (Broselow Tape) is available, you can use it to help determine the proper size.

To achieve a proper mask seal, place the mask over the patient's mouth and nose; avoid compressing the eyes. Using one hand, place your thumb on the mask at the apex and your index finger on the mask at the chin (C-grip). Apply gentle pressure downward on the mask to establish an adequate seal. Maintain the airway by lifting the bony prominence of the chin with the remaining fingers forming an *E* under the jaw; avoid placing pressure on the soft area under the chin. You may use the one-rescuer technique, although the two-rescuer technique will be more effective.

Ventilate according to current standards, obtaining chest rise with each breath. Begin the ventilation and say "squeeze," providing just enough volume to initiate chest rise—be very careful not to overinflate the child's lungs. Allow adequate time for exhalation, saying "release, release." Continue ventilations, saying "squeeze, release, release." To assess adequacy of ventilations, look for adequate chest rise, listen for lung sounds at the third intercostal space, midaxillary line, and assess for clinical improvement (skin color and heart rate).

DEMAND VALVE DEVICE

The **demand valve device,** also called the manually triggered oxygen-powered ventilation device or flow-restricted, oxygen-powered ventilation device, will deliver 100 percent oxygen to a patient at its highest flow rates (40 liters per minute maximum). Flow is restricted to 30 cm H_2O or less to diminish gastric distention that can occur with its use. The device is rugged, compact, and easy to handle. It also includes an easy-to-locate manual control button. In addition, the entire device can be attached to a face mask or a mechanical airway (Figure 13-73 ■).

The complete system consists of high-pressure tubing that connects to an oxygen supply, and a valve that is activated by a push button or lever. When the valve is opened, oxygen flows to the patient. Most of these units also contain an inspiratory release valve that makes them useful in treating spontaneously breathing patients who need high oxygen concentrations. The slight negative pressure created by inhalation

demand valve device *a ventilation device that is manually operated by a push button or lever.*

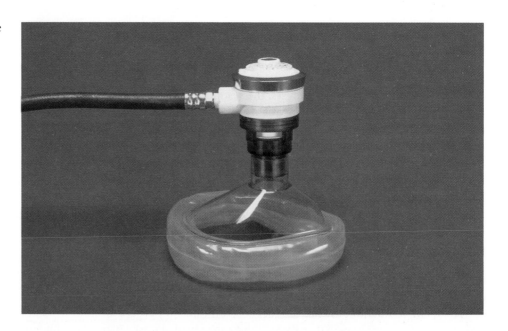

opens the valve. The greater the inspiratory effort, the higher the flow. When inhalation ceases, so does oxygen flow. This helps to decrease the likelihood of overinflation during ventilation of a patient with respiratory effort. The indications for use of oxygen-powered ventilation devices include the need for high-volume, high-oxygen-concentration delivery in awake, compliant patients. You may use it in unconscious patients, but must be extremely cautious, as you cannot measure delivered volumes or feel lung compliance. The demand valve device is easy to use and provides high-oxygen concentrations. However, the demand valve device has several drawbacks. During ventilation, it does not give the rescuer a sense of chest compliance; thus, you must take care not to overinflate the lungs. The high pressures that the device generates may injure the lungs, which can lead to pneumothorax and subcutaneous emphysema. Also, the demand valve resuscitator may open the esophagus, causing gastric distention in patients who have not been intubated. Finally, the demand valve resuscitator's high-flow rate will quickly drain a portable oxygen cylinder. You will have to use another means of ventilatory support if the cylinder requires changing during patient management.

The demand valve resuscitator is not recommended for use with patients under the age of 16. Because of the sudden high pressures that this device can produce, you should use it with extreme caution in intubated patients or those with chest trauma.

AUTOMATIC TRANSPORT VENTILATOR

Several compact mechanical ventilators are available for prehospital care. Designed for convenience and easy use during patient care and transport, these lightweight and durable portable devices offer a number of advantages. They maintain minute volume better than bag-valve devices, and they tolerate temperatures ranging from $-30°$ to $125°$ F with great dependability. In cardiac arrest, the automatic ventilator allows you to interpose chest compressions between mechanical breaths. They are mechanically simple and adapt to a portable oxygen supply.

The compact ventilator typically comes with two or three controls: one for the ventilatory rate, the other for tidal volume (Figure 13-74 ■). It also has a standard 15/22-mm adapter, so that you can attach it to a variety of airway devices. Some of these automatic units deliver controlled ventilation only. Others function as intermittent mandatory ventilators, reverting to controlled mechanical ventilation in patients who are not breathing. Tidal volume in most is adjustable, while the ventilatory rate may be either

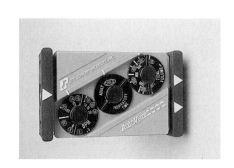

fixed or adjustable. The inspired oxygen concentration is usually fixed at 100 percent, but it may be adjustable.

Many of these ventilators have a pop-off valve that prevents pressure-related injury. When airway pressure exceeds a preset level (typically 60 cmH$_2$O), the valve opens, venting some of the tidal volume. This feature can hinder ventilating patients with cardiogenic pulmonary edema, adult respiratory distress syndrome (ARDS), pulmonary contusion, bronchospasm, or other disorders in which high airway pressures must be overcome. Consider using a bag-valve device if this problem occurs. Also, these devices generally have no alarms to warn of possible tube displacement or barotrauma.

As a rule, you should not use mechanical ventilators in children less than 5 years old, awake patients, or patients with obstructed airways or increased airway resistance, as previously described. Otherwise, when indicated, the device can prove a valuable tool. In intubated patients, the mechanical ventilator allows you to perform other vital tasks. Its disadvantages are that it can be difficult to secure and proper functioning depends on oxygen tank pressure.

Summary

Airway assessment and maintenance is the most critical step in managing any patient. If you do not promptly establish a definitive airway and provide proper ventilation, the patient's outcome will be poor. Frequently reassessing the airway is mandatory to ensure that the patient has not decompensated, requiring additional airway procedures. Successful management of all airways requires the paramedic to follow the proper management sequence.

Basic airway and management skills can make the difference between a successful outcome and a poor patient prognosis. Once you have mastered these basic skills and made them a part of airway management in every patient, you should learn and utilize advanced skills such as intubation, RSI, and cricothyrotomy. You must maintain proficiency in all airway skills, especially the more advanced techniques, through ongoing continuing education, physician medical direction, and testing with each EMS service. If you cannot do this, it is in the patient's best interest to focus on less sophisticated airway skills. If you anticipate that every airway will be complicated, apply basic airway skills before using advanced procedures, and perform frequent reassessments, you will give the patient his best chance for meaningful survival.

You Make the Call

You and your paramedic partner, Preston Connelly, are assigned to District 4, a quiet suburban neighborhood, on a warm Saturday in June. At 2:00 P.M., you are dispatched to care for a choking child at the Happy Hotdog Restaurant on Main Street. On your way to the location, the dispatcher advises you that they are currently giving prearrival instructions to the bystanders at the scene. On arrival, you find a frantic mother who tells you that her 6-year-old son was eating a hotdog and drinking a soda when he started coughing and gasping for air. She keeps yelling for you to do something. Bystanders surround the child and are attempting to perform the Heimlich maneuver without success. On your initial assessment, you find a 6-year-old male lying on the floor, unconscious and apneic, with a pulse rate of 130. There is cyanosis surrounding his lips and fingernail beds, with a moderate amount of secretions coming from his mouth. There are no signs of trauma. You and Preston immediately start management of this child.

1. What is your initial assessment and management of this child?
2. What are the differences between anatomic landmarks in the pediatric patient's airway and the adult's?
3. If you could not maintain the airway with basic mechanical airways, what would be your next course of action?
4. If this patient required rapid sequence intubation because of clenched teeth, what steps would you take to intubate him? (Include drug doses and their proper sequence.)

See Suggested Responses at the back of this book.

Review Questions

1. The depression between the epiglottis and the base of the tongue is called the:
   a. nare.
   b. glottis.
   c. larynx.
   d. vallecula.

2. The average volume of gas inhaled or exhaled in one respiratory cycle is the:
   a. minute volume.
   b. tidal volume.
   c. respiratory rate.
   d. total lung capacity.

3. A drop in blood pressure of greater than 10 torr during inspiration is called:
   a. compliance.
   b. laryngeal spasm.
   c. pulsus paradoxus.
   d. paradoxical breathing.

4. To avoid hypoxia during intubation, limit each intubation attempt to no more than _____ seconds before reoxygenating the patient.
   a. 10
   b. 20
   c. 30
   d. 40

5. _____ is the preferred neuromuscular blocking agent for emergency RSI.
   a. Atracurium
   b. Vecuronium
   c. Pancuronium
   d. Succinylcholine

6. The _____ is the most superior part of the airway.
   a. pharynx
   b. larynx

c. oral cavity

d. nasal cavity

7. The _____ is the only bone in the axial skeleton that does not articulate with any other bone.

   a. femur

   b. hyoid

   c. stapes

   d. patella

8. The _____ comprise(s) the key functional unit of the respiratory system.

   a. hilum

   b. alveoli

   c. bronchi

   d. respiratory bronchioles

9. The paramedic can correct oxygen derangements by:

   a. increasing ventilation.

   b. administering supplemental oxygen.

   c. using intermittent positive pressure ventilation.

   d. all of the above.

10. The _____ is the amount of gas in the tidal volume that remains in air passageways unavailable for gas exchange.

    a. base tidal volume

    b. minute volume

    c. dead-space volume

    d. total lung capacity

11. "Difficulty speaking" defines:

    a. aphagia.

    b. aphonia.

    c. dysphonia.

    d. dysphagia.

12. "An irregular pattern of rate and depth with sudden, periodic episodes of apnea, indicating increased intracranial pressure" describes:

    a. agonal respirations.

    b. Biot's respirations.

    c. Kussmaul's respirations.

    d. Cheyne-Stokes respirations.

13. _____ is often called the "fifth vital sign."

    a. heart rate

    b. blood pressure

    c. pulse oximetry

    d. blood glucose level

14. The visual representation of the expired CO_2 waveform is:

    a. capnogram.

    b. capnograph.

    c. capnometry.

    d. capnography.

15. Which of the following is not a disadvantage of the nasopharyngeal airway?

    a. It isolates the trachea.

    b. It is difficult to suction through.

    c. It is smaller than the oropharyngeal airway.

    d. It may cause severe nosebleeds if inserted too forcefully.

16. Advantages of endotracheal intubation include:
    a. It eliminates the need to maintain a mask seal.
    b. It isolates the trachea and permits complete control of the airway.
    c. It impedes gastric distention by channeling air directly into the trachea.
    d. All of the above.

17. _____ is generally the second-line paralytic when succinylcholine is contraindicated, because it has fewer cardiac and hypotensive side effects than other nondepolarizing agents.
    a. Atracurium
    b. Fentanyl
    c. Vecuronium
    d. Pancuronium

18. Potential indications for blind nasotracheal intubation include:
    a. obesity.
    b. possible spinal injury.
    c. significant angioedema.
    d. all of the above.

19. The _____ can function in either the tracheal or esophageal position.
    a. ET
    b. PtL
    c. LMA
    d. PLA

20. Open cricothyrotomy is contraindicated in children under the age of _____ because the cricothyroid membrane is small and underdeveloped.
    a. 12
    b. 14
    c. 16
    d. 18

See Answers to Review Questions at the back of this book.

Further Reading

American College of Surgeons, Committee on Trauma. *Advanced Trauma Life Support Course: Student Manual.* 5th ed. Chicago, Ill.: American College of Surgeons, 2002.

Bhende, M. S., and D. C. LaLovey. "End-Tidal Carbon Dioxide Monitoring in the Prehospital Setting." *Prehosital Emergency Care* 5 (2001):208–213.

Bledsoe, Bryan E. and Dwayne Clayden. *Prehospital Emergency Pharmacology.* 6th ed. Upper Saddle River, N.J.: Pearson Education/Prentice Hall, 2005.

Kapsner, Christopher E., et al. "The Esophageal Detector Device: Accuracy and Reliability in Difficult Airway Settings." *Prehospital and Disaster Medicine* 11 (1996): 60–62.

Mistovich, Joseph J., Randall W. Benner, and Gregg Margolis. *Prehospital Advanced Cardiac Life Support.* 2nd ed. Upper Saddle River, N.J.: Pearson Education/Prentice Hall, 2004.

Pepe, Paul E., Brian Zachariah, and N. C. Chandra. "Invasive Airway Techniques in Resuscitation." *Annals of Emergency Medicine* 22 (1993): 393–403.

Roberts, James R., and Jerris R. Hedges. *Clinical Procedures in Emergency Medicine.* 4th ed. Philadelphia: W. B. Saunders Company, 2004.

Rosen, Peter, and Roger M. Barkin. *Emergency Medicine Concepts and Clinical Practice.* 5th ed. Philadelphia: W. B. Saunders Company, 2002.

Rumball, C. J., and D. MacDonald. "The PtL, CombiTube, Laryngeal Mask, and Oral Airway: A Randomized Prehospital Comparative Study of Ventilatory Device Effectiveness and Cost-Effectiveness in 470 Cases of Cardiorespiratory Arrest." *Prehospital Emergency Care* 1 (1997): 1–10.

Stewart, Charles E. *Advanced Airway Management.* Upper Saddle River, N.J.: Pearson Education/Prentice Hall, 2002.

Tanigawa, Koichi, and Akio Shigematsu. "Choice of Airway Devices for 12,020 Cases of Nontraumatic Cardiac Arrest in Japan." *Prehospital Emergency Care* 2 (April/June 1998): 96–100.

On the Web

Visit Brady's Paramedic Website at **www.bradybooks.com/paramedic.**

Research in EMS

"Antishock trousers are good." "Antishock trousers are bad." "Intravenous fluids are good." "Intravenous fluids are bad." EMS providers hear these and other similar statements all the time. It can be quite confusing. Furthermore, newspapers and the television news pick up stories from articles in medical journals and report them to the public. How much of these reports can a paramedic believe? Do they apply to all EMS systems? Should they be the basis for changes in prehospital practice?

Research is an increasingly important part of EMS. Many of our ideas about patient care are the result of tradition and have never been evaluated from a scientific standpoint. This is true not just of EMS, but also of medicine in general and emergency medicine in particular. Only in the last few years has anyone paid significant attention to laying the foundation for research-proven quality care in EMS.

This appendix will describe three aspects of research as it applies to EMS. First, it will introduce you to the subject of interpreting research. This will help you understand what to look for in a piece of published research, such as whether to believe the conclusions of the paper and how to apply the research to your EMS system. Second, it will describe what you need to know if you participate in a research project. More and more EMS systems are participating in the research needed to determine how best to care for our patients and to justify what we do. Third, it will list a number of areas where you can learn more about research and how it is interpreted.

UNDERSTANDING RESEARCH

HOW A FIELD ADVANCES

Every area of medicine is rapidly changing. EMS is no exception. One of the ways in which a discipline advances is by common sense. No one has to do a research study to conclude that placing heavy sandbags on the sides of an immobilized patient's head can lead to harm if the patient and backboard must be turned on their sides. In this case, using something sturdy and lightweight makes a great deal more sense. Similarly, it is obvious that glass IV bottles are much more likely to break in a moving ambulance than plastic IV bags. In these cases, common sense guides us in making important decisions.

However, common sense has its limits. Twenty years ago, common sense led us to believe that we could raise the blood pressure of a shock patient by inflating antishock trousers. In fact, it was taught that antishock trousers would potentially autotransfuse two to three units of blood from the lower extremities to the torso. These ideas seemed sound and were based on experiences the military had with gravity suits (G-suits). It was assumed that the same physiological effects would occur in a shock patient when the trousers were applied. Various researchers began to question the effectiveness of the antishock trousers. First, several studies were conducted that addressed the physiological effects of the trousers. Much to the surprise of many, the trousers had very little impact on blood pressure in shock patients. Furthermore, the antishock trousers autotransfused only a very small amount of blood, if any.

Other researchers looked at a much more important and key issue. Do antishock trousers improve patient survival? The research found that the antishock trousers had no beneficial effect on patient survival. In fact, some patients actually did worse when the trousers were applied compared to those who did not have them applied. Because of this research, antishock trousers are no longer routinely used in the prehospital management of hemorrhagic shock.

Several years ago, it was also considered common sense to place a soft cervical collar around the neck of a patient with a suspected cervical-spine injury. That belief is no longer considered valid. Today, common sense tells us that a rigid cervical collar, applied in conjunction with spinal immobilization, does a better job of preventing spine injuries from becoming spinal-cord injuries. It remains to be seen whether this belief will be verified by scientific evidence or if someone will find a better approach.

Sometimes we have to rely on something a little more substantive than common sense, even when we do not have the hard data to make a definitive statement. In this case, we may try to get a consensus of experts in the field. The U.S. DOT's 1998 *EMT-Paramedic: National Standard Curriculum* was developed using this method. A group of team leaders, each responsible for a particular section of the curriculum, discussed the general direction and approach the curriculum should take. Each team leader then discussed more specific information with a group of writing experts (authors) and medical content experts (physicians). Because EMS is such a young field, there was frequently a lack of clear evidence to support certain subjects and interventions. Using this approach, experts discussed and came to agreement on what should and should not be included in this curriculum.

This approach is used often in medicine when there is conflicting and missing information or when there have been many changes in a short time. The American Heart Association (AHA), for example, periodically uses this approach in updating its guidelines for basic and advanced cardiac life support. The AHA has recently augmented its consensus approach with a set of evidence-based guidelines. These guidelines call on participants in the process to evaluate the strength of available evidence by evaluating the nature of the evidence supporting it. The results of a well-conducted study that has a powerful methodology and many study subjects would receive more weight than a case report (a description of what happened to one or a few patients in an emergency department, for example).

Scientific studies are another way of improving the care our patients receive. To many people, this is the best way to advance a field because it allows practitioners to see exactly how an idea was tested. When done well, a piece of research can have a significant impact on many people's lives. EMS has only recently begun to lay this foundation and establish credibility for itself. In recent years, some of the areas that have received attention from EMS researchers include defibrillation, spine immobilization, aeromedical transport (helicopters), triaging of patients to trauma centers, intravenous fluids, endotracheal intubation by EMT-Basics, time saved by use of lights and sirens, and the value of certain advanced life support interventions.

TYPES OF STUDIES

There are four types of scientific studies that you are likely to encounter: descriptive, case-control, cohort, and intervention studies. Each type of study has its strengths and weaknesses.

Descriptive Studies

In a *descriptive study,* researchers do not attempt to change anything or discover the effects of any intervention. Instead, they carefully evaluate a particular subject according to carefully spelled out criteria. This yields a report that describes the current state of affairs in a particular area. For example, an EMS agency may wish to learn how many defibrillators to purchase and where to place them. To accomplish this, they review their run reports for the last 3 years to determine how many cardiac arrests the service had and where those arrests occurred. The results give the organization the information it needs in order to station enough defibrillators in the right places. This will increase the likelihood that a defibrillator will be nearby when a patient goes into cardiac arrest.

Descriptive studies are relatively inexpensive and simple to conduct because they usually involve reviewing a database or conducting a survey. They are limited, though, in their scope and applicability because they typically look only at a single system, which may be very different from other systems, and because like a snapshot it shows conditions at only one particular point in time. A *cross-sectional study,* for example, might look at divorce rates of emergency workers. If the rate were found to be high (or low), we would have the answer to the question we asked. However, we would be left with a lot more questions this study would not be able to answer, such as: Is the divorce rate different because of the work these people do? Or is the rate different because of the kind of person drawn to emergency work?

Because they are very weak in their ability to draw conclusions about cause and effect, descriptive studies are not very useful for investigating hypotheses. Instead, they are better suited for laying the foundation for research in a particular area and for suggesting research questions for the future.

Case-Control Studies

A *case-control study* is an example of *retrospective research,* which looks backward in time. By finding patients who have a particular disease or condition and comparing them to people who do not have the disease or condition, a case-control study can allow investigators to determine which factors place someone at risk for developing the disease. An example of this was a landmark study on the effects of cigarette smoking published in 1950. The investigators looked at the health history, including smoking history, of more than 700 patients hospitalized for lung cancer and compared this to the same information obtained from a large number of patients hospitalized for other conditions. They found that patients with lung cancer were significantly more likely to have smoked than those without lung cancer.[1]

One of the criticisms of case-control studies is a phenomenon called *recall bias.* If you ask someone with lung cancer how long and how much he has smoked, he may, either consciously or unconsciously, give inaccurate answers, depending on whether he believes smoking caused his condition and which answers he believes the investigator wants. He also may not want to admit he was unable to quit smoking and so may be less than completely truthful. Alternatively, he may wish to exaggerate the role smoking played in causing his condition so that others will not imitate him. The person without lung cancer is presumably less likely to be subject to these feelings, but may still be subject to recall bias. Even the most carefully conducted study can fall victim to this kind

[1] Doll, R., and A. B. Hill. "Smoking and Carcinoma of the Lung: Preliminary Report." *British Medical Journal* 2(1950):739.

of distortion, so it is important that researchers take it into consideration and do everything they can to minimize it.

Cohort Studies

Like case-control studies, *cohort studies* look at certain characteristics of study subjects (potential risk factors) and the development of disease. In this case, though, we do not know yet whether the study subjects have the disease we are studying. Instead, we record which potential risk factors patients have or were exposed to and follow them to see which ones develop the disease being studied. This is an example of *prospective research,* where the condition being studied has not yet appeared.

This can be quite time-consuming since many conditions take years to develop. Over a long period of time, study subjects may also move away from the investigators or in other ways be lost to follow-up. This can make such a study quite expensive. Probably one of the best known examples of this type of study is the Framingham Heart Study.[2]

In the early 1950s investigators began studying more than 5,000 middle-age adults without cardiovascular disease in the Framingham, Massachusetts, area. These people have been followed and periodically examined for heart disease. Since the researchers did not (and could not) know at the beginning of the study which patients with which risk factors would develop heart disease, this study has given scientists very strong evidence about the roles of cigarette smoking, cholesterol, and high blood pressure in the development of heart disease.

Intervention Studies

In case-control studies, investigators look at patients who have a disease and determine risk factors for development of the disease. In cohort studies, patients are selected on the basis of whether or not they have been exposed to risk factors and followed for the development of disease. In *experimental* or *intervention studies,* the situation is quite different. In these studies, the investigators determine whether or not a subject is exposed (or treated) instead of depending on nature to determine this. This kind of study, when designed and conducted properly, yields extremely strong evidence about the effects of certain interventions. For this reason, it is often considered the gold standard in research methodology.

The investigators begin, just as they do with case-control and cohort studies, by deciding on a study hypothesis. This consists of an idea that they can test in an objective manner. For instance, a number of years ago, clinicians in King County, Washington, wished to test the hypothesis that EMTs with automated external defibrillators (AEDs) could increase survival from cardiac arrest just as well as EMTs with manual defibrillators.[3] They trained EMTs to use both machines, set up protocols for their use, decided exactly what data they were going to record, and planned how they were going to be able to tell if their hypothesis was correct (through selection of the proper statistical tests). They did this very carefully and planned how to conduct the study so that irrelevant factors were eliminated or minimized.

Since the researchers wanted to find out whether EMTs could operate AEDs, they used just one brand of AED. This eliminated one potential source of confounding. A variable that is not being studied, but which may have an effect on the result, is called a *confounding variable* or *nuisance variable.* In this case, the researchers made sure that no one could say increased (or decreased) survival could be attributed to one brand of AED over another since only one brand of AED was being used.

Whenever possible, researchers performing clinical trials attempt to *randomize* the intervention so that there is less chance of interference from a confounding variable.

---

[2] Dawber, T. R. *The Framingham Study: The Epidemiology of Atherosclerotic Disease.* Cambridge, MA: Harvard University Press, 1980.
[3] Cummins, R. O., M. S. Eisenberg, P. E. Litwin, et al. "Automatic External Defibrillators Used by Emergency Medical Technicians." *Journal of the American Medical Association* 257(1987): 1605–1610.

For example, a number of EMTs in King County had been using manual defibrillators for several years and preferred using them. If they had a choice as to which defibrillator they could use, they might select the manual defibrillator for patients with short down times and the automated defibrillator for long or unknown down times. The researchers took this into account by telling the EMTs to use one of the machines for 75 days and then the other for the next 75 days. Although this is not randomization in the strictest sense of the word, this alternation design, or *alternative time sampling,* is an acceptable means of preventing this type of confounding. Another example is the use of one intervention on even days and another on odd days.

As can be seen in this case, it is not always practical, or even possible, to use truly random sampling. In such cases, *systematic sampling* may be a reasonable alternative. This might include, for example, using the study intervention every second or third day. Although systematic sampling is subject to bias, it is better than *convenience sampling.* Convenience sampling, as the name implies, occurs at the convenience of the investigator, which for example might be only when that person is working. If the investigator is a paramedic with some seniority who gets some choice over when and where he or she works, this could lead to significant bias in subject selection.

All clinical trials compare one group that receives an intervention (the *study group*) against at least one other group that does not receive the intervention being studied (the *control group*). In many studies, the control group receives a placebo, something that resembles the intervention but has no physical effect on the study subject. In drug trials, for instance, a placebo is sometimes a sugar pill. In the case of an AED study, it would have been unethical to deny defibrillation to cardiac-arrest patients in the control group since there was clear evidence that manual defibrillation was saving some lives. So the researchers used manual defibrillation as their control.

Something else researchers attempt to incorporate into their study designs whenever possible is *blinding.* This refers to whether or not someone knows which is being used, a placebo or an active agent. In an *unblinded* study, everyone involved (the patient, researcher, statistician, and so on) knows when the intervention is and is not being used. *Single blinding* occurs when the patient does not know what he is receiving, but the researcher does. *Double blinding* means that neither the patient nor the researcher knows what the patient is receiving. *Triple blinding* is a less commonly used term that refers to the situation where the patient, researcher, and statistician (or principal investigator, who may be functioning in that capacity) do not know whether a patient is receiving the intervention or a placebo.

In the case of a drug study, it can be very important to blind the study subjects and the investigators because of the possibility of *observation bias.* This occurs when, either consciously or unconsciously, someone (either the subject or the investigator) reports an effect because they believe there should be one. This is called the *placebo effect.* Study subjects who receive placebos often report feeling better, even though they did not receive any medication. This effect can occur in as many as a quarter of study subjects and may persist for years afterward. A similar type of bias, known as the *Hawthorne effect,* occurs when outcomes improve during a study just because those participating in the study are aware that experimental attempts are being made to bring about improvement.

In a study where the outcome being studied is as objective as death or survival, there is little or no need for blinding. If, however, a subjective outcome like quality of life after cardiac arrest was being studied, there would be a lot more potential for observation bias. In this case, it would be important to make sure the investigators determining the quality of life do not know which intervention a patient receives, if at all possible.

Another way in which the King County researchers demonstrated good study design was the way they planned their data collection and statistical analysis. Even with randomization, study subjects may differ from the control subjects in important ways.

It thus becomes important for researchers to evaluate the two groups for differences that may confound the results. In this case, they looked at a number of variables, including age, sex, whether or not the arrest was witnessed, initial ECG rhythm, and response times. They found that the two groups were significantly different in a few ways, but they were able to use some sophisticated statistical methods to determine that in this case those differences did not affect patient outcome.

One of the other things they did was to calculate the sample size they would need to detect a difference in survival rates. They calculated that in order to have an 80 percent chance of detecting a difference in survival of more than 15 percent (if a difference truly existed), they would need to have at least 150 patients in each group. This allowed them to plan approximately how long the study would take. The figure of 80 percent is sometimes referred to as the "power of the study" and is directly related to how willing the investigators are to avoid making an error in their conclusions.

There are two types of *statistical error* that researchers can make. A Type I, or alpha, error is accepting a hypothesis when it is false. A Type II, or beta, error is rejecting a hypothesis when it is true. The Type I error rate is set at 0.05, or 5 percent in most research. A commonly accepted Type II error rate is 20 percent or 0.2. The power of a study is equal to $1 - $ beta. Since many studies set beta at 0.2, the power is $1 - 0.2 = 0.8$, or 80 percent to detect a difference at the magnitude specified by the investigators if a difference truly exists. The Type I and Type II error rates have an inverse relationship; that is, the lower the Type I error rate the investigator wishes to have, the higher the Type II error rate the investigator will have to tolerate, all other factors being equal. The reverse is also true.

The Type I error rate, or alpha, receives a great deal of attention in published research. Most investigators set alpha at 0.05. This means the researchers will say there is a difference and consider the study to have statistically significant results only if there is a 5 percent chance or less of getting the results they obtained. Another way of looking at a Type I error rate, or alpha, of 0.05 is that there is only a 5 percent chance of rejecting the study hypothesis when it is false, assuming the hypothesis is true.

A good practice many studies follow is to report not just the acceptable alpha of 0.05, but also the actual probability of getting the results obtained in the study. You may see this written as "$P < .01$." This means the chance of finding such a difference in the study groups is less than 1 percent assuming the hypothesis is true.

Some people have misinterpreted P values in two ways. First, they conclude that because the P value is so small the hypothesis is absolutely proven beyond a shadow of a doubt. This is not true. No study can definitively prove its hypothesis. All a study can do is assign certain probabilities to the conclusions. All studies also make certain assumptions, such as the type of data to be collected, accuracy of the data, and whether or not samples were selected randomly and independently. If these assumptions are violated, the study's conclusions are suspect.

Second, some people conclude that because there is *statistical* significance (because the P value is so small) there must be *clinical* significance. This is not the case. The researcher determines whether or not there is statistical significance by deciding how much Type I error is acceptable. The researcher and the reader must then determine if there is clinical significance by evaluating the effect of this difference on patient care.

For example, suppose a new drug for hypertension is studied. The investigators find statistically significant differences between the blood pressures in the treated and untreated subjects with $P << .01$ (P much less than 1 percent). In other words, if there was no difference between the drug and the control, these results would occur much less than 1 percent of the time. On looking at the data, the reader finds that the experimental drug lowers diastolic blood pressure 0.1 mmHg. Is this a clinically significant difference? Not likely. To see a change that is significant enough to affect patient outcome, the difference would have to be greater.

The Type II error rate, or beta, receives much less attention in most published research. This oversight is unfortunate because in some cases investigators fail to get a large enough sample size and so are unable to find a difference even though it exists. A good way to reduce both error rates is to increase the sample size. This solution can lead to some other problems, though.

With greater sample size comes the difficulties of more data collection, longer times required to conduct the study, and increased expense. Additionally, it may become easier to find differences that are irrelevant. This occurs because a larger sample allows smaller differences to be detected.

Another problem that can arise in clinical trials is violation of protocol. Despite the planning and precautions of the investigators in the King County study, there were some instances in which EMTs used the manual defibrillator when they were supposed to use the AED. In their analysis of the data, they evaluated these cases as a separate group and also with the AED group to which they should have belonged. This is called *intention to treat* analysis and is an appropriate way to manage protocol violations. This approach does increase the difficulty of finding a difference, but this is usually safer than the opposite approach of including these cases in the other treatment group. In this case, when the investigators analyzed the data, they found that the violations did not have an effect on the overall outcome.

In the end, the King County study found that there was no significant difference in survival between the group treated with the manual defibrillator and the group treated with the AED. Since AEDs are less expensive, require less training to operate, are extremely consistent in performance, and can be used in areas where there are fewer cardiac arrests, the investigators concluded that AEDs can make early defibrillation possible for more patients and should be encouraged. This is an example of a study that, because it showed there was no statistically significant difference between two treatments, had great clinical significance.

Table A–1 summarizes the advantages and disadvantages of different types of studies.

Table A–1	Advantages and Disadvantages of Different Types of Studies	
Study Type	**Advantages**	**Disadvantages**
Descriptive	Inexpensive	Not good for testing hypotheses
	Relatively easy to conduct	Very system-specific
	Can be done in relatively short time	
Case Control	Good for testing hypotheses regarding uncommon or rare conditions	Subject to recall bias
	Lays groundwork for cohort and intervention studies	
Cohort	Can provide very strong evidence for effects of risk factors	Not good for uncommon or rare conditions
		Can be very time-consuming
		Expensive
Intervention	Provides strongest kind of evidence research can produce	Expensive
	Can minimize bias through randomization and blinding	Need to protect study subjects may prolong time needed to conduct a study
		Study conditions may not be similar to real-life conditions

COMMON STATISTICAL TESTS

A number of computer programs, including commonly used spreadsheets, are available to calculate statistical tests for researchers and others. This section will briefly describe in layperson's terms a few of the more common tests you will find in reading research papers.

Descriptive Statistics

Descriptive statistics describe the nature of a sample. The most common descriptive statistic you will encounter is the *mean,* or average. It is computed by adding the values and dividing by the number of values involved. This gives a look at the average or typical value of a group of numbers in many cases. The mean is especially well suited when the data are what statisticians call "normally distributed." This means that if you graphed the data, they would form a shape similar to a bell curve described by a particular statistical equation. Height of individuals is an example of a normally distributed variable. Most people have a height close to the average, with a few very short and a few very tall people at each end of the graph.

When the data are not normally distributed, the *median* is a better way of finding a typical value. To compute the median, put the values into numerical order and find the middle value. This is the median, also known as the "fiftieth percentile." For example, if you have seven exam scores, to find the median, you put the scores in order and find the fourth highest (or fourth lowest, since it is the same).

Here is an example of how the median can be more useful than the mean in some situations: In many states the number of emergency calls received by EMS agencies is not normally distributed. There are frequently a few very busy services in urban areas, a good number of moderately busy services, and a larger number of services in rural areas that receive a much smaller number of calls. If you were to compute the mean, or average, it would be skewed by the very busy services, even though there are only a few of them, because they receive such a high number of calls. However, if you computed the median, you would get a smaller number that would better reflect the number of calls received by a typical service.

The mean and the median only tell one part of the story. They are called *measures of central tendency* because they indicate the center of the group in one way or another. A different, but very important, quality to know about a group is how spread out it is, or how dispersed the data are.

There are two closely related measures of this that you are likely to see. The first is called the *variance.* To get it, we take each value and subtract the mean from it. We cannot take the average of these numbers and get anything useful because the negative numbers will cancel out the positive numbers and we will get zero. To overcome this, we multiply each number by itself (square it) and add up the squared numbers. We then divide this sum by the number of values we started with (for reasons statisticians can describe, when we are working with samples, we usually divide by one less than the number of values). This is the variance.

To get the *standard deviation* (SD), the other common measure of dispersion, we take the square root of the variance. Figure A-1 ▨ shows two examples of variance and standard deviation. The standard deviation gives us valuable information about the data. If two groups of data have the same mean, but the second has a standard deviation much larger than the first, the data in the second group are much more spread out than the data in the first group. The SD is also used in many statistical formulas.

Another way we can describe data is to give the *mode.* This is simply the most common value in a set of data. If you graph the data, with the data value on the horizontal axis and the frequency of occurrence on the vertical axis (also known as a frequency distribution), the mode is the value associated with the highest point on the graph.

Examples of Variance and Standard Deviation

To see how the variance and standard deviation can give valuable information about data, consider this example: Two different EMT-P classes take the same midterm exam. The classes are the same size (seven students each) and have the same mean (or average) score, 85%. If we did not look any further, we might think the two classes performed the same on the exam. By looking at the variance and standard deviation, though, we can see that they are actually quite different.

Class 1

	Score	Mean	Score − Mean	(Score − Mean)^2
	78	85	−7	49
	81	85	−4	16
	82	85	−3	9
	84	85	−1	1
	87	85	2	4
	89	85	4	16
	94	85	9	81
Sum	595		0	176

Recall that to get the variance we must find the mean, then find the differences between the scores and the mean, square these differences, add them up, and divide by one less than the number of scores. The mean is included in the second column to make it easier to calculate the difference between each score and the mean. The variance is then 176/6 = 29.3. The standard deviation is the square root of 29.3, which is 5.4.

Class 2

	Score	Mean	Score − Mean	(Score − Mean)^2
	82	85	−3	9
	83	85	−2	4
	84	85	−1	1
	85	85	0	0
	86	85	1	1
	87	85	2	4
	88	85	3	9
Sum	595		0	28

Again, to get the variance, we sum the squared differences in the last column and divide by one less than the number of scores: 28/6 = 4.7. The standard deviation is the square root of 4.7, or 2.2, less than half the standard deviation of the first class.

This implies that the scores in the first class are much more spread out than the scores in the second class. When we graph the scores, we can see that this is true:

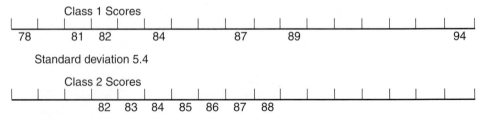

Class 1 Scores

78   81 82   84   87   89   94

Standard deviation 5.4

Class 2 Scores

82 83 84 85 86 87 88

Standard deviation 2.2

Inferential Statistics

As noted earlier, the mean, median, variance, and standard deviation are examples of *descriptive statistics.* They describe the nature of a sample of data taken from a *population,* a group we are interested in.

Descriptive statistics are related to, but quite different from, *inferential statistics.* Here, instead of describing the sample, we wish to draw inferences about the population the sample came from. In this case, we say we are estimating *parameters* of the population. For example, if the sample is of sufficient size and we make certain assumptions about the population and how the sample was selected, we can estimate the mean value of the population from which we drew our sample. Polling organizations commonly use these techniques in reporting results of their surveys. We must keep in mind, however, the phenomenon of *sampling error.* This is the difference between the value obtained from the sample and the value obtained from the population stemming solely from the fact that only a sample of the population was included.

When researchers find that something occurs with a certain frequency, they usually report this proportion as a percentage. For example, survival from cardiac arrest caused by ventricular fibrillation (VF) may be 20 percent in a particular study. But since the study looked at a sample of patients in VF, this proportion is only an estimate and may in reality be higher or lower. Investigators can calculate how much variability exists in this percentage based on the number of observations, the actual data, and how reliable they wish the estimate to be.

This variability (not the same as the variance) can then be added and subtracted to the original proportion to give what is called a *confidence interval.* For example, suppose the investigators calculated the variability in the previous example with 95 percent confidence and found it was 6 percent. Then we would have a 95 percent confidence interval of 20 percent plus or minus 6 percent. This means that, assuming the hypothesis is true, we can be 95 percent confident that the actual rate of survival under the conditions studied was between 14 percent and 26 percent.

Confidence intervals are very important in interpreting the value of the research results. If the confidence interval for a proportion like the previous one included zero, then there would be a real possibility that there is no actual difference between the study group outcome and the control group outcome. We would conclude that the results are not statistically significant and that there is insufficient reason to believe there is a difference between the two groups.

Quantitative and Qualitative Statistics

There are many tests for finding differences between groups. Statisticians frequently classify them into qualitative and quantitative tests. *Qualitative statistics* usually deal with data that are nonnumerical in nature (e.g., female, male) or that are nonnumerical in nature and have been assigned a number indicating ranking or ordering of importance or severity (stage I, II, and III of certain cancers, for example). These are sometimes called *nominal* and *ordinal data.* Finding the mean of such data may be impossible or absurd since they are categorical in nature. *Quantitative statistics,* however, are numerical in nature, such as temperature measured in degrees on a thermometer or height of an individual measured in centimeters or inches. They are sometimes referred to as continuous data.

Other Types of Data

Commonly used tests you may see in research include *t test,* the *analysis of variance (ANOVA),* and the *chi square test.* Which test is used depends to a great extent on the kind of data involved and the kinds of differences the investigators are looking for. We will not describe these tests here, but the interested reader can consult some of the sources listed at the end of this appendix.

Another test you may see is the *odds ratio.* This is used in case-control studies and consists of the odds of having a risk factor, if the condition is present, divided by the odds of having the risk factor, if the condition is not present. Simply put, the odds ratio describes how strong the association is between a risk factor and the condition it is associated with. The larger the risk factor, the stronger the association. When you see an odds ratio, look for the confidence interval. Since an odds ratio of 1 indicates that there is no risk associated with the risk factor, if the confidence interval includes 1, there is no statistically significant risk.

For example, suppose investigators surveyed EMT-P students regarding how much education they had received before enrolling in their course. They wished to test the hypothesis that having at least a college degree is associated with passing the EMT-P certification exam. After the course is over, they perform the proper calculations and determine that the odds ratio is 1.6. This means a student who passes is 1.6 times as likely to have at least a college degree compared to someone who does not pass the exam. The 95 percent confidence interval, though, is 0.8 to 2.4.

This means we are 95 percent confident the true odds ratio lies between 0.8 and 2.4. Since the interval includes 1 (keep in mind an odds ratio of 1 means there is no association), we cannot be 95 percent confident that there really is an association, and so we conclude there is no statistically significant relationship between having at least a college degree and passing the EMT-P exam in this group. However, if the 95 percent confidence interval had been 1.2 to 2.0, an interval that does not include 1, we would have concluded with 95 percent confidence that there is a statistically significant relationship and that a person who passes the EMT-P exam is between 1.2 and 2.0 times as likely to have at least a college degree.

Many other statistical tests are used for different kinds of studies and different kinds of data. The references section at the end of this appendix lists several sources where you can learn more about them.

FORMAT OF A RESEARCH PAPER

When authors submit their findings to a journal, they structure their results in a standardized fashion that allows others to quickly understand what the researchers did and what they found (Table A–2). The first thing to appear after the title and names of the authors is the *abstract.* This is a brief paragraph that summarizes the need for the study, the research methods used, and the results encountered. Many people use the abstract to determine whether or not the paper is one of interest to them and therefore worth reading.

The *introduction* is the first section of the paper itself. This is a brief description of pertinent previously published papers on the subject of the investigation. It should describe why the study was undertaken and what the purpose of the study was or what hypothesis the authors wanted to test.

Next comes the *methods* section. This describes exactly how the authors conducted the study, including what population they wished to study, how subjects were selected

Table A–2	Outline of Research Paper Format
	Abstract
	Introduction
	Methods
	Results
	Discussion
	Summary

(and excluded), and what intervention was performed, if any. There should be enough information for interested readers to repeat the experiment should they so desire. The authors should also describe how they determined the sample size, how much statistical power there was to detect a difference, which statistical tests they used to analyze the data, and what level of significance they chose for their statistical tests.

The *results* come next. Here the researchers provide their data (or a summary of the data), frequently with tables, charts, and graphs to help make sense of the information they gathered. This section presents the data, but does not elaborate on it.

The *discussion* section is where the authors interpret their findings and describe the significance of them. There is usually a description of how this new information fits into the field of study and whether it supports or refutes previous research. There should also be a discussion of the limitations of the study, frequently followed by a call for further research to answer the questions raised by the study.

The *summary,* or conclusion, is a very brief (no more than a few sentences) recap of the main findings of the study.

HOW A RESEARCH PAPER IS PUBLISHED

Once the authors of a study have drafted their paper, they submit it to a scientific journal for publication. Each journal has its own particular rules, but all peer-reviewed journals follow the same general procedure. After receiving the paper, the editor sends it to one or more members of a review board, people who have significant expertise either in the field covered by the journal or a related area, such as statistics or research methodology. The reviewers read the paper and evaluate it for its adherence to standards of research methods, its pertinence to the field, and the potential value it has for practitioners. The reviewers send their comments to the editor, who then decides whether to publish it, send it back for revisions, or reject it. A copy editor may go over it for grammar, spelling, and syntax at some point in the process. Many papers submitted by researchers are not published and some journals have reputations for being very selective.

A note here about the term *abstract:* In the prior section, we mentioned that the first part of a research paper is a brief summary paragraph called the abstract. The term *abstract* more commonly describes a brief form of a longer scientific research paper that is often published before the full research paper. The abstract may be presented at national peer meetings, and responses to the abstract may form the basis for adjustments to the full research paper that is subsequently published. Abstracts are also published and cited in peer review journals.

The peer-review process has recently begun to receive greater attention than it has in the past. This has been the result, ironically enough, of several studies looking at the quality of published papers. A surprisingly large number of papers, when evaluated objectively for adherence to principles of research methodology, have been shown to be deficient. This has led at least one journal, *Annals of Emergency Medicine,* to review and revamp its review procedures.[4] Reviewers now get training in what to look for and how to evaluate papers, and closer attention will be paid to how statistics are used. This may be the beginning of a trend that should improve the quality of the research that is conducted and published.

WHAT TO LOOK FOR WHEN REVIEWING A STUDY

Questions to ask when reviewing a study include the following (Table A–3):

★ *Was the research peer-reviewed?* This is no guarantee of quality, but it at least indicates that experts have reviewed the study and found it to have

[4] Waeckerle, J. F., and M. L. Callaham. "Medical Journals and the Science of Peer Reviewing: Raising the Standard." *Annals of Emergency Medicine* 28(July 1996): 75.

Table A-3	Questions to Ask When Reviewing a Study

- Was the research peer-reviewed?
- Was there a clear hypothesis or study purpose?
- Was the study approved by an institutional review board (IRB) and was it conducted ethically?
- Was the study type appropriate?
- What population were the researchers studying?
- What inclusion and exclusion criteria did the researchers use?
- How did the investigators draw their sample?
- How many groups were patients divided into, and were patients assigned to control and study groups properly?
- Were the control and study groups the proper size?
- Were the effects of confounding variables taken into account?
- What kind of data did the investigators collect, and did they analyze the data with the proper statistical tests?
- Were the results reported properly (e.g., 95 percent confidence interval)?
- How likely is it that the study results would occur by chance alone?
- Are the author's conclusions logical and based on the data?

some merit. Keep in mind that some journals will deliberately publish papers they know to be of lower quality than usual in order to stir up debate about an important subject.

★ *Was there a clear hypothesis or study purpose?* The paper should have a clear description of exactly what the investigators were evaluating and what their study hypothesis was. When a hypothesis is not clearly spelled out, it is very easy for the investigators to draw unjustified conclusions.

★ *Was the study approved by an institutional review board (IRB) and was it conducted ethically?* An IRB is a group of people, usually at a hospital or university, who review study proposals to ensure that patients are protected when they participate in research as study subjects.

★ *Was the study type appropriate?* Not every investigation lends itself to the format of the randomized controlled clinical trial. It may be necessary, for ethical or financial reasons, to use another format. Evaluate whether the questions the investigators asked were well suited to the type of study they conducted.

★ *What population were the researchers studying?* Is the population similar to the one you see?

★ *What inclusion and exclusion criteria did the researchers use?* If the investigators excluded the patients most likely to have a condition or patients very similar to the ones you see, the study may have very little to tell you.

★ *How did the investigators draw their sample?* Did they use true random sampling? Systematic sampling? Alternative time sampling? Convenience sampling?

★ *How many groups were patients divided into, and were patients assigned to control and study groups properly?* The effects of bias and confounding must be taken into account for the study to yield worthwhile results. In particular, ask yourself:

- For case-control and cohort studies, were selection bias and recall bias taken into account?
- For randomized controlled studies, were randomization and blind assignment maintained?

★ *Were the control and study groups the proper size?* Did the investigators describe the sample size necessary to produce sufficient power to avoid a Type II error? What was the power of the study?

★ *Were the effects of confounding variables taken into account?* Did the investigators describe potential confounders and how they prevented them from interfering with the study?

★ *What kind of data did the investigators collect, and did they analyze the data with the proper statistical tests?* There are many tests available and more than one may be appropriate for the conditions at hand. You may need to consult a statistician or researcher to determine whether or not the investigators used the right tests on the data. Did the investigators clearly determine before data collection took place which tests they were going to use? When the data fail to provide statistically significant results, it is very tempting to perform more tests until one shows significant results. This kind of retrospective testing is called *data snooping* or *data dredging*. If one continues to perform statistical tests, eventually one will be significant just by chance alone. This inappropriate use of statistics is to be avoided.

★ *Were the results reported properly?* When a paper includes a proportion or an odds ratio, is there also a 95 percent confidence interval?

★ *How likely is it that the study results would occur by chance alone?* Remember that a *P* value reflects only the odds of seeing the results of a particular piece of research if the study hypothesis is true. A small *P* value may be very impressive, but it does not prove the study hypothesis. Keep in mind also the difference between association and causation. For example, it would be easy to show that the number of drownings increases with sales of ice cream. An inattentive reader might conclude that the sale of more ice cream causes more drownings to occur. In reality, this is an example of association, not causation. Ice cream sales go up when the weather gets warmer, which is also when more people go swimming and drown. This is also an example of confounding.

★ *Are the author's conclusions logical and based on the data?* Occasionally a journal publishes a paper that goes against everything you know. It can then be difficult to determine whether you need to change your approach to a particular problem or consider the paper an aberration. After all, by chance alone, some studies will show statistically significant results that are the result of chance or coincidence. Sometimes, the prudent course is to see if anyone else can replicate the experiment before changing your practice. This is a good example of how you should be very cautious in changing your practice based on just one study. If the conclusion is a real one and not spurious, someone should be able to come up with it, too.

And one more consideration that is very important in EMS research:

★ *How "good" was the EMS system in which the study was done?* This factor can have a profound effect on the validity of a study. As an extreme example, how valid would the results of a study of the impact of AED use be if the time from arrest to First Responder arrival was 15 minutes? In this scenario, there would likely be no survivors, no matter what intervention was used!

APPLYING STUDY RESULTS TO YOUR PRACTICE

Once you have evaluated a study, you are in a better position to determine whether or not it should change your practice. Before you do so, though, you need to consider several factors. Rarely do clinicians make significant changes on the basis of just one study. Since no study can definitively prove a hypothesis, the reader must look at other studies and his own experience in order to construct an informed opinion. If every other study published on a particular topic comes to very different conclusions than the study at hand, the reader has to wonder whether the study was poorly designed, subject to bias of some sort, affected by unknown confounding variables, or just the result of chance. One must evaluate the field and its knowledge base in order to make an informed decision about how to interpret a piece of research.

The clinical significance is another important piece of the puzzle to consider. A P value with lots of zeroes (e.g., $P <0.0001$) may be very impressive, but not very pertinent. Distinguish between the statistical significance and the clinical significance of the study. Was the difference found in the study large enough to make a real difference to patients?

When investigators conduct their experiments, they have the luxury of selecting patients who meet their criteria and excluding patients who do not. In the real world, things are not quite so tidy. Before we can apply the results of a piece of research to a particular patient, we must be sure the patient is similar enough to the study group to benefit from the intervention.

Finally, EMS providers do not function in a vacuum. Before implementing any significant changes in your practice, speak to the management of your organization and especially to your medical director. You are responsible not only to your patients, but also to your bosses and your medical director. Including them in decision making of this nature is essential and will pay off in better patient care overall.

PARTICIPATING IN RESEARCH

Many EMS systems are not content to watch other people advance their field. They have decided to conduct research themselves. They have found that by executing well-designed studies, they can not only improve care in their coverage areas but also improve prehospital care throughout the nation, sharpen the skills of their providers, and rekindle their providers' interest by doing something new and potentially groundbreaking.

Before you participate in such a study, there are certain things you should do and find out (Table A–4). The first step usually is to ask a question. This should involve something of practical importance. Determining the value of a particular intervention (end-tidal CO_2 monitoring, for example) is clearly going to have more impact on EMS than finding out whether ambulances carry 24 four-by-four gauze pads or 48 four-by-four gauze pads.

Once you have focused on the issue and determined exactly what you wish to discover, you can go to the next step. This is where you generate your hypothesis, a statement of exactly what you are going to test. The *null hypothesis* is usually a statement that there is no difference between the groups you are sampling from. The *research* or *alternate hypothesis* is a statement that there is a difference between the groups. This is often, though not always, what you would like to show.

Table A–4	Things to Find Out before You Participate in a Study

- Determine the question.
- Prepare your hypotheses (null hypothesis and research hypothesis).
- Decide what you wish to measure and how you will do it.
- Define the population you are studying.
- Identify the limitations of your study.
- Get the approval of the proper authorities.
- Determine how you will get informed consent from study subjects.
- Gather data, perhaps after conducting pilot trials.
- Analyze the data.
- Determine what you will do with your results (publish, present at a conference, follow-up with more studies).

Once you know what you are evaluating, you need to define the *population* you will be studying, or the group you draw your subjects from and to which you plan to generalize your results.

Closely associated with this step is determining the limitations of your study. This might include limited ability to generalize your results because of the patient-selection methods you used even though you had little or no choice in the methods available to you. Similarly, the population you draw from might be significantly different from other populations.

For example, if you wished to test for improved survival in hypotensive trauma patients, some of whom received antishock trouser treatment and some of whom did not, you would need to describe your EMS and trauma care system very carefully. You might have a primarily urban population with predominantly penetrating trauma, short transport times to Level 1 trauma centers, and experienced paramedics. Your results would have limited applicability to a rural population with predominantly blunt trauma, long transport times to small community hospitals, and less experienced First Responders and EMT-Basics.

The best studies limit themselves to a single question or hypothesis. This is desirable because it allows you to focus better on the question at hand. The downside is that you may not find out everything you wanted to. This is usually considered an acceptable trade-off. No single study can answer every question.

The next step in conducting a study is usually to get approval from an institutional review board (IRB). This allows you to get an outside evaluation of your study methodology and reduces considerably the chance you will be accused of conducting an unethical study. One of the items the IRB will undoubtedly be interested in is the issue of informed consent (consent given by the patient based on full disclosure of information regarding the nature, risks, and benefits of the procedure or study).

Several reports in the media over the last few years have described unethical studies where subjects were not given the opportunity to give or refuse consent because they were not informed of the risks and benefits of participating in the study. In some cases, subjects actually died because they did not receive standard treatment available at the time of the study. These stories have prompted an understandable reluctance on the part of many individuals to participate in research. The U.S. government even came out with standards for government-funded research that describe stringent requirements for informed consent.

A good *principal investigator* (PI), the person who oversees the study, will be familiar with these requirements and will be able to guide you through them. The PI should also gain the approval of other appropriate agencies, including the medical director and the head of the service involved.

After you have determined how to gain informed consent, you need to gather your data. Sometimes a pilot trial is undertaken first so you can find unforeseen obstacles to data gathering. Seemingly trivial matters can become very important (such as whether or not EMS providers have to fill out any more forms). A good PI will meet with the EMS providers who are administering the study intervention and collecting the data. The PI should make sure they know how long the study is expected to last. This allows them to make plans and perhaps reschedule certain activities they had anticipated in the future. The providers collecting data need to know the name of the principal investigator and how to contact him or her. This is usually, though not always, a physician. Many EMS physicians who conduct field research will recruit a field provider to coordinate and assist with data collection.

Other things to tell those who will be participating are the inclusion and exclusion criteria for enrolling patients in the study, the effect of the study on patient care in general, and the risks and potential benefits to patients in the study. Once everyone understands these factors, you will be prepared to go forth with the study.

After you have collected the data and reached your predetermined sample size, it is time to analyze the data. Use the tests you described in your description of the methods for your study. Be very careful about performing additional tests, especially if your results do not show what you hoped or expected. Data snooping is a dangerous activity. If you perform enough statistical tests, you will eventually find one or more that give you "significant" results. Unfortunately, these results may very well be a product of chance rather than your intervention. When multiple statistical tests are planned for the same set of data, statisticians adjust for this with multiple-testing procedures to avoid such false results. Similarly, *post hoc* analysis of subgroups that were not defined before the study can also be dangerous. This can be a good way of generating hypotheses for future studies, but it is not a good basis for drawing conclusions now.

Once you have finished your data analysis, you must decide what to do with your results. If you feel your study addresses a pertinent timely issue, and you think your methods were well thought out and your study was carefully conducted, you should seriously consider submitting them to a peer-reviewed journal. This is the best way to get such information out to the EMS community.

Alternatively, you may decide to present your findings at a conference. This usually involves summarizing your methods and results either orally or in the form of a poster, or both. This is less time-consuming than writing up a paper for publication, but can still get the word out about your results and stimulate others to investigate the same phenomenon.

Do not feel that a "negative" study is worthless. If your study shows no difference in outcome between groups that did and did not receive an intervention, you may have reached important conclusions about the value, or lack of value, of an intervention.

A common result of a well-conducted study is more questions. This frequently stimulates the investigator and others to perform further studies. Once you get involved with researching the answers to questions, you may find yourself a little more skeptical about accepted, untested treatments and more interested in finding out what really works.

LEARNING MORE ABOUT RESEARCH

There are many ways you can learn more about interpreting and conducting research. Two methods in particular are aimed at prehospital providers. In 1994, Ferno-Washington of Wilmington, Ohio, published a manual by James Menegazzi called

Research: The Who, What, Why, When, and How. It is an excellent introduction to this topic and includes the proceedings of the 1992 Winter Assembly of the National Association of EMS Physicians on Research in Prehospital Care Systems. Another excellent source of information for EMS providers is the *EMS Journal Club.* This is a quarterly publication that collects articles of EMS interest from many different journals and summarizes them. It comes with an audiotape of a paramedic and an EMS physician discussing the articles. They describe the good points and the shortcomings of the articles and suggest ways to interpret their results.

A number of peer-reviewed medical journals publish articles regarding prehospital care. Three journals that publish many such articles are *Prehospital Emergency Care, Annals of Emergency Medicine,* and *Academic Emergency Medicine.* Sometimes the *New England Journal of Medicine* and the *Journal of the American Medical Association* also publish articles of an EMS nature. All of these journals should be available at the library of your local hospital or medical school.

The Prehospital Care Research Forum promotes EMS research, and it sponsors an annual supplement to the *Journal of Emergency Medical Services.* This supplement gives selected abstracts from recent EMS studies. The Forum also sponsors oral and poster presentations at the annual *EMS Today* conference.

For the advanced reader who is not afraid of a challenge, there is *Emergency Medical Abstracts.* This is a monthly collection of 40 abstracts of articles pertaining to emergency medicine. Only a few of the articles are directly related to EMS, but for the interested reader the real prize is the audiotape that comes with the abstracts. On the tape, two emergency physicians discuss the abstracts for that month in an educational and frequently humorous fashion. The frequent criticisms of the methodologies used in the articles can enlighten even the most experienced clinician.

An excellent book for those interested in learning about research methodology is *Studying a Study and Testing a Test: How to Read the Medical Literature* by Richard Riegelman and Robert Hirsch. It includes a great deal more information about many of the topics previously discussed.

Probably the most humorous book you will ever see about statistics is *PDQ Statistics* by Geoffrey Norman and David Streiner. This book does not go into detail about how to calculate statistics, but instead concentrates on describing these tests in lay terms so that the reader can gain a fuller understanding of what statisticians do.

Finally, talk to others who have an interest in research. Emergency physicians are an especially good source of information about what is new and how to interpret it. EMS is performed by teams and learning how to do it better is often best done in teams, too.

More information on the sources previously mentioned can be found in the following:

Emergency Medical Abstracts, Center for Medical Education, P.O. Box 600, Creamery, PA 19430. Phone 1–800–458–4779.

EMS Journal Club, Department of Emergency Medicine, SUNY Health Science Center, 750 East Adams Street, Syracuse, NY 13210. Phone 800–755–3675.

Menegazzi, J. *Research: The Who, What, Why, When, and How.* Ferno-Washington, Wilmington, Ohio, 1994.

Norman, G. R., and D. L. Streiner. *PDQ Statistics.* B. C. Decker Inc., 1986.

Riegelman, R. K., and R. P. Hirsch. *Studying a Study and Testing a Test: How to Read the Medical Literature,* Third Edition. Little, Brown and Company, 1996.

Precautions on Bloodborne Pathogens and Infectious Diseases

Prehospital emergency personnel, like all health care workers, are at risk for exposure to bloodborne pathogens and infectious diseases. In emergency situations it is often difficult to take or enforce proper infection control measures. However, as a paramedic, you must recognize your high-risk status. Study the following information on infection control carefully.

Infection control is designed to protect emergency personnel, their families, and their patients from unnecessary exposure to communicable diseases. Laws, regulations, and standards regarding infection control include:

* *Centers for Disease Control and Prevention (CDC) Guidelines.* The CDC has published extensive guidelines on infection control. Proper equipment and techniques that should be used by emergency response personnel to prevent or minimize risk of exposure are defined.
* *The Ryan White Act.* The Ryan White Act of 1990 allows emergency personnel to find out if they were exposed to an infectious disease while rendering patient care. Employers are required to name a "designated officer" to coordinate communications with the treating hospital.
* *Americans with Disabilities Act.* This act prohibits discrimination against individuals with disabilities including those with contagious diseases. It guarantees equal employment opportunities and job protection if the infected individual can perform essential job functions and does not pose a threat to the safety and health of patients and coworkers.
* *Occupational Safety and Health Administration (OSHA) Regulations.* OSHA has enacted a regulation entitled Occupational Exposure to Bloodborne Pathogens that classifies emergency response personnel as being at the greatest risk of occupational exposure to communicable diseases. This regulation requires employers to provide hepatitis B (HBV) vaccinations free of charge, maintain a written exposure control plan, and provide personal protective equipment. These requirements primarily apply to private employers. Applicability to local and state governmental employees varies by locality. Many states have developed their own OSHA plans.
* *National Fire Protection Association (NFPA) Guidelines.* This is a national organization that has established specific guidelines and requirements regarding infection control for emergency response agencies, particularly fire departments and EMS services.

BODY SUBSTANCE ISOLATION PRECAUTIONS AND PERSONAL PROTECTIVE EQUIPMENT

Emergency response personnel should practice body substance isolation (BSI), a strategy that considers ALL body substances potentially infectious. To achieve this, all emergency personnel should utilize personal protective equipment (PPE). Appropriate PPE should be available on every emergency vehicle. The minimum recommended PPE includes the following:

★ *Gloves.* Disposable gloves should be donned by all emergency response personnel BEFORE initiating any emergency care. When an emergency incident involves more than one patient, you should attempt to change gloves between patients. When gloves have been contaminated, they should be removed as soon as possible. To properly remove contaminated gloves, grasp one glove approximately 1 inch from the wrist. Without touching the inside of the glove, pull the glove halfway off and stop. With that half-gloved hand, pull the glove on the opposite hand completely off. Place the removed glove in the palm of the other glove, with the inside of the removed glove exposed. Pull the second glove completely off with the ungloved hand, only touching the inside of the glove. Always wash hands after gloves are removed, even when the gloves appear intact.

★ *Masks and Protective Eyewear.* Masks and protective equipment should be present on all emergency vehicles and used in accordance with the level of exposure encountered. Masks and protective eyewear should be worn together whenever blood spatter is likely to occur, such as during arterial bleeding, childbirth, endotracheal intubation, invasive procedures, oral suctioning, and cleanup of equipment that requires heavy scrubbing or brushing. Both you and the patient should wear masks whenever the potential for airborne transmission of disease exists.

★ *HEPA and N-95 Respirators.* Due to the resurgence of tuberculosis (TB), prehospital personnel should protect themselves from TB infection through use of an N-95 or a high-efficiency particulate air (HEPA) respirator, as approved by the National Institute of Occupational Safety and Health (NIOSH). It should fit snugly and be capable of filtering out the tuberculosis bacillus. An N-95 or HEPA respirator should be worn when caring for patients with confirmed or suspected TB. This is especially true when performing "high-hazard" procedures such as administration of nebulized medications, endotracheal intubation, or suctioning on such a patient.

★ *Gowns.* Gowns protect clothing from blood splashes. If large splashes of blood are expected, such as with childbirth, wear impervious gowns.

★ *Resuscitation Equipment.* Disposable resuscitation equipment should be the primary means of artificial ventilation in emergency care. Such items should be used once, then disposed of.

Remember, the proper use of personal protective equipment ensures effective infection control and minimizes risk. Use ALL protective equipment recommended for any particular situation to ensure maximum protection.

Consider ALL body substances potentially infectious and ALWAYS practice BSI.

Suggested Responses to "You Make the Call"

The following are suggested responses to the "You Make the Call" scenarios presented in each chapter of Paramedic Care, Volume 1, Introduction to Advanced Prehospital Care. *Each represents an acceptable response to the scenario but should not be interpreted as the only correct response.*

Chapter 1

1. *Discuss the vast differences between EMS and paramedic care in the United States, Canada, and other economically developed nations compared with those that exist in some less-developed countries of the world. How should awareness of such differences affect your attitude about your work?*

   While people in the United States, Canada, and other developed countries consider EMS a necessity and benefit from high standards of emergency care, people in some poorer or less-developed countries often do not expect anything more than a ride to the hospital. Rather than feeling smug about our "superiority," however, North American paramedics should feel both privileged and determined to work hard to live up to the high standards we enjoy. There is also an obligation to take part in any opportunities to participate in programs in which information is exchanged between nations and EMS systems in the ongoing effort to raise standards both in the United States and around the world. From those to whom much is given, much is expected.

Chapter 2

1. *Are your stress levels inappropriately high? What are the indications?*

   Yes, stress levels seem inappropriately high. Indications include negativity, irritability, and being argumentative and judgmental (the paramedic is "too new to know much," "arguing *again* with your spouse," "chewing out your partner for bumpy driving"), as well as avoidance behavior (refusing to go to the funeral). Physical signs include tiredness ("yet *another* overtime shift"), improper nutrition ("all you ate all day was glazed doughnuts and fast food"), and ailments ("sour stomach").

2. *Might it be a good idea for you to go to the funeral? Why or why not?*

   Going to a funeral, especially of someone you know, allows for an important sense of closure to the event. Mourning any loss is a recovery process that adds to a person's sense of well-being. Not to mourn can result in an unintended but damaging accumulation of stress due to unresolved grief.

3. *How can you improve stress management in the future?*

   Stress management for the future has to include some problem analysis, including learning your personal stressors, the amount of stress you can take before it becomes a problem, and stress management strategies that work for you. Potential strategies might include regular exercise, more careful attention to diet, regular vacations, reducing financial commitments, avoiding overtime, learning positive thinking methods, and rekindling outside interests.

Chapter 3

1. *Which of the "10 system elements" identified by NHTSA are mentioned in this scenario?*
   - *Transportation*—two modes of transportation were used in this incident, air and ground.

- *Facilities*—by designating special referral centers, prehospital personnel can make transport decisions to medical facilities based on specific patient's needs.
- *Communications*—without a single system of communication, which allows all EMS personnel to communicate with each other, efficiently managing this type of incident would be impossible.
- *Trauma systems*—by having a system of specialized care for trauma patients, patients involved in this incident can be assured of the appropriate care.
- *Medical direction*—an active physician medical director provided online guidance to EMS providers.

2. For what possible reason was the top-priority patient sent so far from the scene?

The top-priority patient may have been sent so far from the scene because, in some cases, the patient's need for special services (such as care for burns) means designating a facility that is not nearby. The ultimate authority for this decision remains with online medical direction.

3. How important was the role the emergency medical dispatcher played in this scenario? Explain.

The role the 911 dispatcher played was extremely important. He or she put the mass-casualty plan into effect and sent the appropriate law enforcement and fire personnel. That is, as a key member of a centralized communications system, he or she directed the movement of resources within the system, while maintaining enough available resources to provide for the rest of the community.

4. How might the EMS system benefit from an evaluation of this incident?

The EMS system would certainly benefit from an evaluation of this incident. Even if everything went smoothly, the evaluation process must continue to improve the response, patient care, and resources management for future incidents. Remember, it can always be done better.

Chapter 4

1. What were your key responsibilities in the above scenario?

Key responsibilities include preparation, response, scene size-up, patient assessment, patient prioritization, patient management, appropriate disposition, patient transfer, documentation, and returning to service.

2. How should you have prepared yourself mentally and physically for this call?

Preparing oneself mentally and physically for a call involves a healthy daily routine including ongoing physical fitness training and stress management.

3. Did you and your partner act professionally? If so, explain how.

Yes, the paramedics acted professionally. Initially, they had to respond to the patient, his wife, and his son. Although the family was being difficult, that did not change the patient-care routine. They did not become rude with the family, or take out their frustrations on the patient. They were self-confident, showed inner strength, self-control, excellent communication skills, and excellent decision-making skills.

Chapter 5

1. How will you counter the arguments the two paramedics made?

Arguments might include the following: The days of simply responding to emergencies and racing to the hospital are over, or should be. EMS goes much deeper than that. No group sees the consequences of emergencies more often than EMS personnel. Being on scene affords us the opportunity to identify needs, injury patterns, interventions, and preventative measures with authority. We are often thought of as high-profile role models and respected members of the community. With such high regard comes the responsibility and opportunity to make a difference.

2. *Why is prevention an important responsibility of being a paramedic?*

As medical professionals, paramedics have the opportunity to assess every scene and situation for information about illness and injury prevention that can impact public health practice as a whole.

3. *List 10 ideas for an illness and injury prevention program that may be appropriate in your area.*

Look at the "Areas of Need" section of this chapter, but do not limit yourself to it. Let your knowledge of your own community guide you.

Chapter 6

1. *You believe that the child needs emergency care, but the child's parents are unavailable. What should you do?*

Begin emergency care under the doctrine of implied consent.

2. *If you decide to treat the child without consent, can you be sued for doing so?*

No. If a responsible person cannot be located, and if the child is suffering from an apparent life-threatening injury or illness, treatment may be rendered under the doctrine of implied consent.

3. *What would you do if the parents returned home and refused to grant permission for treatment?*

Make multiple and sincere attempts to convince the parents to accept care for their child; make certain that they are fully informed about the implications of their decision and the potential risks of refusing care; consult with online medical direction; have them and a disinterested witness, such as a police officer, sign a "release-from-liability" form; advise them that they may call you again for help if necessary; document the entire situation thoroughly on your patient care report.

Chapter 7

1. *What potential benefits are there in yielding to the patient's request (beneficence)?*

The potential benefits in yielding to the patient's request are those involving doing good (beneficence). In this case, that would mean possibly getting to the hospital faster and thereby lessening the time the patient has to suffer severe pain.

2. *What potential harm is there in yielding to the patient's request (nonmaleficence)?*

Possible response: Nonmaleficence refers to the paramedic's obligation to "first, do no harm." In this case, staying within the service's policy restrictions could be described as causing the patient to suffer pain longer than may be necessary. However, if you consider why the policy restricts the use of lights and siren (because they increase the risk of vehicle collision), perhaps the obligation to do no harm is better met by staying within those restrictions and avoiding the risk of further injury or further delay.

3. *How does justice come into play in this situation?*

Possible response: Justice refers to the paramedic's obligation to treat all patients fairly. If the paramedic were to use the emergency lights and siren for Phil Cornock, he would be making an exception to a policy restriction. If he makes this exception, and there are other patients who might benefit by getting to the hospital faster but do not because the paramedics are following the rules, then those patients are not being treated fairly.

4. *How should paramedics in general respond when a patient requests an intervention that is not medically indicated?*

Possible response: In the absence of standards or protocols that fit the situation, the paramedic needs to reason out the problem. He must first state the action in a universal form, then consider the implications or consequences of the action and, finally, compare them to relevant values.

Chapter 8

1. Explain the physiological basis for the patient's apparent dehydration.

As blood glucose levels start to rise, glucose is lost into the urine through the kidneys. This typically occurs when the blood glucose level exceeds 180 mg/dL. The glucose molecules have osmotic properties. Thus, they take water molecules with them into the urine. This phenomenon, called osmotic diuresis, ultimately causes a decrease in intravascular fluid volume resulting in dehydration. This causes tachycardia and ultimately a fall in blood pressure. Also, it is the pathophysiological basis for the polyuria (excessive urination) and polydipsia (excessive thirst) associated with untreated diabetes.

2. Describe the role of insulin in glucose transport into the cell.

Insulin is necessary for the transport of the glucose molecule into the cell. Insulin activates specialized glucose transport proteins present on the surface of the cell. If insulin levels are inadequate, then glucose cannot enter the cell to fuel the various metabolic processes. This causes the cells to shift to a less-effective form of metabolism (anaerobic metabolism), ultimately resulting in the accumulation of acids and ketones. As ketones rise, they are eliminated through the urine and the respiratory tract. When this occurs, the characteristic odor of ketones can often be detected on the breath and in the urine.

3. Prepare a prehospital treatment plan given the information provided.

Prehospital treatment should first address the airway and breathing. If necessary, provide airway and respiratory support. In most cases, the airway will be patent. Supplemental oxygen should be administered via a nonrebreather mask. Then, an IV should be started with an isotonic crystalloid solution such as lactated Ringer's or normal saline. Often the patient will require several liters of fluid to replace lost volume. Later, the patient will require intravenous insulin to move the glucose into the cells for normal metabolic processes. This is often administered in the form of an insulin drip. Blood glucose levels must be constantly monitored to prevent iatrogenic hypoglycemia.

Chapter 9

1. What is dopamine and what is its mechanism of action?

It is a catecholamine that stimulates alpha, beta, and dopaminergic receptors. It was given in moderate dosage, which stimulates the beta receptors more than the others. This increases the force of cardiac contraction, which may increase cardiac output and, subsequently, blood pressure.

2. What was the purpose of the dopamine infusion?

Dopamine was given to increase cardiac output. The patient is suffering from cardiogenic shock with pulmonary edema and needs to have his blood pressure increased. Raising his cardiac output with dopamine is preferable to increasing his peripheral vascular resistance (afterload), because his obvious difficulty overcoming existing afterload is causing the pulmonary edema.

3. What classification of drug is furosemide? What is its mechanism of action?

Furosemide (Lasix) is a loop diuretic. It blocks sodium reabsorption in the ascending loop of Henle. Because water follows sodium, the patient reabsorbs less water and produces more urine. This decreases circulating blood volume.

4. Why was dopamine administered before furosemide?

Because furosemide decreases preload by decreasing circulating volume and, through vasodilation, it may lead to hypotension; therefore, hypotension is a contraindication for furosemide, and blood pressure must be elevated with dopamine before furosemide may be given.

5. What is atropine's mechanism of action? Why was it given before succinylcholine?

Atropine is a parasympatholytic that blocks the effects of acetylcholine at the muscarinic receptors, specifically those at the heart's SA and AV nodes, which regulate heart rate. A side effect of succinylcholine administration is bradycardia (the physical act of intubation may also cause bradycardia). Atropine is therefore given as a prophylactic treatment against expected bradycardia. This bradycardic side effect is most notable in pediatric patients.

6. *What is the purpose of giving lidocaine to this patient?*

Succinylcholine may also lead to an increase in intracranial pressure. Lidocaine can preemptively block that increase by the same mechanism that decreases ventricular ectopy.

7. *Why was midazolam administered before succinylcholine?*

Midazolam is a sedative with amnesic properties. Succinylcholine is a neuromuscular blocker that induces muscular paralysis without affecting consciousness. This would be a very unpleasant sensation, so some type of sedation or anesthesia is given before any neuromuscular blockade.

8. *What are succinylcholine's classification and mechanism of action?*

Succinylcholine is a depolarizing (fasciculating) neuromuscular blocker that is given to induce paralysis. This is most frequently done to facilitate intubation in rapid sequence intubation. It acts by competing with acetylcholine at the $nicotinic_M$ receptors. When succinylcholine binds with these receptors, it causes depolarization much like acetylcholine; however, it remains bound to the receptor and prevents repolarization and subsequent depolarization of the muscle. This in turn prevents muscle contraction and causes paralysis. Pseudocholinesterase, an enzyme similar to acetylcholinesterase, eventually breaks down succinylcholine.

Chapter 10

1. *Before administering aspirin or any other medication orally (p.o.), what major consideration must you be sure of?*

When administering a medication orally, or by way of the mouth and enteral tract, you must make sure that the patient has an adequate level of consciousness and can support his airway. Administering a medication orally to a semiconscious or unresponsive patient who cannot support his airway can cause an airway occlusion and/or aspiration into the lungs. If aspiration occurs, the patient is at risk for an inflammatory response and deadly aspiration pneumonia.

2. *Of the following medications and routes of delivery, which will provide the fastest and most predictable rate of absorption?*

- aspirin—enteral tract
- nitroglycerin—sublingual
- morphine sulfate—IV bolus

The morphine sulfate delivered as an intravenous bolus will provide the most predictable and fastest rate of drug absorption. Any medication delivered directly into the venous circulation will be carried by the blood and quickly reach its target site.

Drug absorption in the enteral tract (aspirin given orally) can adversely be affected by physical activity, emotion, and the presence of food. Absorption via the sublingual route involves passage of the medication (nitroglycerin) through the mucous membranes beneath the tongue. Once it passes through these membranes, the drug can then be circulated via the venous circulation throughout the body. Even though passage is relatively fast, overall absorption does not occur as quickly as when the medication is injected directly into the venous circulation.

3. *When administered sublingually, how is the nitroglycerin absorbed into the body?*

When administering nitroglycerin via the sublingual route, the medication must be absorbed through the mucous membranes beneath the tongue. The area beneath the tongue is extremely rich with blood vessels. Once through the mucous membranes, the nitroglycerin is carried by the venous circulation and systemically distributed throughout the body.

4. *You elect to administer 3 mg of morphine sulfate to the patient. The medication is packaged as 10 mg in 5 mL of solution in a multidose vial. How many milliliters must you administer to give the 3 mg of morphine?*

Using the formula as discussed in the chapter, the drug dosage can be calculated as follows:

$$\frac{5 \text{ mL (volume on hand)} \times 3 \text{ mg (desired dose)}}{10 \text{ mg (dosage on hand)}} = 1.5 \text{ mL}$$

To deliver 3 mg of morphine sulfate, you must administer 1.5 mL of the medication solution.

Using the ratio and proportion method, the amount of drug to administer is calculated as follows:

$$5 \text{ mL}/10 \text{ mg} = X \text{ mL}/3 \text{ mg}$$
$$15/10 = X$$
$$X = 1.5 \text{ mL}$$

Chapter 11

1. *Which interaction among the emergency personnel is nonverbal?*

When the paramedic saw emergency personnel "leaning disgustedly against the bumper," he understood the situation was not critical. Unfortunately, a negative opinion, even when only expressed nonverbally, can create a safety issue because it can irritate the patient's relatives or bystanders, who believed it was necessary and appropriate to call for 911 assistance.

2. *When the patient expresses his prejudice against you, what techniques can you use to begin the process of building trust and rapport?*

Do not be in a hurry to get physically close to a patient like this. In this case, other people are about 12 feet away, in the "public" zone of interpersonal space; stay there while you try to begin the interaction on the most positive note possible. You might begin with an introduction, such as "Well, my name is Kate, and I'd like to help you out with your request, but I'm the only paramedic around right now. I've been asked to check you to see if there's any way we can help you." Once the patient softens, which happens with effective communication, you should ask for permission to enter a closer zone of space; for example, "I can't tell whether your cut will need stitches from here. Would it be okay with you if I came over to check it out more carefully?" Your tone of voice, facial expressions, and body language should all convey sincerity and helpfulness. Other ways to build trust and rapport include finding out and using the patient's name, addressing him properly, and continuing to modulate your voice, using a professional but compassionate tone, and to explain what you are doing and why.

Chapter 12

1. *Do you believe that this is normal behavior for a patient of this age and in this particular situation?*

Yes, it is exactly the type of behavior that should be expected from a patient this age and in this situation.

2. *What is the likely reason for this behavior?*

Adolescents are very concerned with modesty and privacy. The reason for her behavior is likely that her parents and younger sister are in the room with her.

3. *What might you do to make this patient more cooperative?*

If possible, have a "same sex" provider perform the patient assessment. If this is possible, then you might ask the parents and sister to leave the room. If there is no "same sex" provider available, then have the mother stay in the room for the protection of both the patient and the provider, but have her move to a point away from the bed so that answers to your questions cannot be heard. If possible, palpate the abdomen through a thin sheet to further protect the patient's modesty.

Chapter 13

1. *What is your initial assessment and management of this child?*

The assessment begins with the ABCs, and the airway has the highest priority. While your partner prepares the mechanical airways, you should open the airway with the head-tilt/chin-lift maneuver and determine if the child is breathing. Once you establish that the child is not breathing you can perform mouth-to-mouth with a face mask and body fluid precautions, then use the bag-valve mask with 100 percent oxygen. If no air enters the lungs, then use the chest thrust/abdominal thrust and look in the oropharynx for the foreign body. Remove it manually if you can see it. If you cannot see it, you may employ the Magill forceps and the laryngoscope to remove the foreign body. Once it is removed, you should insert either an oropharyngeal (if tolerated) or a nasopharyngeal airway, and use the BVM along with the head-tilt/chin-lift method to assist breathing. If the patient remains apneic, inserting an endotracheal tube is warranted. The patient's size precludes using either the CombiTube or PtL. Once you establish the airway, continuing to assess the patient is essential.

2. *What are the differences between anatomic landmarks in the pediatric patient's airway and the adult's?*

   • Smaller jaw; larger tongue
   • Floppier and rounder epiglottis
   • Softer, more fragile dental ridge and teeth
   • More superior and anterior, funnel shaped larynx
   • Cricoid cartilage is the narrowest part of the airway

3. *If you could not maintain the airway with basic mechanical airways, what would be your next course of action?*

The next step would be intubation to control the airway and manage ventilation. In this patient, use an endotracheal tube of 5.5 mm ($[16 + \text{age}] / 4$) with a noncuffed distal tip. A size 2 or 3 straight blade would be preferred. Confirm placement with visualization of the endotracheal tube's passage through the vocal cords, with auscultation of the chest, and with observation of chest rise with ventilation and of the end-tidal CO_2 detector. If intubating the child is not possible, a needle cricothyrotomy could be performed using transtracheal jet ventilation. Surgical cricothyrotomies should not be performed on children under 12 years old.

4. *If this patient required rapid sequence intubation because of clenched teeth, what steps would you take to intubate him? (Include drug doses and their proper sequence.)*

   • Preoxygenate the patient with BVM at 100 percent.
   • Place on cardiac monitor and pulse oximetry.
   • Obtain IV and assure it is functioning and secure.
   • Prepare the required equipment.
   • Apply the Sellick maneuver.
   • Administer atropine 0.01 to 0.02 mg/kg IV (blocks vagal effects).
   • Administer midazolam (Versed) 0.1 mg/kg IV (sedative).
   • Administer succinylcholine 1.5 to 2 mg/kg IV.

- Watch for jaw relaxation and apnea.
- Intubate the patient.
- Confirm tube placement.
- Inflate the cuff.
- Release the Sellick maneuver.
- Stabilize the tube.

Different types of sedatives may be used instead of midazolam (Versed); atropine is indicated for patients 10 years old or younger.

Answers to Review Questions

The following are the correct answers to the Review Questions presented in each chapter of
Paramedic Care, Volume 1, Introduction to Advanced Prehospital Care.

Chapter 1
1. c
2. d
3. a
4. d
5. c

Chapter 2
1. c
2. c
3. c
4. d
5. d
6. c
7. b
8. b
9. a
10. d

Chapter 3
1. c
2. b
3. a
4. a
5. d
6. d
7. c
8. d
9. d
10. d

Chapter 4
1. b
2. c
3. d
4. a
5. d

6. d
7. c
8. a

Chapter 5
1. c
2. b
3. b
4. c
5. b
6. b

Chapter 6
1. a
2. d
3. b
4. a
5. c
6. c
7. d
8. c
9. d
10. d

Chapter 7
1. b
2. c
3. a
4. a
5. d

Chapter 8
1. a
2. b
3. c
4. b
5. d

6. a
7. d
8. a
9. c
10. c
11. b
12. d
13. b
14. b
15. d
16. d
17. b
18. c
19. a
20. d
21. b
22. c
23. c
24. b
25. c

Chapter 9
1. c
2. b
3. b
4. c
5. b
6. a
7. a
8. b
9. d
10. c
11. c
12. d
13. a
14. c
15. b
16. d

17. *d*
18. *b*
19. *b*
20. *b*

Chapter 10
1. *a*
2. *c*
3. *c*
4. *b*
5. *b*
6. *b*
7. *d*
8. *d*
9. *c*
10. *c*
11. *b*
12. *d*
13. *c*
14. *a*
15. *c*
16. *d*
17. *c*
18. *c*
19. *d*
20. *c*
21. *a*

22. *b*
23. *b*
24. *d*
25. *c*
26. *b*
27. *c*
28. *c*
29. *d*
30. *b*
31. *c*
32. *b*

Chapter 11
1. *c*
2. *c*
3. *b*
4. *a*
5. *b*
6. *b*
7. *a*
8. *c*

Chapter 12
1. *c*
2. *d*
3. *c*

4. *a*
5. *c*
6. *b*
7. *c*
8. *c*

Chapter 13
1. *d*
2. *b*
3. *c*
4. *c*
5. *d*
6. *d*
7. *b*
8. *b*
9. *d*
10. *c*
11. *c*
12. *b*
13. *c*
14. *a*
15. *a*
16. *d*
17. *c*
18. *d*
19. *b*
20. *a*

Glossary

abandonment termination of the paramedic-patient relationship without assurance that an equal or greater level of care will continue.

ABCs airway, breathing, and circulation.

ABO blood groups four blood groups formed by the presence or absence of two antigens known as A and B. A person may have either (type A or type B), both (type AB), or neither (type O). An immune response will be activated whenever a person receives blood containing A or B antigen if this antigen is not already present in his own blood.

acidosis a high concentration of hydrogen ions; a pH below 7.35.

acquired immunity protection from infection or disease that is (a) developed by the body after exposure to an antigen (active acquired immunity) or (b) transferred to the person from an outside source such as from the mother through the placenta or as a serum (passive acquired immunity).

active transport movement of a substance through a cell membrane against the osmotic gradient; that is, from an area of lesser concentration to an area of greater concentration, opposite to the normal direction of diffusion; the use of energy to move a substance.

actual damages refers to compensable physical, psychological, or financial harm.

adenosine triphosphate (ATP) a high-energy compound present in all cells, especially muscle cells; when split by enzyme action it yields energy. Energy is stored in ATP.

adjunct medication agent that enhances the effects of other drugs.

administration tubing flexible, clear plastic tubing that connects the solution bag to the IV cannula.

administrative law law that is enacted by governmental agencies at either the federal or state level. Also called *regulatory law.*

adrenergic pertaining to the neurotransmitter norepinephrine.

advance directive a document created to ensure that certain treatment choices are honored when a patient is unconscious or otherwise unable to express his choice of treatment.

advanced life support (ALS) refers to advanced life-saving procedures such as intravenous therapy, drug therapy, intubation, and defibrillation.

aerobic metabolism the second stage of metabolism, requiring the presence of oxygen, in which the breakdown of glucose (in a process called the Krebs or citric acid cycle) yields a high amount of energy. *Aerobic* means "with oxygen."

affinity force of attraction between a drug and a receptor.

afterload the resistance a contraction of the heart must overcome in order to eject blood; in cardiac physiology, defined as the tension of cardiac muscle during systole (contraction).

agonist drug that binds to a receptor and causes it to initiate the expected response.

agonist-antagonist (partial agonist) drug that binds to a receptor and stimulates some of its effects but blocks others.

AIDS *acquired immunodeficiency syndrome,* a group of signs, symptoms, and disorders that often develop as a consequence of HIV infection.

air embolism air in the vein.

albumin a protein commonly present in plant and animal tissues. In the blood, albumin works to maintain blood volume and blood pressure and provides colloid osmotic pressure, which prevents plasma loss from the capillaries.

alkalosis a low concentration of hydrogen ions; a pH above 7.45.

allergy exaggerated immune response to an environmental antigen.

allied health professions term used to describe members of ancillary health care professions, apart from physicians and nurses, such as paramedics, respiratory therapists, and physical therapists.

alveoli microscopic air sacs where most oxygen and carbon dioxide gas exchanges take place.

ampule breakable glass vessel containing liquid medication.

anabolism the constructive phase of metabolism in which cells convert nonliving substances into living cytoplasm.

anaerobic metabolism the first stage of metabolism, which does not require oxygen, in which the breakdown of glucose (in a process called glycolysis) produces pyruvic acid and yields very little energy. *Anaerobic* means "without oxygen."

analgesia the absence of the sensation of pain.

analgesic medication that relieves the sensation of pain.

anaphylactic shock *see* anaphylaxis.

anaphylaxis a life-threatening allergic reaction; also called *anaphylactic shock.*

anatomy the structure of an organism; body structure.

anchor time set of hours when a night-shift worker can reliably expect to rest without interruption.

anesthesia the absence of all sensations.

anesthetic medication that induces a loss of sensation to touch or pain.

angiocatheter *see* over-the-needle catheter/angiocatheter.

anion an ion with a negative charge—so called because it will be attracted to an anode, or positive pole.

anoxia the absence or near absence of oxygen.

antacid alkalotic compound used to increase the gastric environment's pH.

antagonist drug that binds to a receptor but does not cause it to initiate the expected response.

antibiotic agent that kills or decreases the growth of bacteria.

antibody a substance produced by B lymphocytes in response to the presence of a foreign antigen that will combine with and control or destroy the antigen, thus preventing infection.

anticoagulant drug that inhibits blood clotting.

antidysrhythmic drug used to treat and prevent abnormal cardiac rhythms.

antiemetic medication used to prevent vomiting.

antigen a marker on the surface of a cell that identifies it as "self" or "non-self."

antigen-antibody complex the substance formed when an antibody combines with an antigen to deactivate or destroy it; also called *immune complex.*

antigen-presenting cells (APCs) cells, such as macrophages, that present (express onto their surfaces) portions of the antigens they have digested.

antigen processing the recognition, ingestion, and breakdown of a foreign antigen, culminating in production of an antibody to the antigen or in a direct cytotoxic response to the antigen.

antihistamine medication that arrests the effects of histamine by blocking its receptors.

antihyperlipidemic drug used to treat high blood cholesterol.

antihypertensive drug used to treat hypertension.

antineoplastic agent drug used to treat cancer.

antiplatelet drug that decreases the formation of platelet plugs.

antiseptic cleansing agent that is not toxic to living tissue.

antitussive medication that suppresses the stimulus to cough in the central nervous system.

anxious avoidant attachment a type of bonding that occurs when an infant learns that his caregivers will not be responsive or helpful when needed.

anxious resistant attachment a type of bonding that occurs when an infant learns to be uncertain about whether or not his caregivers will be responsive or helpful when needed.

apnea temporary stop in breathing.

apoptosis response in which an injured cell releases enzymes that engulf and destroy itself; one way the body rids itself of damaged and dead cells.

asepsis a condition free of pathogens.

aspiration inhaling foreign material such as vomitus into the lungs.

assault an act that unlawfully places a person in apprehension of immediate bodily harm without his consent.

assay test that determines the amount and purity of a given chemical in a preparation in the laboratory.

atelectasis alveolar collapse.

atrophy a decrease in cell size resulting from a decreased workload.

aural medication drug administered through the mucous membranes of the ear and ear canal.

authoritarian a parenting style that demands absolute obedience without regard to a child's individual freedom.

authoritative a parenting style that emphasizes a balance between a respect for authority and individual freedom.

autoimmunity an immune response to self-antigens, which the body normally tolerates.

autonomic ganglia groups of autonomic nerve cells located outside the central nervous system.

autonomic nervous system the part of the nervous system that controls involuntary actions.

autonomy a competent adult patient's right to determine what happens to his own body.

B lymphocytes the type of white blood cells that, in response to the presence of an antigen, produce antibodies that attack the antigen, develop a memory for the antigen, and confer long-term immunity to the antigen.

bacteria (singular *bacterium*) single-cell organisms with a cell membrane and cytoplasm but no organized nucleus. They bind to the cells of a host organism to obtain food and support.

bag-valve mask ventilation device consisting of a self-inflating bag with two one-way valves and a transparent plastic face mask.

barotrauma injury caused by pressure within an enclosed space.

basic life support (BLS) refers to basic life-saving procedures such as artificial ventilation and cardiopulmonary resuscitation (CPR).

basophils granular white blood cells that, similarly to mast cells, release histamine and other chemicals that control constriction and dilation of blood vessels during inflammation.

battery the unlawful touching of another individual without his consent.

beneficence the principle of doing good for the patient.

bioassay test to ascertain a drug's availability in a biological model.

bioavailability amount of a drug that is still active after it reaches its target tissue.

bioequivalence relative therapeutic effectiveness of chemically equivalent drugs.

biologic half-life time the body takes to clear one-half of a drug.

biotransformation special name given to the metabolism of drugs.

blood tube glass container with color-coded, self-sealing rubber top.

blood tubing administration tubing that contains a filter to prevent clots or other debris from entering the patient.

blood-brain barrier tight junctions of the capillary endothelial cells in the central nervous system vasculature through which only non-protein-bound, highly lipid-soluble drugs can pass.

body substance isolation (BSI) a strict form of infection control that is based on the assumption that all blood and other body fluids are infectious.

bolus concentrated mass of medication.

bonding the formation of a close personal relationship (as between mother and child), especially through frequent or constant association.

breach of duty an action or inaction that violates the standard of care expected from a paramedic.

bronchi tubes from the trachea into the lungs.

buccal between the cheek and gums.

buffer a substance that tends to preserve or restore a normal acid-base balance by increasing or decreasing the concentration of hydrogen ions.

burette chamber calibrated chamber of Berutrol IV administration tubing that enables precise measurement and delivery of fluids and medicated solutions.

burnout occurs when coping mechanisms no longer buffer job stressors, which can compromise personal health and well-being.

cannula hollow needle used to puncture a vein.

cannulation *see* intravenous access.

capnography a recording or display of the measurement of exhaled carbon dioxide concentrations.

carbon dioxide waste product of the body's metabolism.

cardiac contractile force the strength of a contraction of the heart.

cardiac output the amount of blood pumped by the heart in 1 minute (computed as stroke volume × heart rate).

cardiogenic shock shock caused by insufficient cardiac output; the inability of the heart to pump enough blood to perfuse all parts of the body.

carrier mediated diffusion or facilitated diffusion process in which carrier proteins transport large molecules across the cell membrane.

cascade a series of actions triggered by a first action and culminating in a final action—typical of the actions caused by plasma proteins involved in the complement, coagulation, and kinin systems.

catabolism the destructive phase of metabolism in which cells break down complex substances into simpler substances with the release of energy.

catecholamines epinephrine and norepinephrine, hormones that strongly affect the nervous and cardiovascular systems, metabolic rate, temperature, and smooth muscle.

catheter inserted through the needle/intracatheter Teflon catheter inserted through a large metal stylet.

cation an ion with a positive charge—so called because it will be attracted to a cathode, or negative pole.

cell the basic structural unit of all plants and animals. A membrane enclosing a thick fluid and a nucleus. Cells are specialized to carry out all of the body's basic functions.

cell-mediated immunity the short-term immunity to an antigen provided by T lymphocytes, which directly attack the antigen but do not produce antibodies or memory for the antigen.

cell membrane the outer covering of a cell also called *plasma membrane.*

cellular swelling swelling of a cell caused by injury to or change in permeability of the cell membrane with resulting inability to maintain stable intra- and extracellular fluid and electrolyte levels.

central venous access surgical puncture of the internal jugular, subclavian, or femoral vein.

certification the process by which an agency or association grants recognition to an individual who has met its qualifications.

chemotactic factors chemicals that attract white cells to the site of inflammation, a process called *chemotaxis.*

chemotaxis *see* chemotactic factors.

cholinergic pertaining to the neurotransmitter acetylcholine.

circadian rhythms physiological phenomena that occur at approximately 24-hour intervals.

circulatory overload an excess in intravascular fluid volume.

civil law the division of the legal system that deals with noncriminal issues and conflicts between two or more parties.

cleaning washing an object with cleaners such as soap and water.

clonal diversity the development, by B lymphocyte precursors in the bone marrow, of receptors for every possible type of antigen.

clonal selection the process by which a specific antigen reacts with the appropriate receptors on the surface of immature B lymphocytes, thereby activating them and prompting them to proliferate, differentiate, and produce antibodies to the activating antigen.

closed questions questions that ask for specific information and require only very short or yes-or-no answers. Also called *direct questions*.

closed stance a posture or body position that is tense and suggests negativity, discomfort, fear, disgust, or anger.

coagulation system a plasma protein system, also called the *clotting system*, that results in the formation of a protein called fibrin. Fibrin forms a network that walls off an infection and forms a clot that stops bleeding and serves as a foundation for the repair and healing of a wound.

colloids substances, such as proteins or starches, consisting of large molecules or molecule aggregates that disperse evenly within a liquid without forming a true solution; intravenous solutions containing large proteins that cannot pass through capillary membranes.

common law law that is derived from society's acceptance of customs and norms over time. Also called *case law* or *judge-made law*.

communication the exchange of common symbols—written, spoken, or other kinds such as signing and body language.

compensated shock early stage of shock during which the body's compensatory mechanisms are able to maintain normal perfusion.

competent able to make an informed decision about medical care.

competitive antagonism one drug binds to a receptor and causes the expected effect while also blocking another drug from triggering the same receptor.

complement system a group of plasma proteins (the complement proteins) that are dormant in the blood until activated, as by antigen-antibody complex formation, by products released by bacteria, or by components of other plasma protein systems. When activated, the complement system is involved in most of the events of inflammatory response.

compliance the stiffness or flexibility of the lung tissue.

concentration weight per volume.

confidentiality the principle of law that prohibits the release of medical or other personal information about a patient without the patient's consent.

connective tissue the most abundant body tissue; it provides support, connection, and insulation. Examples: bone, cartilage, fat, blood.

consent the patient's granting of permission for treatment.

constitutional law law based on the U.S. Constitution.

continuous quality improvement (CQI) a program designed to refine and improve an EMS system, emphasizing customer satisfaction.

contraction inward movement of wound edges during healing that eventually brings the wound edges together.

conventional reasoning the stage of moral development during which children desire approval from individuals and society.

cortisol a steroid hormone released by the adrenal cortex that regulates the metabolism of fats, carbohydrates, sodium, potassium, and proteins and also has an anti-inflammatory effect.

cricothyroid membrane membrane between the cricoid and thyroid cartilages of the larynx.

criminal law division of the legal system that deals with wrongs committed against society or its members.

crystalloids substances capable of crystallization. In solution, unlike colloids, they can diffuse through a membrane, such as a capillary wall. Intravenous solutions that contain electrolytes but lack the larger proteins associated with colloids.

cultural imposition the imposition of one's beliefs, values, and patterns of behavior on people of another culture.

cyanosis bluish discoloration.

cytokines proteins, produced by white blood cells, that regulate immune responses by binding with and affecting the function of the cells that produced them or of other, nearby cells.

cytoplasm the thick fluid, or *protoplasm*, that fills a cell.

cytotoxic toxic, or poisonous, to cells.

debridement the cleaning up or removal of debris, dead cells, and scabs from a wound, principally through phagocytosis.

decode to interpret a message.

decompensated shock advanced stages of shock when the body's compensatory mechanisms are no longer able to maintain normal perfusion; also called *progressive shock*.

defamation an intentional false communication that injures another person's reputation or good name.

degranulation the emptying of granules from the interior of a mast cell into the extracellular environment.

dehydration excessive loss of body fluid.

delayed hypersensitivity reaction an allergic response that takes place after the elapse of some time following reexposure to an antigen. Delayed hypersensitivity reactions are usually less severe than immediate reactions.

demand valve device a ventilation device that is manually operated by a push button or lever.

desired dose specific quantity of medication needed.

diapedesis movement of white cells out of blood vessels through gaps in the vessel walls that are created when inflammatory processes cause the vessel walls to constrict.

difficult child an infant, who can be characterized by irregularity of bodily functions, intense reactions, and withdrawal from new situations.

diffusion movement of gas or solute molecules from an area of higher concentration to an area of lower concentration.

dilation enlargement. In reference to the heart, an abnormal enlargement resulting from pathology.

disinfectant cleansing agent that is toxic to living tissue.

disinfecting cleaning with an agent that can kill some microorganisms on the surface of an object.

dissociate separate; break down. For example, sodium bicarbonate, when placed in water, dissociates into a sodium cation and a bicarbonate anion.

diuretic an agent that increases urine secretion and elimination of body water; drug used to reduce circulating blood volume by increasing the amount of urine.

Do Not Resuscitate (DNR) order legal document, usually signed by the patient and his physician, that indicates to medical personnel which, if any, life-sustaining measures should be taken when the patient's heart and respiratory functions have ceased.

dosage on hand the amount of drug available in a solution.

dose packaging medication packages containing a single dose for a single patient.

down-regulation binding of a drug or hormone to a target cell receptor that causes the number of receptors to decrease.

drip chamber clear plastic chamber that allows visualization of the drip rate.

drip rate pace at which the fluid moves from the bag into the patient.

drop former device that regulates the size of drops.

drug chemical used to diagnose, treat, or prevent disease.

drug-response relationship correlation of different amounts of a drug to clinical response.

duration of action length of time the amount of drug remains above its minimum effective concentration.

duty to act a formal contractual or informal legal obligation to provide care.

dynamic steady state homeostasis; the tendency of the body to maintain a net constant composition although the components of the body's internal environment are always changing.

dysplasia a change in cell size, shape, or appearance caused by an external stressor.

dyspnea an abnormality of breathing rate, pattern, or effort.

easy child an infant, who can be characterized by regularity of bodily functions, low or moderate intensity of reactions, and acceptance of new situations.

edema excess fluid in the interstitial space.

efficacy a drug's ability to cause the expected response.

electrolyte a substance that, in water, separates into electrically charged particles.

emancipated minor a person under 18 years of age who is married, pregnant, a parent, a member of the armed forces, or financially independent and living away from home.

embolus foreign particle in the blood.

emergency medical dispatcher (EMD) EMS person responsible for assignment of emergency medical resources to a medical emergency.

emergency medical services (EMS) system a comprehensive network of personnel, equipment, and resources established for the purpose of delivering aid and emergency medical care to the community.

empathy identification with and understanding of another's situation, feelings, and motives.

encode to create a message.

endotoxins molecules in the walls of certain gram-negative bacteria that are released when the bacterium dies or is destroyed, causing toxic (poisonous) effects on the host body.

enema a liquid bolus of medication that is injected into the rectum.

enteral route delivery of a medication through the gastrointestinal tract.

eosinophils granular white blood cells that attack parasites and also help to control and limit the inflammatory response.

epidemiology the study of factors that influence the frequency, distribution, and causes of injury, disease, and other health-related events in a population.

epithelial tissue the protective tissue that lines internal and external body tissues. Examples: skin, mucous membranes, the lining of the intestinal tract.

epithelialization   growth of epithelial cells under a scab, separating it from the wound and providing a protective covering for the healing wound.

erythrocytes   red blood cells, which contain hemoglobin, which transports oxygen to the cells.

Esophageal Tracheal CombiTube (ETC)   dual-lumen airway with a ventilation port for each lumen.

ethics   the rules or standards that govern the conduct of members of a particular group or profession.

ethnocentrism   viewing one's own life as the most desirable, acceptable, or best, and acting in a superior manner to another culture's way of life.

ETT   endotracheal tube.

eustachian tube   a tube that connects the ear with the nasal cavity.

exotoxins   toxic (poisonous) substances secreted by bacterial cells during their growth.

expectorant   medication intended to increase the productivity of cough.

exposure   any occurrence of blood or body fluids coming in contact with non-intact skin, mucous membranes, or parenteral contact (needle stick).

expressed consent   verbal, nonverbal, or written communication by a patient that he wishes to receive medical care.

extension tubing   IV tubing used to extend a macrodrip or microdrip setup.

extracellular fluid (ECF)   the fluid outside the body cells. Extracellular fluid is comprised of intravascular fluid and interstitial fluid.

extrapyramidal symptoms (EPS)   common side effects of antipsychotic medications, including muscle tremors and parkinsonism-like effects.

extravasation   leakage of fluid or medication from the blood vessel that is commonly found with infiltration.

extravascular   outside the vein.

extubation   removing a tube from a body opening.

exudate   substances that penetrate vessel walls to move into the surrounding tissues.

facilitated diffusion   diffusion of a substance such as glucose through a cell membrane that requires the assistance of a "helper," or carrier protein.

false imprisonment   intentional and unjustifiable detention of a person without his consent or other legal authority.

fatty change   a result of cellular injury and swelling in which lipids (fat vesicles) invade the area of injury; occurs most commonly in the liver.

feedback   a response to a message.

fibrinolytic   drug that acts directly on thrombi to break them down; also called *thrombolytic*.

fibroblasts   cells that secrete collagen, a critical factor in wound healing.

filtration   movement of molecules across a membrane from an area of higher pressure to an area of lower pressure; movement of water out of the plasma across the capillary membrane into the interstitial space.

FiO$_2$ concentration of oxygen in inspired air.

first-pass effect   the liver's partial or complete inactivation of a drug before it reaches the systemic circulation.

flail chest   defect in the chest wall that allows a segment to move freely, causing paradoxical chest wall motion.

free drug availability   proportion of a drug available in the body to cause either desired or undesired effects.

French   unit of measurement approximately equal to one-third millimeter.

gag reflex   mechanism that stimulates retching, or striving to vomit, when the soft palate is touched.

gauge   the size of a needle's diameter.

general adaptation syndrome (GAS)   a sequence of stress response stages: stage I, alarm; stage II, resistance or adaptation; stage III, exhaustion.

glottis   liplike opening between the vocal cords.

glucagon   substance that increases blood glucose level.

Good Samaritan laws   laws that provide immunity to certain people who assist at the scene of a medical emergency.

granulation   filling of a wound by the inward growth of healthy tissues from the wound edges.

granulocytes   white cells with multiple nuclei that have the appearance of a bag of granules; also called *polymorphonuclear cells*. Types of granulocytes are neutrophils, eosinophils, and basophils.

granuloma   a tumor or growth that forms when foreign bodies that cannot be destroyed by macrophages are surrounded and walled off.

gtts   drops (Latin *guttae*, drops [*gutta*, drop]).

haptens   molecules that do not trigger an immune response on their own but can become immunogenic when combined with larger molecules.

health care professionals   properly trained and licensed or certified providers of health care.

hematocrit   the percentage of the blood occupied by erythrocytes.

hemoconcentration   elevated numbers of red and white blood cells.

hemoglobin   an iron-based compound that binds with oxygen and transports it to the cells.

hemoglobin-based oxygen-carrying solutions (HBOCs)   intravenous fluids that have the capability to transport oxygen and are compatible with all blood types.

hemolysis   the destruction of red blood cells.

hemostasis   the stoppage of bleeding.

hemothorax   accumulation in the pleural cavity of blood or fluid containing blood.

heparin lock   peripheral IV cannula with a distal medication port used for intermittent fluid or medication infusions. Flushes of heparin solution, which inhibit blood coagulation, are used to maintain patency of the device.

hepatic alteration   change in a medication's chemical composition that occurs in the liver.

high-pressure regulator   regulator used to transfer oxygen at high pressures from tank to tank.

histamine   a substance released during the degranulation of mast cells and also released by basophils that, through constriction and dilation of blood vessels, increases blood flow to the injury site and also increases the permeability of vessel walls.

HIV   *human immunodeficiency virus*, a virus that breaks down the immune defenses, making the body vulnerable to a variety of infections and disorders.

HLA antigens   antigens the body recognizes as self or non-self; present on all body cells except the red blood cells.

hollow-needle catheter   stylet that does not have a Teflon tube but is itself inserted into the vein and secured there.

homeostasis   the natural tendency of the body to maintain a steady and normal internal environment.

Huber needle   needle that has an opening on the side of the shaft instead of the tip.

humoral immunity   the long-term immunity to an antigen provided by antibodies produced by B lymphocytes.

hydrolysis   the breakage of a chemical bond by adding water, or by incorporating a hydroxyl (OH^-) group into one fragment and a hydrogen ion (H^+) into the other.

hydrostatic pressure   blood pressure or force against vessel walls created by the heartbeat. Hydrostatic pressure tends to force water out of the capillaries into the interstitial space.

hypercarbia   excessive pressure of carbon dioxide in the blood.

hyperplasia   an increase in the number of cells resulting from an increased workload.

hypersensitivity   an exaggerated and harmful immune response; an umbrella term for allergy, autoimmunity, and isoimmunity.

hypertonic   having a greater concentration of solute molecules; one solution may be hypertonic to another.

hypertrophy   an increase in cell size resulting from an increased workload.

hypnosis   instigation of sleep.

hypodermic needle   hollow metal tube used with the syringe to administer medications.

hypoperfusion   inadequate perfusion of the body tissues, resulting in an inadequate supply of oxygen and nutrients to the body tissues. Also called *shock*.

hypotonic   having a lesser concentration of solute molecules; one solution may be hypotonic to another.

hypoventilation   reduction in breathing rate and depth.

hypovolemic shock   shock caused by a loss of intravascular fluid volume.

hypoxemia   decreased partial pressure of oxygen in the blood.

hypoxia   oxygen deficiency.

hypoxic drive   mechanism that increases respiratory stimulation when PaO_2 falls and inhibits respiratory stimulation when PaO_2 climbs.

immediate hypersensitivity reaction   a swiftly occurring secondary hypersensitivity reaction (one that occurs after reexposure to an antigen). Immediate hypersensitivity reactions are usually more severe than delayed reactions. The swiftest and most severe such reaction is anaphylaxis.

immune response   the body's reactions that inactivate or eliminate foreign antigens.

immunity   a long-term condition of protection from infection or disease; the body's ability to respond to the presence of a pathogen. *In law*, exemption from legal liability.

immunogens   antigens that are able to trigger an immune response.

immunoglobulins   antibodies; proteins, produced in response to foreign antigens, that destroy or control the antigens.

implied consent   consent for treatment that is presumed for a patient who is mentally, physically, or emotionally unable to grant consent. Also called *emergency doctrine*.

incubation period   the time between contact with a disease organism and the appearance of the first symptoms.

infectious disease   any disease caused by the growth of pathogenic microorganisms, which may be spread from person to person.

inflammation   the body's response to cellular injury; also called the *inflammatory response*. In contrast to the immune response, inflammation develops swiftly, is nonspecific (attacks all unwanted substances in the same way), and is temporary, leading to healing.

informed consent   consent for treatment that is given based on the full disclosure of information.

infusion   liquid medication delivered through a vein.

infusion controller   gravity-flow device that regulates fluid's passage through an electromechanical pump.

infusion pump   device that delivers fluids and medications under positive pressure.

infusion rate speed at which a medication is delivered intravenously.

inhalation drawing of medication into the lungs along with air during breathing.

injection placement of medication in or under the skin with a needle and syringe.

injury intentional or unintentional damage to a person resulting from acute exposure to thermal, mechanical, electrical, or chemical energy or from the absence of such essentials as heat and oxygen.

injury risk a real or potentially hazardous situation that puts people in danger of sustaining injury.

injury-surveillance program the ongoing systematic collection, analysis, and interpretation of injury data essential to the planning, implementation, and evaluation of public health practice.

insufflate to blow into.

insulin substance that decreases the blood glucose level.

interstitial fluid the fluid in body tissues that is outside the cells and outside the vascular system.

intervener physician a licensed physician, professionally unrelated to patients on scene, who attempts to assist EMS providers with patient care.

intracatheter *see* catheter inserted through the needle.

intracellular fluid (ICF) the fluid inside the body cells.

intradermal within the dermal layer of the skin.

intramuscular within the muscle.

intraosseous within the bone.

intravascular fluid the fluid within the circulatory system; blood plasma.

intravenous access surgical puncture of a vein to deliver medication or withdraw blood. Also called *cannulation.*

intravenous fluid chemically prepared solution tailored to the body's specific needs.

intubation passing a tube into a body opening.

involuntary consent consent to treatment granted by the authority of a court order.

ion a charged particle; an atom or group of atoms whose electrical charge has changed from neutral to positive or negative by losing or gaining one or more electrons. (In an atom's normal, nonionized state, its positively charged protons and negatively charged electrons balance each other so that the atom's charge is neutral.)

ionize to become electrically charged or polar.

irreversible antagonism a competitive antagonist permanently binding with a receptor site.

irreversible shock shock that has progressed so far that no medical intervention can reverse the condition and death is inevitable.

ischemia a blockage in the delivery of oxygenated blood to the cells.

isoimmunity an immune response to antigens from another member of the same species, for example, Rh reactions between a mother and infant or transplant rejections; also called *alloimmunity.*

isometric exercise active exercise performed against stable resistance, where muscles are exercised in a motionless manner.

isotonic equal in concentration of solute molecules; solutions may be isotonic to each other.

isotonic exercise active exercise during which muscles are worked through their range of motion.

justice the obligation to treat all patients fairly.

kinin system a plasma protein system that produces bradykinin, a substance that works with prostaglandins to cause pain. It also has actions similar to those of histamine (vasodilation and bronchospasm, increased permeability of the blood vessels, and chemotaxis) but acts more slowly than histamine, thus being more important during later stages of inflammation.

laryngoscope instrument for lifting the tongue and epiglottis in order to see the vocal cords.

larynx the complex structure that joins the pharynx with the trachea.

laxative medication used to decrease the stool's firmness and increase its water content.

leading questions questions framed to guide the direction of a patient's answers.

legislative law law created by law-making bodies such as Congress and state assemblies. Also called *statutory law.*

leukocytes white blood cells, which play a key role in the immune system and inflammatory (infection-fighting) responses.

leukotrienes also called *slow-reacting substances of anaphylaxis (SRS-A);* substances synthesized by mast cells during inflammatory response that cause vasodilation, vascular permeability, and chemotaxis.

liability legal responsibility.

libel the act of injuring a person's character, name, or reputation by false statements made in writing or through the mass media with malicious intent or reckless disregard for the falsity of those statements.

licensure the process by which a governmental agency grants permission to engage in a given occupation to an applicant who has attained the degree of competency required to ensure the public's protection.

life expectancy based on the year of birth, the average number of additional years of life expected for a member of a population.

living will a legal document that allows a person to specify the kinds of medical treatment he wishes to receive should the need arise.

local limited to one area of the body.

Luer sampling needle long, exposed needle that screws into the vacutainer and is inserted directly into the vein.

lumen the tunnel through a tube.

lymphocyte a type of leukocyte, or white blood cell, that attacks foreign substances as part of the body's immune response.

lymphokine a cytokine released by a lymphocyte.

macrodrip tubing administration tubing that delivers a relatively large amount of fluid.

macrophages large white blood cells (matured monocytes) that will ingest and destroy, or partially destroy, invading organisms.

Magill forceps scissor-style clamps with circular tips.

major histocompatibility complex (MHC) a group of genes on chromosome 6 that provide the genetic code for HLA antigens.

malfeasance a breach of duty by performance of a wrongful or unlawful act.

margination adherence of white cells to vessel walls in the early stages of inflammation.

mast cells large cells, resembling bags of granules, that reside near blood vessels. When stimulated by injury, chemicals, or allergic responses, they activate the inflammatory response by degranulation (emptying their granules into the extracellular environment) and synthesis (construction of leukotrienes and prostaglandins).

maturation continuing processes of wound reconstruction that may occur over a period of years after initial healing, as scar tissue is remodeled and strengthened.

maximum life span the theoretical, species-specific, longest duration of life, excluding premature or "unnatural" death.

measured volume administration set IV setup that delivers specific volumes of fluid.

mechanism of injury (MOI) the force or forces that caused an injury.

medical direction medical policies, procedures, and practices that are available to providers either on-line or off-line.

medical director a physician who is legally responsible for all of the clinical and patient-care aspects of an EMS system. Also referred to as *medical direction*.

medically clean careful handling to prevent contamination.

medicated solution parenteral medication packaged in an IV bag and administered as an IV infusion.

medication injection port self-sealing membrane into which a hypodermic needle is inserted for drug administration.

medications/drugs agents used in the diagnosis, treatment, or prevention of diseases.

memory cells cells produced by mature B lymphocytes that "remember" the activating antigen and will trigger a stronger and swifter immune response if reexposure to the antigen occurs.

metabolic acidosis acidity caused by an increase in acid, often because of increased production of acids during metabolism or from causes such as vomiting, diarrhea, diabetes, or medication.

metabolic alkalosis alkalinity caused by an increase in plasma bicarbonate resulting from causes including diuresis, vomiting, or ingestion of too much sodium bicarbonate.

metabolism the total changes that take place during physiological processes.

metaplasia replacement of one type of cell by another type of cell that is not normal for that tissue.

metered dose inhaler handheld device that produces a medicated spray for inhalation.

microdrip tubing administration tubing that delivers a relatively small amount of fluid.

minimum effective concentration minimum level of drug needed to cause a given effect.

minor depending on state law, this is usually a person under the age of 18.

minute volume amount of gas inhaled and exhaled in 1 minute.

misfeasance a breach of duty by performance of a legal act in a manner that is harmful or injurious.

mitosis cell division with division of the nucleus; each daughter cell contains the same number of chromosomes as the mother cell. Mitosis is the process by which the body grows.

modeling a procedure whereby a subject observes a model perform some behavior and then attempts to imitate that behavior. Many believe it is the fundamental learning process involved in socialization.

monoclonal antibody an antibody that is very pure and specific to a single antigen.

monocytes white cells with a single nucleus; the largest normal blood cells. During inflammation, monocytes mature and grow to several times their original size, becoming macrophages.

monokine a cytokine released by a macrophage.

morals social, religious, or personal standards of right and wrong.

Moro reflex occurring when a newborn is startled, arms are thrown wide, fingers spread, and a grabbing motion follows. Also called *startle reflex*.

mucolytic medication intended to make mucus more watery.

mucous membrane lining in body cavities that handles air transport; usually contains small, mucus-secreting cells.

mucus slippery secretion that lubricates and protects airway surfaces.

multiple organ dysfunction syndrome (MODS) progressive impairment of two or more organ systems resulting from an uncontrolled inflammatory response to a severe illness or injury.

muscle tissue tissue that is capable of contraction when stimulated. There are three types of muscle tissue: *cardiac* (myocardium, or heart muscle), *smooth* (within intestines, surrounding blood vessels), and *skeletal,* or *striated* (allows skeletal movement). Skeletal muscle is mostly under voluntary, or conscious, control; smooth muscle is under involuntary, or unconscious, control; cardiac muscle is capable of spontaneous, or self-excited, contraction.

nare nostril.

nasal cannula catheter placed at the nares.

nasal medication drug administered through the mucous membranes of the nose.

nasolacrimal ducts tubular vessels that drain tears and debris from the eyes into the nasal cavity.

nasopharyngeal airway uncuffed tube that follows the natural curvature of the nasopharynx, passing through the nose and extending from the nostril to the posterior pharynx.

nasotracheal route through the nose and into the trachea.

natural immunity inborn protection against infection or disease that is part of the person's or species' genetic makeup.

nature of the illness (NOI) a patient's general medical condition or complaint.

nebulizer inhalation aid that disperses liquid into aerosol spray or mist.

necrosis cell death; a pathological cell change. Four types of necrotic cell change are *coagulative, liquefactive, caseous,* and *fatty. Gangrenous necrosis* refers to tissue death over a wide area.

needle adapter rigid plastic device specifically constructed to fit into the hub of an intravenous cannula.

needle cricothyrotomy surgical airway technique that inserts a 14-gauge needle into the trachea at the cricothyroid membrane.

negative feedback loop body mechanisms that work to reverse, or compensate for, a pathophysiological process (or to reverse any physiological process, whether pathological or nonpathological).

negligence deviation from accepted standards of care recognized by law for the protection of others against the unreasonable risk of harm.

nerve tissue tissue that transmits electrical impulses throughout the body.

net filtration the total loss of water from blood plasma across the capillary membrane into the interstitial space. Normally, hydrostatic pressure forcing water out of the capillary is balanced by oncotic force pulling water into the capillary for a net filtration of zero.

neuroeffector junction specialized synapse between a nerve cell and the organ or tissue it innervates.

neurogenic shock shock resulting from brain or spinal cord injury that causes an interruption of nerve impulses to the arteries with loss of arterial tone, dilation, and relative hypovolemia.

neuroleptanesthesia anesthesia that combines decreased sensation of pain with amnesia while the patient remains conscious.

neuroleptic antipsychotic (literally, *affecting the nerves*).

neuron nerve cell.

neurotransmitter chemical messenger that conducts a nervous impulse across a synapse.

neutrophils granular white blood cells (the most numerous of the white blood cells) that are readily attracted to the site of inflammation where they quickly attack, as well as phagocytose bacteria and other undesirable substances.

noncompetitive antagonism the binding of an antagonist causes a deformity of the binding site that prevents an agonist from fitting and binding.

nonconstituted drug vial/Mix-o-Vial vial with two containers, one holding a powdered medication and the other holding a liquid mixing solution.

nonfeasance a breach of duty by failure to perform a required act or duty.

nonmaleficence the obligation not to harm the patient.

nonverbal communication gestures, mannerisms, and postures by which a person communicates with others; also called *body language.*

nucleus the organelle within a cell that contains the DNA, or genetic material; in the cells of higher organisms, the nucleus is surrounded by a membrane.

ocular medication drug administered through the mucous membranes of the eye.

off-line medical direction refers to medical policies, procedures, and practices that medical direction has set up in advance of a call.

oncotic force a form of osmotic pressure exerted by the large protein particles, or colloids, present in blood plasma. In the capillaries, the plasma colloids tend to pull water from the interstitial space across the capillary membrane into the capillary. Oncotic force is also called *colloid osmotic pressure.*

on-line medical direction occurs when a qualified physician gives direct orders to a prehospital care provider by either radio or telephone.

onset of action the time from administration until a medication reaches its minimum effective concentration.

open cricothyrotomy surgical airway technique that places an endotracheal or tracheostomy tube directly into the trachea through a surgical incision at the cricothyroid membrane.

open stance a posture or body position that is relaxed and suggests confidence, ease, warmth, and attentiveness.

open-ended questions questions that permit unguided, spontaneous answers.

organ a group of tissues functioning together. Examples: heart, liver, brain, ovary, eye.

organ system a group of organs that work together. Examples: the cardiovascular system, formed of the heart, blood vessels, and blood; the gastrointestinal system, comprising the mouth, salivary glands, esophagus, stomach, intestines, liver, pancreas, gallbladder, rectum, and anus.

organelles structures that perform specific functions within a cell.

organism the sum of all the cells, tissues, organs, and organ systems of a living being. Examples: the human organism, a bacterial organism.

oropharyngeal airway semicircular device that follows the palate's curvature.

osmolality the concentration of solute per kilogram of water. *See also* osmolarity.

osmolarity the concentration of solute per liter of water (often used synonymously with *osmolality*).

osmosis movement of solvent in a solution from an area of lower solute concentration to an area of higher solute concentration.

osmotic diuresis greatly increased urination and dehydration due to high levels of glucose that cannot be reabsorbed into the blood from the kidney tubules, causing a loss of water into the urine.

osmotic gradient the difference in concentration between solutions on opposite sides of a semipermeable membrane.

osmotic pressure the pressure exerted by the concentration of solutes on one side of a membrane that, if hypertonic, tends to "pull" water (cause osmosis) from the other side of the membrane.

overhydration the presence or retention of an abnormally high amount of body fluid.

over-the-needle catheter/angiocatheter semiflexible catheter enclosing a sharp metal stylet.

oxidation the loss of hydrogen atoms or the acceptance of an oxygen atom. This increases the positive charge (or lessens the negative charge) on the molecule.

oxygen gas necessary for energy production.

oxygen saturation percentage (SpO$_2$) the saturation of arterial blood with oxygen as measured by pulse oximetry expressed as a percentage.

PA alveolar partial pressure.

Pa arterial partial pressure.

palmar grasp a reflex in the newborn, which is elicited by placing a finger firmly in the infant's palm.

paradoxical breathing assymetrical chest wall movement that lessens respiratory efficiency.

parasympatholytic drug or other substance that blocks or inhibits the actions of the parasympathetic nervous system (also called *anticholinergic*).

parasympathomimetic drug or other substance that causes effects like those of the parasympathetic nervous system (also called *cholinergic*).

parenchyma principle or essential parts of an organ.

parenteral route delivery of a medication outside of the gastrointestinal tract, typically using needles to inject medications into the circulatory system or tissues.

partial agonist *see* agonist-antagonist.

partial pressure the pressure exerted by each component of a gas mixture.

passive transport movement of a substance without the use of energy.

pathogen a microorganism capable of producing infection or disease.

pathology the study of disease and its causes.

pathophysiology the physiology of disordered function; the study of how disease affects normal body processes.

patient interview interaction with a patient for the purpose of obtaining in-depth information about the emergency and the patient's pertinent medical history.

peer review an evaluation of the quality of emergency care administered by an individual, which is conducted by that individual's peers (others of equal rank). Also, an evaluation of articles submitted for publication.

perfusion the supplying of oxygen and nutrients to the body tissues as a result of the constant passage of blood through the capillaries.

peripheral vascular resistance the resistance of the vessels to the flow of blood: increased when the vessels constrict, decreased when the vessels relax.

peripheral venous access surgical puncture of a vein in the arm, leg, or neck.

peripherally inserted central catheter (PICC) line threaded into the central circulation via a peripheral site.

permissive a parenting style that takes a tolerant, accepting view of a child's behavior.

personal protective equipment (PPE) equipment used by EMS personnel to protect against injury and the spread of infectious disease.

pH abbreviation for *potential of hydrogen*. A measure of relative acidity or alkalinity. Since the pH scale is inverse to the concentration of acidic hydrogen ions, the lower the pH the greater the acidity and the higher the pH the greater the alkalinity. A normal pH range is 7.35 to 7.45.

phagocytes cells that have the ability to ingest other cells and substances, such as bacteria and cell debris. All granulocytes and monocytes are phagocytes.

pharmacodynamics how a drug interacts with the body to cause its effects.

pharmacokinetics how a drug is absorbed, distributed, metabolized (biotransformed), and excreted; how drugs are transported into and out of the body.

pharmacology the study of drugs and their interactions with the body.

pharyngo-tracheal lumen airway (PtL) is a two tube system.

pharynx a muscular tube that extends vertically from the back of the soft palate to the superior aspect of the esophagus.

physiological stress a chemical or physical disturbance in the cells or tissue fluid produced by a change in the external environment or within the body.

physiology the functions of an organism; the physical and chemical processes of a living thing.

placental barrier biochemical barrier at the maternal/fetal interface that restricts certain molecules.

plasma the liquid part of the blood.

plasma-level profile describes the lengths of onset, duration, and termination of action, as well as the drug's minimum effective concentration and toxic levels.

plasma protein systems complex sequences of actions triggered by proteins present in the blood. For example, immunoglobulins (antibodies) are plasma proteins. Three plasma protein systems involved in inflammation are the complement system, the coagulation system, and the kinin system.

platelets fragments of cytoplasm that circulate in the blood and work with components of the coagulation system to promote blood clotting. Platelets also release serotonin, a vasoconstrictive substance.

pleura membranous connective tissue covering the lungs.

pneumothorax accumulation of air or gas in the pleural cavity.

postconventional reasoning the stage of moral development during which individuals make moral decisions according to an enlightened conscience.

postganglionic nerves nerve fibers that extend from the autonomic ganglia to the target tissues.

preconventional reasoning the stage of moral development during which children respond mainly to cultural control to avoid punishment and attain satisfaction.

prefilled/preloaded syringe syringe packaged in a tamper-proof container with the medication already in the barrel.

preganglionic nerves nerve fibers that extend from the central nervous system to the autonomic ganglia.

preload the amount of blood delivered to the heart during diastole (when the heart fills with blood between contractions); in cardiac physiology, defined as the tension of cardiac muscle fiber at the end of diastole.

primary care basic health care provided at the patient's first contact with the health care system.

primary immune response the initial development of antibodies in response to the first exposure to an antigen in which the immune system becomes "primed" to produce a faster, stronger response to any future exposures.

primary intention simple healing of a minor wound without granulation or pus formation.

primary prevention keeping an injury from ever occurring.

prodrug (parent drug) medication that is not active when administered, but whose biotransformation converts it into active metabolites.

profession refers to the existence of a specialized body of knowledge or skills.

professionalism refers to the conduct or qualities that characterize a practitioner in a particular field or occupation.

progressive shock *see* decompensated shock.

prostaglandins substances synthesized by mast cells during inflammatory response that cause vasodilation, vascular permeability, and chemotaxis and also cause pain.

protocols the policies and procedures for all components of an EMS system.

prototype drug that best demonstrates the class's common properties and illustrates its particular characteristics.

proximate cause action or inaction of the paramedic that immediately caused or worsened the damage suffered by the patient.

psychoneuroimmunological regulation the interactions of psychological, neurological/ endocrine, and immunological factors that contribute to alteration of the immune system as an outcome of a stress response that is not quickly resolved.

psychotherapeutic medication   drug used to treat mental dysfunction.

pulmonary embolism   blood clot that travels to the pulmonary circulation and hinders oxygenation of the blood.

pulse oximetry   a measurement of hemoglobin oxygen saturation in the peripheral tissues.

pulsus paradoxus   drop in blood pressure of greater than 10 torr during inspiration.

pus   a liquid mixture of dead cells, bits of dead tissue, and tissue fluid that may accumulate in inflamed tissues.

pyrogen   foreign protein capable of producing fever.

quality assurance (QA)   a program designed to maintain continuous monitoring and measurement of the quality of clinical care delivered to patients.

quality improvement (QI)   an evaluation program that emphasizes service and uses customer satisfaction as the ultimate indicator of system performance.

rapid sequence intubation   giving medications to sedate (induce) and temporarily paralyze a patient and then performing orotracheal intubation.

reasonable force   the minimal amount of force necessary to ensure that an unruly or violent person does not cause injury to himself or others.

receptor   specialized protein that combines with a drug resulting in a biochemical effect.

reciprocity   the process by which an agency grants automatic certification or licensure to an individual who has comparable certification or licensure from another agency.

regeneration   regrowth through cell proliferation.

registration   the process of entering your name and essential information within a particular record. In EMS this is done in order for the state to verify the provider's initial certification and to monitor recertification.

repair   healing of a wound with scar formation.

res ipsa loquitur   a legal doctrine invoked by plaintiffs to support a claim of negligence; it is a Latin term that means "the thing speaks for itself."

resolution   the complete healing of a wound and return of tissues to their normal structure and function; the ending of inflammation with no scar formation.

respiration   the exchange of gases between a living organism and its environment.

respiratory acidosis   acidity caused by abnormal retention of carbon dioxide resulting from impaired ventilation.

respiratory alkalosis   alkalinity caused by excessive elimination of carbon dioxide resulting from increased respirations.

respiratory rate   number of times a person breathes in 1 minute.

Rh blood group   a group of antigens discovered on the red blood cells of rhesus monkeys that is also present to some extent in humans.

Rh factor   an antigen in the Rh blood group that is also known as antigen D. About 85 percent of North Americans have the Rh factor (are Rh positive) while about 15 percent do not have the Rh factor (are Rh negative). Rh positive and Rh negative blood are incompatible; that is, a person who is Rh negative can experience a severe immune response if Rh positive blood is introduced, as through a transfusion or during childbirth.

rooting reflex   when an infant's cheek is touched by a hand or cloth, the hungry infant turns his head to the right or left.

rules of evidence   guidelines for permitting a new medication, process, or procedure to be used in EMS.

saline lock   peripheral IV cannula with a distal medication port used for intermittent fluid or medication infusions. Saline is injected into the device to maintain its patency.

scaffolding   a teaching/learning technique in which one builds on what has already been learned.

scope of practice   range of duties and skills paramedics are allowed and expected to perform.

second messenger   chemical that participates in complex cascading reactions that eventually cause a drug's desired effect.

secondary immune response   the swift, strong response of the immune system to repeated exposures to an antigen.

secondary intention   complex healing of a larger wound involving sealing of the wound through scab formation, granulation or filling of the wound, and constriction of the wound.

secondary prevention   medical care after an injury or illness that helps to prevent further problems from occurring.

secretory immune system   lymphoid tissues beneath the mucosal endothelium that secrete substances such as sweat, tears, saliva, mucus, and breast milk; also called the *external immune system* or the *mucosal immune system.*

secure attachment   a type of bonding that occurs when an infant learns that his caregivers will be responsive and helpful when needed.

sedation   state of decreased anxiety and inhibitions.

Sellick maneuver   pressure applied in a posterior direction to the anterior cricoid cartilage; occludes the esophagus.

semipermeable   able to allow some, but not all, substances to pass through. Cell membranes are semipermeable.

septic shock   shock that develops as the result of infection carried by the bloodstream, eventually causing dysfunction of multiple organ systems.

septicemia   the systemic spread of toxins through the bloodstream. Also called *sepsis*.

septum   cartilage that separates the right and left nasal cavities.

serotonin   a substance released by platelets that, through constriction and dilation of blood vessels, affects blood flow to an injured or affected site.

serum   solution containing whole antibodies for a specific pathogen.

sharps container   rigid, puncture-resistant container clearly marked as a biohazard.

shock   *see* hypoperfusion.

side effect   unintended response to a drug.

sinus   air cavity that conducts fluids from the eustachian tubes and tear ducts to and from the nasopharynx.

slander   act of injuring a person's character, name, or reputation by false or malicious statements spoken with malicious intent or reckless disregard for the falsity of those statements.

slow-to-warm-up child   an infant, who can be characterized by a low intensity of reactions and a somewhat negative mood.

solvent   a substance that dissolves other substances, forming a solution.

spike   sharp-pointed device inserted into the IV solution bag's administration set port.

SpO₂   *see* oxygen saturation percentage.

standard of care   the degree of care, skill, and judgment that would be expected under like or similar circumstances by a similarly trained, reasonable paramedic in the same community.

standing orders   preauthorized treatment procedures; a type of treatment protocol.

stem cells   undifferentiated cells in the bone marrow from which all blood cells, including thrombocytes, erythrocytes, and various types of leukocytes, develop; stem cells are also called *hemocytoblasts*.

stenosis   narrowing or constriction.

sterile   free of all forms of life.

sterilizing   use of a chemical or physical method such as pressurized steam to kill all microorganisms on an object.

stock solution   standard concentration of routinely used medications.

stoma   opening in the anterior neck that connects the trachea with ambient air.

stress   a state of physical or psychological arousal to stimulus; a hardship or strain; a physical or emotional response to a stimulus.

stress response   changes within the body initiated by a stressor.

stressor   a stimulus that causes stress.

stroke volume   the amount of blood ejected by the heart in one contraction.

stylet   plastic-covered metal wire used to bend the ETT into a J or hockey-stick shape.

subcutaneous   the layer of loose connective tissue between the skin and muscle.

sublingual   beneath the tongue.

sucking reflex   occurring when an infant's lips are stroked.

suction   to remove with a vacuum-type device.

suppository   medication packaged in a soft, pliable form, for insertion into the rectum.

surfactant   substance that decreases surface tension.

sympatholytic   drug or other substance that blocks the actions of the sympathetic nervous system (also call *antiadrenergic*).

sympathomimetic   drug or other substance that causes effects like those of the sympathetic nervous system (also called *adrenergic*).

synapse   space between nerve cells.

syringe   plastic tube with which liquid medications can be drawn up, stored, and injected.

systemic   throughout the body.

T cell receptor (TCR)   a molecule on the surface of a helper T cell that responds to a specific antigen. There is a specific TCR for every antigen to which the human body may be exposed.

T lymphocytes   the type of white blood cell that does not produce antibodies but, instead, attacks antigens directly.

teachable moments   these occur shortly after an injury, when the patient and observers remain acutely aware of what has happened and may be more receptive to teaching about how similar injury or illness could be prevented in the future.

teratogenic drug   medication that may deform or kill the fetus.

terminal-drop hypothesis   a theory that death is preceded by a 5-year period of decreasing cognitive functioning.

termination of action   time from when the drug's level drops below its minimum effective concentration until it is eliminated from the body.

tertiary prevention   rehabilitation after an injury or illness that helps to prevent further problems from occurring.

therapeutic index   ratio of a drug's lethal dose for 50 percent of the population to its effective dose for 50 percent of the population.

therapy regulator   pressure regulator used for delivering oxygen to patients.

thrombocytes   platelets, which are important in blood clotting.

thrombophlebitis　inflammation of the vein.

thrombus　blood clot.

tidal volume　average volume of gas inhaled or exhaled in one respiratory cycle.

tissue　a group of cells that perform a similar function.

tonicity　solute concentration or osmotic pressure relative to the blood plasma or body cells.

topical medications　material applied to and absorbed through the skin or mucous membranes.

tort　a civil wrong committed by one individual against another.

total body water (TBW)　the total amount of water in the body at a given time.

total lung capacity　maximum lung capacity.

trachea　10 to 12-cm long tube that connects the larynx to the mainstem bronchi.

transdermal　absorbed through the skin.

trauma　a physical injury or wound caused by external force or violence.

trauma center　medical facility that has the capability of caring for the acutely injured patient. Trauma centers must meet strict criteria to use this designation.

triage　a method of sorting patients by the severity of their injuries.

trocar　a sharp, pointed instrument.

trust vs. mistrust　refers to a stage of psychosocial development that lasts from birth to about 1½ years of age.

turgor　normal tension in a cell; the resistance of the skin to deformation. (In a normally hydrated person, the skin, when pinched, will quickly return to its normal formation. In a dehydrated person, the return to normal formation will be slower.)

turnover　the continual synthesis and breakdown of body substances that results in the dynamic steady state.

unit　predetermined amount of medication or fluid.

upper airway obstruction　an interference with air movement through the upper airway.

up-regulation　a drug causes the formation of more receptors than normal.

vaccine　solution containing a modified pathogen that does not actually cause disease but still stimulates the development of antibodies specific to it.

vacutainer　device that holds blood tubes.

vallecula　depression between the epiglottis and the base of the tongue.

venous access device　surgically implanted port that permits repeated access to central venous circulation.

venous constricting band　flat rubber band used to impede venous return and make veins easier to see.

ventilation　the mechanical process that moves air into and out of the lungs.

Venturi mask　high-flow face mask that uses a Venturi system to deliver relatively precise oxygen concentrations.

vial　plastic or glass container with a self-sealing rubber top.

virus　an organism much smaller than a bacterium, visible only under an electron microscope. Viruses invade and live inside the cells of the organisms they infect.

volume on hand　the available amount of solution containing a medication.

years of productive life　a calculation made by subtracting the age at death from 65.

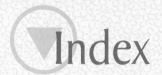

Index

The paramedic index includes entries for all five volumes in the Paramedic Care series. Each reference presents volume number followed by page reference in that volume. The sample entry Abdominal cavity, 4:437 refers to Volume 4, page 437.

rapid sequence intubation, 5:81

special considerations, 5:119–120

suctioning, 5:68–69, 5:71

upper airway obstruction, 5:92–96

ventilation, 5:74

Airway obstruction, 1:523–525, 3:35–37

Airway resistance, 3:13

Airway structures (neck), 4:285

Airway thermal burn, 4:190

Airway trauma, 4:304

AK-Dilate, 1:349

Albumin, 1:193, 1:291

Albuterol, 1:342, 3:39, 3:46, 3:343

Alcohol abuse, 3:450, 3:452–455, 5:193–194

Alcohol intoxication (vehicle collision), 4:35

Alcoholism, 3:452

Aldactone, 1:334

Aldomet, 1:334

Aldosterone, 3:312, 3:388, 4:107

Algorithms, 2:240, 2:241

acute ischemic chest pain, 3:180

acute pulmonary edema, 3:193

asystole, 3:137

bradycardia, 3:102

hypotension, 3:193

hypothermia, 3:509

PEA, 3:140

pediatric asystole treatment, 5:107

pediatric bradycardia treatment, 5:106

resuscitation of newborn, 5:15

shock, 3:193

stroke, 3:280

synchronized cardioversion, 3:168

tachycardia, 3:111

VF/FT, 3:197

ALI, 2:260, 2:261

Alignment of a fracture, 4:247–248

Alkali, 1:196, 3:430

Alkaline agents, 3:430–431

Alkalinizing agents, 3:162

Alkalosis, 1:196

ALL, 3:482, 3:483

All-terrain vehicle (ATV), 4:39–40

Allegra, 1:345

Allergen, 1:256, 3:337

Allergic reaction, 1:298, 1:426, 3:334, 3:337

Allergies, 1:202, 1:253, 1:256

Allergies and anaphylaxis, 3:332–347

airway management, 3:341

allergies, 3:336–338

anaphylaxis, 3:338

assessment, 3:339–341, 3:343, 3:344

hypersensitivity, 3:337

immune system, 3:335–336

management, 3:341–343, 3:343–344

medications, 3:342–343

pathophysiology, 3:334–338

patient education, 3:344

psychological support, 3:343

Allied health professions, 1:86

Allocation of resources, 1:155–156

Alloimmunity, 1:253

Allotypic antigens, 1:234

Alpha, 1:617

Alpha adrenergic antagonists, 1:324

Alpha adrenergic receptors, 1:172

Alpha cells, 3:310, 3:311

Alpha-glucosidase inhibitors, 1:355

Alpha particles, 3:527, 5:440

Alpha radiation, 4:186, 4:187, 5:440, 5:441

Alpha receptors, 3:81–82

Alpha$_1$ agonists, 1:321

Alpha$_1$ antagonists, 1:322, 1:335

Alpha$_1$ receptor, 1:264, 1:321, 1:322

Alpha$_1$ receptor stimulation, 4:107

Alpha$_2$ receptor stimulation, 4:107

Alpha$_2$ receptor, 1:264, 1:321, 1:322

ALS

advanced life support, 1:47, 2:176

Lou Gehrig's disease, 3:292

Alteplase, 1:340, 3:160

Altered mental status, 3:262, 3:273–275

Alternate hypothesis, 1:626

Alternative pathway, 1:244, 1:245

Alternative time sampling, 1:616

Aluminized rescue blankets, 5:386

Alveolar dead space, 3:14, 4:386

Alveolar minute volume (V_{A-min}), 1:522

Alveolar partial pressure, 1:519

Alveolar volume (V_A), 1:522

Alveoli, 1:513–514, 3:9–10

Alzheimer's disease, 1:205, 3:290, 5:179

AMA, 2:297

AMA Drug Evaluation, 1:280

Amantadine, 1:310, 3:574

Ambu laryngeal mask, 1:586

Ambulance, 1:64–66, 5:320

air medical transport, 5:335–340

CAAS guidelines, 5:324

checking, 5:324–326

collisions, 5:328–329, 5:334

deployment, 5:326–327

design, 5:322–323

disinfecting, 5:325

due regard standard, 5:330–331

equipment, 5:323–324

headlights, 5:332

intersections, 5:334

multiple-vehicle responses, 5:332

PAR, 5:326

parking/loading, 5:332–334

police escort, 5:332

response time, 5:326–327

safety, 5:327–335, 5:390

siren, 5:331–332

SOPs, 5:329–330

spotter, 5:328, 5:330

SSM, 5:326

staffing, 5:327

standards, 5:322–324, 5:326–327

traffic congestion, 5:326–327

Ambulance collision, 5:328–329, 5:334

Ambulance design/equipment, 5:322–324

Ambulance response times, 5:326–327

Ambulance volante, 1:49

Amidate, 1:570, 4:323

Aminophylline, 1:343, 3:343

Amiodarone, 1:331, 3:158, 5:85

Amitriptyline, 1:308

AML, 3:482, 3:483

Ammonia, 5:444

Amnesia, 4:297

Amniotic fluid, 3:648

Amniotic sac, 3:648

Ampere, 4:183

Amphetamine sulfate, 1:306

Amphetamines, 1:306

Amphiarthroses, 4:222

Ampule, 1:392, 1:393

Amputation, 4:140, 4:164–165

Amyotrophic lateral sclerosis (ALS), 3:292

Anabolism, 1:179, 3:315

Anaerobic metabolism, 1:177, 1:210, 4:102

Analgesia, 1:302

Analgesics, 1:302, 5:192

Analgesics and antagonists, 1:302–303

Analysis of variance (ANOVA), 1:621

Anamnestic immune response, 1:226

Anaphylactic reactions, 1:255

Anaphylactic shock, 1:217–218, 4:112, 5:103

Anaphylaxis, 1:217, 3:334, 3:338. *See also* Allergies and anaphylaxia

Anastomosis, 3:77

Anatomic dead space, 4:386

Anatomical dead space, 3:14

Anatomical defenses, 1:224

Anatomical regions. *See* Physical examination - anatomical regions

Anatomy, 1:171

abdomen, 4:429–437

brain, 3:253–257, 4:276–278

cardiovascular system, 3:73–79

central nervous system, 3:249–258

diaphragm, 4:382–383

ear, 4:282, 4:283

endocrine system, 3:304–313

eye, 4:282–284

face, 4:280–284

female reproductive system, 3:627–631

head, 4:274–280

heart, 3:73–78

hematology, 3:461–473

kidneys, 3:384–389

lower airway, 1:512–514, 3:8–11, 4:385

Anatomy, *(contd.)*
    lower extremities,
        4:227–228
    muscular system, 4:229–233
    musculoskeletal system,
        4:219–233
    neck, 4:284–285
    neurology, 3:249–261
    pediatric airway, 1:514–515
    peripheral nervous system,
        3:259–260
    placenta, 3:647
    respiratory system,
        1:509–515, 3:5–11
    skin, 3:179–181, 4:130–132
    spinal cord, 3:257–258
    spine, 4:335–344
    thorax, 4:381–392
    upper airway, 1:509–512,
        3:6–8
    upper extremities,
        4:225–227
    urology, 3:384–390
Anchor, 5:415
Anchor time, 1:35
ANDA, 1:284
Androgenic hormones, 3:312
Anectine, 1:318, 4:322, 5:81
Anemia, 3:479–480, 4:91
Anemia of chronic disease,
    3:479
Aneroid sphygmomanometer,
    2:38
Anesthesia, 1:302
Anesthetics, 1:303–304
Aneurysm, 3:199–200, 4:407,
    5:174
Angina pectoris, 3:174–177,
    5:172
Angiocatheter, 1:416
Angioedema, 3:337
Angioneurotic edema, 3:337,
    3:339
Angiotensin, 4:107
Angiotensin converting
    enzyme (ACE), 1:213
Angiotensin I, 1:212–213,
    1:335, 3:313
Angiotensin II, 1:213, 1:335,
    3:313, 3:388, 3:389
Angiotensin II receptor
    antagonists, 1:336
Angle of Louis, 4:382
Angry patient, 2:20–21
Angular impact, 4:37
ANH, 3:313, 3:388
ANI, 2:260, 2:261
Anions, 1:185, 1:186
Anisocoria, 2:65
Anistreplase, 1:340

Antihyperlipidemic, 1:341
Ankle, 2:116–119
Ankle bandage, 4:162, 4:164
Ankle dislocation, 4:260
Ankle strain/sprain,
    4:260–261
*Annals of Emergency
    Medicine,* 1:623, 1:629
Anorexia nervosa, 3:611
ANOVA, 1:621
Anoxia, 1:528
Anoxic hypoxemia, 5:163
ANS, 1:301, 1:311, 1:312,
    3:249, 3:261
ANS medications, 1:310–325
    adrenergic agonists,
        1:323–324
    adrenergic antagonists,
        1:324
    adrenergic receptors,
        1:320–323
    anticholinergics, 1:316–317
    cholinergics, 1:314–316
    ganglionic blocking agents,
        1:317
    ganglionic stimulating
        agents, 1:318
    neuromuscular blocking
        agents, 1:317–318
    parasympathetic nervous
        system, 1:311–318
    skeletal muscle relaxants,
        1:324–325
    sympathetic nervous
        system, 1:318–325
Antacids, 1:347
Antagonist, 1:296
Antegrade depolarization
    wave, 3:99
Antepartum, 3:653, 5:5
Anterior cerebral artery, 3:257
Anterior chest examination,
    2:86–87
Anterior communicating
    artery, 3:257
Anterior cord syndrome,
    4:349
Anterior descending artery,
    3:77
Anterior dislocations of the
    knee, 4:260
Anterior fontanelle, 1:487,
    2:161
Anterior hip dislocation,
    4:256, 4:259
Anterior infarct, 3:218, 3:219
Anterior medial fissure,
    4:340
Anterior pituitary drugs,
    1:351

Anterior pituitary gland,
    3:308–309
Anterograde amnesia, 4:297
Anterolateral infarct,
    3:218–219, 3:220, 3:223
Anthrax, 5:515
Anti-A antibodies, 3:471
Anti-B antigen, 3:471
Anti-inflammatory agents,
    5:192
Antiadrenergic medications,
    1:331
Antianxiety drugs, 1:304
Antiasthmatic medications,
    1:341–344
Antibiotics, 1:358–359, 3:541,
    3:546
Antibodies, 3:335
    antigens, as, 1:234
    defined, 1:225
    functions, 1:233–234
    human antibody
        classifications, 1:234
    immunoglobulins, 1:231
    monoclonal, 1:234–235
Anticholinergic agents,
    5:512
Anticholinergics, 1:316–317,
    1:343, 1:347
Anticoagulants, 1:339–340,
    1:427
Antidepressant, 1:307–308,
    5:190–191
Antidepressant overdose,
    3:432–435
Antidiuresis, 3:388
Antidiuretic hormone
    (ADH), 1:173, 1:190,
    1:213, 1:351, 3:159, 3:308,
    3:388, 4:107
Antidotes (poisoning), 3:421,
    3:422
Antidysrhythmics, 1:329–332,
    3:157–158
Antiemetics, 1:348
Antiepileptic drugs,
    1:305–306
Antifungal/antiviral agents,
    1:359
Antigen, 3:335, 3:471, 3:547
    antibodies, 1:234
    blood group, 1:229–231
    defined, 1:225
    HLA, 1:228–229
    immunogens, 1:226–228
Antigen-antibody binding,
    1:232
Antigen-antibody complex,
    1:233
Antigen-binding sites, 1:232

Antigen-presenting cells
    (APCs), 1:237
Antigen processing, 1:237
Antigenic immunogenicity,
    1:227
Antihistamines, 1:344–345,
    3:342
Antihyperlipidemic agents,
    1:340–341
Antihypertensives, 1:332–338,
    5:189
Antilirium, 1:316
Antineoplastic agents, 1:358
Antiplatelets, 1:339
Antipsychotic medication,
    5:191
Antiseizure drugs, 1:304–305
Antiseizure medications,
    5:192
Antiseptic, 1:374
Antisocial personality
    disorder, 3:612
Antithrombin III, 1:339
Antitussive medications,
    1:345
Anuria, 3:396
Anus, 2:101–102
Anxiety, 3:606
Anxiety disorders, 3:606–608
Anxious avoidant
    attachment, 1:488
Anxious patients, 2:20
Anxious resistant attachment,
    1:488
Aorta, 3:76, 3:77, 4:392, 4:408
Aortic aneurysm, 3:199–200
Aortic aneurysm/rupture,
    4:408–409, 4:421
Aortic dissection, 5:174
Aortic stenosis, 5:8
Aortic valve, 3:75, 3:76
APCs, 1:237
Apgar, Virginia, 3:675
APGAR score, 3:675, 3:676,
    5:9–10
Aphasia, 3:605, 5:231
Aplastic anemia, 3:479
Apnea, 2:36, 3:19
    newborns, 5:27
    primary, 5:6
    secondary, 5:6
Apnea monitors, 5:131
Apneustic center, 1:521
Apneustic respiration, 2:36,
    3:19, 3:20, 3:267
Apocrine glands, 2:50
Aponeurosis, 4:231
Apoptosis, 1:180
Apothecary system of
    measure, 1:451

Appearance, 2:41–42

Appellate courts, 1:115

Appendicitis, 3:371–373

Appendicular skeleton, 4:225

Appendix, 3:372

APR, 5:449

Apraxia, 3:605

Apresoline, 1:336

AquaMEPHYTON, 3:471

Aqueous humor, 4:283

Arachnoid membrane, 3:251, 3:254, 4:276

Arachnoid villi, 4:340

Aralen, 1:359

ARDS, 3:37–39, 3:515–516

Area trauma center, 4:6, 4:7

ARF, 3:396–400

Arfonad, 1:317, 1:337

Arginine vasopressin (AVP), 4:107

Arm, 4:226

Arm strength, 2:149, 2:150

Arrhythmia, 3:98

Arrow (as weapon), 4:63

Arterial blood pressure, 3:389

Arterial gas embolism (AGE), 3:521–522

Arterial hemorrhage, 4:85, 4:141

Arterial partial pressure, 1:519

Arterial PCO₂, 3:15

Arterial puncture, 1:426–427

Arterial system, 3:78–79

Arteries, 2:129, 4:83

Arterio-venous malformation, 5:182

Arterioles, 3:78, 4:83

Arteriosclerosis, 3:199

Arthritis, 4:240–241, 5:237–238

Arthrus reaction, 1:256

Articular surface, 4:221

Articulation disorders, 5:231

Artifacts, 3:86

Artificial pacemaker rhythm, 3:136–139

Artificially acquired immunity, 3:336

Arytenoid cartilage, 1:511

Ascarides, 3:543

Ascending aorta, 3:77

Ascending loop of Henle, 3:385

Ascending reticular activating system, 4:278, 4:279–280

Ascending tracts, 4:340

Ascites, 2:96, 2:98

Asepsis, 1:374

Aseptic meningitis, 5:109

ASHD, 3:177

Asking questions, 2:7–8

Asphyxia, 3:23

Aspirin, 1:339, 3:160, 3:471

Aspirin overdose, 3:435

Assault, 1:130, 5:462–463. *See* Abuse and assault

Assault and battery, 1:130

Assault rifle, 4:63

Assay, 1:282

Assessment. *See* Patient assessment

Assessment-based management, 5:292–319
  accurate information, 5:296–297
  assessment/management choreography, 5:300
  BLS/ALS protocols, 5:297
  differential diagnosis, 5:295
  distracting injuries, 5:298–299
  environmental/personnel considerations, 5:299–300
  equipment, 5:301–302
  history, 5:296, 5:303–304
  initial assessment, 5:303
  inverted pyramid, 5:295
  life-threatening situations, 5:305
  ongoing assessment, 5:304–305
  patient care provider, 5:300
  patient compliance, 5:298
  pattern recognition, 5:297
  personal attitudes, 5:298
  physical exam, 5:296–297, 5:303–305
  practice/rehearsals, 5:308
  presenting the patient, 5:305–307
  scene cover, 5:300
  scene size-up, 5:302
  team leader, 5:300
  trust/credibility, establishing, 5:306
  uncooperative patients, 5:298
  underlying principle, 5:305

Assisted living, 1:499

Asthma, 1:202, 1:341, 3:43–46, 5:96–98, 5:267

Astramorph, 4:264, 4:323

Asystole, 3:135–136, 3:137, 5:107

Asystole algorithm, 3:137

Ata, 3:516

Atarax, 3:342

Ataxic cerebral palsy, 5:239

Ataxic respirations, 3:19, 3:20, 3:267

Atelectasis, 1:514, 4:402

Atherosclerosis, 1:178, 3:199, 3:276

Atherosclerotic heart disease (ASHD), 3:177

Athetosis, 5:239

Athletic musculoskeletal injuries, 4:264, 4:265

Atlas, 4:337

Atom, 1:184

ATP, 1:211

Atracurium, 1:569, 4:322–323

Atria, 3:74, 3:75

Atrial enlargement, 3:232, 3:235

Atrial excitation, 3:91, 3:92

Atrial fib-flutter, 3:112

Atrial fibrillation, 3:113–115

Atrial flutter, 3:112–113

Atrial gallop, 2:92

Atrial natriuretic hormone (ANH), 3:313, 3:388

Atrial septal defect, 5:7

Atrial syncytium, 3:82

Atrial systole, 3:79

Atrioventricular block. *See* AV block

Atrioventricular (AV) bundle, 3:82

Atrioventricular (AV) valves, 3:74, 3:75

Atrophy, 1:175, 2:55

Atropine, 1:317, 1:571, 4:324, 4:374

Atropine sulfate, 3:157, 5:85

Atropisol, 1:349

Atrovent, 1:317, 1:343, 3:46

Attachment, 1:488

ATV crashes, 4:39–40

Atypical angina, 3:174, 3:175

Augmented leads, 3:87, 3:206–209

Aura, 3:281

Aural medication administration, 1:379–380

Auro-Dri Ear Drops, 1:349

Auro Ear Drops, 1:349

Aurocaine 2, 1:349

Auscultation, 2:32–33, 3:27

Authoritarian parents, 1:492

Authoritative parents, 1:492

Auto rollover, 4:33–34

Autocrine signaling, 1:172

Autoimmune disease, 3:467

Autoimmune/isoimmune diseases, 1:257–258

Autoimmunity, 1:253, 1:256–257, 3:548

Automatic collision notification (ACN) system, 2:261–262

Automatic location identification (ALI), 2:260, 2:261

Automatic number identification (ANI), 2:260, 2:261

Automatic transport ventilator, 1:606–607

Automaticity, 3:85

Automobile collisions, 4:22–36, 5:408–414
  air bags, 2:202, 4:26–27, 5:410, 5:492
  child safety seats, 2:202, 4:27–28
  children, 5:117–118
  down-and-under pathway, 4:30
  force, 2:263
  frontal impact, 4:28–30
  lateral impact, 4:30–31
  paper bag syndrome, 4:30
  rear-end impact, 4:32–33
  restraints, 4:25
  rollover, 4:33–34
  rotational impact, 4:31–32
  seat belts, 4:26
  up-and-over pathway, 4:28–30
  vehicle collision analysis, 4:34–36
  vehicle impacts, 4:23–24

Automobile construction (anatomy), 5:411–412

Autonomic dysfunction, 5:175

Autonomic ganglia, 1:311

Autonomic hyperreflexia syndrome, 4:350

Autonomic nervous system (ANS), 1:301, 1:311, 1:312, 3:249, 3:261

Autonomic nervous system disorders, 3:263

Autonomic nervous system medications, 1:310–325. *See also* ANS medications

Autonomic neuropathy, 3:498

Autonomy, 1:147

Autoregulation, 4:279

AV block, 3:115–121, 3:226–227
  complete block, 3:120–121, 3:227
  first-degree, 3:116–117, 3:226

Blistering agents, 5:510
Blood, 1:190–191, 3:461–468. *See also* Hematology
Blood-brain barrier, 1:291, 4:278
Blood clotting abnormalities, 3:484–485
Blood coagulation, 3:469
Blood flow through heart, 1:326, 3:76–77
Blood glucometer, 3:272
Blood glucose, 3:314–316, 3:321–322
Blood glucose determination, 2:48, 3:321–322
Blood group, 1:230
Blood group antigens, 1:229–231
Blood pressure, 1:207, 1:332, 2:35–37, 2:43, 2:44–45, 3:80, 4:103
Blood products, 3:471–472
Blood sampling, 1:437–441
Blood spatter evidence, 5:474
Blood transfusion, 3:472–473, 4:483
Blood tube/tubing, 1:437–438, 1:414–415, 1:422–425
Blood tube sequence, 1:438
Blood types, 3:472
Blood vessel, 1:208, 4:132, 4:133
Blood vessel trauma, 4:304
Blood volume, 3:461
Bloodborne diseases, 3:544, 3:545
Blown outward appearance, 4:70
BLS, 1:47
Blue bloaters, 3:43
Bluish discoloration, 1:528
Blunt abdominal trauma, 5:123
Blunt thoracic trauma, 4:381, 4:393–394
Blunt trauma, 4:16–53
    abdomen, 4:438–439
    automobile collisions, 4:22–36. *See also* Automobile collisions
    blast injuries, 4:40–47. *See also* Blast injuries
    crush injuries, 4:49–50
    falls, 4:47–48
    head, facial, neck region, 4:286
    kinetics, 4:19–21
    law of conservation of energy, 4:20

law of inertia, 4:19
    motorcycle crashes, 4:36–37
    pedestrian collisions, 4:37–38
    recreational vehicle collisions, 4:39–40
    sports injuries, 4:48–49
    thoracic wounds, 4:381, 4:393–394
BMR, 3:496
Body armor, 5:469–470
Body collision, 4:23, 4:24
Body defenses, 1:221–269
    antibodies. *See* Antibodies
    antigens. *See* Antigens
    autoimmune/isoimmune diseases, 1:257–258
    hypersensitivity, 1:253–257
    immune deficiencies, 1:258–260
    immune response, 1:225–239. *See also* Immune response
    inflammatory response, 1:240–253. *See also* Inflammation
    self-defense mechanisms, 1:221–225
    stress and disease, 1:261–269. *See also* Stress
Body dysmorphic disorder, 3:610
Body fluid compartments, 1:181
Body lice, 3:588
Body regions. *See* Physical examination - anatomical regions
Body response to blood loss, 4:106, 4:108–109
Body substance isolation (BSI), 1:24, 1:373–374, 2:177–179, 5:302
Body surface area (BSA), 4:192
Body systems approach, 2:292–293
Body temperature, 2:37, 2:43, 2:45, 3:495–497
Bohr effect, 3:17, 3:463
Boiling point, 5:439
Bolus, 1:389
Bonding, 1:488
Bone aging, 4:228–229
Bone Injection Gun (B.I.G.), 1:444
Bone injury, 4:235–239. *See also* Fractures
Bone marrow, 4:221
Bone repair cycle, 4:239–240

Bone structure, 4:220–222
Bones of foot, 2:116
Bones of human skull, 3:252, 4:275
Booster shot, 1:361, 3:549
Boots, 5:384
Borborygmi, 2:97
Borderline personality disorder, 3:612
Borrowed servant doctrine, 1:122
Botulinum toxin, 5:511
Botulism, 3:438, 3:580
Botulism toxin, 1:222
Bougie, 1:551, 1:552, 4:316
BOW, 3:648
Bowel hemorrhage, 4:91
Bowel injury, 4:442–443
Bowel obstruction, 3:370, 3:371, 5:182
Bowman's capsule, 3:385
Boyle's law, 3:516
BPD, 5:268
Brachial plexus, 3:258, 4:342, 4:343
Brachioradialis, 4:231
Brachioradialis reflex, 2:154, 2:155
Bradycardia, 2:34, 3:97
    algorithm (children), 5:106
    newborns, 5:28
Bradycardia algorithm, 3:102
Bradydysrhythmias, 5:105
Bradypnea, 2:35, 2:36, 3:30
Brain, 2:134, 3:253–257, 4:276–278
Brain abscess, 3:290
Brain attack, 3:275, 5:176. *See also* Stroke
Brain injury, 4:291–298
Brain ischemia, 5:176
Brainstem, 3:254, 3:255, 4:277
Brainstem injury, 4:294
Branch, 5:360–362
Branch directors, 5:361
Brand name, 1:278
Braxton-Hicks contractions, 3:666
Breach of duty, 1:119
Breast cancer, 1:202
Breath sounds, 1:530, 2:85, 3:27–29, 3:149–150
Breathing, 3:23, 5:58–60
    head and neck trauma, 4:307, 4:319
    minute volume, 4:307
    trauma emergencies, 4:471–472
Breathing assessment, 2:194–196

Breathing patterns, 2:35, 2:36
Breech presentation, 3:677, 3:678
Brethine, 1:356
Bretylium, 1:331, 3:157
Bretylol, 1:331
Brevibloc, 1:331
Brian tumors, 3:288–290
Broccoli, 1:20
Bronchi, 1:513, 3:8–9, 4:384
Bronchial arteries, 3:11
Bronchial veins, 3:11
Bronchioles, 3:5, 3:9
Bronchiolitis, 5:98
Bronchitis, 3:42–43, 5:266–267
Bronchophony, 2:86
Bronchopulmonary dysplasia (BPD), 5:268
Bronchospasm, 3:13, 3:339
Broselow tape, 1:288, 2:41
Broviac catheter, 5:276–277
Brown recluse spider, 3:441, 3:442
Brown recluse spider bites, 3:441–442
Brown-Séquard syndrome, 4:350
Brudzinski's sign, 3:572
Bruit, 3:110, 3:268
Bruton agammaglobulinemia, 1:258
BSA, 4:192
BSA-to-weight ratio (children), 5:52
BSI, 1:24, 1:373–374, 2:177–179, 5:302
Buccal medication administration, 1:377, 1:378
Buckle fracture, 5:123
Buffalo hump, 3:327
Buffer system, 1:196
Bulimia nervosa, 3:611
Bulla, 2:53
Bullet entry wounds, 4:70
Bulletproof vests, 5:469–470
Bullet's travel (ballistics), 4:57–61, 4:64
BUN, 3:388
Bundle branch block, 3:140, 3:227–231
Bundle of His, 3:85, 3:116, 3:204
Bundle of Kent, 3:141
Burden nasoscope, 1:578
Burden of proof, 1:119
Burette chamber, 1:414
Burn center, 4:201

Critical decision process, 2:246–248

Critical incident stress debriefing (CISD), 1:38

Critical incident stress management (CISM), 1:38, 5:373

Critically life-threatening conditions, 2:239

Crixivan, 1:359

Crohn's disease, 1:204, 3:366–367

Cromolyn, 1:343

Cromolyn sodium, 3:343

Cross-sectional study, 1:614

Cross tolerance, 1:298

Croup, 3:578, 5:92–94

Crowded frequencies, 5:483

Crowning, 3:669, 3:673

Crumple zone, 4:30, 4:31

Crush injury, 4:49–50, 4:136, 4:137, 4:148–149, 4:166–169

Crush points, 5:493

Crush syndrome, 4:136, 4:148

Crushing trauma, 4:87

Crust, 2:55

Crying, 2:21

"Crystal" (meth), 5:465

Crystalloids, 1:193, 1:409

Crystodigin, 1:337

CSF pH, 1:521

CTZ, 1:348

Cullen's sign, 2:96, 2:208, 3:355

Cultural considerations, 3:374
  analgesia, 3:480
  blood loss and transfusion, 4:483
  cardiovascular disease, 3:72
  cholecystitis, 3:374
  Christian Scientists, 5:243
  communication, 1:477–479
  diabetes, 3:314
  elderly/impoverished populations, 1:104, 5:154
  folk remedies, 1:279
  gastroenterology, 3:374
  glaucoma, 5:229
  hair, 2:54–55
  Hispanic families, 1:478
  Hmong people, 5:213
  immunization of at-risk populations, 1:105
  infant baptism, 5:35
  metric system, 1:449
  nails, 2:56
  physical exam, 2:30
  prenatal care, 3:654
  religious/cultural beliefs, 1:126

responses to death, 1:30
responses to illness/injury, 1:145
smoking, 3:39

Cultural imposition, 1:478

Culvert, 5:405

Cumulative effect, 1:298

Current, 4:183

Current of injury, 3:214

Cushing's disease, 1:352

Cushing's reflex, 4:297, 4:298

Cushing's syndrome, 3:327–328

Cushing's triad, 3:271, 4:297

Customer satisfaction, 1:69

Cutting the umbilical cord, 5:12, 5:13

CVD, 3:71. See also Cardiology

CX, 5:510

Cyanide antidote, 3:429

Cyanide antidote kit, 4:205

Cyanide exposure, 5:444–445

Cyanide poisoning, 3:428

Cyanide toxicity, 4:205

Cyanocobalamin, 1:363

Cyanosis, 1:528

Cyanotic spell, 5:104

Cyclobenzaprine, 1:324

Cyclophosphamide, 1:358

Cyclosporidium infection, 3:361

Cyst, 2:53, 3:637

Cystic fibrosis (CF), 5:240, 5:268

Cystic medial necrosis, 3:200

Cystine stones, 3:407

Cystitis, 3:409, 3:637

cyt, 1:167

Cytochrome oxidase, 5:444

Cytokines, 1:237, 1:249

Cytomegalovirus, 5:229–230

Cytoplasm, 1:168

Cytoskeleton, 1:166, 1:168

Cytosol, 1:168

Cytotoxic T cells, 1:236

Cytoxan, 1:358

D₅W, 1:194, 1:410

D₅₀W, 1:355

D post, 5:411

DAI, 4:294

Daily stress, 1:37

Dalton's law, 3:516

Dam, 5:400

Damage pathway (penetrating trauma), 4:64–66

DAN, 3:523

Dandruff, 2:54

Dangerous crowds, 5:463

"Dangerous" placard, 5:433

Dantrium, 1:325

Dantrolene, 1:325

Date rape drug, 3:452, 5:218

DC countershock, 3:112

DCAP-BTLS, 2:203

Dead space volume (V$_D$), 1:522, 4:386

Deafness, 5:226–229

Death and dying, 1:29–33, 1:501

Death in the field, 1:135

Debridement, 1:251

Decadron, 3:343

Deceleration injury, 4:393, 4:403

Decerebrate posture, 3:269

Deci-, 1:450

Decision making. See Clinical decision making

Decision-making algorithm. See Algorithms

Decompensated shock, 1:213, 4:110–111, 5:100–101

Decompensation, 1:173

Decompression illness, 3:519–521

Decontamination, 3:420–421, 5:445–449

Decontamination methods, 3:553–554

Decontamination of equipment, 1:27–28

Decorticate posture, 3:269

Decubitus ulcers, 5:183–184

Decubitus wounds, 5:256

Deep frostbite, 3:511

Deep pitting edema, 2:133

Deep venous thrombosis (DVT), 3:201

Deerfly fever, 5:515

Defamation, 1:124

Defendant, 1:115

Defense wounds, 4:66

Defensive strategies, 1:33

Defibrillation, 3:162–166

Defibrillator, 3:162

Degenerative disk disease, 3:295

Degenerative joint disease, 4:240

Degenerative neurological disorders, 3:290–294
  ALS, 3:292
  Alzheimer's disease, 3:290
  Bell's palsy, 3:292
  central pain syndrome, 3:292
  dystonia, 3:291

MD, 3:291

MS, 3:291

myoclonus, 3:292

Parkinson's disease, 3:291–292

polio, 3:293

spina bifida, 3:292–293

Degloving injury, 4:139, 4:140

Degranulation, 1:242–243, 3:337

Dehydration, 1:183, 3:503, 5:111

Deka-, 1:450

Delayed effects, 5:442

Delayed hypersensitivity, 1:236, 3:337

Delayed hypersensitivity reactions, 1:254

DeLee suction trap, 5:10, 5:17

Delirium, 3:605, 5:177–178

Delirium tremens (DTs), 3:454

Delivery, 3:671–683. See also Pregnancy
  abnormal presentations, 3:677–680
  APGAR score, 3:675, 3:676
  breech presentation, 3:677, 3:678
  cephalopelvic disproportion, 3:680
  field, 3:671–674
  limb presentation, 3:678
  maternal complications, 3:681–683
  meconium staining, 3:681
  multiple births, 3:680
  neonatal care, 3:674–677
  neonatal resuscitation, 3:675–677
  normal (vertex position), 3:672–673
  occiput posterior position, 3:678–680
  precipitous, 3:680–681
  prolapsed cord, 3:677–678, 3:679
  shoulder dystocia, 3:681

Delta cells, 3:310, 3:311

Delta wave, 3:141

Deltoid, 1:403, 1:404, 4:230, 4:231

Delusions, 3:606

Demand pacemaker, 3:136, 3:138

Demand valve resuscitator, 1:605–606

Demargination, 3:464

Dementia, 3:605, 5:178–179

Dendrites, 3:250

Dental injury, 4:300, 4:327
Deontological method, 1:146
Depakote, 1:305, 1:309
Dependent personality disorder, 3:612
Depersonalization, 3:611
Depo-Provera, 3:634
Depolarization, 3:83–84
Depolarization impulse, 3:99
Deposition, 1:116
Depression, 2:21, 3:608–609, 5:194–195
Dermatologic drugs, 1:362
Dermatome, 3:257, 3:259, 4:343
Dermatome chart, 2:151, 2:152, 3:352
Dermis, 4:131–132, 4:179–180
Descending colostomy, 5:282
Descending loop of Henle, 3:385
Descending tracts, 4:340
Descriptive statistics, 1:619
Descriptive studies, 1:614
Desensitization, 3:345
Desensitization techniques, 1:255
Desipramine, 1:308
Desired dose, 1:453
Desmopressin, 1:351
Destination log, 5:368–369
Detached retina, 2:66
Detailed physical examination, 2:221–228. *See also* Physical exam
Devascularization, 4:220
Developmental stages. *See* Life-span development
Developmentally disabled patients, 5:235–236
Dexamethasone, 3:343
Dexedrine, 1:306
Dextran, 1:193, 1:409
Dextroamphetamine, 1:306
Dextromethorphan, 1:345
Dextrose, 4:324
Diabetes, 1:352–355, 3:314–317, 5:180
  adult onset, 3:317
  cultural considerations, 3:314
  emergencies, 3:318
  gestational, 1:353, 3:665–666
  glucose metabolism, 3:315–316
  hyperglycemic agents, 1:350
  hypoglycemic agents, 1:350
  IDDM, 1:353, 3:317

insulin preparations, 1:353–354
  NIDDM, 1:353, 1:355, 3:317
  peripheral circulation, 5:255
  pregnancy, 3:665–666
  regulation of blood glucose, 3:316
  type I, 3:317
  type II, 3:317
Diabetes insipidus, 3:308
Diabetes mellitus. *See* Diabetes
Diabetic ketoacidosis, 3:318–320, 5:112, 5:113
Diabetic retinopathy, 5:229
Diabetogenic effect of pregnancy, 3:665
Diabinese, 1:355
Diagnostic and Statistical Manual of Mental Disorders, Fourth Edition (DSM-IV), 3:604
Dialysate, 3:404
Dialysis, 3:403–405
Dialysis shunts, 5:277
Diamox, 3:524
Diapedesis, 1:247, 3:464
Diaphragm, 3:5, 3:12, 3:18, 3:73, 3:634, 4:382–383
Diaphragmatic excursion, 2:83–85
Diaphragmatic hernia, 5:27–28
Diaphragmatic injury, 4:440
Diaphragmatic perforation, 4:409
Diaphragmatic rupture, 4:409
Diaphragmic hernia, 5:8
Diaphysis, 4:220
Diapid, 1:351
Diarrhea, 1:348
  children, 5:111
  newborns, 5:33–34
Diarthroses, 4:222
Diastole, 2:88, 3:79
Diastolic blood pressure, 2:35, 4:103
Diazepam, 1:570, 3:161, 3:285, 3:620, 4:264, 4:323
Diazoxide, 1:355
Dibenzyline, 1:324
DIC, 3:485–486
Diencephalon, 3:254
Diesel hybrid ambulance, 1:66
Diet-induced thermogenesis, 3:494
Diet supplements, 1:362–363
Differential diagnosis, 5:295

Differential field diagnosis, 2:5, 2:242
Differentiation, 1:168
Difficult child, 1:489
Diffuse axonal injury (DAI), 4:294
Diffuse injuries, 4:294
Diffusion, 1:186–188, 1:289, 1:519, 3:15–16
DiGeorge syndrome, 1:258
Digestion, 1:349
Digestive system, 2:93, 2:94
Digestive tract, 4:430, 4:431
Digibind, 5:190
Digital communications, 2:267–268
Digital intubation, 1:563–566, 4:315–316
Digitalis, 3:161–162, 5:190
Digitalis glycosides, 1:337
Digitoxin, 1:337
Digoxin, 1:331, 1:332, 1:337–338, 3:161–162, 5:190
Digoxin toxicity, 5:190
Dihydropyridines, 1:336
Dilantin, 1:305, 1:330
Dilatation, 3:668
Dilation, 1:175
Diltiazem, 1:331, 1:338, 3:113, 3:162
Dimenhydrinate, 1:345
Diphenhydramine, 1:307, 1:310, 1:345, 3:342
Diphtheria-pertussis-tetanus (DPT), 3:576
Diphtheria-tetanus toxoid (Td), 3:583
Diphtheria-tetanus toxoid, pertussis (DTP), 3:583
Diplegic patients, 5:239
Diplomacy, 1:91
Diprivan, 1:570
Dipyridamole, 1:339, 3:471
Direct-acting cholinergic, 1:314–316
Direct brain injury, 4:291–292
Direct pressure, 4:88
Direct questions, 1:472
Direct vasodilators, 1:336–338
Directed intubation, 4:316–317
Dirty bomb, 5:508
Dirty radiation accidents, 3:529
Disabled patients. *See* Challenged patient
Disaster management, 5:371

Disaster mental health services, 1:38, 5:373
Disaster plan, 1:67
Discovery, 1:116
Disease
  causes, 1:200–221
  defenses, 1:221–269. *See also* Body defenses
  family history, 1:201–205
  genetic, 1:200
  infectious agents, 1:221–223
Disease - causes and pathophysiology, 1:200–221
  clinical factors, 1:201
  epidemiological factors, 1:201
  family history, 1:201–205
  genetic diseases, 1:200
  hypoperfusion, 1:205–221. *See also* Shock
Disease period, 3:546
Disentanglement, 5:393–394
Disinfectants, 1:374
Disinfecting/disinfection, 1:27, 3:553–554
Disk injury, 3:295
Dislocation, 4:235. *See also* Musculoskeletal trauma
Dislocation of the patella, 4:260
Dislodged teeth, 4:327
Disopyramide, 1:330
Disorganized schizophrenia, 3:606
Dispatch information, 4:463–464
Dispatching system, 1:57–58
Disposable equipment, 1:27, 1:28
Dissecting aortic aneurysm, 3:199–200
Disseminated intravascular coagulation (DIC), 3:485–486
Dissociative disorders, 3:611
Distal tubule, 3:385
Distancing, 1:474
Distracting injuries, 5:298–299
Distraction, 4:347
Distraction injury, 4:346
Distress, 1:33
Distributive shock, 4:111–112, 5:102
Disturbance in executive functioning, 3:605
Diuresis, 3:316, 3:387
Diuretics, 1:199, 1:333–334, 4:321–322, 5:189

decontamination, 1:27–28
disposable, 1:27, 1:28
drawing blood, 1:437–438
endotracheal intubation, 1:546–551
hazmat protection, 5:449–451
hypodermic needle, 1:391
IO access, 1:443–444
oral administration, 1:385–386
physical exam, 2:37–40
PPE, 5:383–385
rescue operations, 5:382–386
resuscitation, 1:25
suctioning, 1:597–598
syringes and needles, 1:390–391
vehicle stabilization, 5:413
venous access, 1:408–417
Erectile dysfunction, 1:357
Erector spinae muscles, 4:384
ERG, 4:466, 5:512, 5:435
Erosion, 2:54
ERV, 1:523, 3:14, 4:385
Erythema, 4:135
Erythroblastosis fetalis, 3:472
Erythrocytes, 1:191, 3:389, 3:462
Erythromycin (PCE), 3:587
Erythropoiesis, 3:464
Erythropoietin, 3:313, 3:389, 3:464, 4:108
Eschar, 4:193, 4:194
Eschmann tracheal tube introducer, 1:551
Eskalith, 3:609
Esmolol, 1:331
Esophageal detector device (EDD), 1:536, 1:537
Esophageal gastric tube airway (EGTA), 1:587
Esophageal intubation, 1:555
Esophageal obturator airway (EOA), 1:587
Esophageal rupture, 4:410
Esophageal Tracheal CombiTube (ETC), 1:580–582
Esophageal varices, 3:358–359, 4:91, 5:182
Esophagus, 3:6, 4:389, 4:392
Estimated date of confinement (EDC), 3:651
Estradiol, 1:355
Estrogen, 1:355, 3:312
ETC, 1:580–582

ETCO$_2$, 1:532, 3:31, 4:113
ETCO$_2$ detector/detection, 1:532–536, 2:46, 2:47, 3:33–34, 3:272
Ethical decision making, 1:145–146, 1:149
Ethical relativism, 1:145
Ethical responsibilities, 1:113–114
Ethics, 1:86–87, 1:142–161
allocation of resources, 1:155–156
code of ethics, 1:88, 1:146
confidentiality, 1:153–155
conflict resolution, 1:148–151
consent, 1:155
decision making, 1:145–146, 1:149
defined, 1:144
elderly patients, 5:145–147
fundamental principles, 1:147–148
fundamental questions, 1:146–147
individual practice, and, 1:146
law, and, 1:144, 1:145
obligation to provide care, 1:156–157
professional relations, 1:157–158
religion, and, 1:144–145
research, 1:159. See also Research in EMS
resuscitation attempts, 1:151–153
teaching, 1:157
testing, 1:150–151
Ethmoid bone, 3:252, 4:274, 4:275
Ethmozine, 1:330
Ethnocentrism, 1:477
Ethosuximide, 1:305
Ethylene glycol ingestion, 3:453
Etomidate, 1:570, 4:323
ETT, 1:548–550. See also Endotracheal intubation
Eukaryotes, 1:166
Eupnea, 2:36
Eustachian tube, 1:510, 4:46, 4:283
Eustress, 1:33
Evaporation, 3:495
Evidence-based medicine (EBM), 1:70–71
Evisceration, 4:440
Evisceration care, 4:453
Ex-Lax, 1:347

Examining the patient. See Field examination; Physical examination
Examples of colostomy stoma locations, 5:282
Excitability, 3:84
Exclusionary zone, 5:438, 5:439
Excoriation, 2:54
Excretion, 1:169
Exertional heatstroke, 3:502
Exertional metabolic rate, 3:496
Exit wound, 4:71
Exocrine glands, 1:172, 3:303
Exotoxin, 3:438, 3:541
Expectorants, 1:345
Experimental studies, 1:615–618
Expiration, 3:12–13
Expiratory reserve volume (ERV), 1:523, 3:14, 4:385
Explosion, 4:40
Explosive agents, 5:505–506
Explosive/flammable limits, 5:439
Explosives, 5:505
Exposure, 1:28
Expressed consent, 1:125
Extension, 4:223
Extension injury, 4:345
Extension tubing, 1:413
Extensor carpi, 4:231
Extensors, 2:110
External auditory canal, 3:252
External cardiac pacing, 3:167–171
External hemorrhage, 4:88–89
External hemorrhoids, 3:369
External immune system, 1:235
External jugular vein, IV access, 1:420–422
External oblique, 4:231
External respiration, 4:384
External urinary tract device, 5:279
Extracellular fluid (ECF), 1:181
Extramedullary hematopoiesis, 3:461
Extraocular muscles, 2:61
Extrapyramidal symptoms (EPS), 1:307
Extrauterine, 5:6
Extravasation, 1:425
Extravascular space, 4:183
Extremities, 4:68
children, 5:52, 5:123

lower, 4:227–228
physical exam, 2:105–123
upper, 4:225–227
Extrication/rescue unit, 5:369
Extrinsic pathway, 1:245, 1:246
Exudate, 1:247
Eye
anatomy, 4:282–284
drugs, 1:349
head injury, 4:299, 4:326–327
physical exam, 2:60–67
Eye contact, 1:471, 2:6
Eye protection, 5:383
Eyedrop administration, 1:378–379
Eyewear, 1:24
EZ-IO, 1:444, 1:445

Face, 4:280–284. *See also* **Head, facial, and neck trauma**
Face mask, 1:602
Facial bones, 2:57, 2:58, 4:274, 4:275, 4:281
Facial dislocations/fractures, 4:300–301
Facial injury, 4:299–304
dislocations/fractures, 4:300–301
dislodged teeth, 4:327
ear injury, 4:302, 4:326
eye injury, 4:302, 4:326–327
nasal injury, 4:301–302
neck injury, 4:303–304
soft-tissue injury, 4:299–300
Facial nerve, 2:138, 2:141, 2:146, 3:260, 4:279, 4:280
Facial paralysis, 3:266–267
Facial soft-tissue injury, 4:299–300
Facilitated diffusion, 1:188, 1:289, 3:387
Facilities unit, 5:360
Facsimile machine (fax), 2:268
Factitious disorders, 3:610–611
Factor VIII, 3:485
Failsafe franchise, 1:72
Fainting, 3:285, 5:175
Fall, 4:47–48
children, 5:116–117
elderly persons, 5:152–153
Fallopian tubes, 3:630–631
Fallout, 5:507
False assurance, 1:474
False imprisonment, 1:130
False labor, 3:666

Head injury, *(contd.)*
geriatric patients, 5:200
scalp avulsion, 4:325–326
scalp injury, 4:287–288,
4:289
skull fracture, 4:288–291
Head lice, 3:588–589
Head-tilt/chin-lift maneuver,
1:538–539, 2:191, 5:57
Head-to-toe approach, 2:292
Headache, 3:286–288
Healing, 1:251–252
Health care proxy, 1:132
Health Insurance Portability
and Accountability Act
(HIPAA), 1:123, 1:124
Health maintenance
organization (HMO),
1:156
Hearing aids, 5:228
Hearing-impaired patients,
1:477, 2:22
Hearing impairment,
5:226–229
Hearing protection, 5:383
Heart, 2:87, 2:88, 3:73–78,
4:390–392
Heart disease. *See* Cardiology
Heart failure, 3:183–188,
5:173
Heart rate, newborn, 5:18
Heart rate calculator rulers,
3:97
Heart sounds, 2:89, 2:91, 2:92,
3:150
Heart valves, 3:74–76
Heat cramps, 3:499, 3:500
Heat disorders, 3:494–504
dehydration, 3:503
elderly persons, 5:187–188
fever, 3:503–504
heat cramps, 3:499, 3:500
heat exhaustion, 3:499–501
heat stroke, 3:500,
3:501–503
hyperthermia, 3:497–499
mechanisms of heat
gain/loss, 3:494–495
temperature regulation,
3:495–497
Heat escape lessening
position (HELP), 5:397
Heat exhaustion, 3:499–501
Heat illness, 3:497
Heat stress, 5:451
Heat stroke, 3:500, 3:501–503,
5:187–188
Heavy metal toxicity,
3:437–438
Hecto-, 1:450

Heel-to-shin testing, 2:149,
2:151
HEENT, 2:18
Heimlich maneuver, 1:587
Helicobacter pylori, 3:361,
3:363
Helicopter, 1:63, 1:64
air medical transport,
5:335–340. *See* also Air
medical transport
hazardous terrain rescue,
5:418
rural emergencies, 5:487
Helicopter landing zone,
5:339
Helmet, 5:383
Helmet removal, 4:365–366
Helminths (worms), 3:543
HELP, 5:397
Helper T cells, 1:235, 1:236,
1:238
Hematemesis, 3:357
Hematochezia, 3:360, 4:97
Hematocrit, 1:191, 3:464
Hematologic disorders, 1:203
Hematology, 3:458–489
anemia, 3:479–480
blood clotting
abnormalities, 3:484–485
blood products, 3:471–472
blood transfusion,
3:472–473
blood types, 3:472
cardiorespiratory system,
3:478
cultural considerations,
3:480
defined, 3:460
DIC, 3:485–486
gastrointestinal system,
3:477
general management, 3:478
genitourinary effects, 3:478
hemophilia, 3:484–485
hemostasis, 3:469–471
history, 3:474–475
leukemia, 3:482–483
leukopenia, 3:482
lymphatic system, 3:476
lymphoma, 3:483
multiple myeloma, 3:486
musculoskeletal system,
3:477–478
nervous system, 3:475
neutropenia, 3:482
physical exam, 3:475–478
plasma, 3:461
platelet abnormalities,
3:484–485
platelets, 3:468

polycythemia, 3:481–482
red blood cells (RBCs),
3:462–464
red blood cell diseases,
3:479–482
scene size-up/initial
assessment, 3:474
sickle cell anemia,
3:480–481
skin, 3:475–476
thrombocytopenia, 3:484
thrombocytosis, 3:484
von Willebrand's disease,
3:485
white blood cell diseases,
3:482–483
white blood cells (WBCs),
3:464–468
Hematoma, 4:89, 4:136
Hematopoiesis, 3:461
Hematopoietic system, 3:461
Hemiblocks, 3:230–231
Hemochromatosis, 1:203
Hemoconcentration, 1:441
Hemodialysis, 3:404
Hemodilution, 3:514
Hemoglobin, 1:191, 1:411,
3:16, 3:462, 3:464
Hemoglobin-based oxygen-
carrying solutions
(HBOCs), 1:193,
1:410–411
Hemolysis, 1:441, 3:464
Hemolytic anemia, 3:479
Hemolytic disease of the
newborn, 1:230, 1:258,
3:472
Hemolytic transfusion
reaction, 3:472–473
Hemolytic uremic syndrome,
3:580
Hemophilia, 1:203, 3:484–485
Hemophilia A, 3:484
Hemophilia B, 3:484
Hemopneumothorax, 4:403
Hemoptysis, 3:24, 4:405,
5:268
Hemopure, 1:193, 1:411
Hemorrhage, 4:81–101. *See
also* Bleeding
acute/chronic, 4:91
arterial, 4:85
assessment, 4:94–98
blood, 4:84
capillary, 4:85
circulatory system, 4:81–84
clotting process, 4:85–88
control, method of,
4:88–91, 4:100, 4:157–160
crush injuries, 4:101

defined, 4:81
external, 4:88–89
gaping wounds, 4:100–101
head injuries, 4:99–100
heart, 4:81, 4:82
internal, 4:89–91
management, 4:98–101
neck wounds, 4:100
nosebleed, 4:90–91
postpartum, 3:682
pressure points, 4:100
rapid trauma assessment,
4:96–97
soft-tissue wounds,
4:157–160
special populations (i.e.,
elderly, infant, etc.),
4:93–94
splinting, 4:99
stages of, 4:91–93
stopping the bleeding,
4:88–91, 4:100
tourniquet, 4:89, 4:90
transport considerations,
4:101
vascular system, 4:82–84
venous, 4:85
Hemorrhage classification,
4:84–87
Hemorrhage control,
4:88–91, 4:100, 4:157–160
Hemorrhage management,
4:98–101
Hemorrhagic strokes, 3:276
Hemorrhoids, 3:369–370
Hemostasis, 3:469–471
Hemostatic agents, 1:338–340
Hemothorax, 1:520, 3:18,
4:403, 4:421
Henry's law, 3:517
HEPA respirator, 1:24, 1:26,
3:567
Heparin, 1:339, 3:471
Heparin lock, 1:432–434
Hepatic alteration, 1:387
Hepatitis, 3:376–377,
3:562–565
Hepatitis A (HAV), 3:376,
3:562–563
Hepatitis A vaccine, 1:361
Hepatitis B (HBV), 3:376,
3:553, 3:563–564
Hepatitis B vaccine, 1:361
Hepatitis C (HCV),
3:376–377, 3:564
Hepatitis D (HDV), 3:377,
3:564
Hepatitis E (HEV), 3:377,
3:564–565
Hepatomegaly, 5:173

Infectious disease, (contd.)
preventing disease transmission, 3:591–592
protozoa, 3:543
public health agencies, 3:539
public health principle, 3:538–539
rabies, 3:581–583
recovery, 3:552–553
reporting requirements, 3:538, 3:555
response, 3:551
RSV, 3:575–576
rubella, 3:575
SARS, 3:569–570
scabies, 3:589–590
sinusitis, 3:578
skin diseases, 3:588
STDs, 3:584–588. See also Sexually transmitted diseases (STDs)
sterilization, 3:554
tetanus, 3:549, 3:583
tuberculosis (TB), 3:565
virus, 3:541–542
worms, 3:543
Infectious disease control officer (IDCO), 3:550
Infectious disease exposure, 3:555–556
Infectious disease exposure procedure, 1:29
Infectious injury, 1:177
Inferential statistics, 1:621
Inferior infarct, 3:219, 3:220
Inferior vena cava, 3:76
Inferior wall infarct, 3:224
Inferolateral infarct, 3:219
Infertility agents, 1:356–357
Infiltration, 1:448
Inflammation, 1:240–253
acute response, 1:241–242
cellular components, 1:247–248
chronic inflammatory responses, 1:249–250
defined, 1:240
functions, 1:241
geriatric patients, 1:253
immune response, contrasted, 1:240
local inflammatory responses, 1:250
mast cells, 1:242–243
medications, 1:358–362
neonates, 1:253
overview, 1:224
phases of, 1:240–241

plasma protein systems, 1:244–247
resolution and repair, 1:251–252
systemic responses of acute, 1:249
wound healing, 4:142–143
Inflammation sequence, 1:247
Inflammatory bowel disorder (IBD), 3:364–367
Inflammatory injury, 1:178
Inflammatory process, 3:468
Inflammatory response, 1:224. See also Inflammation
Influenza, 3:573–574
Influenza vaccine, 1:362
Information officer (IO), 5:359
Informed consent, 1:125
Infranodal block, 3:119–120
Infusion controller, 1:436
Infusion pump, 1:436–437
Infusion rates, 1:456–457
Ingested toxins, 3:422–424
Ingestion, 3:418
INH, 1:359
Inhalation, 1:380, 3:418–419
Inhalation injury, 4:189–190, 4:204
Inhaled toxins, 3:424–425
Initial assessment, 2:186–200
airway assessment, 2:190–194
AVPU, 2:189–190
breathing assessment, 2:194–196
circulation assessment, 2:196–199
general impression, 2:187–188
mental status, 2:188
priority determination, 2:197–200
Initial education, 1:59
Initial immune response, 1:225
Injected toxins, 3:440–448
Injection, 1:380, 3:419
Injection injury, 4:149–150
Injurious genetic factors, 1:178–179
Injurious nutritional imbalances, 1:178
Injurious physical agents, 1:178
Injury, 1:98
Injury current, 3:214

Injury prevention, 1:96–109
areas in need, 1:103–104
definitions, 1:99
EMS provider commitment, 1:101–103
geriatric patients, 1:104
immunization of at-risk populations, 1:105
infants/children, 1:103–104
organizational commitment, 1:99–101
prevention strategies, 1:105–107
work hazards, 1:104
Injury risk, 1:98
Injury-surveillance program, 1:98
Innate immunity, 3:335
Inner circle, 5:393
Innominate, 4:227
Insect bites/stings, 3:441–444
Insecticides, 5:444
Insensible loss, 1:183
Insertion, 4:229
Inspection, 2:29–30
Inspiration, 3:12
Inspiratory capacity, 3:14, 4:386
Inspiratory reserve volume (IRV), 1:523, 3:14, 4:385
Institutional elder abuse, 5:210
Institutional review board (IRB), 1:148, 1:627
Insulin, 1:353, 3:311, 3:315, 4:102, 4:107
Insulin-dependent diabetes mellitus (IDDM), 1:353, 3:317. See also Diabetes
Insulin preparations, 1:353–354
Insulin shock, 3:318–319, 3:323–324
Intal, 1:343
Integrity, 1:89
Intention to treat analysis, 1:618
Interatrial septum, 3:74, 3:75
Interbrain, 3:254
Intercalated discs, 3:82, 3:83
Intercostal muscles, 3:11, 4:383, 4:384
Intercostals, 4:231
Interference, 1:298
Interferon, 1:249
Interleukin (IL), 1:249
Interleukin-1 (IL-1), 1:238, 1:249

Intermediate-level disinfection, 3:553–554
Intermittent explosive disorder, 3:613
Internal carotid arteries, 3:257, 4:278
Internal hemorrhage, 4:89–91
Internal hemorrhoids, 3:369–370
Internal (systemic) immune system, 1:231
Internal losses, 1:183
Internal mammary vessels, 4:392
Internal oblique, 4:231
Internal respiration, 4:384
Internal urinary catheter, 5:279
Interneurons, 4:343
Internodal atrial pathways, 3:85
Interpersonal justifiability test, 1:151
Interpersonal relationism, 1:39
Interpersonal zones, 1:469
Interpolated beat, 3:129
Interpreter, 1:478
Interrogators, 1:116
Interstitial fluid, 1:181
Interstitial nephritis, 3:398
Intervener physician, 1:55
Intervention studies, 1:615–618
Interventricular septum, 3:74, 3:75
Intervertebral disk, 4:336
Interviewing techniques, 1:471–474
Intestinal adhesion, 3:370, 3:372
Intestinal hernia, 3:371
Intestinal intussusception, 3:370, 3:371
Intestinal volvulus, 3:370, 3:372
Intimate zone, 1:469
Intoxicated patient, 2:21
Intoxication (vehicle collision), 4:35
Intracellular fluid (ICF), 1:181
Intracerebral hemorrhage, 3:277, 4:294, 5:176
Intracranial hemorrhage, 3:275–281, 4:292–293. See also Stroke
Intracranial perfusion, 4:295–296

Macule, 2:52
MAF, 1:249
Magill forceps, 1:552
Magnesium, 1:186, 1:332, 3:82, 5:506
Mainstem bronchi, 3:8–9
Major basic protein (MBP), 3:466
Major depressive episode, 3:608
Major elements, 1:184
Major histocompatibility complex (MHC), 1:229
Making decisions. *See* Clinical decision making
Malaria, 1:359
Malathion, 5:509
Male genitalia, 2:100–101
Male reproductive system, 1:357, 2:96
Male urethra, 3:389
Malfeasance, 1:119
Malignant tumors, 3:289
Malleolus, 4:227, 4:228
Malleus, 4:283
Mallory-Weiss tear, 3:357, 5:182
Malnutrition, 5:156
Malpractice suits, 1:554, 2:301
Mammalian diving reflex, 3:514, 5:402
Management staff, 5:358
Mandatory reporting requirements, 1:117
Mandible, 3:252, 4:275, 4:280
Mandibular dislocations, 4:300
Mandibular fracture, 4:300
Manhole, 5:405
Manic, 3:609
Manic-depressive illness, 1:205, 3:609
Mannitol, 1:334, 3:275
Manometer, 2:39
Manual airway maneuvers, 1:538–542
Manual cervical immobilization, 4:361–362
Manual immobilization, 4:354
Manually triggered oxygen-powered ventilation device, 1:605
MAOI, 1:308–309
MAOI overdose, 3:433–434
MAP, 4:278
March fractures, 4:238, 4:261
Marfan's syndrome, 3:199

Marginal artery, 3:77
Margination, 1:247
Marijuana, 3:451
Marine animal injection, 3:447–448
Marinol, 1:349
Mark I kit, 5:510
Mask, 1:24, 3:567
Mass, 4:20
Mass casualty incident, 348. *See also* Medical incident management
Masseter, 4:231
MAST (medical anti-shock trouser), 4:120
Mast cell, 1:242–243, 3:337
Mast cell degranulation and synthesis, 1:242–243
MAST program,1:63–64
Mastoid process, 3:252, 4:275
MAT, 3:107–108
Material safety data sheet (MSDS), 5:436, 5:437
Maternal-fetal circulation, 3:652
Math, 1:449–458. *See also* Medical mathematics
Maturation, 1:168, 1:252
Maxilla, 4:280
Maxillary bone, 3:252, 4:275
Maxillary fracture, 4:300
Maximum life-span, 1:496
MBP, 3:466
McBurney point, 3:373
MCI, 5:348. *See also* Medical incident management
MCL₁, 3:87, 3:152, 3:155
MD, 3:291, 5:241, 5:269
MDI, 1:381–383
MDMA, 3:452, 5:218
MDR-TB, 3:565
Meals on Wheels, 5:149
Mean, 1:619
Mean arterial pressure (MAP), 4:278
Measured volume administration set, 1:414, 1:422, 1:423
Measures of respiratory function, 1:522–523
Mebendazole, 1:359
Mecamylamine, 1:317
Mechanical airway, 1:542
Mechanical immobilization, 4:354
Mechanism of injury (MOI), 1:80, 2:185–186
Mechlorethamine, 1:358
Meconium, 5:10, 5:26

Meconium-stained amniotic fluid, 5:26–27
Meconium staining, 3:681
MED COM, 5:370
Medevac, 5:335
Medi-Port, 5:277
Median, 1:619
Median nerve, 3:258, 4:342
Mediastinum, 3:5, 4:389
Medic alert bracelet anaphylactic reactions, 3:345
hemophiliac, 3:485
Medicaid, 5:147
Medical anti-shock trouser (MAST), 4:120
Medical calculations, 1:452–458
converting prefixes, 1:454
dosage - oral medications, 1:453–454
dosage - parenteral medications, 1:455
fluid volume over time, 1:456–457
infants/children, 1:457–458
infusion rates, 1:456–457
weight-dependent dosages, 1:455–456
Medical direction, 1:54–55
Medical direction physician (medical director), 1:54, 1:122, 2:255, 2:264–265
Medical gynecological emergencies, 3:636–639
Medical helicopters, 5:335–340. *See also* Helicopters
Medical history, 2:2–25. *See also* History taking
Medical incident management, 5:344–377
C-FLOP, 5:351
command, 5:352–357
command staff, 5:358–360
common problems, 5:372
communications, 5:355, 5:370
disaster management, 5:371
division of operations functions, 5:361–362
EOC, 5:351
extrication/rescue unit, 5:369
green treatment unit, 5:367
IC, 5:352
incident size-up, 5:353–354
incident stabilization, 5:353
mental health support, 5:359–360, 5:373

morgue, 5:366
on-scene physicians, 5:368
preplanning, drills, critique, 5:372–373
property conservation, 5:354
red treatment unit, 5:367
regulations/standards, 5:349–351
rehabilitation unit, 5:369–370
resource utilization, 5:356
rest home - command structure, 5:374
staging area, 5:355, 5:368
START system, 5:363–365
supporting units, 5:357–361
toolbox theory, 5:362
transport unit, 5:368–369
treatment, 5:366–368
triage, 5:362–366
windshield survey, 5:352
yellow treatment unit, 5:367
Medical mathematics, 1:449–458
apothecary system of measure, 1:451
calculations, 1:452–458. *See also* Medical calculations
household system of measure, 1:451
metric system, 1:449–452
temperature, 1:452–453
weight conversion, 1:451
Medical record, 1:137. *See* Documentation
Medical supply unit, 5:360
Medically clean, 1:374
Medicare, 5:147
Medication. *See also* Pharmacology
alkalinizing agents, 3:162
antidysrhythmics, 3:157–158
beta-blockers, 3:162
calcium channel blockers, 3:162
cardiovascular disease, 3:156–162
children, 5:84–86
combative patient, 4:374
elderly persons, 5:150–151
fibrinolytic agents, 3:160–161
head and neck injury, 4:321–325
musculoskeletal trauma, 4:263–265
myocardial ischemia, 3:159–160

Motor aphasia, 5:231
Motor system, 2:146–151
Motor vehicle actions. *See* Automobile collisions
Motor vehicle construction, 5:411–412
Motor vehicle fatalities, 4:35
Motor vehicle laws, 1:117
Motorcycle crashes, 4:36–37
Mountain climbing/biking. *See* Hazardous terrain rescues
Mountain sickness, 3:523–526
Mourning, 1:30
Mouth, 2:73–78. *See also* Head, facial, and neck trauma
Mouth droop, 3:267
Mouth-to-mask ventilation, 1:603
Mouth-to-mouth ventilation, 1:603
Mouth-to-nose ventilation, 1:603
Mouth-to-stoma technique, 1:596–597
Moving spinal injury patient, 4:366–373
    diving injury immobilization, 4:372–373
    final patient positioning, 4:370
    four-count, 4:366
    log roll, 4:367
    long spine board, 4:371–372
    orthopedic stretcher, 4:368
    rapid extrication, 4:370
    rope-sling slide, 4:368
    straddle slide, 4:368
    vest-type immobilization device, 4:368–370
MRSA, 3:590
MS, 1:205, 3:291, 5:240–241
MS-ABC, 2:245
MSDS, 5:436, 5:437
MSE, 3:603–604
Mucolytics, 1:345
Mucosal immune system, 1:235
Mucoviscidosis, 5:240
Mucus, 1:510
Multi-infarct dementia, 5:178
Multifactorial disorders, 1:200
Multifocal atrial tachycardia (MAT), 3:107–108
Multifocal seizures, 5:31
Multigravida, 3:653
Multipara, 3:653

Multiple births, 3:680
Multiple-casualty incident (MCI), 5:348. *See also* Medical incident management
Multiple drug resistant tuberculosis (MDR-TB), 3:565
Multiple myeloma, 3:486
Multiple organ dysfunction syndrome (MODS), 1:219–221
Multiple personality disorder, 3:611
Multiple sclerosis, 1:205
Multiple sclerosis (MS), 1:205, 3:291, 5:240–241
Multiple symptoms, patients with, 2:20
Multiple system failure, 5:150
Multiplex communications system, 2:267
Mumps, 3:574–575
Munchausen syndrome, 3:611
Murder, 5:462–463
Murmur, 2:92
Murphy's sign, 3:375
Muscarinic cholinergic antagonists, 1:317
Muscarinic receptors, 1:314, 1:315
Muscle, 4:230, 4:231
Muscle cramp, 4:234
Muscle fatigue, 4:234
Muscle spasm, 4:234
Muscle strength, 2:148–150
Muscle tissue, 1:169, 1:170
Muscle tone, 2:148, 4:233
Muscles of the arm, 2:107
Muscular/connective tissue care, 4:254
Muscular dystrophy (MD), 3:291, 5:241, 5:269
Muscular injury, 4:233–234
Muscular strength, 1:17
Muscular system, 4:230, 4:231
Muscular tissue/structure, 4:229–233
Musculocutaneous nerve, 3:258, 4:342
Musculoskeletal system, 4:219–233. *See also* Musculoskeletal trauma
    bone aging, 4:228–229
    bone structure, 4:220–222
    elderly persons, 5:166–167, 5:184–185
    joint structure, 4:222–224
    ligaments, 4:223
    lower extremity, 4:227–228

    muscular tissue/structure, 4:229–233
    physical exam, 2:102–128
    skeletal organization, 4:224–228
    skeletal tissue/structure, 4:220
    upper extremity, 4:225–227
Musculoskeletal trauma, 4:216–269
    anatomy/physiology, 4:219–233. *See also* Musculoskeletal system
    ankle injuries, 4:261
    assessment, 4:241–246
    bone injury, 4:235–239. *See also* Fractures
    bone repair cycle, 4:239–240
    clavicular fracture, 4:257
    compartment syndrome, 4:234, 4:245
    elbow injuries, 4:262
    femur fracture, 4:255–256
    finger injuries, 4:262–263
    foot injuries, 4:261
    fracture care, 4:253
    general considerations, 4:239
    geriatric injuries, 4:238–239
    hip dislocation, 4:256, 4:259
    humerus fracture, 4:257–258
    immobilization, 4:248–249
    inflammatory/degenerative conditions, 4:240–241
    injury management, 4:246–249
    injury prevention, 4:219
    joint care, 4:253–254
    joint injury, 4:235
    knee injuries, 4:259–260
    limb alignment, 4:247–248
    medications, 4:263–265
    muscular/connective tissue care, 4:254
    muscular injury, 4:233–234
    neurovascular function, 4:249
    open wounds, 4:247
    pediatric injuries, 4:238, 4:265
    pelvis fracture, 4:254–255
    psychological support, 4:266
    radius/ulna, 4:258
    refusal/referral incidents, 4:266
    scene size-up, 4:241
    shoulder injuries, 4:261

    six Ps (assessment), 4:243–244
    soft/connective tissue injuries, 4:263
    sports injuries, 4:246, 4:265
    tibular/fibular fracture, 4:257
    wrist/hand injuries, 4:262
Mushroom poisoning, 3:439–440
Mustard gas, 5:510
Mustargen, 1:358
Mutual-aid agreement, 1:66, 5:361
Myasthenia gravis, 1:258, 5:242–243, 5:269
Myeloblasts, 3:465
Myelomeningocele SB, 3:293
Myocardial aneurysm/rupture, 4:407–408
Myocardial contusion, 4:405–406, 4:421
Myocardial infarction (MI), 1:177, 3:177–182, 3:214–215
    algorithm, 3:180
    cardiac enzymes, 3:181–182
    causes, 3:178
    ECG, 3:218–226
    elderly persons, 5:172–173
    field assessment, 3:178–179
    lead groupings, 3:218–221
    management, 3:180–182
    right ventricular infarction, 3:221, 3:225–226
    sequence, 3:95
    silent MI, 5:173
    surgical treatment, 3:182
Myocardial injury, 3:214
Myocardial ischemia, 3:159–160, 3:214
Myocardium, 3:74, 4:391
Myoclonic seizures, 5:31
Myoclonus, 3:292
Myoglobin, 3:182
Myometrium, 3:629–630
Myotome, 4:343
Myxedema, 3:326–327
Myxedema coma, 3:326, 3:327

N. meningitidis, 3:571
N95 respirators, 1:24, 1:26, 3:566–567
Nabilone, 1:349
Nails, 2:55–57
Nalbuphine, 1:303, 3:160, 4:265
Naloxone, 1:302, 3:274, 4:324, 5:23

Protropin, 1:351
Proventil, 1:342, 3:46, 3:343
Proximal fractures of the femur, 4:256
Proximal tubule, 3:385
Proximate cause, 1:120
Prozac, 1:308
Pruritus, 5:183
PSAP, 2:260
Pseudo-instinctive, 2:244
Pseudoseizures, 3:282
Psilocybin, 3:451
Psoriasis, 2:56, 5:183
PSVT, 3:108–112, 3:125
Psychiatric and behavioral disorders, 3:596–623
  anxiety disorders, 3:606–608
  biological causes, 3:599–600
  bipolar disorder, 3:609–610
  cognitive disorders, 3:605
  delirium, 3:605
  dementia, 3:605
  depression, 3:608–609
  dissociative disorders, 3:611
  DSM-IV, 3:604
  eating disorders, 3:611–612
  elderly persons, 5:194–196
  factitious disorders, 3:610–611
  general treatment principles, 3:615
  geriatric patients, 3:614–615
  impulse control disorders, 3:613
  medical causes, 3:600
  medical conditions, 3:615–616
  medication, 3:604
  mood disorders, 3:608–610
  MSE, 3:603–604
  panic attack, 3:606–607
  patient restraint, 3:617–621
  pediatric patients, 3:615
  personality disorders, 3:612–613
  phobia, 3:607
  post-traumatic stress syndrome, 3:607–608
  psychological care, 3:616–617
  psychosocial causes, 3:600
  scene size-up/initial assessment, 3:601–603
  schizophrenia, 3:605–606
  sociocultural causes, 3:600
  somatoform disorders, 3:610
  substance-related disorders, 3:610
  suicide, 3:613–614
  treatment, 3:615–617
  violent patients, 3:617–621
Psychiatric disorders, 1:205
Psychogenic amnesia, 3:611
Psychological dependence, 3:449
Psychological first aid, 1:38
Psychological stress, 1:267
Psychomotor seizure, 3:282
Psychoneuroimmunological regulation, 1:262
Psychotherapeutic medications, 1:306–309
Psyllium, 1:347
PTCA, 3:183
PTH, 3:309–310
PtL, 1:582–584
PTU, 1:352
Pubic lice, 3:588
Pubis, 4:227
Public distance, 1:469
Public health. See Infectious diseases
Public health agencies, 3:539
Public health principle, 3:538–539
Public information officer (PIO), 5:359
Public safety answering point (PSAP), 2:260
Public utility model, 1:72
Publicly funded resources, 5:147
PUD, 1:204–205, 1:346–347, 3:362–363
Pudendum, 3:627
Puerperium, 3:668
Pulmonary agents, 5:511
Pulmonary arteries, 3:10, 3:76
Pulmonary blast trauma, 4:45–46
Pulmonary capillaries, 3:9
Pulmonary circulation, 1:517, 1:518
Pulmonary contusion, 4:403–405
Pulmonary drug administration, 1:380–384
  endotracheal tube, 1:384
  MDI, 1:381–383
  nebulizer, 1:380–381, 1:382
Pulmonary edema, 3:186–187, 5:171, 5:193
Pulmonary embolism (PE), 1:448, 3:184, 3:200, 3:56–57, 3:682–683, 5:170–171
Pulmonary hilum, 4:384
Pulmonary injuries, 4:399–405
Pulmonary irritants, 5:444
Pulmonary occlusion, 3:202
Pulmonary overpressure, 3:518
Pulmonary overpressure accidents, 3:521
Pulmonary respiration, 3:17–18
Pulmonary veins, 3:10, 3:76
Pulmonic valve, 3:75, 3:76
Pulmonology, 3:2–63
  abnormal breath sounds, 3:28–29
  abnormal respiratory patterns, 3:19–20
  airway obstruction, 3:35–37
  alveoli, 3:9–10
  anatomy, 3:5–11
  ARDS, 3:37–39
  asthma, 3:43–46
  bronchi, 3:8–9
  bronchitis, 3:42–43
  carbon monoxide inhalation, 3:55–56
  children, 5:90–99
  chronic bronchitis, 3:42–43
  CNS dysfunction, 3:59
  COPD, 3:39
  diagnostic testing, 3:30–34
  diffusion, 3:15–16
  dysfunction of spinal cord/respiratory muscles, 3:60
  elderly persons, 5:162–163, 5:168–172, 5:198
  emphysema, 3:40–42
  history, 3:24–25
  hyperventilation syndrome, 3:58–59
  inspiration/expiration, 3:12–13
  larynx, 3:7–8
  lung cancer, 3:53–54
  lung volumes, 3:13–14
  lungs, 3:10
  management principles, 3:35
  nasal cavity, 3:6–7
  obstructive lung disease, 3:39–40
  pathophysiology, 3:18–20
  perfusion, 3:16–18
  pharynx, 3:7
  physical exam, 3:25–29
  physiological processes, 3:11–18
  pneumonia, 3:50–51
  pulmonary/bronchial vessels, 3:10–11
  pulmonary embolism, 3:56–57
  risk factors, 3:4–5
  SARS, 3:51–52
  spontaneous pneumothorax, 3:57–58
  toxic inhalation, 3:54–55
  trachea, 3:8
  upper airway obstruction, 3:35–37
  URI, 3:46–50
  ventilation, 3:11–15, 3:18–20
  vital signs, 3:29–30
Pulse (children), 5:65, 5:66
Pulse oximeter, 1:531, 3:272
Pulse oximetry, 1:531–532, 2:45–46, 3:30–31, 4:197
Pulse pressure, 2:36
Pulse quality, 2:34
Pulse rate, 2:33, 2:200
Pulse rhythm, 2:33
Pulse sites, 2:34
Pulseless electrical activity (PEA), 3:139, 3:140, 5:107–108
Pulseless electrical activity (PEA) algorithm, 3:140
Pulsus alternans, 3:187
Pulsus paradoxus, 1:529, 3:187, 4:407
Pump failure, 3:178
Puncture, 4:135, 4:138
Punitive damages, 1:120
Pupil, 3:266, 4:283
Pure Food and Drug Act of 1906, 1:280
Purified protein derivative (PPD) skin test, 3:565–566
Purkinje fibers, 3:85
Purkinje system, 3:85
Purpura, 2:51, 3:475, 3:476
Purulent otitis, 2:72
Pus, 1:250
Pustule, 2:53
PVC, 3:129–131
Pyelonephritis, 3:409
Pyramid, 3:384, 3:385
Pyrexia, 3:503
Pyridoxine, 1:363
Pyrogen, 1:222, 3:503
Pyrogenic reaction, 1:426
Pyromania, 3:613
Pyruvic acid, 1:211

Q fever, 5:516
QA, 1:67–70
QF, 3:527

QI program, 1:67–70
QNB, 5:512
QRS axis, 3:210
QRS complex, 3:90, 3:93, 3:98
QRS interval, 3:94, 3:95, 3:206
QT interval, 3:94, 3:206
Quadriceps, 2:119, 2:120
Quadriceps femoris, 4:231
Quadriceps reflex, 2:155, 2:157
Quadrigeminy, 3:129
Qualitative statistics, 1:621
Quality assurance (QA), 1:67–70
Quality factor (QF), 3:527
Quality improvement (QI) program, 1:67–70
Quality of respiration, 2:35
Quantitative statistics, 1:621
Questioning techniques, 1:471–472
Questions, asking, 2:7–8
Questran, 1:341
Quick-look paddles, 3:152
Quinidex, 1:330
Quinidine, 1:330, 3:113, 3:115

R. Adams Cowley Shock Trauma Center, 1:67, 4:7
R-R interval, 3:97
Rabbit ear, 3:228
Rabbit fever, 5:515
Rabies, 3:581–583
Raccoon eyes, 2:222, 4:288–289, 4:290
Race. *See* Cultural considerations
RAD, 3:527
Rad, 4:188
Radial nerve, 3:258, 4:342
Radiation, 3:495
Radiation absorbed dose (RAD), 3:527
Radiation accidents, 3:529
Radiation burns, 4:185–189, 4:210–212
Radiation emergencies, 3:526–530
Radiation exposure, 5:506–508
Radio band, 2:257
Radio communication, 2:258, 2:266–268, 2:271–272
Radio dead spots, 5:482, 5:483
Radio frequency, 2:257
Radioactive contamination, 5:508
Radioactive iodine (^{131}I), 1:352

Radioactive warning labels, 3:530
Radioisotope, 3:526, 3:527
Radionuclide, 3:526
Radius, 4:226
Radius/ulna fracture, 4:258
RAE, 3:25, 3:231
Railroad accidents, 5:431
Rales, 1:530, 2:85, 3:29
Ranitidine, 1:346, 3:342
Rape, 5:217
Rapid axis determination, 3:212
Rapid extrication, 4:370
Rapid intervention team, 5:370
Rapid isotonic infusion, 4:503
Rapid medical assessment, 2:220
Rapid plasmin reagin (RPR) test, 3:586
Rapid sequence intubation (RSI), 1:568–572, 4:317, 5:81
Rapid transport, 4:485
Rapid trauma assessment, 2:203–210
Rappel, 5:415
Rapport, 2:5–11
Raptures of the deep, 3:518, 3:522
RAS, 3:256
Rattlesnake bites, 3:444–446
Raynaud's phenomenon, 1:255
Re-bleeding, 4:146
Reabsorption, 3:385, 3:386
Reach-throw-row-go, 5:397
Reactive airway disease, 5:267
Rear-end collision, 4:32–33
Reasonable force, 1:130–131
Reasonably foreseeable, 1:120
Reassurance, 2:20
Rebound tenderness, 4:443
Recall bias, 1:614
Receiving facilities, 1:66
Receiving facility, 1:82–83
Recent memory, 2:137
Receptor, 1:172, 1:295
Receptor-mediated drug actions, 1:296
Reciprocal/reciprocity, 1:59, 3:219
Recirculating currents, 5:398, 5:399
Recombivax (HB), 3:263
Recompression, 3:520
Reconstruction, 1:251–252
Record keeping, 1:84. *See* Documentation

Recreational emergencies (rural EMS), 5:496–498
Recreational vehicle collisions, 4:39–40
Rectal administration, 1:387–390
Rectal thermometer, 2:45
Rectus abdominis, 4:231
Rectus femoris, 1:404, 1:405, 4:231
Red blood cell diseases, 3:479–482
Red blood cells (RBCs), 3:462–464
Red bone marrow, 4:221
Red reflex, 2:65–66
Red skin rash, 1:528
Red treatment unit, 5:367
Reduced nephron mass, 3:400
Reduced renal mass, 3:400
Reduction, 4:253–254
Reentrant pathways, 1:329
Refer/release incidents, 4:172
Referred pain, 3:352, 3:391–392
Reflex response, 4:344
Reflexes, 1:487, 2:153–157, 3:257, 4:343, 4:344
Refractory period, 3:95
Refusal of care, 2:296–298, 4:481, 4:483, 5:243, 5:244
Refusal of care documentation checklist, 2:297
Refusal of care form, 2:298
Refusal of service, 1:127–128, 1:129
Refusal of Treatment and Transportation form, 5:244
Regeneration, 1:251
Regional trauma center, 4:6, 4:7
Registration, 1:59
Regitine, 1:324
Reglan, 1:348
Regulatory law, 1:115
Rejection, 3:468
Relative refractory period, 3:95
Release from liability form, 1:121, 1:127
Release from responsibility form, 2:298
Relenza, 3:574
Religious organizations, 5:148
REM (roentgen equivalent in man), 3:527
REM sleep, 1:304
Remodeling, 4:143

Remote memory, 2:137
Removal of pinch-point injury patient, 5:494–495
Renal, 3:383
Renal ARF, 3:397–398
Renal calculi, 3:405–408
Renal dialysis, 3:403
Renal disorders. *See* Urology and nephrology
Renal excretion, 1:292–293
Renal kidney failure, 1:204
Renal pelvis, 3:384
Renin, 1:335, 3:313, 3:389, 4:107
Renin-angiotensin system, 1:212
ReoPro, 1:339
Repair, 1:251
Reperfusion, 3:176
Repetitive PVCs, 3:129
Repolarization, 3:84
Reporting requirements, 1:117
Reproductive system
  female, 1:355–357, 2:95, 3:627–631
  male, 1:357, 2:96, 2:100–101
Request for document production, 1:116
RES, 3:547
Res ipsa loquitor, 1:119, 1:120
Rescue awareness and operations, 5:378–423. *See also* Medical incident management
  assessment, 5:391
  automobile collisions, 5:408–414
  cave-ins/structural collapses, 5:407–408
  confined-space rescues, 5:404–408
  disentanglement, 5:393–394
  hazardous atmosphere rescues, 5:404–408
  hazardous terrain rescues, 5:414–420. *See also* Hazardous terrain rescues
  highway rescues, 5:408–414
  motor vehicle accidents, 5:408–414
  paramedic, role of, 5:381
  patient access, 5:390
  patient fears, 5:393
  patient packaging, 5:394–395
  phase 1 (arrival/size-up), 5:388
  phase 2 (hazard control), 5:389–390

Split S$_2$, 2:89, 2:92
Splitting, 2:92
SpO$_2$, 1:531, 3:31
Spondylosis, 5:200
Spongy (cancellous) bone, 4:221
Spontaneous abortion, 3:659
Spontaneous pneumothorax, 3:57–58
Sports injuries, 1:104, 4:48–49, 4:246, 4:265
Sports medicine, 1:11
Spotter, 5:328, 5:330
Spouse abuse, 5:206–209
Sprain, 4:235. *See also* Musculoskeletal trauma
SRS, 4:26, 5:410
SRS-A, 1:243, 3:338
SSM, 5:326
SSRI, 1:308
SSRI overdose, 3:434
ST segment, 3:94–96, 3:206
Stab wound, 4:394, 4:416, 4:438, 4:440
Stabbings, 4:63
Stable angina, 3:174
Stadol, 1:303
Staff functions, 5:358
Stage 1 hemorrhage, 4:92
Stage 2 hemorrhage, 4:92
Stage 3 hemorrhage, 4:92–93
Stage 4 hemorrhage, 4:92, 4:93
Stages of labor, 3:668–670
Stages of life. *See* Life-span development
Stages of loss, 1:30
Staging area, 5:355, 5:368
Staging officer, 5:368
Stance, 1:470
Standard deviation (SD), 1:619, 1:620
Standard of care, 1:119
Standards
  ambulance design/equipment, 5:322–324
  ambulance response times, 5:326–327
  consensus, 5:351
  hospice, 5:286
Standing orders, 1:55, 2:240
Standing posture, 1:22
Standing takedown, 4:364–365
Stapes, 4:283
Staphylococcal enterotoxin B (SEB), 5:511
Starling's hypothesis, 1:189
Starling's law of the heart, 3:80, 3:185, 4:82

START system, 5:363–365
State court system, 1:115
Statewide EMS Technical Assessment Program, 1:51–52
Statistical error, 1:617
Statistical significance, 1:617
Statistical tests, 1:619–622
  descriptive statistics, 1:619
  inferential statistics, 1:621
  other types of data, 1:621–622
  quantitative/qualitative statistics, 1:621
Status asthmaticus, 3:46, 5:98
Status epilepticus, 3:284–285, 5:108
Statute of limitations, 1:121
Statutory law, 1:115
Steady-state metabolism, 3:496
Stem cells, 1:231
Step 2 Nit Removal System, 3:589
Step-by-step procedure. *See* Procedure
Sterile/sterilization, 1:27, 1:374, 3:554
Sterile dressings, 4:150
Sternal fracture/dislocation, 4:397–398, 4:417–418
Sternoclavicular dislocation, 4:417–418
Sternocleidomastoid, 4:230, 4:231, 4:383, 4:384
Sternum, 4:382
Steroidal hormones, 3:312
Stethoscope, 2:37–38
Stimate, 1:351
Stimulant laxatives, 1:347
Stingray (marine-acquired infection), 3:447–448
Stock solution, 1:452
Stokes-Adams syndrome, 5:175
Stokes basket stretcher, 5:416–417
Stoma, 1:596, 5:131
Stoma sites, patients with, 1:596–597
Stopping the bleeding, 4:88–91, 4:100
STP, 3:451
Straddle injury, 3:639
Straddle slide, 4:368
Strain, 4:235. *See also* Musculoskeletal trauma
Strainers, 5:398–400
Street crime, 5:462–463
Street gangs, 5:463–464

Strep throat, 3:578
Streptase, 1:340
Streptokinase, 1:340
Stress, 1:261
Stress and stress management, 1:33–38, 1:261–269
  coping, 1:266–269
  disaster mental health services, 1:38
  disease, 1:268
  GAS, 1:261–262
  immune system, 1:266
  mental health services, 1:38
  neuroendocrine regulation, 1:263–266
  phases of stress response, 1:34
  shift work, 1:35
  signs of stress, 1:35, 1:36
  specific EMS stresses, 1:37
  stressors, 1:33
  technique for managing stress, 1:35–37
Stress response, 1:262–263
Stressor, 1:33, 1:261
Stretch receptors, 1:521, 3:15
Stretcher day, 5:324
Stretching, 1:18
Stridor, 1:530, 2:85, 3:28
Stroke, 3:275–281
  algorithm, 3:280
  assessment, 3:278
  elderly persons, 5:176–177, 5:186–188
  fibrinolytic therapy, 3:279
  management, 3:279–281
  TIA, 3:278–279
  types, 3:275–277
Stroke volume, 1:207, 2:89, 3:79–80, 4:81–84
Structural collapses, 4:42, 4:43, 4:167, 5:407–408
Structural hierarchy of body, 1:169
Structural lesions, 3:261
Struvite stones, 3:407
Study designs
  case-control studies, 1:614–615
  cohort studies, 1:615
  descriptive studies, 1:614
  intervention studies, 1:615–618
Study group, 1:616
Studying a Study and Testing a Test: How to Read the Medical Literature (Riegelman/Hirsch), 1:629
Stuttering, 5:232

Stylet, 1:550–551
Styloid process, 3:252, 4:275
Subarachnoid hemorrhage, 3:277, 5:176
Subarachnoid space, 3:251, 3:254
Subcapital femoral neck fracture, 5:199
Subconjunctival hemorrhage, 4:303, 4:304
Subcutaneous emphysema, 2:205, 3:26
Subcutaneous injection, 1:399–403
Subcutaneous injection sites, 1:401
Subcutaneous tissue, 4:132, 4:180
Subdural hematoma, 4:293
Subdural space, 3:251, 3:254
Subendocardial infarction, 3:177, 3:215, 3:217
Subjective narrative, 2:291–292
Sublingual medication administration, 1:376, 1:377
Subluxation, 4:235
Substance abuse and overdose, 3:448–455
  addiction, withdrawal, 3:448–449
  alcohol abuse, 3:450, 3:452–455
  amphetamines, 3:451
  barbiturates, 3:450, 3:452
  benzodiazepines, 3:451, 3:452
  cocaine, 3:450
  date rape drug, 3:452
  ecstasy, 3:452
  elderly persons, 5:192–194
  hallucinogens, 3:451
  marijuana, 3:451
  narcotics, 3:450
  sedatives, 3:451
Substance-related disorders, 3:610
Subtle seizures, 5:30
Succinylcholine, 1:318, 1:569, 4:322, 5:81
Sucking reflex, 1:487
Suctioning, 1:597–600, 5:68–69, 5:71
Suctioning catheters, 1:598
Sudden infant death syndrome (SIDS), 5:125–126
Sudoriferous glands, 4:131
Suicidal patients, 3:421

Suicide, 3:613–614, 4:300, 5:195–196
Suicide attempts, 4:70, 4:300
Sulfonylureas, 1:355
Sulfur mustard (HD), 5:510
Sumatriptan, 3:287
Sumer (Mesopotamia), 1:47
Summation, 1:298
Sunburn, 4:191
Superficial burn, 4:191, 4:199
Superficial frostbite, 3:511
Superheated steam, 4:190
Superior sagittal sinus, 4:277
Superior vena cava, 3:76
Supine hypotensive syndrome, 3:664, 3:665, 4:435
Supplemental restraint system (SRS), 4:26, 5:410
Supplies. See Equipment and supplies
Suppository, 1:389
Suppressor T cell, 1:236, 1:238
Suppressor T cell dysfunction, 1:257
Supraclavicular nerve, 3:258, 4:342
Suprapubic catheters, 5:279
Supraventricular tachycardia, 5:104–105
Surface-absorbed toxins, 3:425
Surface absorption, 3:419
Surface water rescues, 5:396–404
  basic rescue technique, 5:397
  body recovery, 5:402
  cold-protective response, 5:402
  drowning/near-drowning, 5:401
  flat water, 5:400–404
  foot/extremity pins, 5:400
  hypothermia, 5:397
  in-water patient immobilization, 5:402–404
  moving water, 5:397–400
  recirculating currents, 5:398, 5:399
  self-rescue techniques, 5:400
  strainers, 5:398–400
  submerged victims, 5:402
  water temperature, 5:397
Surfactant, 3:10, 3:514
Surfactant laxatives, 1:347
Surgical airways, 1:587
Surgical cricothyrotomy, 4:318, 4:319

Surgical mask, 5:383
Surgical menopause, 3:632
Surgically implanted medication delivery systems, 5:277
Survival, 3:195
Suspensions, 1:294
Sutures, 4:274
SWAT-Medics, 5:471
SWAT team, 5:469
Sweat test, 5:240
Sweating, 3:496, 3:499
Swift-water rescue, 5:397–400
Swimmer's ear, 5:227
Symmetrel, 1:310, 3:574
Sympathetic chain ganglia, 1:319
Sympathetic ganglia, 1:318, 1:319
Sympathetic nervous system, 1:318–320, 3:81–82, 3:249, 3:261
Sympathetic postganglionic fibers, 1:319
Sympathetic receptors, 1:320–324
Sympatholytics, 1:321
Sympathomimetic agents, 3:158–159
Sympathomimetics, 1:321
Synapse, 1:311, 3:251
Synaptic signaling, 1:172
Synaptic terminals, 3:250
Synarthroses, 4:222
Synchronized cardioversion, 3:164, 3:167, 3:168
Synchronized cardioversion algorithm, 3:168
Syncope, 3:283, 3:285–286, 5:175
Syncytium, 3:82
Synergism, 1:298, 5:443
Synovial capsule, 4:223–224
Synovial fluid, 4:224
Synovial joint, 2:103, 2:104, 4:222
Synthesis, 1:243
Synthroid, 1:351
Syphilis, 3:585–586
Syringe, 1:390–391
Syringe-type infusion pump, 1:436
Syrup, 1:295
Syrup of ipecac, 3:421
System financing, 1:71–72
System integration, 1:171–174
System status management (SSM), 5:326
Systematic sampling, 1:616

Systemic effects, 5:443
Systemic immune system, 1:231
Systemic inflammation, 3:468
Systemic lupus erythematosis (SLE), 1:258, 3:467
Systemic lymphocytes, 1:235
Systems of documentation, 2:294–296. See also Documentation
Systems of measurement, 1:449–458. See also Medical mathematics
Systole, 2:88, 3:79
Systolic blood pressure, 2:35, 4:103

T_3, 3:309
T_4, 3:309
T cell, 1:235, 1:236, 1:238, 3:467, 3:547
T cell receptor (TCR), 1:238
T lymphocytes, 1:226, 1:231, 3:547
T test, 1:621
T wave, 3:90
T2, 5:511
Tabun, 5:509
Tachycardia, 2:34, 3:23, 3:97
Tachycardia algorithm, 3:111
Tachydysrhythmias, 3:99, 5:104–105
Tachyphylaxis, 1:298
Tachypnea, 2:35, 2:36, 3:30
Tactical emergency medical service (TEMS), 1:61–62, 5:458, 5:471
Tactile fremitus, 3:26
Tadalafil, 1:357
Tagamet, 1:346, 3:342
Talwin, 1:303
Tambocor, 1:330
Tamiflu, 3:574
Tandem walking, 2:150
Target heart rate, 1:18
Tavist, 1:345
TB, 1:359, 3:565
TB skin test, 3:565–566
TBW, 1:180–182
Tc cells, 1:236
TCAs, 1:291, 1:308
TCR, 1:238
Td, 1:361, 3:583
Td boosters, 1:361
Td cells, 1:236
Teachable moments, 1:98
Teaching, 1:157
Teaching Resource for Instructors in Prehospital Pediatrics (TRIPP), 5:42

Teamwork, 1:91
Technique. See Procedure
Teflon catheter, 1:416
Tegretol, 1:305, 1:309, 3:292
Telangiectasia, 2:53
Television, 1:492
Temperature, 2:37, 2:43, 2:45
Temperature regulation, 3:495–497
Tempered glass, 5:412
Temporal bone, 3:252, 4:274, 4:275
Temporal lobe seizure, 3:282
Temporalis, 4:231
Temporary cavity, 4:65
Temporomandibular joint (TMJ), 2:57, 2:59
TEMS, 1:61–62, 5:458, 5:471
10-code system, 2:256
Ten Commandments, 1:146
Tendon, 2:232, 4:133, 4:224
Tendonitis, 4:240
Tenecteplase, 3:161
Teniae coli, 3:367, 3:368
Tension headache, 3:286
Tension lines, 4:134
Tension pneumothorax, 1:556, 3:18, 3:58, 4:401–403, 4:419–421
Tentorium cerebelli, 4:277
Tentorium incisura, 4:277
Teratogenic drug, 1:287
Terbutaline, 1:324, 1:356, 3:39
Teres major, 4:230
Teres minor, 4:230
Terfenadine, 1:345
Terminal bronchioles, 3:9
Terminal-drop hypothesis, 1:499
Terminal hair, 2:53
Terminally ill patients, 5:244, 5:285–288
Termination of action, 1:299
Termination of resuscitation, 3:196–198
Terrestrial-based triangulation, 2:261
Terrorism, 5:428, 5:432, 5:502–521
  biological agents, 5:513–517
  biotoxins, 5:511
  blast injuries, 4:40–47. See also Blast injuries
  chemical agents, 5:508–513
  encephalitis-like agents, 5:516
  explosive agents, 5:505–506
  incapacitating agents, 5:512
  incendiary agents, 5:506
  nerve agents, 5:509–510

Venous blood sampling, 1:437–441
Venous constricting band, 1:417
Venous hemorrhage, 4:85, 4:141
Venous return, 4:105
Venous star, 2:51
Venous system, 3:79, 4:83–84
Ventilation, 1:602–607, 3:11–15, 3:18–20. *See also* Airway management
  automatic transport ventilator, 1:606–607
  bag valve devices, 1:603–605
  BMV, 1:603–605
  demand valve device, 1:605–606
  home ventilators, 5:273, 5:276
  mouth-to-mask, 1:603
  mouth-to-mouth, 1:603
  mouth-to-nose, 1:603
  pediatric patients, 1:605
Ventilation/perfusion mismatch, 1:520
Ventolin, 1:342, 3:46, 3:343
Ventricles, 3:74, 3:75
Ventricular aneurysm, 3:178
Ventricular conduction disturbances, 3:139–140
Ventricular ectopic, 3:129
Ventricular enlargement, 3:231, 3:232, 3:236
Ventricular escape beat, 3:128
Ventricular escape rhythm, 3:128–129
Ventricular fibrillation (VF), 3:134–135, 3:197
Ventricular fibrillation/pulseless ventricular tachycardia (VF/FT) 3:197, 5:107 algorithm, 3:197
Ventricular gallop, 2:92
Ventricular pacemaker, 3:136
Ventricular repolarization, 3:94
Ventricular septal defect, 5:7
Ventricular syncytium, 3:82
Ventricular tachycardia (VT), 3:131–134, 3:197
Ventricular tachycardia with a pulse, 5:105
Venturi mask, 1:602
Venules, 3:79
Verapamil, 1:331, 1:338, 3:158, 3:162
  atrial defibrillation, 3:115
  PSVT, 3:112
Verbal de-escalation, 3:618

Vermox, 1:359
Versed, 1:570, 4:323
Vertebrae, 2:126, 4:335–339
Vertebral arteries, 3:257, 4:278
Vertebral body, 4:335, 4:336
Vertebral column, 3:253, 4:335–337
Vertebrobasilar system, 3:256
Vertebrochondral ribs, 4:382
Vertex position (normal delivery), 3:672–673
Vertical technical rescue, 5:414–415
Vertigo, 5:177
Very high frequency (VHF), 2:272
Vesicants, 5:510
Vesicles, 1:168, 2:53
Vest-type immobilization device, 4:368–370
Vestibule, 3:627, 3:628
Veterans Administration (VA), 5:147
VF, 3:134–135, 3:197
VF/VT algorithm, 3:197
VHF, 2:272, 5:516
Viagra, 1:357
Vials, 1:392–397
Vibramycin, 3:587
Vibration sense, 2:151, 2:152
Viewmax laryngoscope blade, 1:550
Vinblastine, 1:358
Vincristine, 1:358
Vinyl tarps, 5:386
Viokase, 1:349
Violent patients, 3:617–621
Violent street incidents, 5:462–464
Viral hemorrhagic fever (VHF), 5:516
Viral hepatitis, 3:562–563
Viral meningitis, 5:109
Viral rhinitis, 3:574
Virazole, 3:576
Virus, 1:222–223, 3:541–542
Visceral motor nerves, 3:259
Visceral pain, 3:351, 3:391
Visceral pericardium, 3:74
Visceral pleura, 3:10
Visceral sensory nerves, 3:259
Vistaril, 3:342
Visual acuity card, 2:60
Visual acuity wall chart, 2:60
Visual field abnormalities, 2:64
Visual impairment, 5:229–231
Vital capacity, 3:14, 4:386
Vital signs

blood pressure, 2:35–37, 2:43, 2:44–45, 3:80
body temperature, 2:37, 2:43, 2:45
head and neck trauma, 4:311
increased ICP, 3:271
infants, 1:484–485
infants/children, 5:60, 5:65
late adulthood, 1:496
neurology, 3:271
newborns, 5:14, 5:18
normal, 1:485, 2:34, 4:488
pediatric, 2:162
pregnancy, 3:656
pulmonology, 3:29–30
pulse, 2:33–34, 2:42–44
renal/urologic disorders, 3:395
respiration, 2:35, 2:43, 2:44
shock, 3:271
spinal trauma, 4:357, 4:359
taking/calculating, 2:42–45
trauma emergencies, 4:478–479
Vital statistics, 2:41
Vitamin A, 1:363
Vitamin B_1, 1:363, 3:274
Vitamin B_2, 1:363
Vitamin B_6, 1:363
Vitamin B_9, 1:363
Vitamin B_{12}, 1:363
Vitamin C, 1:362, 1:363
Vitamin D, 1:362, 1:363
Vitamin deficiencies, 1:259
Vitamin E, 1:363
Vitamin K, 1:363, 3:471
Vitreous humor, 4:283
Vocal cords, 1:512, 3:6, 4:285
Voice production disorders, 5:232
Volatility, 5:509
Voltage, 4:183
Volume expanders, 5:24
Volume on hand, 1:453
Volvulus, 3:370, 3:372
Vomiting
  children, 5:110
  newborns, 5:33
Vomiting center, 1:348
von Willebrand's disease, 3:485
von Willebrand's factor (VWF), 3:485
VRE, 3:590
Vulva, 3:627
VWF, 3:485
VZIG, 3:571
VZV, 1:223, 3:570

Wandering atrial pacemaker, 3:106–107
Warfarin, 1:340, 3:471
Warm zone, 5:438, 5:439
Warning placards, 5:432–434
Warning signs, 5:405
Washout, 4:109
Waste removal, 1:209–210
Water, 1:180–183
Water moccasin (snake bite), 3:444–446
Water rescues, 5:396–404. *See also* Surface water rescues
Water solubility, 5:440
Watercraft crashes, 4:39
WBCs, 1:248, 3:464–468
Weakness and dizziness, 3:288
Weapons, 4:61–63
  arrow, 4:63
  assault rifle, 4:63
  handgun, 4:61–62
  knife, 4:63
  rifle, 4:62–63
  shotgun, 4:63
Weapons of mass destruction (WMD), 5:432, 5:504. *See also* Terrorism
Weber test, 2:69
Weight-dependent dosages, 1:455–456
Weight lifting, 1:17
Weiner, A. S., 3:472
Well-being of paramedic, 1:14–43
  addictions/habits, 1:21
  back injuries, 1:21–23
  death and dying, 1:29–33
  decontamination of equipment, 1:27–28
  general safety considerations, 1:38–40
  handwashing, 1:25–27
  infection control practices, 1:23–29
  interpersonal relationism, 1:39
  lifting technique, 1:21, 1:23
  nutrition, 1:18–20
  physical fitness, 1:17–23
  post-exposure procedures, 1:28, 1:29
  posture, 1:21, 1:22
  PPE, 1:24–26
  roadway safety, 1:39–40
  stress, 1:33–38
  vaccinations, 1:27
Wenckebach phenomenon, 3:117–119, 3:226–227
Wernicke's syndrome, 3:274
Wet dressings, 4:151
Wet drowning, 3:513